The SAGES Manual of Contemporary Indications and Management of Hepatic and Biliary Diseases

Adnan Alseidi
Mihir M. Shah • Trang Nguyen
Editors

The SAGES Manual of Contemporary Indications and Management of Hepatic and Biliary Diseases

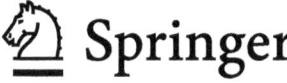

Editors
Adnan Alseidi
Hepato-Pancreato-Biliary (HPB)
Surgery and Endocrine Surgery
University of California, San Francisco
San Francisco, CA, USA

Mihir M. Shah
Surgery
MedStar Health and MedStar Washington Hospital Center
Washington, DC, USA

Trang Nguyen
Division of Surgical Oncology
Washington University in St. Louis
St Louis, MO, USA

ISBN 978-3-032-04822-6   ISBN 978-3-032-04823-3   (eBook)
https://doi.org/10.1007/978-3-032-04823-3

© Society of American Gastrointestinal 2025

This work is subject to copyright. All rights are solely and exclusively licensed by the Publisher, whether the whole or part of the material is concerned, specifically the rights of translation, reprinting, reuse of illustrations, recitation, broadcasting, reproduction on microfilms or in any other physical way, and transmission or information storage and retrieval, electronic adaptation, computer software, or by similar or dissimilar methodology now known or hereafter developed.

The use of general descriptive names, registered names, trademarks, service marks, etc. in this publication does not imply, even in the absence of a specific statement, that such names are exempt from the relevant protective laws and regulations and therefore free for general use.

The publisher, the authors and the editors are safe to assume that the advice and information in this book are believed to be true and accurate at the date of publication. Neither the publisher nor the authors or the editors give a warranty, expressed or implied, with respect to the material contained herein or for any errors or omissions that may have been made. The publisher remains neutral with regard to jurisdictional claims in published maps and institutional affiliations.

This Springer imprint is published by the registered company Springer Nature Switzerland AG
The registered company address is: Gewerbestrasse 11, 6330 Cham, Switzerland

If disposing of this product, please recycle the paper.

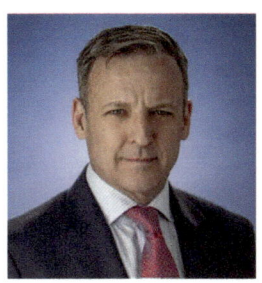

On behalf of the editors and the SAGES HPB/Solid Organ/Safe Chole committee, we dedicate this manual to Dr. Sean P Cleary, who's untimely passing in 2025 has shaken so many in the field. Anyone who knew Dr. Cleary or worked with him knows how dedicated and passionate he was to improve the care of all surgical patients. Specifically, Dr. Cleary devoted his surgical career to the advancement of minimally invasive techniques of the HPB system, and many who contributed to this very work did so on the shoulders of Dr. Cleary's teaching, mentorship, and leadership. There is no doubt that his impact will transcend time, and his legacy will live on in all those who have been touched by his life and friendship.

Foreword

It is a true pleasure to introduce The SAGES *Manual: Hepatic and Biliary Diseases*, a project that reflects what can happen when great minds, clinical experience, and cross-societal collaboration come together with purpose.

This book is the result of a focused and thoughtful effort by the Solid Organ/HPB Committee of the Society of American Gastrointestinal and Endoscopic Surgeons (SAGES), with key contributions from members of the Americas Hepato-Pancreato-Biliary Association (AHPBA). Over the years, SAGES and AHPBA have partnered on several important educational initiatives, and this *Manual* illustrates again the successful and high-impact collaborations between the members of both societies. This seamless partnership reflects the evolving spirit of collegiality and knowledge-sharing in modern surgical practice, transcending institutional and geographical boundaries.

Guided by the editorial leadership of Dr. Mihir M. Shah, Dr. Trang Nguyen, and Dr. Adnan Alseidi, this manual brings together a team of exceptional contributors—leaders in hepatobiliary surgery who share their time, knowledge, and practical insights. The Manual doesn't just cover the "what" of liver surgery but also the "how" and "why" behind the decisions we make every day in and outside of the operating room.

What sets this work apart is its accessibility. It doesn't try to be everything to everyone—instead, it delivers focused, high-yield content with an emphasis on real-world application. Readers will find this book to be not only an academic resource but also a reliable companion in clinical decision-making. Whether you're a trainee just stepping into the world of HPB surgery or a seasoned expert looking for a refresher or second opinion, this manual was designed with you in mind.

On behalf of all those involved in its creation, I am proud to present *The SAGES Manual: Hepatic and Biliary Diseases* as a reflection of excellence in surgical collaboration, scholarship, and education. It is our hope that this book will serve as a trusted resource for current and future generations of surgeons, and contribute meaningfully to the ongoing advancement of hepatobiliary care.

We hope you enjoy the read—and more importantly, let it support the great work you do every day.

Miami Cancer Institute Herbert Wertheim College of Medicine, Florida International University Miami, FL, USA	Horacio J. Asbun

Disclaimer for Society of American Gastrointestinal and Endoscopic Surgeons (SAGES) Manual

The contents of this manual are intended exclusively for educational and informational purposes only, and nothing contained within constitutes medical advice. Neither this manual nor its contents have been subject to formal peer-review. The information provided herein does not represent, nor should it be interpreted as, the official position, view, or endorsement of the Society of American Gastrointestinal and Endoscopic Surgeons (SAGES) or its governing body. This manual is not intended for use in diagnosing or treating any health problem, condition, or disease. Individuals seeking personal medical advice should consult an appropriate licensed professional.

Neither SAGES, nor its officers, directors, employees, members, nor any of the contributors to this manual, make any representation or warranty, express or implied, regarding the accuracy, completeness, fitness for any intended purpose, or suitability of the information contained herein for any specific use or function. Neither access to, nor use of, this manual creates or implies any physician-patient relationship, and reliance on any information provided, contained, or implied herein is solely at the user's own risk.

Contents

Part I Gall Bladder

1 **Gallbladder Malignancy**........................ 3
Núria Lluís, Domenech Asbun, and Eduardo A. Vega

2 **Pre-malignant Gallbladder Lesions** 35
Kevin M. Turner, Aaron M. Delman,
and Gregory C. Wilson

3 **Intraoperative Management of Incidental
Neoplastic Findings (Gallbladder)**................ 45
Holly V. Spitzer and Daniel W. Nelson

Part II Biliary Disease

4 **Intraductal Papillary Neoplasm of the Bile
Duct (IPNB)**................................. 61
Lyonell B. Kone, Thomas M. Fishbein,
and Timothy J. Kennedy

5 **Intrahepatic Cholangiocarcinoma**................ 71
Emilie A. K. Warren and Shishir K. Maithel

6 **Extrahepatic Cholangiocarcinoma** 87
Ranish K. Patel and Flavio G. Rocha

Part III Liver

7 Hepatic Pre-malignant Lesions 113
Fatima Mustansir and Juan M. Sarmiento

8 Hepatocellular Carcinoma 127
Guido Fiorentini and Sean P. Cleary

9 Surgical Management of Colorectal Liver Metastases 147
Gloria Y. Chang, Nicole M. Nevarez, and Georgios Karagkounis

10 Neuroendocrine Liver Metastasis 193
Pranay S. Ajay and David A. Kooby

11 Non-CR, Non-NE Liver Metastases 215
David Henault, Hala Muaddi, and Chaya Shwaartz

Part IV Basic Procedures

12 Positions and Access 275
Fabio Giannone, Oronzo Ligurgo, and Patrick Pessaux

13 Instrumentation and Approaches for Parenchymal Transection 299
Ana Luiza Mandelli Gleisner and Sumaya Abdul Ghaffar

14 Robotic Approaches to Hepatic Transection 335
Miho Akabane, Brendan Visser, and Kazunari Sasaki

15 Hemostasis and Basics of Hemorrhage Control 349
Alice Zhu, Brittany Greene, and Shiva Jayaraman

16 Assessment of the Hepatic Remnant and Preoperative Imaging 367
Matthew Dixon, Jordan Tasse, and Sam Pappas

17 Hilar Dissection 389
Federico Gaudenzi, Taiga Wakabayashi, and Go Wakabayashi

Part V Basic Maneuvers Procedure

18 Liver Mobilization and Ultrasound................ 411
James M. McDermott, Jonathan C. Delong,
and Monica M. Dua

19 Minimally Invasive Pringle Maneuvers 433
Hemasat Alkhatib, Ali M. Kara, Ahmad Abou Abbass,
and Kevin El-Hayek

**20 Intraoperative Cholangiography, Choledochoscopy,
and Fluorescent Cholangiography** 439
Domenech Asbun, Levan Tsamalaidze,
and Horacio Asbun

Part VI Partial Hepatectomy (Non-anatomical) – Procdure

21 Liver Core Needle Biopsies and Wedge Resection... 465
Tyler D. Robinson and Erin W. Gilbert

**22 Inferior Partial Hepatectomy and Superior Partial
Hepatectomy** 481
Aleksandr Kalabin, John Martinie, and Erin Baker

**23 Anatomic Metastasectomy/Segmentectomy
and Left Lateral Sectionectomy**................... 495
Gabriella Lionetto, Avril Kaye Coley,
and Cristina R. Ferrone

Part VII Major Hepatectomy

24 Open Right and Left Hepatectomy............... 515
Daniel W. Nelson and Ching-Wei D. Tzeng

**25 Major Hepatectomy: MIS Left Hepatectomy
and Right Hepatectomy** 533
Christine Chung, Camilla Gomes,
Paige-Ashley Campbell, and Adnan Alseidi

26 Right Posterior Sectionectomy, Anterior Sectionectomy, and Central Hepatectomy 543
Chase J. Wehrle, Alejandro Pita, Jaekeun Kim, and Choon Hyuck David Kwon

27 Extended Hepatectomy........................ 561
Peter J. Altshuler and Shareef M. Syed

Part VIII Biliary Procedures

28 Bile Duct Resection and Reconstruction............ 581
Caitlin A. McIntyre and Alice C. Wei

29 Radical Cholecystectomy 595
Elizabeth L. Carpenter and Timothy E. Newhook

30 Portal Lymphadenectomy: Technical Pearls and Pitfalls 615
Hop S. Tran Cao, Reed I. Ayabe, and Ahad M. Azimuddin

Part IX Locoregional Hepatic Therapies

31 Surgical Microwave Ablation of the Liver 635
Sushruta Nagarkatti, Aleksandr Kalabin, John B. Martinie, and David A. Iannitti

32 Nonthermal Ablation 657
Yasmin Essaji, Christine Chung, Lauren M. Wancata, and Scott Helton

33 Hepatic Artery Infusion Pump: Open and Robotic Techniques for Placement............ 677
Mengyuan Liu and T. Peter Kingham

Index.. 689

Contributors

Ahmad Abou Abbass South Orange County Surgical Medical Group, Mission Viejo, CA, USA

Pranay S. Ajay Division of Surgical Oncology, Department of Surgery, Emory University School of Medicine, Atlanta, GA, USA

Miho Akabane Division of Abdominal Transplant, Department of Surgery, Stanford University Medical Center, Stanford, CA, USA

Hemasat Alkhatib Department of General Surgery, The MetroHealth System, Cleveland, OH, USA

Adnan Alseidi Department of Surgery, University of California, San Francisco, San Francisco, CA, USA

Peter J. Altshuler Division of Transplant Surgery, Department of Surgery, University of California San Francisco, San Francisco, CA, USA

Domenech Asbun Division of Hepatobiliary and Pancreas Surgery, Miami Cancer Institute, Miami, FL, USA

Horacio Asbun Division of Hepatobiliary and Pancreas Surgery, Miami Cancer Institute, Miami, FL, USA

Reed I. Ayabe Division of Hepatobiliary and Pancreas Surgery, Department of Surgery, University of California Irvine, Irvine, CA, USA

Ahad M. Azimuddin Department of Surgical Oncology, The University of Texas MD Anderson Cancer Center, Houston, TX, USA

Division of Hepatobiliary and Pancreas Surgery, Department of Surgery, University of California Irvine, Irvine, CA, USA

Department of Surgery, Northwestern University Feinberg School of Medicine, Chicago, USA

Erin Baker Charlotte, NC, USA

Paige-Ashley Campbell Department of Surgery, University of California, San Francisco, San Francisco, CA, USA

Elizabeth L. Carpenter San Antonio Military Medical Center, San Antonio, TX, USA

Gloria Y. Chang Department of Surgery, Division of Surgical Oncology, University of Texas Southwestern Medical Center, Dallas, TX, USA

Christine Chung Virginia Mason Medical Center, Seattle, WA, USA

Department of Surgery, Virginia Mason Franciscan Health, Seattle, WA, USA

Sean P. Cleary Department of Surgery, University of Toronto, Toronto, CA, USA

Avril Kaye Coley Department of Surgery, Massachusetts General Hospital, Harvard Medical School, Boston, MA, USA

Aaron M. Delman Department of Surgery, University of Cincinnati College of Medicine, Cincinnati, OH, USA

Jonathan C. Delong Department of Surgery, University of Tennessee Medical Center Knoxville, Knoxville, TN, USA

Matthew Dixon Division of Surgical Oncology, Rush University Medical Center, Chicago, IL, USA

Monica M. Dua Department of Surgery, Stanford University, Stanford, CA, USA

Contributors

Kevin El-Hayek Department of General Surgery, The MetroHealth System, Cleveland, OH, USA

Case Western Reserve University School of Medicine, Cleveland, OH, USA

Yasmin Essaji Department of Surgery, McMaster University, Hamilton, ON, Canada

Cristina R. Ferrone Department of Surgery, Cedars Sinai Medical Center, Los Angeles, CA, USA

Guido Fiorentini Hepatobiliary and Pancreas Surgery Division, Mayo Clinic, Rochester, MN, USA

Thomas M. Fishbein Department of Surgery, MedStar Georgetown, Washington, DC, USA

Federico Gaudenzi Center for Advanced Treatment of Hepatobiliary and Pancreatic Diseases, Ageo Central General Hospital, Saitama, Japan

Sumaya Abdul Ghaffar Department of Surgery, University of Colorado, Aurora, CO, USA

Fabio Giannone Department of Visceral and Digestive Surgery, University Hospital of Strasbourg, Strasbourg, France

Erin W. Gilbert Department of Surgery, Louisiana State University Health & Science University, New Orleans, LA, USA

Ana Luiza Mandelli Gleisner Department of Surgery, University of Colorado, Aurora, CO, USA

Camilla Gomes Department of Surgery, University of California, San Francisco, San Francisco, CA, USA

Brittany Greene Division of General Surgery, Department of Surgery, University of Toronto, Toronto, ON, Canada

HPB Surgery Service, Division of General Surgery, St. Joseph's Health Centre, Unity Health Toronto, Toronto, ON, Canada

Scott Helton Department of Surgery, Virginia Mason Franciscan Health, Seattle, WA, USA

David Henault HPB Surgical Oncology, University Health Network, University of Toronto, Toronto, ON, Canada

David A. Iannitti Atrium Health/Carolinas Medical Center, Charlotte, NC, USA

Shiva Jayaraman Division of General Surgery, Department of Surgery, University of Toronto, Toronto, ON, Canada

HPB Surgery Service, Division of General Surgery, St. Joseph's Health Centre, Unity Health Toronto, Toronto, ON, Canada

Aleksandr Kalabin Atrium Health/Carolinas Medical Center, Charlotte, NC, USA

Ali M. Kara Department of General Surgery, The MetroHealth System, Cleveland, OH, USA

Georgios Karagkounis Department of Surgery, Division of Surgical Oncology, University of Texas Southwestern Medical Center, Dallas, TX, USA

Department of Surgery, Colorectal Service, Memorial Sloan Kettering Cancer Center, New York, NY, USA

Timothy J. Kennedy Division of Surgical Oncology, Department of Surgery, MedStar Georgetown, Washington, DC, USA

Jaekeun Kim Department of Liver Transplantation, Cleveland Clinic Foundation, Cleveland, OH, USA

Department of General Surgery, Section of HPB Surgery, Cleveland Clinic Foundation, Cleveland, OH, USA

T. Peter Kingham Department of Surgery, Memorial Sloan Kettering Cancer Center, New York, NY, USA

Lyonell B. Kone Division of Surgical Oncology, Department of Surgery, Winship Cancer Institute, Emory University, Atlanta, GA, USA

David A. Kooby Division of Surgical Oncology, Department of Surgery, Emory University School of Medicine, Atlanta, GA, USA

Choon Hyuck David Kwon Department of Liver Transplantation, Cleveland Clinic Foundation, Cleveland, OH, USA

Department of General Surgery, Section of HPB Surgery, Cleveland Clinic Foundation, Cleveland, OH, USA

Oronzo Ligurgo Department of Visceral and Digestive Surgery, University Hospital of Strasbourg, Strasbourg, France

Gabriella Lionetto Department of Surgery, Unit of General and Pancreatic Surgery, University of Verona Hospital Trust, Verona, Italy

Mengyuan Liu Department of Surgery, Memorial Sloan Kettering Cancer Center, New York, NY, USA

Núria Lluís Division of Hepatobiliary and Pancreas Surgery, Miami Cancer Institute, Miami, FL, USA

Shishir K. Maithel Division of Surgical Oncology, Department of Surgery, Northwestern University, Atlanta, GA, USA

John B. Martinie Atrium Health/Carolinas Medical Center, Charlotte, NC, USA

James M. McDermott Department of Surgery, Stanford University, Stanford, CA, USA

Caitlin A. McIntyre Department of Surgery, Brigham and Women's Hospital, Boston, MA, USA

Hala Muaddi Department of General Surgery, University of Toronto, Toronto, Canada

Fatima Mustansir Department on Surgery, Washington University, St. Louis, MO, USA

Sushruta Nagarkatti University of Tennessee, Health Sciences Center, Memphis, TN, USA

Daniel W. Nelson Department of Surgery, University of Tennessee Health Science Center College of Medicine - Chattanooga, Chattanooga, Chattanooga, TN, USA

Department of Surgical Oncology, The University of Texas M.D. Anderson Cancer Center, Houston, TX, USA

Nicole M. Nevarez Department of Surgery, Division of Surgical Oncology, University of Texas Southwestern Medical Center, Dallas, TX, USA

Timothy E. Newhook Department of Surgical Oncology, The University of Texas MD Anderson Cancer Center, Houston, TX, USA

Sam Pappas Division of Surgical Oncology, Rush University Medical Center, Chicago, IL, USA

Ranish K. Patel Division of Surgical Oncology, Knight Cancer Institute, Oregon Health and Science University, Portland, OR, USA

Patrick Pessaux Department of Visceral and Digestive Surgery, University Hospital of Strasbourg, Strasbourg, France

Alejandro Pita Department of Liver Transplantation, Cleveland Clinic Foundation, Cleveland, OH, USA

Tyler D. Robinson Mercy Medical Group, Sacramento, CA, USA

Flavio G. Rocha Division of Surgical Oncology, Knight Cancer Institute, Oregon Health and Science University, Portland, OR, USA

Juan M. Sarmiento Department of Surgery, Emory University, Atlanta, GA, USA

Kazunari Sasaki Division of Abdominal Transplant, Department of Surgery, Stanford University Medical Center, Stanford, CA, USA

Chaya Shwaartz HPB Surgical Oncology, University Health Network, University of Toronto, Toronto, ON, Canada

Holly V. Spitzer Department of Surgery, William Beaumont Army Medical Center, El Paso, TX, USA

Shareef M. Syed Division of Transplant Surgery, Department of Surgery, University of California San Francisco, San Francisco, CA, USA

Jordan Tasse Department of Interventional Radiology, Rush University Medical Center, Chicago, IL, USA

Hop S. Tran Cao Department of Surgical Oncology, The University of Texas MD Anderson Cancer Center, Houston, TX, USA

Levan Tsamalaidze Division of Hepatobiliary and Pancreas Surgery, Miami Cancer Institute, Miami, FL, USA

Kevin M. Turner Department of Surgery, University of Cincinnati College of Medicine, Cincinnati, OH, USA

Ching-Wei D. Tzeng Department of Surgical Oncology, The University of Texas M.D. Anderson Cancer Center, Houston, TX, USA

Eduardo A. Vega Department of Surgery, Hepato-Pancreato-Biliary Surgery, Boston Medical Center Brighton, Boston University School of Medicine, Boston, MA, USA

Brendan Visser Section of Hepatobiliary and Pancreatic Surgery, Division of General Surgery, Department of Surgery, Stanford University Medical Center, Stanford, CA, USA

Go Wakabayashi Center for Advanced Treatment of Hepatobiliary and Pancreatic Diseases, Ageo Central General Hospital, Saitama, Japan

Taiga Wakabayashi Center for Advanced Treatment of Hepatobiliary and Pancreatic Diseases, Ageo Central General Hospital, Saitama, Japan

Lauren M. Wancata Department of Surgery, Virginia Mason Franciscan Health, Seattle, WA, USA

Emilie A. K. Warren Division of Surgical Oncology, Department of Surgery, Emory University, Atlanta, GA, USA

Chase J. Wehrle Department of Liver Transplantation, Cleveland Clinic Foundation, Cleveland, OH, USA

Department of General Surgery, Section of HPB Surgery, Cleveland Clinic Foundation, Cleveland, OH, USA

Alice C. Wei Department of Surgery, Hepatopancreatobiliary Service, Memorial Sloan Kettering Cancer Center, New York, NY, USA

Gregory C. Wilson Department of Surgery, Division of Surgical Oncology, University of Cincinnati College of Medicine, Cincinnati, OH, USA

Alice Zhu Division of General Surgery, Department of Surgery, University of Toronto, Toronto, ON, Canada

Part I
Gall Bladder

# Gallbladder Malignancy

Núria Lluís, Domenech Asbun, and Eduardo A. Vega

Introduction

Gallbladder cancer (GBC) is the most common biliary tract cancer and the sixth most common gastrointestinal cancer worldwide [1]. GBC shows significant geographic variation in incidence, being particularly common in certain countries such as Chile and India, and in native American communities [2]. Gallstones and gallbladder polyps are considered local risk factors, whereas gender, diabetes, obesity, and parity are considered systemic risk factors for GBC [1–3]. Globally, it is responsible for 1.7% of all cancer mortality. An upward trend in incidence has been detected which, fortunately, has been accompanied by a decrease in mortality [3]. Its incidence increases with age and is more common among women [2]. GBC is an aggressive disease that is often diagnosed at an advanced stage similar to other biliary tract cancers. Currently, 80% of all patients with GBC are diagnosed with metastatic or locoregional advanced disease. According to the American Society of Clinical Oncology, the overall 5-year survival is approximately 19% [3].

Surgery with curative intent is the only method to cure. According to a comprehensive review from 2015, approximately 20% of patients with GBC were candidates for curative surgery [1]. The procedures performed range from simple cholecystectomy to multi-visceral resection [4]. Most early-stage GBCs are detected incidentally after cholecystectomy. Today, even with resection of all apparent disease, there is a high rate of early recurrence [5]. However, the role of adjuvant, neoadjuvant, and palliative chemo and/or radiotherapy remains to be established. This chapter will review the epidemiology, risk and causative factors, common clinical presentations, and therapeutic options for GBC.

Epidemiology and Risk Factors

According to Global Cancer Observatory estimates [6], in 2020 there were 115,949 newly diagnosed cases of GBC worldwide (0.6% of all new cancer cases), and 84,695 deaths reported (0.9% of all deaths). In the United States, approximately 3700 new cases are identified each year [7]. There are stark differences in incidence within different populations globally. The highest incidence of GBC is found in Chilean Mapuche Indian women (27.3 cases per 100,000 population annually) followed by women living in India (22 cases per 100,000 population annually), and natives of North America (7.1 cases per 100,000 population annually) [8]. Further differences are observed based on socioeconomic status. Global data from 2018 suggests that incidence and mortality are increasing in developed countries, possibly due to increase in risk factors (see below) [3]. Within these countries, rates of GBC are particularly high in areas of lower socioeconomic status. This suggests that limited access to health care results in decreased rate of screening and cholecystectomy for gallstone disease, potentially leading to higher rate of GBC [9].

Multiple risk factors for the development of GBC have been identified. Gallbladder adenomatous polyps are one such risk factor, as they have the potential for malignant transformation. Although the majority of gallbladder polyps are benign cholesterol polyps, they are difficult to distinguish from adenomatous polyps on preoperative workup [1]. Hence, it is important to identify those polyps with high-risk features in order to recommend a prophylactic cholecystectomy and avoid the potential risk of GBC development. Clinical guidelines recommend a cholecystectomy for gallbladder polyps >10 mm if the patient is fit for and accepts surgery [10]. Increased polyp size is also important: the larger the adenomatous polyp, the greater the risk of malignancy, which can reach 45–67% in polyps between 10 and 15 mm [11]. If the patient has no risk factors for gallbladder malignancy and a 6–9 mm polyp, or has risk factors and a ≤5 mm polyp, follow-up ultrasound is recommended at 6 months, 1 year, and annually up to 5 years [10]. If the patient has no risk factors for malignancy and a polyp ≤5 mm, follow-up at 1 year, 3 years, and 5 years is recommended [10]. When patients have polyps and gallbladder stones with a thickened gallbladder wall or a progressive increase in the size of gallbladder polyps, they are candidates for a prophylactic cholecystectomy [12]. If a cholecystectomy is not performed, surveillance is recommended for the following risk factors: patient >50 years, history of primary sclerosing cholangitis, Indian ethnicity, or presence of a sessile polyp (including focal gallbladder wall thickening >4 mm) [10].

Obesity has also been related to GBC. A linear trend in deaths with increased body mass index has been observed. Specifically, the relative risk of death for a body mass index of ≥ 30.0 kg/m^2 is 2.44 (95% CI, 1.73–3.44) [13]. Pooled analysis of 19 prospective cohort studies including patients from the United States, Europe, Asia, and Australia showed that being overweight was associated with an increased risk of developing GBC [14]. Conversely, a recent meta-analysis showed that high physical activity was associated with a lower risk of GBC (risk ratio, 0.79; 95% CI, 0.64–0.98). Engaging in moderate physical activity was also observed to be a protective factor [15].

Similar to obesity, diabetes has also been associated with GBC. According to a large systematic review on the temporal pattern of GBC, the relative risk of diabetes-associated incidence of GBC has increased since the year 2000 in comparison to previous decades [16]. However, it is not clear whether the association of type 2 diabetes and cancer mortality is causal, or it reflects the impact of other concomitant confounding factors, such as obesity. Multiple studies have analyzed survival data in diabetic patients with GBC and have produced mixed conclusions. A meta-analysis of multiple cohorts with a total population of 32 million revealed that type 2 diabetes is linked to a higher incidence of GBC, but is not associated with increased mortality from this malignancy [17]. On the contrary, a recent meta-analysis of eight cohorts showed that GBC mortality was higher in diabetic than nondiabetic patients (hazard ratio, 1.10; 95% CI, 1.06–1.14; $P < 0.001$) [18]. Therefore, there is no clear evidence to support increased mortality in these patients.

The presence of gallbladder stones is one of the main risk factors for the development of GBC. Up to 75–90% of GBCs occur in the context of cholelithiasis. A meta-analysis of seven cohort studies and 23 case-control studies from around the world showed that the presence of gallstones was associated with an increased risk of GBC (odds ratio, 7.26; 95% CI, 4.33–12.18), as was gallstone size >1 cm (odds ratio, 1.88; 95% CI, 1.10–3.22) [3]. Indeed, the odds ratio increased to 10.1 in patients with gallstones >3 cm [19]. This association was confirmed in a study that compared gallstones in patients with benign disease vs GBC. Gallstones from patients with GBC were more numerous, larger, and weighed more than those from patients with benign disease [20].

Until recently, tobacco smoking was not known to be a predisposing factor for GBC. A meta-analysis of 20 studies, however, found that smokers had a higher risk of GBC than never-smokers [21]. The risk increased linearly with intensity and duration of smoking and, after 20 years of quitting, decreased to match the risk of never-smokers.

Regarding the impact of infectious processes on the susceptibility of developing GBC, data from a series of patients from

Chile, and the meta-analysis of 22 published studies of patients from Asia, Latin America, Europe, and the United States showed a positive association between chronic biliary infection with Salmonella typhi and GBC [22]. However, the pathogenesis remains unknown. Chronic Helicobacter infection (H. pylori, H. bilis) has also been associated with GBC [23].

Lastly, several studies have suggested that parity, age when giving birth, and sex hormones may play a role in the development of GBC in the mother. A meta-analysis of 13 case-control studies demonstrated that parity and parity number were associated with increased risk of GBC [24]. In fact, gallstones are strongly associated with higher parity in women [25].

In summary, the evidence provided supports a relationship between gallstone disease, diabetes, obesity, tobacco smoking, chronic biliary infection by certain pathogens, and parity with GBC. Such findings suggest a multifactorial pattern in which each component may play a role in influencing tumor onset and development. For this reason, the adoption of healthy lifestyle habits seems to be a sound recommendation to decrease the risk of GBC, especially in areas with an endemically high incidence.

Genetics, Immunology, and Pathogenesis

To understand how GBC carcinogenesis occurs, it is important to determine the evolutionary sequence from benign to malignant lesions of gallbladder epithelium. A recent study characterized the genetic changes during progression from normal epithelium to low-grade and high-grade biliary intraepithelial neoplasia (BilIN) and GBC in tissue samples obtained from the same patients [26]. The findings revealed that GBC can evolve through this pathway (adenoma/dysplasia/carcinoma) or be independent of the BilIN pathway through initial extensive loss of heterozygosity and accumulation of mutations [26] (Fig. 1.1).

As with many diseases, several GBC-associated genetic polymorphisms were initially identified but lost relevance in subsequent studies [27]. An early meta-analysis of 40 studies that included 80 candidate gene variants and 173 polymorphisms [27]

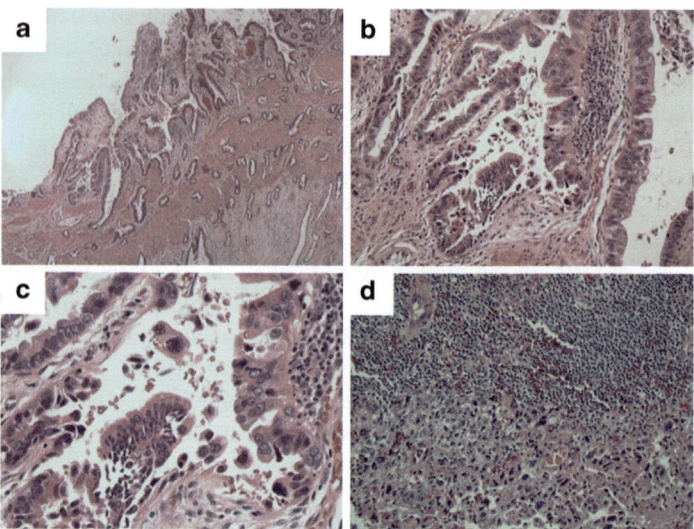

Fig. 1.1 Gallbladder carcinoma histology patterns: (**a**) Normal mucosal glands and high-grade dysplasia, H&E stain, × 40. (**b/c**) Gall bladder adenocarcinoma, highly pleomorphic neoplastic cells. Both H&E stain, C- × 100, D- ×400. (**d**) Metastatic gall bladder carcinoma, high grade to the lymph node, H&E stains, G- × 100, H- × 400. (Courtesy of Dr. Aleksandr Perepletchikov at Saint Elizabeth's Medical Center, Boston, MA, USA)

found no association between any of these polymorphisms and GBC susceptibility. Nevertheless, a recent genome-wide association study in a large cohort of patients [28] suggested a strong association between one or more loci of the ABCB4 and ABCB1 gene regions (involved in hepatobiliary phospholipid transmembrane transport) with risk of GBC in India, a country with a high incidence of this malignancy.

In support of another genetic association with biliary tract tumors, recent studies suggest that intrahepatic cholangiocarcinoma is correlated with epigenetic changes, while extrahepatic carcinoma and GBC are driven by mutations in TP53 and other cell cycle genes [29]. In geographical areas where there is a high prevalence of GBC, it is recognized that physiological and environmental variables such as genetics, gallstone presence, dysregulated inflammation, and exposure to aflatoxin [30], as well as ethnicity may facilitate the accumulation of genetic and epigenetic alterations that promote the progression of premalignant lesions to invasive cancer. A recent epigenome-wide association study identified three stages of increased methylation in gallbladder carcinogenesis: early, present in gallbladder lithiasis and low-grade epithelial dysplasia; intermediate, found in high-grade dysplasia; and late, in GBC [31]. An understanding of this progression serves to further strengthen the aforementioned surgical and screening interventions in small but potentially premalignant lesions of the gallbladder.

A recent study [32] demonstrated that poor survival in GBC was associated with an immunosuppressive microenvironment and T-cell dysfunction. Improved survival was associated with the opposite features. These findings suggest that the aggressiveness of GBC depends on both somatic genetic characteristics and the microenvironment and immune profiles of the tumor [32].

The studies presented here suggest that to date there appear to be no genetic polymorphisms associated with, or relevant to, GBC. During carcinogenesis, somatic genetic aberrations, epigenetic changes consistent with increased methylation, and decreased immunity in the tumor microenvironment coexist. Finally, the scant evidence suggests that malignancy can evolve along one of two paths: progression through the adenoma, dysplasia, carcinoma sequence; or, independently, by extensive loss of heterozygosity and accumulation of mutations.

Clinical Presentation

GBC typically presents in one of three clinical scenarios: 1) it is discovered postoperatively in the gallbladder specimen after cholecystectomy for presumed benign disease namely incidental GBC (IGBC); 2) it is suspected preoperatively based primarily on imaging abnormalities; or 3) it is identified intraoperatively upon finding malignant-appearing tissue. The percentage distribution of these clinical scenarios varies according to geographic location, the incidence of GBC in the area, and the usual referral patterns in the local health system.

Incidental GBC

Most resectable GBCs are diagnosed incidentally after elective or emergency cholecystectomy. An increase in cholecystectomies in younger patients and advances in preoperative imaging have led to earlier diagnosis of GBC in recent decades [33]. Approximately 1% of cholecystectomy specimens for benign disease are found to harbor malignancy [34]. It is essential to carry out a complete histological mapping of the gallbladder specimen, regardless of its macroscopic appearance, to ensure a correct diagnosis of the tumor category and to guarantee that there are no suspicious lesions left to be explored [34] (Fig. 1.2).

However, some clinical features may increase our suspicion of GBC. The presence of risk factors such as obesity, diabetes, mul-

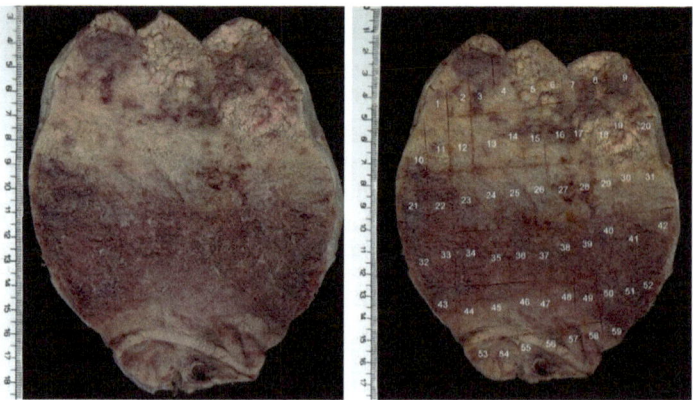

Fig. 1.2 Mapping the gallbladder: The challenges in detecting GBC in this setting prompt the need for performing a complete and detailed histological examination of the cholecystectomy specimen, regardless of gallbladder gross appearance. Mapping of the gallbladder (GB) specimen is crucial to avoid missing cancer and to correctly diagnose the T category (Courtesy of Dr. Xabier De Arextabala at Clinica Alemana Santiago, Santiago, Chile)

tiple stones or stones >1 cm or larger, current or past smoking, and parity should raise the suspicion of occult GBC. One study identified that patients with incidental GBC were older and had undergone more preoperative imaging tests [35]. On ultrasonography, the gallbladder wall was thickened with no peri-vesicular fluid collections. They had a larger common bile duct diameter, and a higher alkaline phosphatase level. A higher rate of conversion from laparoscopic to open surgery was also noted [35, 36].

Once GBC is detected on pathologic examination after cholecystectomy, the next steps are critical [37, 38]. The manual of the American Joint Committee on Cancer (AJCC), 8th edition [39], defines T1a if the tumor invades the lamina propria, and T1b if it invades the muscular layer of the gallbladder. It defines T2 if the tumor invades the connective tissue on the peritoneal (T2a) or hepatic (T2b) side of the gallbladder, respectively, without extension to the peritoneal serosa or the liver. National Comprehensive Cancer Network (NCCN) guidelines [40] recommend different pathways for incidental GBC: (1) for T1a tumors with negative margins, observation would be the primary treatment; (2) if cystic lymph node is positive, the postoperative workup would include imaging studies and optional staging laparoscopy, and the primary treatment would be neoadjuvant therapy followed by oncologic extended resection (OER, see below); and (3) for patients with T1b or greater, and/or patients with T1a and positive margins, postoperative workup and primary treatment would be similar to a positive cystic node if the tumor is considered resectable, or palliation for unresectable tumors.

The cystic duct resection margin has special significance. Invasion of the cystic duct margin worsens the overall survival of patients undergoing OER. In addition, patients with a positive cystic margin benefit from common bile duct resection [41]. In both scenarios, the influence of the positive cystic margin is evident even in patients without residual cancer after resection.

Invasion of the cystic lymph node also influences therapeutic decision-making. A study in patients with incidental GBC showed that cystic duct lymph node positivity was associated with poorer disease-free survival [42]. In addition, positivity of the cystic node was associated with positivity of lymph nodes around the common bile duct and hepatic hilum (so-called D1 lymph node stations) but did not predict the status of the lymph nodes located next to the common hepatic artery or around the pancreas (D2 lymph nodes) [42]. Therefore, the state of the cystic duct lymph node cannot discourage the performance of OER in patients with incidental GBC.

Historically, patients with incidentally found GBC during laparoscopic cholecystectomy were recommended to have port sites excised upon reoperation. This is no longer recommended and should only be performed in selected cases [37].

Suspected Before Surgery or Non-incidental Gallbladder Cancer

Non-incidental GBC refers to malignancy diagnosed before cholecystectomy. This can be difficult, as GBC is often asymptomatic or causes symptoms that mimic gallstone disease. However, more atypical and possibly concerning symptoms include constant right upper quadrant abdominal pain, weight loss, anorexia, and possible jaundice. On physical examination, a mass may be palpable in the right upper quadrant of the abdomen and can be an ominous sign of advanced disease.

Standard abdominal ultrasound is the most common modality used to diagnose gallstone disease, yet it has poor diagnostic performance to diagnose GBC. Recent evidence suggests that contrast-enhanced ultrasonography improves the performance of conventional and Doppler ultrasonography in the differential diagnosis of benign and malignant gallbladder lesions [43]. The risk of GBC in patients with gallbladder wall calcifications, also known as porcelain gallbladder, is lower than previously thought. Prophylactic cholecystectomy is appropriate for fit patients, and surveillance should be considered for patients with relevant co-morbidities [44].

In patients with suspected GBC, computed tomography (CT) and/or magnetic resonance imaging (MRI) should be performed to evaluate tumor penetration through the gallbladder wall, suspicious lesions in the liver and regional and distant lymph nodes, as well as invasion of adjacent organs and large vessels [45]. GBC can be detected as a focal thickening of the gallbladder wall, a mass, or a polyp. It often coexists with benign biliary disease and is difficult to identify in the setting of acute or chronic cholecystitis, especially xanthogranulomatous cholecystitis. Irregular margins, invasion of adjacent structures, and abnormal lymphadenopathy are suspicious signs [45]. Another method for early GBC detection is utilizing diffusion-weighted MRI, which can help delineate neoplastic tissue. In the gallbladder, diffusion-weighted MRI can help distinguish wall thickening from polyps or malignant lesions. A meta-analysis of eight studies endorsed its utilization for the differential diagnosis of gallbladder malignancy [46], although it usually complements ultrasonography and conventional MRI. In addition, ^{18}F-FDG positron emission tomography (PET) and PET/CT are useful in the evaluation of the primary tumor (AUC, 0.88) [47] and lymph node metastasis in patients with GBC [48] (Fig. 1.3).

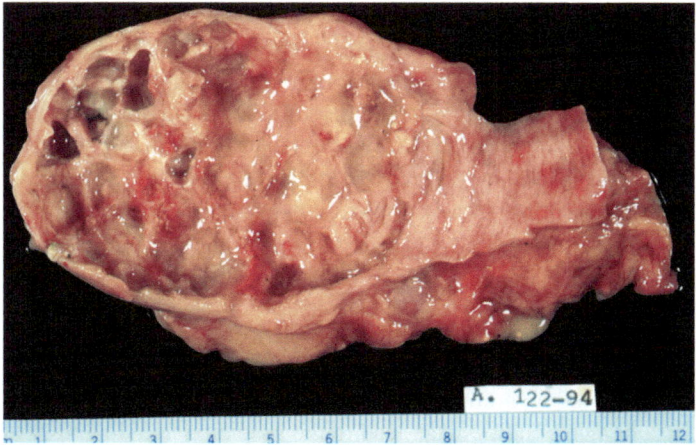

Fig. 1.3 Chronic cholecystitis: For Western GBC, detecting small lesions is particularly difficult due to the high proportion of flat tumors that are embedded in chronically inflamed gallbladder walls as shown in the picture. (Courtesy of Dr. Xabier De Aretxabala and Dr. Marcelo Vivanco at Clinica Alemana Santiago, Santiago, Chile)

Regarding tumor markers, several studies have suggested that serum carbohydrate antigen (CA) 19-9 may be useful in the diagnosis of GBC. A recent meta-analysis of 27 studies conducted in Asia over the past 25 years quantified an area under the curve of 0.89 (95% CI, 0.86–0.92) for the diagnosis of GBC [49]. Nevertheless, caution is recommended since the cut-off levels vary between studies.

When GBC is suspected on imaging and a tissue sample to confirm the diagnosis is not available, referral to a center with expertise in hepato-pancreato-biliary (HPB) surgery is in the best interest of the patient [34]. The 3-year disease-specific survival of patients with T2b GBC was better after initial oncologic resection in a center specialized in HPB surgery than after incidental finding of the tumor in index cholecystectomy performed without oncological criteria [50].

Several studies suggest that the initial non-oncologic gallbladder resection for undiagnosed GBC (index cholecystectomy) does not have a negative impact on survival [34]. However, there are emerging data that suggests index cholecystectomy for undiagnosed GBC may actually have a deleterious effect on survival, especially for T2b tumors located on the hepatic side of the gallbladder [50]. Hence the importance of thorough preoperative assessment of patients with features suspicious of GBC. According to NCCN recommendations, staging laparoscopy may be considered when GBC is suspected. Primary treatment is OER (see below) if the tumor is resectable; biopsy and supportive treatment if unresectable [40].

Intraoperative Discovery of Gallbladder Cancer

At times, intraoperative findings during cholecystectomy planned for a benign condition can lead to the suspicion and diagnosis of GBC. These include the presence of masses or abnormal areas of thickening within the gallbladder wall, or findings of malignant-appearing hepatic or peritoneal lesions. Given this scenario, intraoperative ultrasonography can accurately estimate the depth of tumor invasion in the gallbladder wall. Despite the low diagnostic sensitivity of frozen samples, core needle biopsy can complement the diagnosis in some cases before committing to an OER. If the center does not have an expert team in HPB surgery, it is preferable not to proceed with cholecystectomy, and instead take a biopsy and refer the patient to a center that has the staff, skills, and knowledge needed to deal with this condition in a multidisciplinary approach [40]. If the center has an expert team in HPB surgery, intraoperative staging and biopsy are performed. From here on, the operation is similar to that described below.

Oncologic Extended Resection in Gallbladder Cancer

OER is the recommended treatment for patients with GBC stage T1b or more advanced, without evidence of disseminated disease. OER involves resection of the gallbladder as well as *en-bloc* resection of the gallbladder fossa. Also, according to NCCN recommendations [40], OER stands for: (1) hepatic resection that usually includes segments IVb and V, or beyond if necessary to obtain negative margins; (2) lymph node dissection of the hepatoduodenal ligament; and (3) optional bile duct resection to obtain negative margins, but it will not be performed routinely. It is not considered appropriate to excise the port sites as it would be useless in disseminated disease.

The new AJCC classification subdivides stage T2 GBC into stage T2a for those arising from the peritoneal surface of the gallbladder, and stage T2b for tumors that grow on the hepatic side, without invading the liver. All T2 tumors invade the peri-muscular connective tissue of the gallbladder, but not beyond. A pioneer study showed that T2b GBCs had higher rates of vascular, neural, and lymph node invasion than those located on the peritoneal side [51]. Furthermore, patients with T2b GBCs achieved a lower overall survival rate 3 and 5 years after OER than patients with tumor located on the peritoneal side. Multivariable analysis demonstrated an association between location on the hepatic side and worse survival [51]. In fact, the location on the hepatic side of the gallbladder predicted recurrence in the liver and distant lymph nodes after radical resection. These data support the idea that tumor location on the hepatic or peritoneal side of the gallbladder predicts the pattern of recurrence and survival after OER of stage T2 GBC (Fig. 1.4).

The magnitude of liver resection is a controversial issue. A meta-analysis of 15 retrospective studies [52], which included a 1332 tumors in stage T2a, and 199 tumors in stage T2b, showed that liver resection improved the overall survival of patients in stage T2b [52]. Gallbladder fossa excision is routinely performed for small-sized T1b, T2a, and T2b GBCs; and IVb/V bi-segmentectomy for larger T2b and T3 tumors with an epicenter in the liver. Note that resection of a large volume of liver parenchyma is not useful if the portal bifurcation is predictably close. Therefore, we favor a IVb/V bi-segmentectomy not for oncological purposes but to achieve a clean R0 margin, with minimum risk of intraoperative hemorrhagic events and/or bile leaks. The rationality of the aforementioned can be supported by the mode by which GBC spreads in the liver. A retrospective analysis was conducted of 42 consecutive patients who underwent resection for

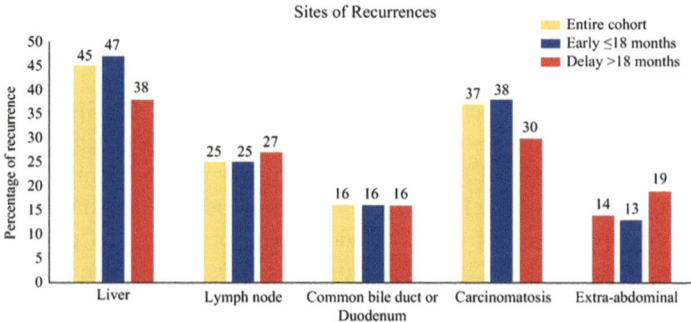

Fig. 1.4 Recurrence in GBC. This bar graphic showed the initial site of recurrence and recurrence patterns (early ≤18 m vs delay >18 m) of gallbladder cancer after OER for 484 patients. (Adapted from: Fig. 1. Vega et al. [5])

GBC. The mode of hepatic spread was classified into 3 patterns: direct invasion through the gallbladder bed, portal tract invasion, and hepatic metastatic nodules. Thirty-five (83%) of the patients had portal track invasion or metastatic nodule in the liver (Fig. 1.5).

There is controversy as to whether the extrahepatic bile duct should be removed. A recent meta-analysis of 12 retrospective studies [54] showed no differences in overall and progression-free survival between patients with or without extrahepatic bile duct

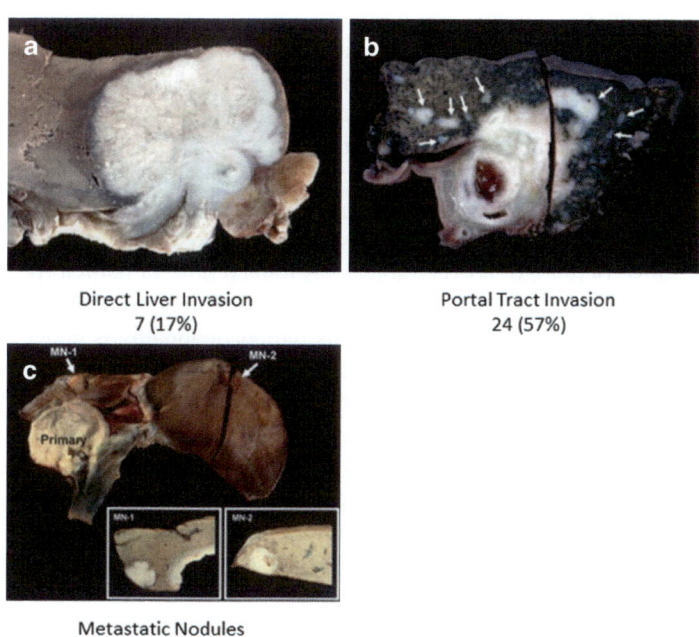

Direct Liver Invasion
7 (17%)

Portal Tract Invasion
24 (57%)

Metastatic Nodules
11 (26%)

Fig. 1.5 Mode of hepatic spread from GBC. 42 consecutive patients underwentresection for gallbladder carcinoma with hepatic involvement verified histologically. Direct liver invasion accounted for only 17% of cases, while portal tract invasion (with or without direct liver invasion) and metastatic nodules in the liver accounted for 83%. (Adapted from: Fig. 1. Wakai et al. [53])

resection. Most strikingly, subgroup analysis of patients in stages T2N0, T3N0, or with positive lymph nodes also showed no improvement in survival after extrahepatic bile duct resection [54]. A bias of this meta-analysis was the inclusion of a high proportion of patients who had advanced tumors undergoing extrahepatic bile duct resection [54]. As such, we do not recommend routine extrahepatic bile duct excision. However, it may be necessary in select patients with a positive cystic duct margin near its insertion to the common bile duct, or if an extended resection is otherwise needed for negative margins.

Adequate lymphadenectomy is important during OER. Inadequate lymphadenectomy is associated with worse outcomes [55–58]. Most current guidelines from the NCCN and the Americas Hepato-Pancreato-Biliary Association (AHPBA) recommend that at least six lymph nodes be harvested to ensure adequate lymphadenectomy [55, 56]. The extent of lymphadenectomy has been a point of debate. Current guidelines recommend dissection of the portal lymph nodes as standard of care, but recommend against routine extended lymphadenectomy (celiac or para-aortic) as this is not associated with improved outcomes [55, 56]. However, in cases where suspicious lymphadenopathy is noticed beyond the portal nodes, or if there is inadequate lymph node yield from portal lymphadenectomy, dissection into other locoregional lymphatic basins may be appropriate [55]. Unfortunately, studies exploring lymph node resection during OER find that surgeons often have inadequate lymphadenectomy, which may have a significant effect on survival [58–60].

Prognostic Factors After Oncologic Extended Resection

The finding of residual cancer after OER for incidental GBC, both in countries with high and low incidence of this disease, is associated with poor progression-free survival even in patients with negative resection margins [61]. These patients are generally good candidates for adjuvant therapy, outlined below. Regarding the

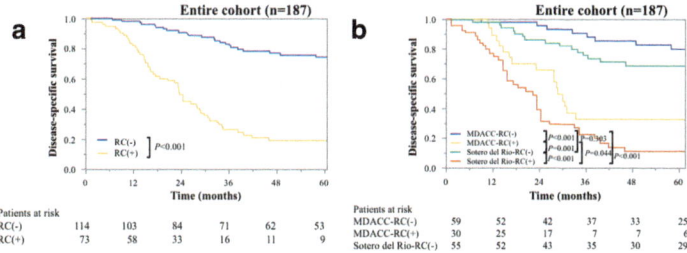

Fig. 1.6 Residual cancer (RC) or residual disease impact. (**a**) Comparison of disease-specific survival (DSS) between patients with and without RC. (**b**) Comparison of DSS between centers with and without RC. (Adapted from: Figs. 2a and 3c. Vinuela et al. [61])

tumor stage, a large international study showed that only T3 and T4 stage disease increases likelihood of recurrence after OER [5] (Fig. 1.6).

Surveillance After Oncologic Extended Resection

The risk of recurrence is highest immediately after OER and decreases with time. In fact, it peaks at 8 months, and more than 80% of recurrences occur within 18 months after OER [5]. Current NCCN guidelines [56] recommend surveillance imaging every 3–6 months for 2 years, followed by imaging every 6–12 months for up to 5 years. However, the risk of recurrence varies according to the stage of GBC found in OER. In fact, it is six times higher for stage III–IV than for stage I–II [5], suggesting that follow-up after OER should be stage-specific. Thus, for patients with stage I-II GBC, we recommend imaging every 6 months for 2 years, followed by annual studies for up to 5 years. For patients with stage III-IV GBC, we recommend imaging and tumor markers every 3 months for 18 months, followed by every 6 months for up to 3 years, and annually for up to 6 years [34]. (Fig. 1.7).

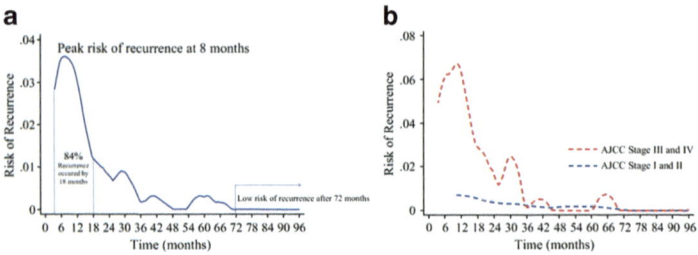

Fig. 1.7 Change in recurrence risk. The figure shows the hazard function made by plotting the incidence rate at any point of time since surgery according to time after OER for GBC overall (**a**) and by stage group (**b**). (Adapted from: Fig. 2. Vega et al. [5])

Minimally Invasive Techniques and Indications

Until recently, radical resection of GBC was performed using an open approach, but some studies have evaluated the feasibility of laparoscopy. A meta-analysis including 18 retrospective studies showed that laparoscopy was similar to the open approach in terms of free resection margin status, recurrence rate, and overall survival [62]. However, most of these studies focused on cases of patients in the early stages of the disease. The suitability of laparoscopy in advanced stages needs to be further evaluated. In addition to the overall comparisons between open and laparoscopic approaches for patients with GBC, it is important to compare outcomes ranked by tumor stage. A meta-analysis of 14 studies showed that patients in stages T1-T3 achieved equal or better survival after laparoscopic surgery compared to the open approach. The analysis, however, was limited by the retrospective nature of the studies [63]. A minimally invasive approach to OER appears feasible and safe in experienced hands. However, a low threshold for choosing an open approach should be maintained, particularly when resection may include adjacent structures or organs.

Adjuvant Treatment

Adjuvant treatment regimens for GBC have often been co-evaluated in phase III trials seeking to determine the therapeutic effect of these regimens on biliary tract malignancies in general [64, 65]. Thus, current treatment regimens for GBC are deduced from series that included not only GBC but also other biliary malignancies such as intrahepatic, perihilar, and extrahepatic cholangiocarcinoma (Table 1.1). The ABC-02 trial [66] showed that the combination of gemcitabine and cisplatin was better than gemcitabine alone in advanced or metastatic biliary tract cancer. These results have since been extrapolated to the adjuvant setting. The PRODIGE trial [67] compared the combination of gemcitabine and oxaliplatin with surveillance, and found no survival benefit of the combined chemotherapeutic agents, although it was criticized for having an underpowered design. The BILCAP trial [68] compared capecitabine versus observation in biliary tract cancers. It showed an overall survival benefit for patients receiving capecitabine that was statistically significant in the per-protocol analysis, but not the intention-to-treat analysis. It serves as the basis for the current recommendation of adjuvant capecitabine in GBC. Recently, long-term outcomes of the BILCAP trial [70] have confirmed that adjuvant treatment with capecitabine can improve overall survival of resected patients and should be considered as the standard of care. Finally, the BCAT clinical trial [69] failed to show a beneficial effect with adjuvant gemcitabine. Although the results are mixed, capecitabine is still considered a first-line agent for GBC patients who qualify for adjuvant therapy.

The role of adjuvant radiotherapy remains to be defined. The meta-analysis of pooled results from 14 retrospective studies [71] showed that adjuvant radiotherapy reduced the risk of death and the risk of recurrence compared to surgery alone. Furthermore, subgroup analysis showed that radiation therapy increased survival in patients with positive lymph nodes and R1 resection. These data suggested that adjuvant radiation therapy may be ben-

Table 1.1 Phase III randomized clinical trials in patients with biliary tract cancers

	ABC-02 [66]	PRODIGE [67]	BILCAP [68]	BCAT [69]
Year of publication	2010	2019	2019	2018
Recruitment period	February 2002–October 2008	July 2009–February 2014	March 2006–December 2014	September 2007–January 2011
Setting (centers, n)	Multicenter (37)	Multicenter (33)	Multicenter (44)	Multicenter (48)
Country	United Kingdom	France	United Kingdom	Japan
Patients, n	410	196	447	225
Pathology	Locally advanced or metastatic cholangiocarcinoma, GBC, or ampullary cancer	Resected biliary tract cancers (intra-, extra-hepatic cholangiocarcinoma, GBC)	Resected biliary tract cancers (cholangiocarcinoma, muscle-invasive GBC)	Resected perihilar and distal cholangiocarcinoma NO GBC
Treatment arms	Cisplatin + gemcitabine vs gemcitabine alone	Gemcitabine + oxaliplatin vs surveillance	Capecitabine vs observation	Gemcitabine vs observation
End-point	Overall survival	Relapse-free survival	Overall survival	Overall survival

Follow-up	8.2 months	46.5 months (96% CI, 42.6–49.3)	60 months (IQR, 37–60)	79.4 months
Overall survival	11.7 months vs 8.1 months (hazard ratio, 0.64; 95% CI, 0.52–0.80)	75.8 months vs 50.8 months (log-rank P = 0.74)	51.1 months vs 36.4 months (hazard ratio P = 0.097)	62.3 months vs 63.8 months (hazard ratio P = 0.964)
Progression-free survival	8.0 months vs 5.0 months (P < 0.001)	30.4 months vs 18.5 months (P = 0.48)	24.4 months vs 17.5 months (P = 0.033)	36.9 months vs 39.9 months (P = 0.693)
Adverse events	Similar, except more neutropenia in the cisplatin + gemcitabine group	Grade 3: 62% vs 18%; grade 4: 11% vs 3% (P = <0.001)	In the capecitabine group, grade 3: 44%; grade 4: 1%	In the gemcitabine group, grade 3/4: Transient non-hematological
Clinical trial information	ClinicalTrials.gov number, NCT00262769	EudraCT, number 2008-004560-39	EudraCT, number 2005-003318-13	UNIM, number ID 000000820

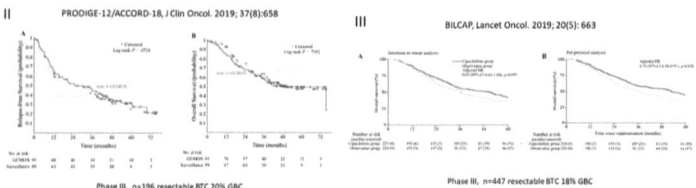

Fig. 1.8 Phase III randomized controlled trials in patients with biliary tract cancers. Survival curves from randomized controlled trials in patients with cancer of the gallbladder (I = 36%, II = 20%, III = 18%) and other locations of the biliary tract (i.e., intrahepatic, perihilar, and extrahepatic cholangiocarcinoma) [66–68]. See Table 1.1 for further details

eficial, especially in high-risk patients. Furthermore, a recent meta-analysis of 21 nonrandomized studies [72] showed that adjuvant external beam radiation therapy, given at doses between 45 and 50.4 Gy, reduced the risk of locoregional recurrence but did not modify the appearance of distant metastases (Fig. 1.8).

Role of Immunotherapy (PD-L1 Inhibitors)

At the somatic level, about 20 aberrant genes have been described in GBC among the approximately 200 genes known to be involved in DNA repair and maintenance of genetic stability [73]. An association was found between the presence of these DNA aberrations and a higher rate of mutation in GBC. Recently, therapies targeting mutations in certain genes such as FGFR, and BRAF, or targeting checkpoint inhibitors such as programmed death-ligand 1 (PD-L1) to trigger a patient's immune response have emerged [74]. In addition, mainly low-positive expression of PD-L1 was detected in 15.6% of GBCs [73]. One study found that increased expression of PD-L1 in tumor and immune cells during late tumorigenesis was a negative predictor of response to immunotherapy in a subset of Western patients with GBC [75]. These findings provide the basis for the future use of immune checkpoint inhibitors to treat patients with GBC. An ongoing study [76] has shown that the addition of durvalumab, a PD-L1 inhibitor, with gemcitabine and cisplatin improves the overall survival of patients with biliary tract cancer. However, to determine whether this therapeutic regimen specifically benefits patients with GBC, data on tumor type and genetic profile would have to be available.

Palliative Treatment

To date, the strongest evidence for palliative chemotherapy comes from the ABC-02 trial, which showed that the combination of gemcitabine and cisplatin was superior to gemcitabine alone in prolonging survival, without increasing toxicity, in patients with advanced or metastatic biliary tract cancer [66]. However, palliative treatment of advanced GBC is not well established. A meta-analysis of 58 studies [77], grouping 1986 patients with metastatic GBC, demonstrated that a high proportion of therapeutic administrations included gemcitabine, either alone or in combination with cisplatin or oxaliplatin. In patients with advanced GBC who received chemotherapy, disease-free survival (4.8 months, 95% CI 4.3 – 5.2) and overall survival (8.3 months, 95% CI 7.6–8.9) were shorter than in patients treated for other biliary malignancies. Improved chemotherapeutic agents or therapeutic regimens that favorably impact the survival of patients with advanced or metastatic GBC are needed.

New therapeutic targets for GBC are being sought. Amplification of the human epidermal growth factor receptor (HER2/neu) gene and overexpression of the protein is associated with a worse prognosis in certain malignancies, a finding that has promoted blockade of these receptors with monoclonal antibodies as a conventional treatment in tumors with HER2/neu overexpression. A large study [78] found that 14% of patients with advanced GBC had both HER2/neu overexpression and worse overall survival, suggesting that this subgroup of patients could benefit from treatment with inhibitors of the HER2/neu pathway. Trastuzumab was the first humanized recombinant monoclonal antibody against HER2, but several biosimilars have recently been approved. One of them, called trastuzumab-*pkrb*, showed promising results in patients with advanced GBC in a recent pilot study [79].

Summary

The increasing incidence of GBC seems to be associated with environmental and lifestyle factors. More incidental GBCs are discovered as more cholecystectomies are performed. Tumors in stage T1b and above require OER, which should be performed in centers with experience in HPB surgery. Although surgical resection is the mainstay of treatment with curative intent, adjuvant chemotherapy and radiotherapy have been shown to improve outcomes. Ongoing research is necessary to find novel ways to combat this aggressive malignancy.

Summary box of the consensus of the American Hepato-Pancreato-biliary Association [55]

1. Evaluate 3 sections of the gallbladder specimen and the cystic duct margin
2. Perform a cholecystectomy for polyps >1.0 cm
3. Determine surgical staging by diagnostic laparoscopy
4. Perform a lymphadenectomy and obtain ~6 lymph nodes and other suspicious areas
5. *En bloc* resection of adjacent liver parenchyma for stages T1b and T2
6. Execute OER in incidental GBC for stages T1b, T2, and T3
7. Perform routine portal lymphadenectomy
8. Resect the bile duct in selected patients if needed to obtain R0 margin
9. Consider neoadjuvant chemotherapy clinical trials for stages T3/T4 or N1
10. Consider adjuvant chemotherapy after R0 resection in stages T2–T4 with N1 nodes or RC

Abbreviations: *OER* oncologic extended resection, *RC* residual cancer

Acknowledgments We would like to thank Dr. Ariana M. Chirban for her valuable editorial support.

References

1. Kanthan R, Senger J-L, Ahmed S, Kanthan SC. Gallbladder cancer in the 21st century. J Oncol. 2015;2015:967472. https://doi.org/10.1155/2015/967472.
2. Misra S, Chaturvedi A, Misra NC, Sharma ID. Carcinoma of the gallbladder. Lancet Oncol. 2003;4(3):167–76. https://doi.org/10.1016/s1470-2045(03)01021-0.
3. Huang J, Patel HK, Boakye D, et al. Worldwide distribution, associated factors, and trends of gallbladder cancer: a global country-level analysis: global epidemiology of gallbladder cancer. Cancer Lett. 2021;521:238–51. https://doi.org/10.1016/j.canlet.2021.09.004.
4. Okumura K, Gogna S, Gachabayov M, et al. Gallbladder cancer: historical treatment and new management options. World J Gastrointest Oncol. 2021;13(10):1317–35. https://doi.org/10.4251/wjgo.v13.i10.1317.
5. Vega EA, Newhook TE, Kawaguchi Y, et al. Conditional recurrence-free survival after oncologic extended resection for gallbladder cancer: an international multicenter analysis. Ann Surg Oncol. 2021;28(5):2675–82. https://doi.org/10.1245/s10434-021-09626-3.
6. Sung H, Ferlay J, Siegel RL, et al. Global cancer statistics 2020: GLOBOCAN estimates of incidence and mortality worldwide for 36 cancers in 185 countries. CA Cancer J Clin. 2021;71(3):209–49. https://doi.org/10.3322/caac.21660.
7. Henley SJ, Weir HK, Jim MA, Watson M, Richardson LC. Gallbladder cancer incidence and mortality, United States 1999–2011. Cancer Epidemiol Biomarkers Prev. 2015;24(9):1319–26. https://doi.org/10.1158/1055-9965.EPI-15-0199.
8. Hundal R, Shaffer EA. Gallbladder cancer: epidemiology and outcome. Clin Epidemiol. 2014;6(1):99–109. https://doi.org/10.2147/CLEP.S37357.
9. Serra I, Calvo A, Báez S, Yamamoto M, Endoh K, Aranda W. Risk factors for gallbladder cancer. An international collaborative case-control study. Cancer. 1996;78(7):1515–7. https://doi.org/10.1097/00008469-200302000-00004.
10. Wiles R, Thoeni RF, Barbu ST, et al. Management and follow-up of gallbladder polyps: joint guidelines between the European Society of Gastrointestinal and Abdominal Radiology (ESGAR), European Association for Endoscopic Surgery and other interventional techniques (EAES), International society of digestive surgery–European Federation (EFISDS) and European society of gastrointestinal endoscopy (ESGE). Eur Radiol. 2017;27(9):3856–66. https://doi.org/10.1007/s00330-017-4742-y.
11. Elmasry M, Lindop D, Dunne DFJ, Malik H, Poston GJ, Fenwick SW. The risk of malignancy in ultrasound detected gallbladder polyps: a

systematic review. Int J Surg. 2016;33(Pt A):28–35. https://doi.org/10.1016/j.ijsu.2016.07.061.
12. Choi SY, Kim TS, Kim HJ, et al. Is it necessary to perform prophylactic cholecystectomy for asymptomatic subjects with gallbladder polyps and gallstones? J Gastroenterol Hepatol. 2010;25(6):1099–104. https://doi.org/10.1111/j.1440-1746.2010.06288.x.
13. Calle EE, Rodriguez C, Walker-Thurmond K, Thun MJ. Overweight, obesity, and mortality from cancer in a prospectively studied cohort of U.S. adults. N Engl J Med. 2003;348(17):1625–38. https://doi.org/10.1056/NEJMoa021423.
14. Campbell PT, Newton CC, Kitahara CM, et al. Body size indicators and risk of gallbladder cancer: pooled analysis of individual-level data from 19 prospective cohort studies. Cancer Epidemiol Biomarkers Prev. 2017;26(4):597–606. https://doi.org/10.1158/1055-9965.EPI-16-0796.
15. Xie F, You Y, Huang J, et al. Association between physical activity and digestive-system cancer: an updated systematic review and meta-analysis. J Sport Heal Sci. 2021;10(1):4–13. https://doi.org/10.1016/j.jshs.2020.09.009.
16. Ling S, Brown K, Miksza JK, et al. Risk of cancer incidence and mortality associated with diabetes: a systematic review with trend analysis of 203 cohorts. Nutr Metab Cardiovasc Dis. 2021;31(1):14–22. https://doi.org/10.1016/j.numecd.2020.09.023.
17. Ling S, Brown K, Miksza JK, et al. Association of type 2 diabetes with cancer: a meta-analysis with bias analysis for unmeasured confounding in 151 cohorts comprising 32 million people. Diabetes Care. 2020;43(9):2313–22. https://doi.org/10.2337/dc20-0204.
18. Jing C, Wang Z, Fu X. Effect of diabetes mellitus on survival in patients with gallbladder cancer: a systematic review and meta-analysis. BMC Cancer. 2020;20(1):1–8. https://doi.org/10.1186/s12885-020-07139-y.
19. Diehl AK. Gallstone size and the risk of gallbladder cancer. JAMA. 1983;250(17):2323–6. http://www.ncbi.nlm.nih.gov/pubmed/6632129
20. Roa I, Ibacache G, Roa J, Araya J, De Aretxabala X, Muñoz S. Gallstones and gallbladder cancer-volume and weight of gallstones are associated with gallbladder cancer: a case-control study. J Surg Oncol. 2006;93(8):624–8. https://doi.org/10.1002/jso.20528.
21. Lugo A, Peveri G, Gallus S. Should we consider gallbladder cancer a new smoking-related cancer? A comprehensive meta-analysis focused on dose–response relationships. Int J Cancer. 2020;146(12):3304–11. https://doi.org/10.1002/ijc.32681.
22. Koshiol J, Wozniak A, Cook P, et al. Salmonella enterica serovar Typhi and gallbladder cancer: a case–control study and meta-analysis. Cancer Med. 2016;5(11):3235–310. https://doi.org/10.1002/cam4.915.
23. Rawla P, Sunkara T, Thandra KC, Barsouk A. Epidemiology of gallbladder cancer. Clin Exp Hepatol. 2019;5(2):93–102. https://doi.org/10.5114/ceh.2019.85166.

24. Guo P, Xu C, Zhou Q, et al. Number of parity and the risk of gallbladder cancer: a systematic review and dose–response meta-analysis of observational studies. Arch Gynecol Obstet. 2016;293(5):1087–96. https://doi.org/10.1007/s00404-015-3896-6.
25. Ko CW, Beresford SAA, Schulte SJ, Matsumoto AM, Lee SP. Incidence, natural history, and risk factors for biliary sludge and stones during pregnancy. Hepatology. 2005;41(2):359–65. https://doi.org/10.1002/hep.20534.
26. Lin J, Peng X, Dong K, et al. Genomic characterization of co-existing neoplasia and carcinoma lesions reveals distinct evolutionary paths of gallbladder cancer. Nat Commun. 2021;12(1):1–11. https://doi.org/10.1038/s41467-021-25012-9.
27. Srivastava K, Srivastava A, Sharma KL, Mittal B. Candidate gene studies in gallbladder cancer: a systematic review and meta-analysis. Mutat Res. 2012;728(1-2):67–79. https://doi.org/10.1016/j.mrrev.2011.06.002.
28. Mhatre S, Wang Z, Nagrani R, et al. Common genetic variation and risk of gallbladder cancer in India: a case-control genome-wide association study. Lancet Oncol. 2017;18(4):535–44. https://doi.org/10.1016/S1470-2045(17)30167-5.
29. Wardell CP, Fujita M, Yamada T, et al. Genomic characterization of biliary tract cancers identifies driver genes and predisposing mutations. J Hepatol. 2018;68(5):959–69. https://doi.org/10.1016/j.jhep.2018.01.009.
30. Koshiol J, Gao YT, Dean M, et al. Association of Aflatoxin and Gallbladder Cancer. Gastroenterology. 2017;153(2):488–494.e1. https://doi.org/10.1053/j.gastro.2017.04.005.
31. Brägelmann J, Barahona Ponce C, Marcelain K, et al. Epigenome-wide analysis of methylation changes in the sequence of gallstone disease, dysplasia, and gallbladder cancer. Hepatology. 2021;73(6):2293–310. https://doi.org/10.1002/hep.31585.
32. Nepal C, Zhu B, O'Rourke CJ, et al. Integrative molecular characterisation of gallbladder cancer reveals micro-environment-associated subtypes. J Hepatol. 2021;74(5):1132–44. https://doi.org/10.1016/j.jhep.2020.11.033.
33. Butte JM, Matsuo K, Gnen M, et al. Gallbladder cancer: differences in presentation, surgical treatment, and survival in patients treated at centers in three countries. J Am Coll Surg. 2011;212(1):50–61. https://doi.org/10.1016/j.jamcollsurg.2010.09.009.
34. Vega EA, Mellado S, Salehi O, Freeman R, Conrad C. Treatment of resectable gallbladder cancer. Cancers (Basel). 2022;14(6):1–16. https://doi.org/10.3390/cancers14061413.
35. Goussous N, Maqsood H, Patel K, et al. Clues to predict incidental gallbladder cancer. Hepatobiliary Pancreat Dis Int. 2018;17(2):149–54. https://doi.org/10.1016/j.hbpd.2018.02.001.
36. Pitt SC, Jin LX, Hall BL, Strasberg SM, Pitt HA. Incidental gallbladder cancer at cholecystectomy: when should the surgeon be suspicious?

Ann Surg. 2014;260(1):128–33. https://doi.org/10.1097/SLA.0000000000000485.
37. Feo CF, Ginesu GC, Fancellu A, et al. Current management of incidental gallbladder cancer: a review. Int J Surg. 2022;98(Jan):106234. https://doi.org/10.1016/j.ijsu.2022.106234.
38. Søreide K, Guest RV, Harrison EM, Kendall TJ, Garden OJ, Wigmore SJ. Systematic review of management of incidental gallbladder cancer after cholecystectomy. Br J Surg. 2019;106(1):32–45. https://doi.org/10.1002/bjs.11035.
39. Giannis D, Cerullo M, Moris D, et al. Validation of the 8th edition American joint commission on cancer (AJCC) gallbladder cancer staging system: prognostic discrimination and identification of key predictive factors. Cancers (Basel). 2021;13(3):1–15. https://doi.org/10.3390/cancers13030547.
40. NCCN clinical practice guidelines in oncology (NCCN guidelines®). Hepatobiliary Cancers, version 2.2022. Accessed August 24, 2022. https://www.nccn.org/guidelines/recently-published-guidelines.
41. Vega EA, Vinuela E, Sanhueza M, et al. Positive cystic duct margin at index cholecystectomy in incidental gallbladder cancer is an important negative prognosticator. Eur J Surg Oncol. 2019;45(6):1061–8. https://doi.org/10.1016/j.ejso.2019.01.013.
42. Vega EA, Vinuela E, Yamashita S, et al. Extended lymphadenectomy is required for incidental gallbladder cancer independent of cystic duct lymph node status. J Gastrointest Surg. 2018;22(1):43–51. https://doi.org/10.1007/s11605-017-3507-x.
43. Behzadmehr R, Salarzaei M. Is contrast enhanced ultrasonography an accurate way to diagnose gallbladder adenoma? A systematic review and meta-analysis. J Med Imag Radiat Sci. 2021;52(1):127–36. https://doi.org/10.1016/j.jmir.2020.09.014.
44. Schnelldorfer T. Porcelain gallbladder: a benign process or concern for malignancy? J Gastrointest Surg. 2013;17(6):1161–8. https://doi.org/10.1007/s11605-013-2170-0.
45. Klimkowski SP, Fung A, Menias CO, Elsayes KM. Gallbladder imaging interpretation pearls and pitfalls: ultrasound, computed tomography, and magnetic resonance imaging. Radiol Clin North Am. 2022;60(5):809–24. https://doi.org/10.1016/j.rcl.2022.05.002.
46. Kuipers H, Hoogwater FJH, Holtman GA, van der Hoorn A, de Boer MT, de Haas RJ. Clinical value of diffusion-weighted MRI for differentiation between benign and malignant gallbladder disease: a systematic review and meta-analysis. Acta Radiol. 2021;62(8):987–96. https://doi.org/10.1177/0284185120950115.
47. Annunziata S, Pizzuto DA, Caldarella C, Galiandro F, Sadeghi R, Treglia G. Diagnostic accuracy of fluorine-18-fluorodeoxyglucose positron emission tomography in gallbladder cancer: a meta-analysis. World J

Gastroenterol. 2015;21(40):11481–8. https://doi.org/10.3748/wjg.v21. i40.11481.
48. Hwang JP, Lim I, Na II, et al. Prognostic value of SUVmax measured by fluorine-18 fluorodeoxyglucose positron emission tomography with computed tomography in patients with gallbladder cancer. Nucl Med Mol Imaging. 2014;48(2):114–20. https://doi.org/10.1007/s13139-013-0255-z.
49. Zhou X. Meta-analysis of the diagnostic performance of serum carbohydrate antigen 19-9 for the detection of gallbladder cancer. Int J Biol Markers. 2022;37(1):81–9. https://doi.org/10.1177/17246008211068866.
50. Vega EA, Vinuela E, Okuno M, et al. Incidental versus non-incidental gallbladder cancer: index cholecystectomy before oncologic re-resection negatively impacts survival in T2b tumors. HPB. 2019;21(8):1046–56. https://doi.org/10.1016/j.hpb.2018.12.006.
51. Shindoh J, De Aretxabala X, Aloia TA, et al. Tumor location is a strong predictor of tumor progression and survival in T2 gallbladder cancer: an international multicenter study. Ann Surg. 2015;261(4):733–9. https://doi.org/10.1097/SLA.0000000000000728.
52. Alrawashdeh W, Kamarajah SK, Gujjuri RR, et al. Systematic review and meta-analysis of survival outcomes in T2a and T2b gallbladder cancers. HPB. 2022;24(6):789–96. https://doi.org/10.1016/j.hpb.2021.12.019.
53. Wakai T, et al. Mode of hepatic spread from gallbladder carcinoma: an immunohistochemical analysis of 42 hepatectomized specimens. Am J Surg Pathol. 2010;34(1):65–74.
54. Lv TR, Liu F, Hu HJ, et al. The role of extra-hepatic bile duct resection in the surgical management of gallbladder carcinoma. A first meta-analysis. Eur J Surg Oncol. 2022;48(3):482–91. https://doi.org/10.1016/j.ejso.2021.11.131.
55. Aloia TA, Járufe N, Javle M, et al. Gallbladder cancer: expert consensus statement. HPB. 2015;17(8):681–90. https://doi.org/10.1111/hpb.12444.
56. National Comprehensive Cancer Network (NCCN) Guidelines, version 2.2022. Biliary Tract Cancers: Gallbladder Cancer.
57. Widmann B, Warschkow R, Beutner U, et al. Effect of lymphadenectomy in curative gallbladder cancer treatment: a systematic review and meta-analysis. Langenbeck's Arch Surg. 2020;405(5):573–84. https://doi.org/10.1007/s00423-020-01878-z.
58. Kemp Bohan PM, O'Shea AE, Ellis OV, et al. Rates, predictors, and outcomes of portal lymphadenectomy for resectable gallbladder cancer. Ann Surg Oncol. 2021;28(6):2960–72. https://doi.org/10.1245/s10434-021-09667-8.
59. Leigh NL, Solomon D, Feingold D, et al. Staging gallbladder cancer with lymphadenectomy: the practical application of new AHPBA and AJCC guidelines. HPB. 2019;21(11):1563–9. https://doi.org/10.1016/j.hpb.2019.03.372.

60. Salehi O, Vega EA, Mellado S, et al. High-quality surgery for gallbladder carcinoma: rare, associated with disparity, and not substitutable by chemotherapy. J Gastrointest Surg. 2022;26(6):1241–51. https://doi.org/10.1007/s11605-022-05290-4.
61. Vinuela E, Vega EA, Yamashita S, et al. Incidental gallbladder cancer: residual cancer discovered at oncologic extended resection determines outcome: a report from high- and low-incidence countries. Ann Surg Oncol. 2017;24(8):2334–43. https://doi.org/10.1245/s10434-017-5859-6.
62. Lv TR, Yang C, Regmi P, et al. The role of laparoscopic surgery in the surgical management of gallbladder carcinoma: a systematic review and meta-analysis. Asian J Surg. 2021;44(12):1493–502. https://doi.org/10.1016/j.asjsur.2021.03.015.
63. Nakanishi H, Miangul S, Oluwaremi TT, Sim BL, Hong SS, Than CA. Open versus laparoscopic surgery in the management of patients with gallbladder cancer: a systematic review and meta-analysis. Am J Surg. 2022;224(1):348–57. https://doi.org/10.1016/j.amjsurg.2022.03.002.
64. Gamboa AC, Maithel SK. The landmark series: gallbladder cancer. Ann Surg Oncol. 2020;27(8):2846–58. https://doi.org/10.1245/s10434-020-08654-9.
65. Allen MJ, Knox JJ. A review of current adjuvant and neoadjuvant systemic treatments for cholangiocarcinoma and gallbladder carcinoma. Hepatoma Res. 2021;7:73. https://doi.org/10.20517/2394-5079.2021.98.
66. Valle J, Wasan H, Palmer DH, et al. Cisplatin plus gemcitabine versus gemcitabine for biliary tract cancer. N Engl J Med. 2010;362(14):1273–81. https://doi.org/10.1056/NEJMoa0908721.
67. Edeline J, Benabdelghani M, Bertaut A, et al. Gemcitabine and oxaliplatin chemotherapy or surveillance in resected biliary tract cancer (Prodige 12-accord 18-Unicancer GI): a randomized phase III study. J Clin Oncol. 2019;37(8):658–67. https://doi.org/10.1200/JCO.18.00050.
68. Primrose JN, Neoptolemos J, Palmer DH, et al. Capecitabine compared with observation in resected biliary tract cancer (BILCAP): a randomised, controlled, multicentre, phase 3 study. Lancet Oncol. 2019;20(5):663–73. https://doi.org/10.1016/S1470-2045(18)30915-X.
69. Ebata T, Hirano S, Konishi M, et al. Randomized clinical trial of adjuvant gemcitabine chemotherapy versus observation in resected bile duct cancer. Br J Surg. 2018;105(3):192–202. https://doi.org/10.1002/bjs.10776.
70. Bridgewater J, Fletcher P, Palmer DH, et al. Long-term outcomes and exploratory analyses of the randomized phase III BILCAP study. J Clin Oncol. 2022;40(18):2048–57. https://doi.org/10.1200/JCO.21.02568.
71. Kim BH, Kwon J, Chie EK, et al. Adjuvant Chemoradiotherapy is associated with improved survival for patients with resected gallbladder carcinoma: a systematic review and meta-analysis. Ann Surg Oncol. 2018;25(1):255–64. https://doi.org/10.1245/s10434-017-6139-1.

72. Choi SH, Rim CH, Shin IS, Yoon WS, Koom WS, Seong J. Benefit of adjuvant radiotherapy for gallbladder cancer: a comparability-based meta-analysis. Hepatol Int. 2022;16(3):712–27. https://doi.org/10.1007/s12072-022-10343-6.
73. Abdel-Wahab R, Yap TA, Madison R, et al. Genomic profiling reveals high frequency of DNA repair genetic aberrations in gallbladder cancer. Sci Rep. 2020;10(1):1–8. https://doi.org/10.1038/s41598-020-77939-6.
74. Hu ZI, Lim K-H. Evolving paradigms in the systemic treatment of advanced gallbladder cancer: updates in year 2022. Cancers (Basel). 2022;14(5):1–16. https://doi.org/10.3390/cancers14051249.
75. Albrecht T, Brinkmann F, Albrecht M, et al. Programmed death Ligand-1 (PD-L1) is an independent negative prognosticator in Western-world gallbladder cancer. Cancers (Basel). 2021;13(7):1–18. https://doi.org/10.3390/cancers13071682.
76. Oh D-Y, Ruth He A, Qin S, et al. Durvalumab plus gemcitabine and cisplatin in advanced biliary tract cancer. NEJM Evid. 2022;1:EVIDoa2200015. https://doi.org/10.1056/evidoa2200015.
77. Azizi AA, Lamarca A, McNamara MG, Valle JW. Chemotherapy for advanced gallbladder cancer (GBC): a systematic review and meta-analysis. Crit Rev Oncol Hematol. 2021;163(August 2020):103328. https://doi.org/10.1016/j.critrevonc.2021.103328.
78. Roa I, de Toro G, Schalper K, de Aretxabala X, Churi C, Javle M. Overexpression of the HER2/neu gene: a new therapeutic possibility for patients with advanced gallbladder cancer. Gastrointest Cancer Res. 2014;7(2):42–8.
79. Jeong H, Jeong JH, Kim K-P, et al. Feasibility of HER2-targeted therapy in advanced biliary tract cancer: a prospective pilot study of Trastuzumab biosimilar in combination with gemcitabine plus cisplatin. Cancers (Basel). 2021;13(2):1–12. https://doi.org/10.3390/cancers13020161.

Pre-malignant Gallbladder Lesions

Kevin M. Turner, Aaron M. Delman, and Gregory C. Wilson

Introduction

While gallbladder cancer (GBC) is a rare malignancy in the United States, affecting just over 12,000 persons per year, prognosis remains poor, especially for those with unresectable disease [1]. In the minority of patients who present with resectable disease, survival outcomes are significantly improved, with up to two-thirds of patients surviving to 5 years [2]. Early diagnosis is paramount to success with this deadly disease. Increasing awareness by surgeons of pre-malignant gallbladder lesions promises to lead to earlier interventions when surgical resection remains feasible to stop the malignant transformation. However, inherent challenges in identifying a rare cancer when the "precursor" lesion (i.e., gallbladder polyp) is relatively common have proved difficult to overcome. Therefore, a complete understanding of the optimal management of these lesions is needed for all surgeons

K. M. Turner · A. M. Delman
Department of Surgery, University of Cincinnati College of Medicine, Cincinnati, OH, USA

G. C. Wilson (✉)
Department of Surgery, Division of Surgical Oncology, University of Cincinnati College of Medicine, Cincinnati, OH, USA
e-mail: wilsong3@ucmail.uc.edu

operating on the gallbladder to optimize outcomes and prevent mortality due to GBC.

Gallbladder Polyps

Gallbladder polyps (GP) are defined as raised projections of the gallbladder wall into the lumen. They are immobile and display no acoustic shadowing, differentiating them from calculi. Moreover, a mass that is infiltrating and large is considered a cancer and treated as such. Most GPs remain asymptomatic, but some can cause symptoms of biliary colic or acute cholecystitis if they occlude the cystic duct. They are most commonly found on transabdominal ultrasound (TAUS), occurring in 0.3–9.5% of studies, but can also be seen on gross pathologic evaluation of gallbladder specimens [3]. The sensitivity and specificity for TAUS reported in a recent Cochrane review is very good at 0.84 (95%CI: 0.59–0.95) and 0.96 (95%CI: 0.92–0.98), respectively [4]. The Achilles heel of this modality is a high false positive rate and a low positive predictive value due to the low prevalence of GPs. However, the ubiquitous nature of this modality combined with its low cost, low risk profile, and high sensitivity still makes it first-line for evaluating suspected GPs. Additional diagnostic modalities, including high-resolution ultrasound, endoscopic ultrasound, and diffusion weighted MRI, among others, may be appropriate at expert institutions, but require more research prior to broad dissemination [5].

GPs can be divided into two categories: true polyps and pseudopolyps. The former are also called adenomatous polyps and are seen in the clear minority following cholecystectomy for GPs, occurring in only 0.4–15.9% of specimens [6–9]. Pseudopolyps include cholesterol polyps, inflammatory polyps, and adenomyomatosis [10]. In the case of clear reverberations or "comet tail artifact" seen on TAUS of suspected GPs, the lesion is classified as a pseudopolyp and requires no further intervention (Fig. 2.1) [5]. However, not all pseudopolyps display these findings and therefore require further evaluation. TAUS does not perform as well differentiating true polyps from

2 Pre-malignant Gallbladder Lesions

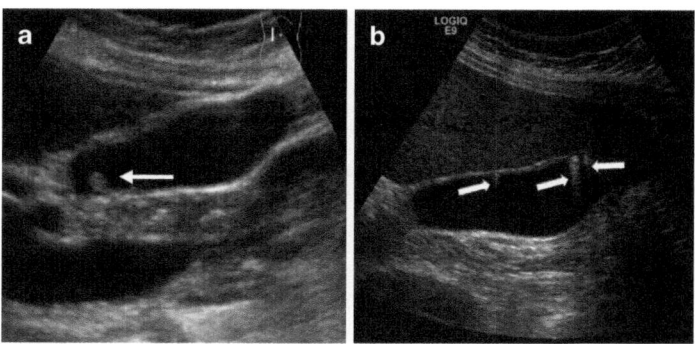

Fig. 2.1 Selected images from two different patients show (**a**) a true gallbladder polyp and (**b**) a pseudo-polyp demonstrating posterior reverberation or "comet-tail" artifact. (Figure and legend adopted from [5]. Publisher: SpingerLink)

pseudopolyps, with a summary sensitivity and specificity of 0.68 (95%CI: 0.44–0.85) and 0.79 (95%CI: 0.57–0.95), respectively [4].

The management of GPs is designed to allow for early intervention to prevent the development of malignancy, while also lowering the rate of unnecessary cholecystectomies and associated risks (i.e., surgical site infection, bile leak, bile duct injury). Unfortunately due to their rare nature and subsequent difficulty designing prospective studies, the majority of data to date on GPs is based on retrospective series. Therefore, current management is in line with consensus guidelines adopted by the European Society of Gastrointestinal and Abdominal Radiology (ESGAR), European Association for Endoscopic Surgery and other Interventional Techniques (EAES), International Society of Digestive Surgery-European Federation (EFISDS), and the European Society of Gastrointestinal Endoscopy (ESGE), first published in 2017 and updated in 2022 [3, 5]. The guidelines primarily use polyp size on TAUS and risk factors for GBC to delineate need for cholecystectomy, follow-up imaging, or no additional follow-up (Fig. 2.2). Polyp size is the predominant factor because of the known increased risk of malignancy with larger polyps. The decision for surgical intervention is always taken in context with

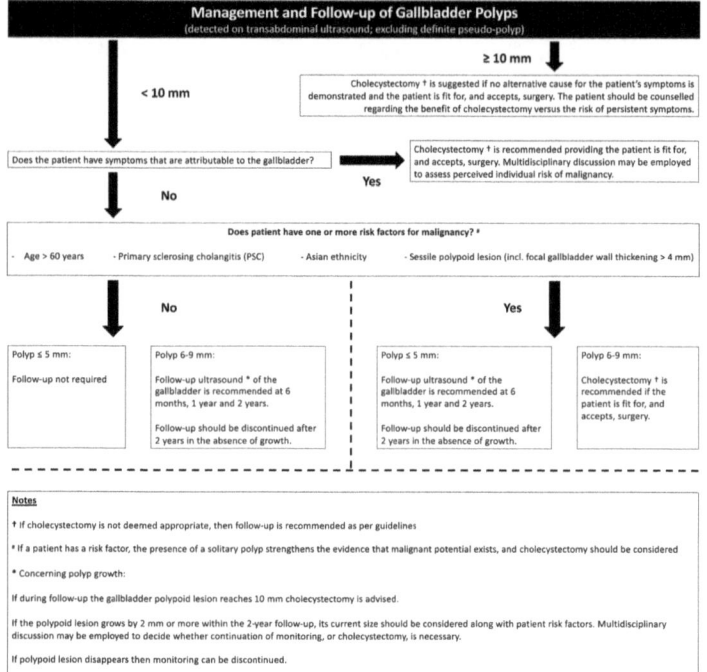

Fig. 2.2 Management algorithm for gallbladder polyps. (Figure adopted from [5]. Publisher: SpingerLink)

the fitness of the patient to undergo surgery. For patients with multiple lesions, guidelines are based on the largest polyp.

Any symptomatic patient is recommended for cholecystectomy. GP size is divided into three categories: ≥10 mm, 6–9 mm, and <5 mm. Patients are described as non-high risk and high risk based on the following: Age >60, primary sclerosing cholangitis, Asian ethnicity, and sessile polyp. Solitary polyps strengthen the argument for cholecystectomy but alone does not classify a patient as high-risk. Cholecystectomy is indicated for any lesion ≥10 mm or those high-risk patients with a 6–9 mm polyp. Follow-up imaging with TAUS at 6 months, 1 year, and 2 years is recommended for high-risk patients with polyps <5 mm and non-high-risk patients with polyps 6–9 mm. In those patients without risk factors and lesions <5 mm, no follow-up is required. On follow-up imaging, cholecystectomy is indicated if the lesion ≥10 mm. Individualized patient discussions should be had for polyps that grow ≥2 mm on follow-up imaging. If the polyp disappears, monitoring should be discontinued.

Numerous studies have questioned the utility of current recommendations with respect to GP size and growth on serial imaging. Metman et al. showed in a series of 108 patients who underwent cholecystectomy for GPs with a mean pre-operative diameter of 10 mm that only 3% had true adenomas on final pathology [8]. In an elegant study out of the Kaiser Permanente Northern California system, Szpakowski et al. suggested that GP growth by 2 mm was part of the natural history of the lesion and the rate of GBC was similar with and without GPs [11]. Despite these findings, polyp size remains the benchmark factor to guide the management of these lesions.

Dysplastic Precursors of Gallbladder Cancer

The major precursor lesions of GBC can be broken down into two main forms: [1] Flat/Non-Tumoral Forming Dysplasia and [2] Tumoral Forming Dysplasia. The former accounts for the majority of GBC with coexisting precursor lesions, while tumoral forming dysplasia is found in only 5–23% of invasive carcinomas [12]. GBC can also develop independently of precursor lesions in up to half of the cases and is associated with more aggressive disease [13].

Flat/Non-tumoral Forming Dysplasia

Similar to the pathogenesis of Barrett's Esophagus and pancreatic intraepithelial neoplasia, the stepwise microscopic dysplasia (<1 cm) associated with GBC is termed biliary intraepithelial neoplasms (BilIN). These lesions are indistinguishable from the surrounding mucosa grossly. As in other organs of the digestive tract, BilIN is categorized by increasing cytologic atypia into BilIN-1, BilIN-2, and BilIN-3 [14]. While the first two are of little clinical significance, BilIN-3 is equivalent to "carcinoma in situ" and requires extensive sampling to rule out co-existing invasive disease [15]. It is particularly difficult to determine high-grade BilIN from invasive disease in a Rokitansky-Aschoff sinus, requiring experienced pathologic review [12]. Research has suggested the dysplasia–carcinoma progression is a stepwise approach, with early KRAS mutations and overexpression of p53 reserved for later in disease progression, often in invasive disease [16]. However, the presence of BilIN independent of invasive disease is extremely rare. In those rare cases where it is isolated, cholecystectomy with negative margins is curative of even high-grade dysplasia (BilIN-3). However, optimal management of cholecystectomy specimens with margins involved by BilIN remains unknown, due to the infrequent nature of this finding.

Tumoral Forming Dysplasia

Intracholecystic papillary neoplasms (ICPN) of the gallbladder is a relatively new pathologic entity used to describe exophytic pre-invasive neoplasms that measure ≥1 cm [14]. These lesions are akin to the more recognizable intraductal papillary mucinous neoplasms of the pancreas. Predominantly found in older females, they represent a terminology meant to unify the confusing lexicon of exophytic precursor gallbladder lesions existing in the literature, while emphasizing the fact that subcentimeter lesions are rarely of clinical importance. IPCN represents the adenoma–carcinoma sequence of GBC, similar to the progression seen in colon cancer and reportedly found in 6.4% of all GBCs [17]. Syndromic occurrences in Gardner's and Puetz-Jeghers have been reported [12]. IPCNs are classified based on the cell type and marked by hallmark genes: (a) biliary (50%, MUC1); (b) gastric (foveolar [16%, MUC5AC] and pyloric [20%, MUC6]); (c) intestinal (8%, CK20/CDX2/MUC2); (d) oncocytic (6%, MUC1). In contrast to flat dysplasia, mass-forming dysplasia can be seen in the absence of invasive disease, reportedly in up to half of cases [15, 17]. Moreover, survival outcomes were dramatically better for invasive IPCNs with a median overall survival of 35 months, compared to convention GBC at 9 months [17]. While infrequently encountered, IPCNs represent a pathologic entity with a chance for prolonged survival and even cure when detected in a preinvasive state [12]. In general when these lesions are encountered, cholecystectomy is recommended so that complete histologic examination can be performed and the underlying invasive component identified or excluded.

Porcelain Gallbladder

Porcelain gallbladder is defined as calcifications of the gallbladder due to an idiopathic etiology, though chronic cholecystitis, alterations in calcium metabolism, and intramural hemorrhage have all been suggested as potential mechanisms [18–20]. This finding is exceedingly rare, reported in between 0.01% and 0.2% of patients with gallbladder disease, most often occurring in the elderly [21, 22]. A majority of patients remain asymptomatic with the finding detected incidentally on abdominal imaging, though patients may present with right upper quadrant pain due to gallstone or gallbladder disease. While early reports suggested very high rates of associated GBC, contemporary studies have shown a much weaker association, with malignancy found between 0% and 5% of all porcelain gallbladders [21, 23, 24]. Two subtypes have been proposed due to their differential risk of malignancy: complete intramural calcification and selective mucosal calcification [25]. Reports have shown malignancy rates up to 7% of all gallbladders with selective mucosal calcification, while the risk of malignancy is much lower or even absent with complete intramural calcification [24, 26–28].. Based on the low risk of malignancy found in patients with porcelain gallbladders, a shared decision-making process should be conducted for all patients regarding the need for cholecystectomy.

Conclusion

In conclusion, increasing awareness of pre-malignant lesions of the gallbladder has greatly increased our understanding of these lesions with the hope of lowering the mortality of GBC. Polyps are the most frequently recognized lesions whose management is based on retrospective evidence of increasing risk of malignancy with increasing size and the presence of risk factors. Due to a lack of level one evidence, 10 mm remains the cutoff after which cholecystectomy is recommended, with earlier intervention reserved for those at high-risk for GBC. Improved understanding of the pathogenesis of GBC has led to the classification of non-tumor and tumoral dysplasia, with the latter described as IPCNs, a clinically detectable lesion that can mandate resection to prevent malignant transformation. Finally, recent literature has shown that a porcelain gallbladder does not carry the same malignancy risk as once prescribed, with the risk of malignancy mostly limited to those with selective mucosal calcification. All surgeons operating on the gallbladder should have an understanding of these lesions to offer guideline-appropriate care and optimize outcomes in this population.

References

1. Society. AC. Cancer Facts & Figures 2022. https://www.cancer.org/content/dam/cancer-org/research/cancer-facts-and-statistics/annual-cancer-facts-and-figures/2022/2022-cancer-facts-and-figures.pdf. Accessed 17 Aug 2022.
2. American Cancer Society. Survival rates for gallbladder cancer. https://www.cancer.org/cancer/gallbladder-cancer/detection-diagnosis-staging/survival-rates.html. Accessed 17 Aug 2022.
3. Wiles R, Thoeni RF, Barbu ST, et al. Management and follow-up of gallbladder polyps: joint guidelines between the European Society of Gastrointestinal and Abdominal Radiology (ESGAR), European Association for Endoscopic Surgery and other interventional techniques (EAES), International Society of Digestive Surgery—European federation (EFISDS) and European Society of Gastrointestinal Endoscopy (ESGE). Eur Radiol. 2017;27(9):3856–66.

4. Wennmacker SZ, Lamberts MP, Di Martino M, Drenth JP, Gurusamy KS, van Laarhoven CJ. Transabdominal ultrasound and endoscopic ultrasound for diagnosis of gallbladder polyps. Cochrane Database Syst Rev. 2018;8:CD012233.
5. Foley KG, Lahaye MJ, Thoeni RF, et al. Management and follow-up of gallbladder polyps: updated joint guidelines between the ESGAR, EAES, EFISDS and ESGE. Eur Radiol. 2022;32(5):3358–68.
6. Farinon AM, Pacella A, Cetta F, Sianesi M. "Adenomatous polyps of the gallbladder" adenomas of the gallbladder. HPB Surg. 1991;3(4):251–8.
7. Ito H, Hann LE, D'Angelica M, et al. Polypoid lesions of the gallbladder: diagnosis and followup. J Am Coll Surg. 2009;208(4):570–5.
8. Metman MJH, Olthof PB, van der Wal JBC, van Gulik TM, Roos D, Dekker JWT. Clinical relevance of gallbladder polyps; is cholecystectomy always necessary? HPB (Oxford). 2020;22(4):506–10.
9. Sarkut P, Kilicturgay S, Ozer A, Ozturk E, Yilmazlar T. Gallbladder polyps: factors affecting surgical decision. World J Gastroenterol. 2013;19(28):4526–30.
10. Christensen AH, Ishak KG. Benign tumors and pseudotumors of the gallbladder. Report of 180 cases. Arch Pathol. 1970;90(5):423–32.
11. Szpakowski JL, Tucker LY. Outcomes of gallbladder polyps and their association with gallbladder cancer in a 20-year cohort. JAMA Netw Open. 2020;3(5):e205143.
12. Bal MM, Ramadwar M, Deodhar K, Shrikhande S. Pathology of gallbladder carcinoma: current understanding and new perspectives. Pathol Oncol Res. 2015;21(3):509–25.
13. Nakanuma Y, Sugino T, Nomura Y, et al. Association of precursors with invasive adenocarcinoma of the gallbladder: a clinicopathological study. Ann Diagn Pathol. 2022;58:151911.
14. Nagtegaal ID, Odze RD, Klimstra D, et al. The 2019 WHO classification of tumours of the digestive system. Histopathology. 2020;76(2):182–8.
15. Adsay NV. Neoplastic precursors of the gallbladder and extrahepatic biliary system. Gastroenterol Clin N Am. 2007;36(4):889–900. vii
16. Hsu M, Sasaki M, Igarashi S, Sato Y, Nakanuma Y. KRAS and GNAS mutations and p53 overexpression in biliary intraepithelial neoplasia and intrahepatic cholangiocarcinomas. Cancer. 2013;119(9):1669–74.
17. Adsay V, Jang KT, Roa JC, et al. Intracholecystic papillary-tubular neoplasms (ICPN) of the gallbladder (neoplastic polyps, adenomas, and papillary neoplasms that are >/=1.0 cm): clinicopathologic and immunohistochemical analysis of 123 cases. Am J Surg Pathol. 2012;36(9):1279–301.
18. Cornell CM, Clarke R. Vicarious calcification involving the gallbladder. Ann Surg. 1959;149(2):267–72.
19. Fowler WF. Calcareous changes of the gall-bladder wall. Ann Surg. 1923;78(5):623–7.

20. Phemister DB, Rewbridge AG, Rudisill H. Calcium carbonate gall-stones and calcification of the gall-bladder following cystic-duct obstruction. Ann Surg. 1931;94(4):493–516.
21. Schnelldorfer T. Porcelain gallbladder: a benign process or concern for malignancy? J Gastrointest Surg. 2013;17(6):1161–8.
22. Towfigh S, McFadden DW, Cortina GR, et al. Porcelain gallbladder is not associated with gallbladder carcinoma. Am Surg. 2001;67(1):7–10.
23. DesJardins H, Duy L, Scheirey C, Schnelldorfer T. Porcelain gallbladder: is observation a safe option in select populations? J Am Coll Surg. 2018;226(6):1064–9.
24. Khan ZS, Livingston EH, Huerta S. Reassessing the need for prophylactic surgery in patients with porcelain gallbladder: case series and systematic review of the literature. Arch Surg. 2011;146(10):1143–7.
25. Shimizu M, Miura J, Tanaka T, Itoh H, Saitoh Y. Porcelain gallbladder: relation between its type by ultrasound and incidence of cancer. J Clin Gastroenterol. 1989;11(4):471–6.
26. Berk RN, Armbuster TG, Saltzstein SL. Carcinoma in the porcelain gallbladder. Radiology. 1973;106(1):29–31.
27. Kane RA, Jacobs R, Katz J, Costello P. Porcelain gallbladder: ultrasound and CT appearance. Radiology. 1984;152(1):137–41.
28. Stephen AE, Berger DL. Carcinoma in the porcelain gallbladder: a relationship revisited. Surgery. 2001;129(6):699–703.

Intraoperative Management of Incidental Neoplastic Findings (Gallbladder)

Holly V. Spitzer and Daniel W. Nelson

Introduction

With an incidence ranging from 0.14% to 2.8% worldwide [1–4], gallbladder carcinoma represents the 6th most common malignancy in the world and the single most common cancer of the biliary tract [1, 5]. It is an aggressive cancer with most patients presenting with locally advanced or metastatic disease at the time of diagnosis [1–4]. Prognosis is generally poor with only 16–18% of patients surviving to 5 years [1, 6, 7]. Carcinoma is thought to develop from chronic inflammation of the gallbladder, which can result from cholelithiasis, morbid obesity, autoimmune disease, and occupational exposures [1].

While 30–40% of gallbladder cancer cases are diagnosed clinically during routine evaluation for abdominal pain or abnormal liver function tests, the majority of cases are incidentally discovered, either during or following cholecystectomy for apparent

H. V. Spitzer
Department of Surgery, William Beaumont Army Medical Center, El Paso, TX, USA

D. W. Nelson (✉)
Department of Surgery, University of Tennessee Health Science Center College of Medicine - Chattanooga, Chattanooga, TN, USA

benign biliary disease [4, 8]. In fact, among all cholecystectomies, incidental gallbladder cancer is identified in up to 3% of resections for presumed benign gallbladder disorders [8, 9]. Laparoscopic cholecystectomy is the second most commonly performed abdominal surgery worldwide. Consequently, incidental gallbladder cancer is being encountered with increasing frequency [9].

Incidental gallbladder cancer presents a uniquely challenging scenario, as management guidelines are poorly established and numerous controversies remain. Although challenging, incidentally discovered gallbladder cancer is usually diagnosed at an earlier pathologic stage and is associated with a twofold improved survival compared to preoperatively diagnosed cases [8, 9]. In this chapter, we review current recommendations for the management of unsuspected or incidentally discovered gallbladder cancer, in two common scenarios:

- Intraoperative concern for gallbladder cancer identified during cholecystectomy for benign biliary disease or other intra-abdominal procedures.

- Postoperatively diagnosed gallbladder cancer identified on final histopathology following cholecystectomy for benign biliary disease.

Intraoperative Concern for Gallbladder Cancer

While performing a cholecystectomy or other intra-abdominal procedure, one may suspect gallbladder cancer based on a number of factors, including difficult dissection, presence of lymphadenopathy, visible masses or lesions on the gallbladder, liver or on the peritoneum, isolated segmental thickening of the gallbladder wall, sclerotic mucosa or abnormal mucosal appearance, presence of polyps, or palpable masses within the specimen following removal [9, 10]. Gallbladder cancer has been identified intraoperatively during cholecystectomy for a wide range of suspected benign biliary pathologies. The preoperative diagnosis and surgical indications have not been shown to predict intraoperative discovery of gallbladder cancer [3].

Suspicion may be aroused immediately upon visualization of the gallbladder or early during cholecystectomy (prior to ligation of the cystic duct or artery). In this situation, the most prudent course of action would be to perform intraoperative staging and discontinue the procedure with plans for referral to a center with hepatobiliary expertise for complete staging evaluation and definitive management [11]. Intraoperative staging should include careful inspection of the peritoneum, omentum, and viscera for metastasis [12]. It should also include evaluation of the lymph node basins, including the celiac axis and superior mesenteric artery, retroperitoneum, and hepatoduodenal ligament for overt lymphadenopathy [12]. Consideration of intraoperative biopsy has been recommended, but should be approached with caution as this may increase the risk of local recurrence and peritoneal carcinomatosis associated with perforation [4, 9].

The National Comprehensive Cancer Network (NCCN) guidelines do provide recommendations for consideration of definitive management at the time of discovery with radical cholecystectomy consisting of either anatomic segment 4b and 5 liver resection or non-anatomic partial or wedge liver resection and lymphadenectomy, if hepatobiliary expertise is readily available (Fig. 3.1) [9, 13]. However, some caveats to this approach should be considered. First, in this situation, preoperative consent was likely limited to cholecystectomy and may not have included possible hepatic resection and lymphadenectomy, as this was not anticipated. As both hepatic resection and lymphadenectomy carry increased risk of morbidity [12, 14–17], preoperative discussion of this possibility is an important component of informed consent. Second, proceeding with radical cholecystectomy without staging poses the risk of performing a non-therapeutic, morbid operation for patients who would have been deemed unresectable due to the presence of distant metastases, which can be discovered in over 25% of patients [8]. Finally, incomplete resection is associated with significantly reduced overall and disease-free survival, so resection should not be attempted unless R0 resectability is certain [8].

Some centers have endorsed routinely opening and inspecting all gallbladder specimens after extraction, with the intention to

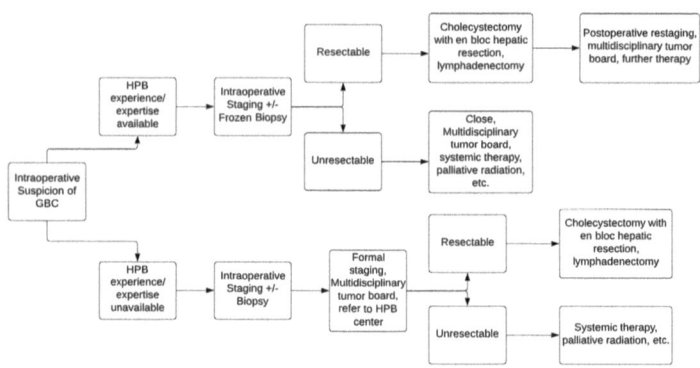

Fig. 3.1 Management of incidental gallbladder cancer identified intraoperatively [9, 12]

identify gallbladder cancer at initial operation [9]. This potentially would allow for immediate oncologic resection, rather than delayed re-resection. This is in response to data suggesting that the presence of residual disease after initial resection is associated with shorter disease-free survival and overall survival [8]. If suspicion for gallbladder cancer is aroused following removal of the gallbladder specimen from the abdomen, a full-thickness tissue biopsy of the extracted gallbladder may be obtained and sent for pathologic frozen section evaluation. Diagnosis from frozen biopsy has been shown to be congruent with final pathologic reports, supporting its use to accurately diagnose gallbladder cancer, and may assist with expediting initial diagnostic and staging information [18]. Although frozen section has been shown to prolong operative time, this has not been shown to affect outcomes [18]. If the frozen biopsy returns consistent with gallbladder cancer, intraoperative staging should be completed and the presence of hepatobiliary expertise should guide next steps (Fig. 3.1). If the biopsy demonstrates adenocarcinoma and suggests that disease is confined to the mucosa, the patient can be considered surgically complete [4, 9, 11, 13, 19]. If hepatobiliary expertise is present and the biopsy is suggestive of extension beyond the mucosa, then hepatic resection and lymphadenectomy may reasonably follow during the same procedure [9, 13], with the caveats discussed above.

If the surgeon elects to proceed with hepatic resection and lymphadenectomy at the initial procedure, principles of resectability must be prioritized. These principles are also priorities of re-resection and are discussed later in this chapter. However, some unique considerations exist in this setting. In particular, for the patient to benefit from initial resection, an R0 resection must be achieved [9]. Multivisceral resection is reasonable in this pursuit [9]. En bloc resection should be performed, if possible, to avoid transection of the tumor and potential seeding [12]. Factors associated with failed initial R0 resection include difficult dissection, perforation, lymphadenopathy, hepatic-sided tumor, T3 and T4 tumor, and presence of lymphovascular or perineural invasion [12, 20].

Regardless of whether resection is performed at the time of discovery or at a future date, any patient diagnosed with gallbladder cancer should undergo complete staging evaluation and be discussed in a multidisciplinary setting [4, 9, 13, 18, 19, 21, 22].

Postoperative Pathologic Diagnosis of Gallbladder Cancer

Any patient found to have gallbladder cancer after cholecystectomy should undergo a complete staging evaluation. This should include clinical evaluation with history and physical, laboratory evaluation consisting of liver function testing and tumor markers (CA 19-9, CEA), and computed tomography (CT) of the chest, abdomen, and pelvis [13]. Positron emission tomography (PET) may be considered, but is not necessary in all cases [11].

Pathologic evaluation should include reporting of the area of the gallbladder involved. In particular, T2 tumors involving the hepatic side of the gallbladder are associated with worse overall survival, and are associated with concurrent occult nodal disease, vascular invasion, microscopic invasion of the liver, and subsequent hepatic recurrence [12, 23]. This is thought to be related to diffuse lymphatics and vascularity in the area, facilitating drainage to the portal venous system [24, 25]. Importantly, the significance of peritoneal side and hepatic side location is reflected in the American Joint Committee on Cancer (AJCC) 8th edition staging system, with hepatic side T2 tumors receiving a T2b designation, while T2 tumors on the peritoneal side are designated T2a [13]. This delineation is primarily prognostic, but should be considered during staging, as patients with hepatic side disease may require more extensive re-resection and may have occult nodal or metastatic disease at the time of diagnosis.

Patients who are diagnosed based on pathologic evaluation of the gallbladder specimen postoperatively can be divided into three major groups that drive further management decisions: T1a tumors with negative margins, ≥T1b tumors, and T1a tumors with a positive cystic duct margin and/or a positive cystic duct node (Fig. 3.2).

Patients with T1a tumors are considered surgically complete after simple cholecystectomy, as long as resection margins are negative on final pathology [3, 4, 6, 8–10, 13, 19]. These patients have a near 100% 5-year survival rate [4, 9, 11, 19]. Regardless, these patients should still be discussed at a multidisciplinary tumor board and undergo complete postoperative staging with cross-sectional imaging of the chest, abdomen, and pelvis. Negative occurrences at the initial procedure, including gallbladder perforation, should be considered and result in re-stratification of these patients due to increased risk of peritoneal and port-site metastasis [4, 9].

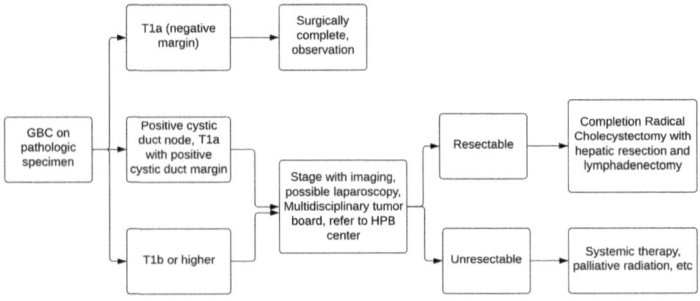

Fig. 3.2 Management of incidental gallbladder cancer identified postoperatively [9, 12]

Patients with tumors invading the muscularis mucosa (T1b) or further should be evaluated for resectability, after postoperative staging [4, 9–13, 19]. Consideration of resectability should revolve around the ability to achieve an R0 resection, which is closely correlated with outcomes [8, 9]. Invasion of adjacent organs, including the liver, colon, duodenum, stomach, and pancreas, is not a contraindication to resection so long as R0 resection is possible. Extensive lymphatic spread involving the celiac and mesenteric axes signals unresectable disease, but more localized lymphatic spread, including the peripancreatic and hepatoduodenal stations, is not a contraindication to resection [8, 9].

Among T1a tumors, some findings should prompt consideration for re-resection. Detection of metastasis in the cystic duct node is a marker of concomitant disease in second-tier nodes and should be interpreted as evidence of more advanced disease [26]. In addition, T1a tumors with positive resection margins also represent a high risk of residual disease and are independently associated with increased risk of local recurrence and reduced survival [8, 13]. Therefore, in both cases, formal partial liver resection and lymphadenectomy is recommended.

Once the decision to proceed with resection has been made, several factors should be considered, including hepatic resection, lymphadenectomy, and bile duct resection. En bloc resection without transection of the tumor should be a priority, if possible. Although some studies demonstrate no advantage to radical cholecystectomy for T1b tumors, 10% of these tumors will have positive nodal disease, so regional lymphadenectomy and partial liver resection are still considered key management components for these tumors [4, 9, 19]. All tumors invading into the perimuscular connective tissue (T2) or further (>T2) should proceed to radical cholecystectomy, to include hepatic resection and lymphadenectomy [9, 13, 19].

Although a radical cholecystectomy has historically required formal anatomic resection of segments 4b and 5 of the liver, this has not been shown to be superior to wedge resection, so long as an R0 resection is achieved [9, 12, 14–17, 19, 27]. Therefore, in patients without hepatoduodenal invasion or visible extension of tumor, a parenchyma-sparing non-anatomic wedge resection of 2–3 cm of the gallbladder bed is a reasonable approach [9, 12,

19]. However, in patients with clearly visible extension into the liver, a formal liver resection may be warranted to achieve a complete resection. Residual tumor is a predictor of worsened survival and should be avoided [16, 17, 28, 29] but this must be weighed against the increased morbidity associated with major hepatic resection [14, 16, 17].

All radical cholecystectomies should include a regional lymphadenectomy, to include the cystic duct and portal lymph nodes with a goal of resecting at least 6 nodes to allow for optimal staging and prognostication [9, 19]. Although gallbladder cancer is traditionally believed to spread from the cystic nodal station, along the common bile duct with progression through the portal nodes to the third level nodes, it has also been shown to spread directly to third level nodes (celiac, superior mesenteric, and para-aortic) [9, 24, 26]. This finding has led to consideration of extended radical lymphadenectomy in patients with T2 or higher disease [9]. However, some authors argue that nodal disease at the third level represents distant metastasis and caution against extended lymphadenectomy and the associated morbidity [12].

An additional consideration during resection of gallbladder cancer is resection of the common bile duct. Numerous studies have demonstrated increased perioperative morbidity with routine bile duct resection without associated survival benefit [14, 16, 30, 31]. Bile duct resection should be performed only if neoplastic disease involves the cystic duct stump [16].

As previously mentioned, local invasion of surrounding organs is not a contraindication to resection, so long as R0 resection can be achieved [9]. However, multivisceral resection is associated with increased morbidity and mortality [32]. Therefore, before undertaking resection, the surgeon must have performed thorough staging to be certain of the possibility of R0 resection.

Remaining Controversies

Some controversies remain in the management of gallbladder cancer. These include staging laparoscopy, port-site resection, timeline to re-resection, as well as the optimal surgical approach, whether through a minimally invasive or traditional open approach.

Staging laparoscopy has been shown to be an effective tool for the detection of peritoneal dissemination and detection of otherwise occult nodal disease [11, 19, 33]. Detection of disseminated disease by staging laparoscopy has reduced non-therapeutic laparotomies in numerous trials [12, 34]. Gaujoux and Allen reported that staging laparoscopy may prevent futile laparotomy in as many as 1/3 of patients previously thought to be resectable after standard imaging-based staging [35].

Rates of port site metastasis and peritoneal metastasis are closely associated with perforation [19]. Known disseminated cancer is a contraindication to resection [13]. Historically, possibility of occult port site metastasis was managed with port site excision. However, port site excision has not been shown to improve survival [36, 37]. Fuks, et al. demonstrated equivalent 1-, 3-, and 5-year survival, regardless of port-site resection and showed that both port-site metastasis and poor survival were closely associated with R1 and R2 resection [36]. To help reduce port site metastasis, some technical details should be routinely observed during the index operation to reduce the risk of perforation and seeding, including meticulous dissection, use of endoscopic bag for specimen retrieval, and desufflation with trocars in situ.

Ideal time to re-resection is controversial. Studies have demonstrated that disease stage is a much greater determinant of overall prognosis than time to definitive resection [4, 9, 19, 38]. Barreto et al. demonstrated that the association initially demonstrated between overall survival and delay to re-resection disappeared after adjusting for stage of disease [38]. Urgent re-resection (less than 4 weeks interval) is associated with unresolved inflammation from the index procedure and has not been shown to improve outcomes [4, 9, 19].

As minimally invasive techniques have expanded in surgery for benign disease, these techniques have also expanded in surgery for malignancy. Although observational studies have not demonstrated a significant difference in survival or recurrence-based outcomes between minimally invasive and open re-

resections [11, 39–42], a recent expert consensus statement cautions against broad implementation of minimally invasive techniques for re-resection, citing learning curve and lack of long-term data as factors that should restrict use of these approaches [43, 44]. Length of surgery is longer with minimally invasive approaches [39, 44]. However, minimally invasive approaches are associated with reduced blood loss and reduced length of stay [39–41]. Minimally invasive re-resection carries a theoretically increased risk of port site metastasis, but this has not been borne out [39]. As the field continues to grow, it is likely that minimally invasive techniques will become more widely accepted for use in the resection of gallbladder cancer [44].

Conclusion

Unlike many other cancers, which are diagnosed after the development of symptoms or through screening, gallbladder cancer is most frequently diagnosed incidentally, complicating the usual coordinated response and workup of neoplastic disease. Although it is rare, the incidence of the disease has been increasing as laparoscopic cholecystectomy has become more common. As such, all general surgeons should be familiar with the basic tenants of management of this complex disease, including intraoperative and postoperative staging, determinants of resectability, and general management. As with other neoplastic diseases, oncologic principles, including complete staging and multidisciplinary care, should be priorities for these patients.

References

1. Rawla P, Sunkara T, Thandra KC, Barsouk A. Epidemiology of gallbladder cancer. Clin Exp Hepatol. 2019;5(2):93–102. https://doi.org/10.5114/ceh.2019.85166.
2. Dorobisz T, Dorobisz K, Chabowski M, et al. Incidental gallbladder cancer after cholecystectomy: 1990 to 2014. Onco Targets Ther. 2016;9:4913–6. https://doi.org/10.2147/OTT.S106580.

3. Nitta T, Kataoka J, Ohta M, et al. Surgical strategy for suspected early gallbladder carcinoma including incidental gallbladder carcinoma diagnosed during or after cholecystectomy. Ann Med Surg (Lond). 2018;33:56–9. https://doi.org/10.1016/j.amsu.2018.07.009.
4. Soreide K, Guest RV, Harrison EM, Kendall TJ, Garden OJ, Wigmore SJ. Systematic review of management of incidental gallbladder cancer after cholecystectomy. Br J Surg. 2019;106(1):32–45. https://doi.org/10.1002/bjs.11035.
5. Hundal R, Shaffer EA. Gallbladder cancer: epidemiology and outcome. Clin Epidemiol. 2014;6:99–109. https://doi.org/10.2147/CLEP.S37357.
6. Aloia TA, Jarufe N, Javle M, et al. Gallbladder cancer: expert consensus statement. HPB (Oxford). 2015;17(8):681–90. https://doi.org/10.1111/hpb.12444.
7. Smith GC, Parks RW, Madhavan KK, Garden OJ. A 10-year experience in the management of gallbladder cancer. HPB (Oxford). 2003;5(3):159–66. https://doi.org/10.1080/13651820310000037.
8. Qadan M, Kingham TP. Technical aspects of gallbladder cancer surgery. Surg Clin North Am. 2016;96(2):229–45. https://doi.org/10.1016/j.suc.2015.12.007.
9. Cavallaro A, Piccolo G, Di Vita M, et al. Managing the incidentally detected gallbladder cancer: algorithms and controversies. Int J Surg. 2014;12(Suppl 2):S108–19. https://doi.org/10.1016/j.ijsu.2014.08.367.
10. Kanthan R, Senger JL, Ahmed S, Kanthan SC. Gallbladder cancer in the 21st century. J Oncol. 2015;2015:967472. https://doi.org/10.1155/2015/967472.
11. Leal JNV, Brendan C. Chapter 42: Who to resect for gallbladder cancer and how extensive should the resection be? In: Quyen Chu CV, Zibari G, Orloff S, Williams M, Gimenez M, editors. Hepato-pancreato-biliary and transplant surgery: practial management of dilemmas. Beaux Books Publishing; 2018. p. 337–43.
12. Cherkassky L, D'Angelica M. Gallbladder cancer: managing the incidental diagnosis. Surg Oncol Clin N Am. 2019;28(4):619–30. https://doi.org/10.1016/j.soc.2019.06.005.
13. Hepatobiliary: Biliary Tract Cancers: Gallbladder Cancer (Version 2.2022). https://www.nccn.org/professionals/physician_gls/pdf/hepatobiliary.pdf. Accessed 31 July 2022.
14. Fuks D, Regimbeau JM, Le Treut YP, et al. Incidental gallbladder cancer by the AFC-GBC-2009 study group. World J Surg. 2011;35(8):1887–97. https://doi.org/10.1007/s00268-011-1134-3.
15. Pawlik TM, Choti MA. Biology dictates prognosis following resection of gallbladder carcinoma: sometimes less is more. Ann Surg Oncol. 2009;16(4):787–8. https://doi.org/10.1245/s10434-009-0319-6.
16. Pawlik TM, Gleisner AL, Vigano L, et al. Incidence of finding residual disease for incidental gallbladder carcinoma: implications for re-resec-

tion. J Gastrointest Surg. 2007;11(11):1478–86.; discussion 1486–7. https://doi.org/10.1007/s11605-007-0309-6.
17. Shih SP, Schulick RD, Cameron JL, et al. Gallbladder cancer: the role of laparoscopy and radical resection. Ann Surg. 2007;245(6):893–901. https://doi.org/10.1097/SLA.0b013e31806beec2.
18. Chan BKY, Carrion-Alvarez L, Telfer R, et al. Surgical management of suspected gallbladder cancer: the role of intraoperative frozen section for diagnostic confirmation. J Surg Oncol. 2022;125(3):399–404. https://doi.org/10.1002/jso.26726.
19. Feo CF, Ginesu GC, Fancellu A, et al. Current management of incidental gallbladder cancer: a review. Int J Surg. 2022;98:106234. https://doi.org/10.1016/j.ijsu.2022.106234.
20. Ramos E, Lluis N, Llado L, et al. Prognostic value and risk stratification of residual disease in patients with incidental gallbladder cancer. World J Surg Oncol. 2020;18(1):18. https://doi.org/10.1186/s12957-020-1794-2.
21. Cho JY, Han HS, Yoon YS, Ahn KS, Kim YH, Lee KH. Laparoscopic approach for suspected early-stage gallbladder carcinoma. Arch Surg. 2010;145(2):128–33. https://doi.org/10.1001/archsurg.2009.261.
22. Yamaguchi K, Chijiiwa K, Saiki S, Shimizu S, Tsuneyoshi M, Tanaka M. Reliability of frozen section diagnosis of gallbladder tumor for detecting carcinoma and depth of its invasion. J Surg Oncol. 1997;65(2):132–6. https://doi.org/10.1002/(sici)1096-9098(199706)65:2<132::aid-jso11>3.0.co;2-7.
23. Kim WJ, Lim TW, Park PJ, Choi SB, Kim WB. Clinicopathological differences in T2 gallbladder cancer according to tumor location. Cancer Control. 2020;27(1):1073274820915514. https://doi.org/10.1177/1073274820915514.
24. Fahim RB, Mc DJ, Richards JC, Ferris DO. Carcinoma of the gallbladder: a study of its modes of spread. Ann Surg. 1962;156:114–24. https://doi.org/10.1097/00000658-196207000-00021.
25. Nagahashi M, Shirai Y, Wakai T, Sakata J, Ajioka Y, Hatakeyama K. Perimuscular connective tissue contains more and larger lymphatic vessels than the shallower layers in human gallbladders. World J Gastroenterol. 2007;13(33):4480–3. https://doi.org/10.3748/wjg.v13.i33.4480.
26. Vega EA, Vinuela E, Yamashita S, et al. Extended lymphadenectomy is required for incidental gallbladder cancer independent of cystic duct lymph node status. J Gastrointest Surg. 2018;22(1):43–51. https://doi.org/10.1007/s11605-017-3507-x.
27. Hueman MT, Vollmer CM Jr, Pawlik TM. Evolving treatment strategies for gallbladder cancer. Ann Surg Oncol. 2009;16(8):2101–15. https://doi.org/10.1245/s10434-009-0538-x.
28. Duffy A, Capanu M, Abou-Alfa GK, et al. Gallbladder cancer (GBC): 10-year experience at memorial Sloan-Kettering Cancer Centre

(MSKCC). J Surg Oncol. 2008;98(7):485–9. https://doi.org/10.1002/jso.21141.
29. Jensen EH, Abraham A, Habermann EB, et al. A critical analysis of the surgical management of early-stage gallbladder cancer in the United States. J Gastrointest Surg. 2009;13(4):722–7. https://doi.org/10.1007/s11605-008-0772-8.
30. Araida T, Higuchi R, Hamano M, et al. Should the extrahepatic bile duct be resected or preserved in R0 radical surgery for advanced gallbladder carcinoma? Results of a Japanese Society of Biliary Surgery Survey: a multicenter study. Surg Today. 2009;39(9):770–9. https://doi.org/10.1007/s00595-009-3960-6.
31. Higuchi R, Ota T, Araida T, Kobayashi M, Furukawa T, Yamamoto M. Prognostic relevance of ductal margins in operative resection of bile duct cancer. Surgery. 2010;148(1):7–14. https://doi.org/10.1016/j.surg.2009.11.018.
32. Hasselgren K, Sandstrom P, Gasslander T, Bjornsson B. Multivisceral resection in patients with advanced abdominal Tumors. Scand J Surg. 2016;105(3):147–52. https://doi.org/10.1177/1457496915622128.
33. Agarwal AK, Kalayarasan R, Javed A, Gupta N, Nag HH. The role of staging laparoscopy in primary gall bladder cancer—an analysis of 409 patients: a prospective study to evaluate the role of staging laparoscopy in the management of gallbladder cancer. Ann Surg. 2013;258(2):318–23. https://doi.org/10.1097/SLA.0b013e318271497e.
34. D'Angelica M, Fong Y, Weber S, et al. The role of staging laparoscopy in hepatobiliary malignancy: prospective analysis of 401 cases. Ann Surg Oncol. 2003;10(2):183–9. https://doi.org/10.1245/aso.2003.03.091.
35. Gaujoux S, Allen PJ. Role of staging laparoscopy in peri-pancreatic and hepatobiliary malignancy. World J Gastrointest Surg. 2010;2(9):283–90. https://doi.org/10.4240/wjgs.v2.i9.283.
36. Fuks D, Regimbeau JM, Pessaux P, et al. Is port-site resection necessary in the surgical management of gallbladder cancer? J Visc Surg. 2013;150(4):277–84. https://doi.org/10.1016/j.jviscsurg.2013.03.006.
37. Maker AV, Jarnagin WR. Port-site resection in the surgical management of incidental gallbladder cancer: a still inconclusive question: a reply. Ann Surg Oncol. 2017;24(Suppl 3):647–8. https://doi.org/10.1245/s10434-017-6227-2.
38. Barreto SG, Pawar S, Shah S, Talole S, Goel M, Shrikhande SV. Patterns of failure and determinants of outcomes following radical re-resection for incidental gallbladder cancer. World J Surg. 2014;38(2):484–9. https://doi.org/10.1007/s00268-013-2266-4.
39. Agarwal AK, Javed A, Kalayarasan R, Sakhuja P. Minimally invasive versus the conventional open surgical approach of a radical cholecystectomy for gallbladder cancer: a retrospective comparative study. HPB (Oxford). 2015;17(6):536–41. https://doi.org/10.1111/hpb.12406.

40. Navarro JG, Kang I, Hwang HK, Yoon DS, Lee WJ, Kang CM. Oncologic safety of laparoscopic radical cholecystectomy in pT2 gallbladder cancer: a propensity score matching analysis compared to open approach. Medicine (Baltimore). 2020;99(20):e20039. https://doi.org/10.1097/MD.0000000000020039.
41. Regmi P, Hu HJ, Chang-Hao Y, et al. Laparoscopic surgery for oncologic extended resection of T1b and T2 incidental gallbladder carcinoma at a high-volume center: a single-center experience in China. Surg Endosc. 2021;35(12):6505–12. https://doi.org/10.1007/s00464-020-08146-7.
42. Vega EA, De Aretxabala X, Qiao W, et al. Comparison of oncological outcomes after open and laparoscopic re-resection of incidental gallbladder cancer. Br J Surg. 2020;107(3):289–300. https://doi.org/10.1002/bjs.11379.
43. Han HS, Yoon YS, Agarwal AK, et al. Laparoscopic surgery for gallbladder cancer: an expert consensus statement. Dig Surg. 2019;36(1):1–6. https://doi.org/10.1159/000486207.
44. Yoon YS, Han HS, Agarwal A, et al. Survey results of the expert meeting on laparoscopic surgery for gallbladder cancer and a review of relevant literature. Dig Surg. 2019;36(1):7–12. https://doi.org/10.1159/000486208.

Part II

Biliary Disease

Intraductal Papillary Neoplasm of the Bile Duct (IPNB)

Lyonell B. Kone, Thomas M. Fishbein, and Timothy J. Kennedy

Definition and Significance

Intraductal papillary neoplasm of the bile duct (IPNB) is the terminology endorsed by the 2019 World Health Organization (WHO) classification system [1]. First introduced in the 2010 WHO classification, IPNB and IPNB with invasive carcinoma encompass several previously distinct entities, including papillary cholangiocarcinoma (CCA), mucin-producing CCA, mucin hypersecreting bile duct tumor, intraductal papillary mucinous neoplasm of the bile duct, biliary papilloma or papillomatosis, papillary adenocarcinoma of the bile duct, and intraductal growth-type CCA [2].

L. B. Kone
Division of Surgical Oncology, Department of Surgery, Winship Cancer Institute, Emory University, Atlanta, GA, USA

T. M. Fishbein
Department of Surgery, MedStar Georgetown, Washington, DC, USA

T. J. Kennedy (✉)
Division of Surgical Oncology, Department of Surgery, MedStar Georgetown, Washington, DC, USA
e-mail: timothy.kennedy@medstar.net

IPNB is defined as a macroscopic "exophytic growth in a dilated bile duct with villous/papillary neoplastic epithelia with tubular components covering fine fibrovascular stalk" [3]. It is recognized as one of the three main pre-invasive lesions that can progress to an invasive carcinoma of the bile duct, alongside biliary intraepithelial neoplasia (a flat microscopic lesion) and mucinous cystic neoplasm (which lacks communication with the biliary tree and contains ovarian-type stroma) [4, 5]. It is worth noting that IPNB grading encompasses a full spectrum of disease from adenoma, low-grade dysplasia, high-grade dysplasia, carcinoma in-situ, and IPNB with invasive carcinoma.

Invasive carcinoma arising from IPNB generally carries a more favorable prognosis than invasive CCA, making early identification, histologic classification, and timely management essential. It is a recently defined disease category, and data on clinicopathologic features and outcomes are evolving.

Classification

Analogous to intraductal papillary mucinous neoplasms of the pancreas (IPMNs), IPNBs have been classified into four histologic subtypes: intestinal type consists of stratified columnar cells with goblet cells, gastric type consists of columnar cells with abundant mucin and clear cytoplasm, pancreatobiliary type consists of columnar cells with eosinophilic cytoplasm and round nuclei, and oncocytic type is a variant of the pancreatobiliary type [6].

The Japan-Korea Collaborative Study on IPNB introduced a clinically meaningful subclassification—adopted in the 2019 WHO guidelines—based on pathologic and prognostic features: [7]

- Type 1, Classical Type, is histologically similar to IPMN, often produces mucin, is intra-hepatic, associated with gastric or intestinal subtypes, demonstrates low/intermediate grade dysplasia (20%), and associated invasive cancer (50%).

- Type 2, typically located in the extra-hepatic bile duct, rarely produces mucin and associated with pancreatobiliary or intestinal subtypes, and frequently associated with an invasive cancer (90%) [7].

Epidemiology

IPNB is more common in males, with a male-to-female ratio ranging from 2:1 to 3:2, and a median age of presentation between 60 and 66 years [8]. IPNB is more prevalent in East Asian countries including China, Korea, and Japan [9]. Notably, IPNB represents 9.9–30% of bile duct tumors in Asian countries, but only 7–11% of bile duct tumors in Western countries. Wu et al. reported a decreased incidence of invasive IPNB in the United States between 1970 and 2014 using the SEER database [10]. A plausible explanation for the decreased incidence is lead-time bias, as enhanced imaging techniques and their widespread application have likely increased early detection and surgical resection of non-invasive IPNB, thereby decreasing the incidence of invasive IPNB. It will be interesting to see how the prevalence and frequency of both non-invasive and invasive IPNB evolves over time with the increased recognition of this disease entity, and with a unifying definition by the WHO.

Risk Factors

IPNB is considered a disease spectrum progressing from benign to dysplasia to carcinoma in-situ to invasive cancer with chronic inflammation as a potential driver. Hepatolithiasis is thought to play a role in initiation of cholangiocarcinomatosis [11], and has a strong association with IPNB [12]. Other reported associations include liver parasites, primary sclerosing cholangitis, and hepatocellular carcinoma. Despite its close embryologic and histologic feature to IPMN, IPNB and IPMN very rarely occur in the same patient [2].

Diagnostics

Clinical presentation ranges from right upper quadrant pain, jaundice, and cholangitis to incidental detection. Tumor markers, such as CEA, is elevated in 25% of patients, and CA 19-9 in 40% of patients [2]. Both ultrasound, CT-scan, MRI/MRCP, and cholangiography have been used in the diagnosis of IPNB. Ultrasound has a reported sensitivity of 41%, with 50% for CT scan and the highest for MRI/MRCP at 65.5% [10]. On CT scan, IPNB tend to be isointense or hyperintense on late arterial phase with occasional rim enhancement of the base of the lesion. On MRI, IPNB are hypointense in T1, and hyperintense in T2. MRI findings of visible intraductal mass, tumor size >2.5 cm, multiplicity of the tumor, bile duct wall thickening, and invasion of adjacent organs are predictors of IPNB with associated invasive carcinoma [13]. Combined CT and MRI modality has a reported accuracy of 83–88% in distinguishing IPNB from cholangiocarcinoma with intraductal papillary growth [14].

There are four radiologic subtypes of IPNB: [10]

1. Masses with proximal ductal dilation—flat or fungating intraductal mass with upstream dilation and no mucin.
2. Disproportionate dilation without mass—superficial spreading IPNB without sizeable intraductal mass with biliary dilation secondary to excessive mucin.
3. Mass with proximal and distal dilation—IPNB causes proximal dilation from tumor obstruction and distal dilation from mucin production, a characteristic feature only of IPNB.
4. Cystic lesion—focal aneurysmal dilation of a bile duct.

Management

Preoperative evaluation may include ERCP for cytology, mucin detection, or biliary decompression in jaundiced patients. Cholangioscopy aids in assessing lesion extent and surgical planning. Surgical resection with negative margins is the cornerstone of treatment, using techniques similar to those for CCA—ranging from bile duct resection to liver or pancreatic resection and biliary reconstruction. Regional lymphadenectomy is essential for accurate staging. Liver transplant is generally not considered a first option for IPNB, but it remains an option, specifically for cases with limited future liver remnant. Lluis et al. report 5 patients that underwent liver transplant for IPNB, two were performed as a first option, and three were performed as salvage transplant due to liver failure from prior IPNB resection [15]. For non-surgical candidates, endoscopic ablative therapies such as electrocoagulation, radiofrequency ablation, or argon plasma coagulation may offer palliation with its attendant risks [16].

Prognosis

Long-term survival data after resection remains heterogenous due to utilization of different terminology, classification, and inclusion criteria. The degree of dysplasia and invasion is the most common stratification used when comparing survival. In a cohort of 146 patients, Luvira et al. reported a 1-, 3-, and 5-year overall survival (OS) of 84%, 64%, and 47%. The reported median survival for low-grade/high-grade dysplasia was 8.4 years, for carcinoma in situ was 5.6 years, for micro-invasive carcinoma was 4.2 years, and for macro-invasive carcinoma was 2 years. On multivariable analysis both positive lymph node (HR 4.1, $p < 0.001$) and positive (R1 or R2) resection margins (HR 1.8, $p = 0.011$) were associated with worse OS [17]. While the gastric, intestinal, and pancreatobiliary subtypes appear to have similar survival rates (~70% 5-year OS) [6], the oncocytic subtypes appears to have improved survival rates (92% 5-year OS, 100% Recurrence Free Survival) [18] (Table 4.1). A meta-analysis by Zeng et al. identified prognostic factors associated with worse survival—extra-hepatic tumor location, subclassification type 2, R1 margin status, elevated CA 19–9, tumor multiplicity, and adjacent organ invasion [19].

The larger, more contemporary, study by the Japan-Korea Collaborative, which included 771 IPNB patients, reported a 1-,

Table 4.1 Case series with proportion of IPNB subtypes, grading, and long-term outcomes

Study	N	Classification (N)	Dysplasia (%), Carcinoma (%)	Survival
[12]	124	N/A	LGD: 27% HGD: 14% CIS: 12% IC: 48%	5-year OS: LGD/HGD: 100% CIS: 17% IC: 14%
[10]	138	N/A	L/IGD: 12% HGD: 39% IC: 49%	5-year OS: 69%
Luvira et al. (2017)	146	N/A	A: 5% LGD/HGD: 12% CIS: 23% IC(micro):34% IC(macro): 27%	1-, 3-, 5-year OS: 84%, 64%, 47% Median survival: (LGD/HGD) 8.4 years, (CIS) 5.6 years, (IC-micro) 4.2 years, (IC-macro) 2 years
[21]	21	N/A	LGD/HGD: 38% CIS/IC: 62%	Mean survival: All: 44 months LGD/HGD: 56 months CIS/IC: 38 months
[6]	112	G: 17% IT: 49% PB: 30% O: 5%	L/IGD: 3% IC: 97%	5-year OS: All: 72%, no differences btw 4 subtypes R1: 25%
Uemura et al. (2020)	83	Type 1: 45% Type 2: 55%	N/A	5-year DSS: All: 79% Type 1: 90% Type 2: 69% N1 vs. N0: 44 vs. 84%
[7]	771	Type 1: 67% Type 2: 33%	L/IGD, HGD, IC: Type 1: 10% 40%, 50% Type 2: 1%, 6%, 94%	1-,5-,10-year OS: Type 1: 96%, 75%, 59% Type 2: 95%, 51%, 27%

(continued)

Table 4.1 (continued)

Study	N	Classification (N)	Dysplasia (%), Carcinoma (%)	Survival
[15]	85	G:9% IT:20% PB:69% O:1%	LGD:25% HGD:16.5% CIS:13% IC:42%	1-,5-,10-year OS: 92%, 63%, 31%
[20]	43	N/A	LGD/HGD: 47% IC: 53%	1-,5-,10-year OS: 87%, 49%, 32%
[18]	127	G:12% IT:47% PB:31% O:10%	LGD, HGD/IC: G: 60%,40% IT:18%,82% PB: 3%, 97% O: 0%, 100%	5-year OS / RFS: G: 85% / 80% IT: 71% / 65% PB: 59% / 47% O: 92%/ 100%

Annotation: *G* gastric, *IT* intestinal, *PB* pancreatobiliary, *O* oncocytic, *A* adenoma, *L/IGD* low/intermediate-grade dysplasia, *HGD* high-grade dysplasia, *IC* invasive carcinoma, *DSS* disease-specific survival, *RFS* recurrence-free survival, *OS* overall survival

5-, and 10-year survival rate of 96%, 75%, and 59% for Type 1 IPNB; and 95%, 51%, and 27% for Type 2 IPNB, respectively [7]. Other studies reporting survival data are included in Table 4.1 [8, 12, 18, 20–22].

Future Directions

Accurate classification of IPNB is crucial to optimize patient outcomes. Molecular profiling is a promising frontier. In 2019, Yang et al. used next-generation sequencing on 37 resected IPNBs and identified three distinct molecular signatures: [23]

- Group 1 is consistent with Type 1 IPNB and has frequent KRAS, GNAS, and RNF43 mutations.
- Group 2 is consistent with Type 2 intestinal IPNB, and has frequent KRAS mutations but rare GNAS mutation, and MUC2 expression.
- Group 3 is also consistent with Type 2 IPNB but notable for having CTNNB1 mutation and a lack of KRAS, GNAS, and RNF43 mutations.

These findings suggest a role for genomics in stratifying oncologic risk and potentially guiding treatment. Future studies may focus on using cholangioscopy-derived biopsy, mucin, or bile samples for molecular diagnosis and subtype classification. Ultimately, insights gained from studying these distinct pathways in a larger patient population may help guide treatment and potentially targeted therapies.

References

1. Basturk O, Nakanuma Y, Aishima S, et al. The WHO classification of tumours Editoral board, WHO classification of tumours of digestive system. Lyon: International Agency for Research on Cancer; 2019.
2. Mocchegiani F, Vincenzi P, Conte G, et al. Intraductal papillary neoplasm of the bile duct: the new frontier of biliary pathology. World J Gastroenterol. 2023;29(38):5361–73.
3. Nakanuma Y, Uesaka K, Kakuda Y, et al. Intraductal papillary neoplasm of bile duct: updated Clinicopathological characteristics and molecular and genetic alterations. J Clin Med. 2020;9(12):3991.
4. Quigley B, Reid MD, Pehlivanoglu B, et al. Hepatobiliary mucinous cystic neoplasms with ovarian type stroma (so-called "hepatobiliary cystadenoma/cystadenocarcinoma"): Clinicopathologic analysis of 36 cases illustrates rarity of carcinomatous change. Am J Surg Pathol. 2018;42(1):95–102.
5. Hucl T. Precursors to cholangiocarcinoma. Gastroenterol Res Pract. 2019;2019:1389289.
6. Kim JR, Lee KB, Kwon W, Kim E, Kim SW, Jang JY. Comparison of the clinicopathologic characteristics of intraductal papillary neoplasm of the bile duct according to morphological and anatomical classifications. J Korean Med Sci. 2018;33(42):e266.
7. Kubota K, Jang JY, Nakanuma Y, et al. Clinicopathological characteristics of intraductal papillary neoplasm of the bile duct: a Japan-Korea collaborative study. J Hepatobiliary Pancreat Sci. 2020;27(9):581–97.
8. Park HJ, Kim SY, Kim HJ, et al. Intraductal papillary neoplasm of the bile duct: clinical, imaging, and pathologic features. AJR Am J Roentgenol. 2018;211(1):67–75.
9. Wu RS, Liao WJ, Ma JS, Wang JK, Wu LQ, Hou P. Epidemiology and outcome of individuals with intraductal papillary neoplasms of the bile duct. World J Gastrointest Oncologia. 2023;5(5):843–58.
10. Zen Y, Jang KT, Ahn S, et al. Intraductal papillary neoplasms and mucinous cystic neoplasms of the hepatobiliary system: demographic differ-

ences between Asian and Western populations, and comparison with pancreatic counterparts. Histopathology. 2014;65(2):164–73.
11. Jan YY, Chen MF, Wang CS, Jeng LB, Hwang TL, Chen SC. Surgical treatment of hepatolithiasis: long-term results. Surgery. 1996;120(3):509–14.
12. Yeh TS, Tseng JH, Chiu CT, et al. Cholangiographic spectrum of intraductal papillary mucinous neoplasm of the bile ducts. Ann Surg. 2006;244(2):248–53.
13. Lee S, Kim MJ, Kim S, Choi D, Jang KT, Park YN. Intraductal papillary neoplasm of the bile duct: assessment of invasive carcinoma and long-term outcomes using MRI. J Hepatol. 2019;70(4):692–9.
14. Liu Y, Zhong X, Yan L, Zheng J, Liu Z, Liang C. Diagnostic performance of CT and MRI in distinguishing intraductal papillary neoplasm of the bile duct from cholangiocarcinoma with intraductal papillary growth. Eur Radiol. 2015;25(7):1967–74.
15. Lluis N, Serradilla-Martin M, Achalandabaso M, et al. Intraductal papillary neoplasms of the bile duct: a European retrospective multicenter observational study (EUR-IPNB study). Int J Surg. 2023;109(4):760–71.
16. Arai J, Kato J, Toda N, et al. Long-term survival after palliative argon plasma coagulation for intraductal papillary mucinous neoplasm of the bile duct. Clin J Gastroenterol. 2021;14(1):314–8.
17. Luvira V, Pugkhem A, Bhudhisawasdi V, et al. Long-term outcome of surgical resection for intraductal papillary neoplasm of the bile duct. J Gastroenterol Hepatol. 2017;32(2):527–33.
18. Chun J, Sung YN, An S, Hong SM. Oncocytic type has distinct immunohistochemical and recurrence-free survival than other histologic types of the intraductal papillary neoplasm of the bile duct. Hum Pathol. 2024;148:72–80.
19. Zeng D, Li B, Cheng N. Prognostic factors for intraductal papillary neoplasm of the bile duct following surgical resection: a systematic review and meta-analysis. Surg Today. 2025;55(2):131–43.
20. Wu X, Li B, Zheng C. Clinicopathologic characteristics and long-term prognosis of intraductal papillary neoplasm of the bile duct: a retrospective study. Eur J Med Res. 2023;28(1):132.
21. Wu X, Li B, Zheng C, et al. Intraductal papillary neoplasm of the bile duct: a single-center retrospective study. J Int Med Res. 2018;46(10):4258–68.
22. Uemura S, Higuchi R, Yazawa T, et al. Prognostic factors for surgically resected Intraductal papillary neoplasm of the bile duct: a retrospective cohort study. Ann Surg Oncol. 2021;28(2):826–34.
23. Yang CY, Huang WJ, Tsai JH, et al. Targeted next-generation sequencing identifies distinct clinicopathologic and molecular entities of intraductal papillary neoplasms of the bile duct. Mod Pathol. 2019;32(11):1637–45.

Intrahepatic Cholangiocarcinoma

Emilie A. K. Warren and Shishir K. Maithel

Epidemiology

Cholangiocarcinoma (CCA), stratified into intrahepatic cholangiocarcinoma (iCCA) and extrahepatic cholangiocarcinoma (eCCA), is a rare malignancy, accounting for 15% of all primary liver cancers and 3% of all gastrointestinal cancers, and occurring at an age-standardized incidence of <3 per 100,000 inhabitants globally per year [1, 2]. There is substantial geographical variation in incidence, with significantly higher rates seen in Japan, South Korea, Thailand, Chile, and Bolivia. In the United States, the incidence of iCCA is higher in males, adults over the age of 45, and Hispanic individuals, and these groups also had lower survival rates [3]. For iCCA specifically, mortality rates have been increasing worldwide, ranging from 0.2 to 2.5 per 100,000 person-years, with the highest rates seen in Hong Kong and Western Europe and the lowest rates in Latin America and Eastern Europe [4].

E. A. K. Warren
Division of Surgical Oncology, Department of Surgery,
Emory University, Atlanta, GA, USA
e-mail: emilie.warren@emory.edu

S. K. Maithel (✉)
Division of Surgical Oncology, Department of Surgery,
Northwestern University, Atlanta, GA, USA
e-mail: smaithe@emory.edu

© The Author(s), under exclusive license to Springer Nature Switzerland AG 2025
A. Alseidi et al. (eds.), *The SAGES Manual of Contemporary Indications and Management of Hepatic and Biliary Diseases*, https://doi.org/10.1007/978-3-032-04823-3_5

Most of the known risk factors for CCA are associated with chronic inflammation of the biliary epithelium and bile stasis. These include primary sclerosing cholangitis, choledochal cysts, and Caroli's disease (congenital dilatation of intrahepatic bile ducts), and are associated with the development of either iCCA or eCCA [5, 6]. Cirrhosis, non-alcoholic fatty liver disease, and hepatitis B, however, are more strongly associated with development of iCCA. In Southeast Asia, infections with liver flukes *Clonorchis sinensi or Opisthorchi viverrini* are a major cause of CCA [7]. Humans become infected upon consumption of undercooked fish carrying the larval parasite, which mature and migrate through the ampulla of Vater to inhabit the biliary tract, where they can live for many years. The mechanical damage to the biliary epithelium caused by these flukes promotes a chronic inflammatory state that is believed to be a major factor in tumorigenesis [8]. Nevertheless, despite all of these known associations, it should be noted that most cases of CCA do not have an identifiable risk factor.

Pathophysiology

iCCA can originate from any point along the intrahepatic biliary tree, from bile ductules to segmental bile ducts. By gross examination, three main growth patterns have been described: mass-forming, periductal-infiltrating, and intraductal-growing (Fig. 5.1) [9, 10]. The mass-forming type presents as a solid nodular lesion in the hepatic parenchyma; they can be quite large and central necrosis is common. The periductal-infiltrating type spreads along the portal tracts, causing strictures of the affected bile ducts and dilatation of the peripheral ones. The intraductal-growing type presents as a papillary tumor within a variably dilated bile duct lumen and represents the malignant progression of an intraductal papillary neoplasm of the bile duct (IPNB). These three growth patterns can also sometimes overlap in variable combinations.

Histologically, iCCA can be subdivided into four different categories: conventional (bile duct), bile ductular, intraductal neoplasm, and rare variants [11]. Conventional iCCAs can be further classified into small duct or large duct type according to the size of the affected bile ducts [12–14]. Small duct type arises in small

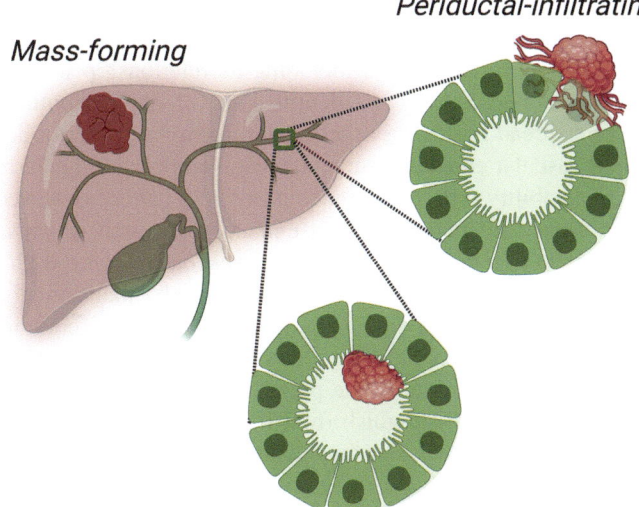

Fig. 5.1 Growth patterns of iCCA: mass-forming, periductal-infiltrating, and intraductal-growing

intrahepatic bile ducts and is believed to be derived from cuboidal cholangiocytes; this type typically develops in the background of chronic viral hepatitis or cirrhosis and is characterized by a mass-forming growth pattern. Large duct type arises in large intrahepatic bile ducts, considered to be derived from columnar cholangiocytes and peribiliary glands; it typically develops in the setting of primary sclerosing cholangitis or liver fluke infection and usually follows the periductal-infiltrating growth pattern.

Diagnosis and Staging

During the early stages of disease, iCCAs are typically asymptomatic. Symptoms of advanced disease can include abdominal pain, malaise, nausea, anorexia, weight loss, and less frequently, jaundice. While ultrasonographic surveillance for hepatocellular carcinoma (HCC) in patients with cirrhosis often enables iCCA diagnosis at an earlier stage in these patients, CT and MRI are the standard modalities for diagnosis and staging, providing an evaluation of the primary tumor, including its relationship with adjacent structures, as well as identification of any abdominal or thoracic spread [15]. Cross-sectional imaging has superior detection of vascular enhancement and, thus, is important in determining resectability. The most frequent imaging pattern observed in iCCA is arterial peripheral rim enhancement with progressive contrast enhancement and absence of washout in delayed phases [16]. Peripheral washout and delayed central enhancement can also be seen. In MRIs obtained with gadoxetic acid (commonly marketed as Eovist in the United States, Promovist in Europe), the washout should be read in the portal venous phase instead of in delayed phases to distinguish from HCC in cirrhotic livers [17]. Histopathological analysis is mandatory to confirm the diagnosis, which is based on the WHO classification of biliary tract cancer showing an adenocarcinoma or mucinous carcinoma, with tubular and/or papillary structures and a variable fibrous stroma [18, 19]. ^{18}FDG-PET imaging is an adjunct tool for lymph node staging and identification of distant metastasis [20].

CCA is staged according to the TNM system from the American Joint Committee on Cancer (AJCC), now in the 8th edition (Fig. 5.2) [21, 22]. Stages IA and IB are distinguished by a tumor size threshold of 5 cm; intrahepatic vasculature invasion or multifocal disease defines stage II. Stage III is classified by any lymphatic spread, perforation of the visceral peritoneum, or invasion of local extrahepatic structures. The presence of any distant metastasis specifies stage IV. Based on a retrospective study of over 600 patients who underwent resection of iCCA, independent prognostic factors for recurrence and survival included the presence of multiple tumors, tumor size >5 cm, lymph node involvement, and extrahepatic invasion [23]. In this same study, however, there was no prognostic difference between patients with T2 versus T3 tumors, suggesting that the current T-staging system may not accurately reflect iCCA biology. Future versions of the AJCC TNM classification will require refinement of this definition. Based on data from the NCI Surveillance, Epidemiology, and End Results Program (SEER), localized disease carries a 5-year sur-

5 Intrahepatic Cholangiocarcinoma

Primary tumor (T)	
Tx	Primary tumor cannot be assessed
T0	No evidence of tumor
Tis	Carcinoma in situ (intraductal)
T1a	Solitary tumor ≤ 5 cm, without vascular invasion
T1b	Solitary tumor >5 cm, without vascular invasion
T2	Solitary tumor with intrahepatic vascular invasion or multiple tumors with or without vascular invasion
T3	Tumor perforates the visceral peritoneum
T4	Tumor involves local extrahepatic structures by direct invasion
Regional lymph nodes (N)	
NX	Regional lymph nodes cannot be assessed
N0	No regional lymph node metastasis
N1	Regional lymph node metastasis present
Distant Metastasis (M)	
M0	No distant metastasis
M1	Distant metastasis present

Stage	T	N	M
0	Tis	N0	M0
IA	T1a	N0	M0
IB	T1b	N0	M0
II	T2	N0	M0
IIIA	T3	N0	M0
IIIB	T4	N0	M0
	Any T	N1	
IV	Any T	Any N	M1

Fig. 5.2 Staging of intrahepatic cholangiocarcinoma, according to the AJCC 8th edition TNM system

vival rate of 23%, which drops to 9% with regional disease, and 3% for distant disease [24].

Management

Figure 5.3 summarizes the recommended management of patients diagnosed with CCA according to current guidelines. A detailed discussion of that management schema follows in the text below.

Resectable Disease

Surgical resection is the mainstay of treatment for patients who present with resectable disease; a negative-margin resection offers the patient the best chance for prolonged survival [25]. For iCCA, a non-anatomic or anatomic segmental or major hepatic resection with concomitant portal lymphadenectomy is recommended. Technical and oncologic considerations must be taken into

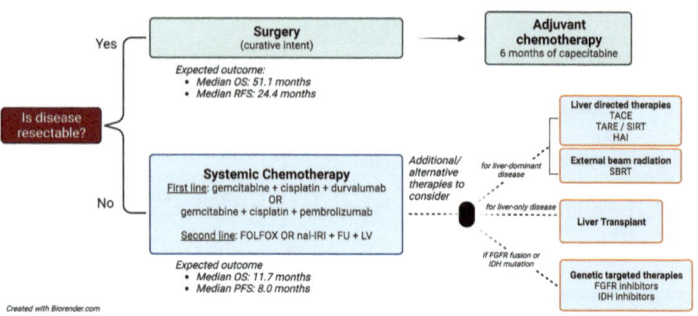

Fig. 5.3 Clinical decision tree for the management of patients with intrahepatic cholangiocarcinoma. *OS* overall survival, *RFS* recurrence-free survival, *PFS* progression-free survival, *FOLFOX* folinic acid, 5-fluorouracil and oxaliplatin, *nal-IRI* nanoliposomal irinotecan, *FU* fluorouracil, *LV* leucovorin, *TACE*: transarterial chemoembolization, *TARE* transarterial radioembolization, *SIRT* selective internal radiation therapy, *HAI* hepatic arterial infusion, *SBRT* stereotactic body radiation therapy, *FGFR* fibroblast growth factor receptor; IDH: isocitrate dehydrogenase

account when evaluating a patient for resection. The absence of extensive vascular invasion of the portal vein and/or hepatic artery, paraceliac and/or retropancreatic nodal disease, extrahepatic organ invasion, and distant metastasis are crucial criteria to assess when determining resectability. In high-risk patients (multicentric disease, high CA 19-9, questionable vascular invasion, or suspicion of peritoneal disease), a staging laparoscopy can be utilized to determine resectability and rule out occult metastasis [26]. The AJCC 8th edition recommends the removal of at least 6 lymph nodes to provide adequate nodal stage [22].

If a major hepatectomy is indicated, the surgeon must determine if the future liver remnant (FLR) has adequate inflow, outflow, and biliary drainage. The liver has a remarkable regenerative capacity for functional recovery after hepatectomy. In patients with healthy livers, 80% of the liver volume can be resected with a meaningful recovery [27, 28]. Pre-operative volumetric analysis aids in predicting sFLR function, which can be done using predictive mathematical models or cross-sectional imaging, including CT and 3D CT volumetry [29, 30]. Portal vein embolization is one strategy to optimize FLR function and expand the patient population eligible for resection. By occluding the branch of the portal vein to the intended surgical specimen, portal vein embolization allows for hypertrophy of the FLR, increasing its volume an average of 10–15% [31, 32]. Studies have shown there is no significant increase in morbidity or mortality following hepatectomy in patients who received such an embolization [33, 34].

The BILCAP trial, a randomized phase III multicenter trial, recently published the results of 447 patients who underwent curative-intent resection and were randomized to 6 months of oral capecitabine versus observation [35]. There was a significant improvement in median overall survival (OS) (53 vs 36 months, $p = 0.028$) and median recurrence-free survival (RFS) (26 vs 16 months, $p = 0.0093$) in the capecitabine group compared to observation in the per-protocol analysis, but the intent-to-treat analysis did not reach statistical significance for the primary outcome of OS. The BILCAP trial has largely informed current consensus guidelines favoring adjuvant chemotherapy with 6 months of capecitabine for resected biliary tract malignancies [36]. Another phase III study (ACTICCA-1) is currently underway comparing gemcitabine/cisplatin to capecitabine in the adjuvant setting (NCT02170090). A large retrospective analysis of over 3500 patients showed a possible clinical benefit with adjuvant radiation for iCCA, but there have been no clinical trials to date [37].

Currently, there are no formal recommendations for neoadjuvant therapy in the NCCN guidelines or ASCO clinical practice guidelines. Neoadjuvant treatment has the potential to eradicate micrometastatic disease, downsize tumors, and improve patient selection for resection. A retrospective study of 186 patients compared neoadjuvant therapy in locally advanced unresectable disease to upfront surgery in resectable disease [38]. Short- and long-term outcomes were equivalent between the two groups, and notably, 53% of the initially unresectable tumors were able to undergo resection after receiving chemotherapy, suggesting that neoadjuvant treatment may be an effective means of downstaging. Nevertheless, randomized controlled clinical trials are needed. A completed phase II single-arm multi-institutional trial, NEO-

GAP, demonstrated the feasibility of administering neoadjuvant gemcitabine, cisplatin, and nab-paclitaxel for high-risk but technically resectable iCCA (NCT03579771) [39].

Unresectable Disease

The ABC-02 trial, first published in 2010, established the use of chemotherapies cisplatin plus gemcitabine for the treatment of advanced CCA [40]. The current standard of care now includes the addition of immunotherapy with durvalumab or pembrolizumab to cisplatin and gemcitabine, based on the TOPAZ-1 trial or KEYNOTE-966 trial, respectively [41, 42]. After progression on first-line chemotherapy, FOLFOX (folinic acid, fluorouracil, and oxaliplatin) or nal-IRI (liposomal irinotecan) plus fluorouracil and leucovorin are recommended as second-line standard of care chemotherapy [43, 44].

Patients with liver-predominant disease can be considered for liver-directed therapies. Options include transarterial chemoembolization (TACE) or transarterial radioembolization (TARE) with yttrium-90 microspheres, also referred to as selective internal radiation therapy (SIRT). Several retrospective studies have reported clinical benefit with TACE [45–47]. For TARE/SIRT, the recent phase II clinical trial MISPHEC included 41 patients, and showed a radiographic response rate of 39% and a median OS of 22 months [48]. Hepatic arterial infusion (HAI) therapy is also an option at some centers. A phase II trial of 38 patients who received HAI therapy with floxuridine in combination with systemic chemotherapy reported a striking radiographic response rate of 58% and a median OS of 25 months [49]. A major limitation of HAI therapy is the limited availability of oncologists experienced with its use outside of select institutions. Given the lack of prospective comparative trials, any of these directed therapies are viable options for liver-only advanced disease. Choice of therapy is largely dependent on individual institution experience.

Other options for local therapy include external beam radiation, such as stereotactic body radiation therapy (SBRT), which has shown preliminary efficacy in unresectable iCCA based on single-arm, phase II studies [50, 51]. Data from the clinical trials ABC-07 and EudraCT 2014–003656-31 using SBRT in combination with systemic chemotherapy are greatly anticipated.

In most centers, intrahepatic cholangiocarcinoma is considered a formal contraindication to liver transplantation. However, in a retrospective multicenter international cohort study, patients with cirrhosis who underwent transplantation and were found to have a small iCCA ($\leq$2 cm) had a reported 5-year survival rate of 65% and recurrence rate of 18%; those with larger tumors (>2 cm) or multifocal disease had a 5-year survival rate of 45% but recurrence was much higher at 61% [52]. A small series of 6 patients with locally advanced iCCA received neoadjuvant chemotherapy followed by liver transplantation, with a reported 5-year OS of 83% and RFS of 50% [53]. These studies indicate that a select group of iCCA patients can benefit from liver transplantation and protocols for transplanting iCCA are slowly emerging at select institutions.

Molecular profiling of CCA in recent years has revealed potentially targetable genetic alterations [54]. The most frequent mutations are *FGFR* fusions, most commonly *FGFR2* fusions (reported incidence of 10—16%) and *IDH1* mutations (reported incidence of 8—18%) [55, 56]. Within large duct type iCCAs, there is also an increased frequency of mutations in the *KRAS* and *TP53* genes [13].

Retrospective analysis of patients has shown that presence of an *FGFR* genetic aberration is associated with presentation at an earlier stage, an indolent disease course, and longer OS [57]. Several phase II studies in locally advanced or metastatic CCA patients with *FGFR* alterations have demonstrated durable objective responses to an FGFR inhibitor, with an overall response rate ranging from 14% to 42% and a median progression-free survival (PFS) of 5.6–9 months [58–63]. In the FIGHT-202 phase II trial, only patients with specifically FGFR2 fusions or rearrangements demonstrated clinical response to FGFR therapy [64]; in the majority of other trials, only patients with aberrations in *FGFR2* were included. Therefore, the presence of an *FGFR2* fusion is currently considered the most "actionable" of the *FGFR* family. The Food and Drug Administration (FDA) has granted accelerated approval for FGFR inhibitors pemigatinib and futibatinib, pending confirmatory studies, for the treatment of patients with chemorefractory CCA that harbors an *FGFR2* fusion or rearrangement. Multiple phase III studies using FGFR inhibition in the first-line setting are ongoing (NCT04093362, NCT03656536).

In patients with advanced CCA harboring an *IDH1* mutation who progressed on previous therapy, the phase III trial ClarIDHy compared ivosidenib, a small molecule inhibitor of mDH1, to placebo. There was a significant improvement in median PFS (2.7 vs. 1.4 months, $P < 0.0001$) and a favorable benefit in median OS (10.3 vs. 7.5 months, $P = 0.09$) with targeted therapy [65, 66]. In the last year, the FDA approved ivosidenib for the treatment of chemorefractory CCA with an *IDH1* mutation. The horizon is bright for the future treatment of cholangiocarcinoma as we better understand the molecular makeup of these tumors and learn to personalize therapy.

References

1. Kocarnik JM, Compton K, Dean FE, Fu W, Gaw BL, Harvey JD, et al. Cancer incidence, mortality, years of life lost, years lived with disability, and disability-adjusted life years for 29 cancer groups from 2010 to 2019 a systematic analysis for the global burden of disease study 2019. JAMA Oncol. 2022;8(3):420–44.
2. Banales JM, Marin JJG, Lamarca A, Rodrigues PM, Khan SA, Roberts LR, et al. Cholangiocarcinoma 2020: the next horizon in mechanisms and management. Nat Rev Gastroenterol Hepatol. 2020;17(9):557–88.
3. Antwi SO, Mousa OY, Patel T. Racial, ethnic, and age disparities in incidence and survival of intrahepatic cholangiocarcinoma in the United States; 1995–2014. Ann Hepatol. 2018;17(4):604–14.
4. Bertuccio P, Malvezzi M, Carioli G, Hashim D, Boffetta P, El-Serag HB, et al. Global trends in mortality from intrahepatic and extrahepatic cholangiocarcinoma. J Hepatol. 2019;71(1):104–14.
5. Khan SA, Tavolari S, Brandi G. Cholangiocarcinoma: epidemiology and risk factors. Liver Int. 2019;39(S1):19–31.
6. Brindley PJ, Bachini M, Ilyas SI, Khan SA, Loukas A, Sirica AE, et al. Cholangiocarcinoma. Nat Rev Dis Prim. 2021;7:1.
7. Sithithaworn P, Yongvanit P, Duenngai K, Kiatsopit N, Pairojkul C. Roles of liver fluke infection as risk factor for cholangiocarcinoma. J Hepatobiliary Pancreat Sci. 2014;21(5):301–8.

8. Suttiprapa S, Sotillo J, Smout M, Suyapoh W, Chaiyadet S, Tripathi T, et al. Opisthorchis viverrini proteome and host–parasite interactions. Adv Parasitol. 2018;102:45–72.
9. Lim JH. Cholangiocarcinoma: morphologic classification according to growth pattern and imaging findings. AJR Am J Roentgenol. 2003;181(3):819–27.
10. Nakanuma Y, Sato Y, Harada K, Sasaki M, Xu J, Ikeda H. Pathological classification of intrahepatic cholangiocarcinoma based on a new concept. World J Hepatol. 2010;2(12):419–27.
11. Kendall T, Verheij J, Gaudio E, Evert M, Guido M, Goeppert B, et al. Anatomical, histomorphological and molecular classification of cholangiocarcinoma. Liver Int. 2019;39(S1):7–18.
12. Liau JY, Tsai JH, Yuan RH, Chang CN, Lee HJ, Jeng YM. Morphological subclassification of intrahepatic cholangiocarcinoma: etiological, clinicopathological, and molecular features. Mod Pathol. 2014;27(8):1163–73.
13. Hayashi A, Misumi K, Shibahara J, Arita J, Sakamoto Y, Hasegawa K, et al. Distinct Clinicopathologic and genetic features of 2 histologic subtypes of intrahepatic Cholangiocarcinoma. Am J Surg Pathol. 2016;40:1021–30.
14. Komuta M, Govaere O, Vandecaveye V, Akiba J, Van Steenbergen W, Verslype C, et al. Histological diversity in cholangiocellular carcinoma reflects the different cholangiocyte phenotypes. Hepatology. 2012;55(6):1876–88.
15. Joo I, Lee JM, Yoon JH. Imaging diagnosis of intrahepatic and perihilar cholangiocarcinoma: recent advances and challenges. Radiology. 2018;288(1):7–23.
16. Rimola J, Forner A, Reig M, Vilana R, De Lope CR, Ayuso C, et al. Cholangiocarcinoma in cirrhosis: absence of contrast washout in delayed phases by magnetic resonance imaging avoids misdiagnosis of hepatocellular carcinoma. Hepatology. 2009;50(3):791–8.
17. Choi S, Lee S, Kim S, Park S, Park S, Kim K, et al. Intrahepatic cholangiocarcinoma in patients with cirrhosis: differentiation from hepatocellular carcinoma by using gadoxetic acid-enhanced MR imaging and dynamic CT. Radiology. 2017;282(3):771–81.
18. Hamilton S, Aaltonen L, editors. World Health Organization classification of tumours. Pathology and genetics of tumours of the digestive system. 3rd ed. Lyon: IARC Press; 2000.
19. Ishak K, Goodman Z, Stocker J. Atlas of tumor pathology: tumors of the liver and intrahepatic bile ducts. Washington, DC: Armed Forces Institute of Pathology; 2001.
20. Lamarca A, Barriuso J, Chander A, McNamara MG, Hubner RA, ÓReilly D, et al. 18F-fluorodeoxyglucose positron emission tomography (18FDG-PET) for patients with biliary tract cancer: systematic review and meta-analysis. J Hepatol. 2019;71(1):115–29.

21. Amin MB, Edge SB, Greene FL, Byrd DR, Brookland RK, Washington MK, et al. AJCC cancer staging manual. 8th ed. Springer; 2016.
22. Chun YS, Pawlik TM, Vauthey JN. 8th edition of the AJCC cancer staging manual: pancreas and hepatobiliary cancers. Ann Surg Oncol. 2018;25(4):845–7.
23. Kang SH, Hwang S, Lee YJ, Kim KH, Ahn CS, Moon DB, et al. Prognostic comparison of the 7th and 8th editions of the American joint committee on cancer staging system for intrahepatic cholangiocarcinoma. J Hepatobiliary Pancreat Sci. 2018;25(4):240–8.
24. Survival Rates for Bile Duct Cancer [Internet]. American Cancer Society 2023 [Cited 2023 Aug 5]. Available from: https://www.cancer.org/cancer/types/bile-duct-cancer/detection-diagnosis-staging/survival-by-stage.html.
25. Cherqui D, Tantawi B, Alon R, Piedbois P, Rahmouni A, Dhumeaux D, et al. Intrahepatic Cholangiocarcinoma: results of aggressive surgical management. Arch Surg (Chicago 1960). 1995;130(10):1073–8.
26. Weber SM, Ribero D, O'Reilly EM, Kokudo N, Miyazaki M, Pawlik TM. Intrahepatic Cholangiocarcinoma: expert consensus statement. HPB. 2015;17(8):669–80.
27. Abdalla EK, Barnett CC, Doherty D, Curley SA, Vauthey JN. Extended hepatectomy in patients with hepatobiliary malignancies with and without preoperative portal vein embolization. Arch Surg (Chicago 1960). 2002;137(6):675–81.
28. Vauthey JN, Pawlik TM, Abdalla EK, Arens JF, Nemr RA, Wei SH, et al. Is extended hepatectomy for hepatobiliary malignancy justified? Ann Surg. 2004;239(5):722–32.
29. Saito S, Yamanaka J, Miura K, Nakao N, Nagao T, Sugimoto T, et al. A novel 3D hepatectomy simulation based on liver circulation: application to liver resection and transplantation. Hepatology. 2005;41(6):1297–304.
30. Yamanaka J, Saito S, Fujimoto J. Impact of preoperative planning using virtual segmental volumetry on liver resection for hepatocellular carcinoma. World J Surg. 2007;31(6):1249–55.
31. Ribero D, Abdalla EK, Madoff DC, Donadon M, Loyer EM, Vauthey JN. Portal vein embolization before major hepatectomy and its effects on regeneration, resectability and outcome. Br J Surg. 2007;94(11):1386–94.
32. Shindoh J, Truty MJ, Aloia TA, Curley SA, Zimmitti G, Huang SY, et al. Kinetic growth rate after portal vein embolization predicts posthepatectomy outcomes: toward zero liver-related mortality in patients with colorectal liver metastases and small future liver remnant. J Am Coll Surg. 2013;216(2):201–9.
33. Farges O, Belghiti J, Kianmanesh R, Regimbeau JM, Santoro R, Vilgrain V, et al. Portal vein embolization before right hepatectomy: prospective clinical trial. Ann Surg. 2003;237(2):208–17.
34. Ethun CG, Maithel SK. Determination of resectability. Surg Clin North Am. 2016;96(2):163–81.

35. Primrose JN, Neoptolemos J, Palmer DH, Malik HZ, Prasad R, Mirza D, et al. Capecitabine compared with observation in resected biliary tract cancer (BILCAP): a randomised, controlled, multicentre, phase 3 study. Lancet Oncol. 2019;20(5):663–73.
36. Shroff RT, Kennedy EB, Bachini M, Bekaii-Saab T, Crane C, Edeline J, et al. Adjuvant therapy for resected biliary tract cancer: ASCO clinical practice guideline. J Clin Oncol. 2019;37(12):1015–27.
37. Shinohara ET, Mitra N, Guo M, Metz JM. Radiation therapy is associated with improved survival in the adjuvant and definitive treatment of intrahepatic cholangiocarcinoma. Int J Radiat Oncol Biol Phys. 2008;72(5):1495–501.
38. Le Roy B, Gelli M, Pittau G, Allard MA, Pereira B, Serji B, et al. Neoadjuvant chemotherapy for initially unresectable intrahepatic cholangiocarcinoma. Br J Surg. 2018;105(7):839–47.
39. Maithel SK, Keilson JM, Cao HST, Rupji M, Mahipal A, Lin BS, et al. NEO-GAP: a single-arm, phase II feasibility trial of neoadjuvant gemcitabine, cisplatin, and nab-paclitaxel for resectable, high-risk intrahepatic cholangiocarcinoma. Ann Surg Oncol. 2023;30(11):6558–66.
40. Valle J, Wasan H, Palmer DH, Cunningham D, Anthoney A, Maraveyas A, et al. Cisplatin plus gemcitabine versus gemcitabine for biliary tract cancer. N Engl J Med. 2010;362(14):1273–81.
41. Oh DY, Ruth He A, Qin S, Chen LT, Okusaka T, Vogel A, et al. Durvalumab plus gemcitabine and cisplatin in advanced biliary tract cancer. NEJM Evid. 2022;1(8).
42. Kelley RK, Ueno M, Yoo C, Finn RS, Furuse J, Ren Z, et al. Pembrolizumab in combination with gemcitabine and cisplatin compared with gemcitabine and cisplatin alone for patients with advanced biliary tract cancer (KEYNOTE-966): a randomised, double-blind, placebo-controlled, phase 3 trial. Lancet. 2023;401(10391):1853–65.
43. Lamarca A, Palmer DH, Wasan HS, Ross PJ, Ma YT, Arora A, et al. Second-line FOLFOX chemotherapy versus active symptom control for advanced biliary tract cancer (ABC-06): a phase 3, open-label, randomised, controlled trial. Lancet Oncol. 2021;22(5):690–701.
44. Hyung J, Kim I, Kim KP, Ryoo BY, Jeong JH, Kang MJ, et al. Treatment with liposomal Irinotecan plus fluorouracil and Leucovorin for patients with previously treated metastatic biliary tract cancer: the phase 2b NIFTY randomized clinical trial. JAMA Oncol. 2023;9(5):692–9.
45. Kiefer MV, Albert M, McNally M, Robertson M, Sun W, Fraker D, et al. Chemoembolization of intrahepatic cholangiocarcinoma with cisplatinum, doxorubicin, mitomycin C, ethiodol, and polyvinyl alcohol. Cancer. 2011;117(7):1498–505.
46. Vogl TJ, Naguib NNN, Nour-Eldin NEA, Bechstein WO, Zeuzem S, Trojan J, et al. Transarterial chemoembolization in the treatment of patients with unresectable cholangiocarcinoma: results and prognostic factors governing treatment success. Int J Cancer. 2012;131(3):733–40.

47. Park SY, Kim JH, Yoon HJ, Lee IS, Yoon HK, Kim KP. Transarterial chemoembolization versus supportive therapy in the palliative treatment of unresectable intrahepatic cholangiocarcinoma. Clin Radiol. 2011;66(4):322–8.
48. Edeline J, Touchefeu Y, Guiu B, Farge O, Tougeron D, Baumgaertner I, et al. Radioembolization plus chemotherapy for first-line treatment of locally advanced intrahepatic cholangiocarcinoma: a phase 2 clinical trial. JAMA Oncol. 2020;6(1):51–9.
49. Cercek A, Boerner T, Tan BR, Chou JF, Gönen M, Boucher TM, et al. Assessment of hepatic arterial infusion of floxuridine in combination with systemic gemcitabine and oxaliplatin in patients with unresectable intrahepatic cholangiocarcinoma: a phase 2 clinical trial. JAMA Oncol. 2020;6(1):60–7.
50. Ohkawa A, Mizumoto M, Ishikawa H, Abei M, Fukuda K, Hashimoto T, et al. Proton beam therapy for unresectable intrahepatic cholangiocarcinoma. J Gastroenterol Hepatol. 2015;30(5):957–63.
51. Hong TS, Wo JY, Yeap BY, Ben-Josef E, McDonnell EI, Blaszkowsky LS, et al. Multi-institutional phase II study of high-dose hypofractionated proton beam therapy in patients with localized, unresectable hepatocellular carcinoma and intrahepatic cholangiocarcinoma. J Clin Oncol. 2016;34(5):460–8.
52. Sapisochin G, Facciuto M, Rubbia-Brandt L, Marti J, Mehta N, Yao FY, et al. Liver transplantation for "very early" intrahepatic cholangiocarcinoma: international retrospective study supporting a prospective assessment. Hepatology. 2016;64(4):1178–88.
53. Lunsford KE, Javle M, Heyne K, Shroff RT, Abdel-Wahab R, Gupta N, et al. Liver transplantation for locally advanced intrahepatic cholangiocarcinoma treated with neoadjuvant therapy: a prospective case-series. Lancet Gastroenterol Hepatol. 2018;3(5):337–48.
54. Warren EAK, Maithel SK. Molecular pathology for cholangiocarcinoma: a review of actionable genetic targets and their relevance to adjuvant & neoadjuvant therapy, staging, follow-up, and determination of minimal residual disease. Hepatobiliary Surg Nutr. 2023;13(1):29.
55. Churi CR, Shroff R, Wang Y, Rashid A, Kang HSC, Weatherly J, et al. Mutation profiling in cholangiocarcinoma: prognostic and therapeutic implications. PLoS One. 2014;9(12).
56. Boscoe AN, Rolland C, Kelley RK. Frequency and prognostic significance of isocitrate dehydrogenase 1 mutations in cholangiocarcinoma: a systematic literature review. J Gastrointest Oncol. 2019;10(4):751–65.
57. Jain A, Borad MJ, Kelley RK, Wang Y, Abdel-Wahab R, Meric-Bernstam F, et al. Cholangiocarcinoma with FGFR genetic aberrations: a unique clinical phenotype. JCO Precis Oncol. 2018;2:1–12.
58. Voss MH, Hierro C, Heist RS, Cleary JM, Meric-Bernstam F, Tabernero J, et al. A phase I, open-label, multicenter, dose-escalation study of the oral selective FGFR inhibitor debio 1347 in patients with advanced solid

tumors harboring FGFR gene alterations. Clin Cancer Res. 2019;25(9):2699–707.
59. Park JO, Feng YH, Chen YY, Su WC, Oh DY, Shen L, et al. Updated results of a phase IIa study to evaluate the clinical efficacy and safety of erdafitinib in Asian advanced cholangiocarcinoma (CCA) patients with FGFR alterations. J Clin Oncol. 2019;37(Suppl 15):4117.
60. Javle M, Roychowdhury S, Kelley RK, Sadeghi S, Macarulla T, Weiss KH, et al. Infigratinib (BGJ398) in previously treated patients with advanced or metastatic cholangiocarcinoma with FGFR2 fusions or rearrangements: mature results from a multicentre, open-label, single-arm, phase 2 study. Lancet Gastroenterol Hepatol. 2021;6(10):803–15.
61. Droz Dit Busset M, Shaib W, Mody K, Personeni N, Damjanov N, Harris W, et al. Derazantinib for patients with intrahepatic cholangiocarcinoma harboring FGFR2 fusions/ rearrangements: primary results from the phase II study FIDES-01. Ann Oncol. 2021;32(S5):2021.
62. Mazzaferro V, El-Rayes BF, Droz dit Busset M, Cotsoglou C, Harris WP, Damjanov N, et al. Derazantinib (ARQ 087) in advanced or inoperable FGFR2 gene fusion-positive intrahepatic cholangiocarcinoma. Br J Cancer. 2019;120(2):165–71.
63. Goyal L, Meric-Bernstam F, Hollebecque A, Morizane C, Valle JW, Karasic TB, et al. Updated results of the FOENIX-CCA2 trial: efficacy and safety of futibatinib in intrahepatic cholangiocarcinoma (iCCA) harboring FGFR2 fusions/rearrangements. J Clin Oncol. 2022;40(Suppl 16):4009.
64. Abou-Alfa GK, Sahai V, Hollebecque A, Vaccaro G, Melisi D, Al-Rajabi R, et al. Pemigatinib for previously treated, locally advanced or metastatic cholangiocarcinoma: a multicentre, open-label, phase 2 study. Lancet Oncol. 2020;21(5):671–84.
65. Abou-Alfa GK, Macarulla T, Javle MM, Kelley RK, Lubner SJ, Adeva J, et al. Ivosidenib in IDH1-mutant, chemotherapy-refractory cholangiocarcinoma (ClarIDHy): a multicentre, randomised, double-blind, placebo-controlled, phase 3 study. Lancet Oncol. 2020;21(6):796–807.
66. Zhu AX, Macarulla T, Javle MM, Kelley RK, Lubner SJ, Adeva J, et al. Final overall survival efficacy results of Ivosidenib for patients with advanced cholangiocarcinoma with IDH1 mutation: the phase 3 randomized clinical ClarIDHy trial. JAMA Oncol. 2021;7(11):1669–77.

Extrahepatic Cholangiocarcinoma

6

Ranish K. Patel and Flavio G. Rocha

Etiology, Incidence, and Prognosis

Cholangiocarcinoma is the most common primary malignancy of the biliary tract, originating from ductal epithelia along the biliary tree, exclusive of the gallbladder and ampulla of Vater. In the United States alone, cholangiocarcinoma accounts for approximately 5000 deaths every year, with a reported annual incidence of 1 per 100,000 people. The incidence of cholangiocarcinoma appears to be increasing worldwide, most predominantly in endemic regions of Southeast Asia [1]. This cancer is further classified into two major subtypes: intrahepatic (ICC) and extrahepatic cholangiocarcinoma (ECC), with ECCs representing 2/3 of cholangiocarcinomas. However, the incidence of ICC has been increasing corresponding to a decrease in cancer of unknown primary (CUP) likely due to more frequent molecular profiling of liver tumors.

R. K. Patel · F. G. Rocha (✉)
Division of Surgical Oncology, Knight Cancer Institute, Oregon Health and Science University, Portland, OR, USA
e-mail: rochaf@ohsu.edu

ECCs are further subdivided into perihilar and distal tumors, with perihilar lesions accounting for 60–70% of all ECCs. Overall prognosis remains poor, with an estimated 5-year overall survival rate of 11% for all patients diagnosed with ECC [2]. The incidence rate has been difficult to characterize as all cholangiocarcinomas have historically been grouped together with primary gallbladder malignancies. Earlier data suggest a stable or decreasing incidence of ECC worldwide, though more recent work suggests a rising incidence of ECC worldwide [3–5].

Risk Factors and Pathophysiology

While most patients develop ECC sporadically, with no specific identifiable risk factor, it appears that the risk of development of cholangiocarcinoma strongly correlates with various chronic inflammatory states of the biliary tree. Primary sclerosing cholangitis (PSC) is a biliary inflammatory disorder that represents a major risk factor toward the development of cholangiocarcinoma. It remains the most common risk factor for cholangiocarcinoma in Western countries, with an approximately 40-fold increased risk of developing extrahepatic cholangiocarcinoma in those with PSC, and at significantly younger ages when compared to those who develop cholangiocarcinoma sporadically [4]. Congenital biliary abnormalities, such as Caroli syndrome or choledochal cysts, significantly increase risk of development of cholangiocarcinoma, with a reported incidence of cholangiocarcinoma in those with unresected choledochal cysts as high as 15%-20% [1, 6]. While no clear underlying carcinogenic mechanism has been delineated, chronic inflammation secondary to biliary stasis, pancreatic secretion reflux, or abnormalities in bile salt transporter proteins have been implicated [7]. In Southeast Asia, where the incidence of cholangiocarcinoma is the highest, chronic biliary ductal inflammation secondary to liver flukes *Clonorchis sinensis* and *Opisthorchis viverrini* endemics is associated with a fivefold risk of developing malignancy [8]. Other notable risk factors for cholangiocarcinoma include choledocholithiasis, cirrhosis, type

II diabetes, hepatitis B and C, and toxic exposures such as thorium dioxide (Thorotrast), asbestos, smoking, and excessive alcohol use [9, 10].

Clinical Presentation

ECCs are generally asymptomatic during earlier stages of disease. As disease progresses, patients most commonly present with manifestations of progressive biliary obstruction, such as jaundice, pruritus, steatorrhea, acholic stools, and dark urine. Other common, though non-specific, symptoms include right upper quadrant abdominal pain, fatigue, anorexia, nausea, and weight loss. It is important to note, however, that clinical presentations can vary depending upon the anatomic location of the ECC. For example, patients with perihilar ECC resulting in unilobar biliary obstruction may not present until later stages of disease, as the contralateral hepatic lobe can hypertrophy and compensate; however, distal ECC may present in earlier stages of disease as a result of earlier complete biliary outflow obstruction. Interestingly, patients rarely present with ascending cholangitis initially as a consequence of ECC [7, 11].

Histologic and Anatomic Classification, and Staging

The vast majority (~90%) of cholangiocarcinomas are adenocarcinomas, and can be categorized into three histologic subtypes. *Sclerosing tumors* are most common, tend to occur in the proximal biliary tree, and characteristically spread longitudinally in a sub-epithelial manner along the bile ducts. Histologically, this can result in microscopic tumor extension that can account for as much as 1–2 cm of spread outside of the macroscopic lesion, which can make obtaining satisfactory surgical margins difficult and contribute to poor surgical and oncologic outcomes [12–15]. *Nodular tumors* are the second most common, and tend to occur distally within the biliary tree, and preferentially project into the biliary lumen; they are however, aggressive and highly invasive

[14, 15]. *Papillary tumors* are the least common, and while they too expand into the ductal lumen and tend to occur distally, they tend to be less invasive, and thus ultimately have better resectability rates and prognosis [14, 15].

Anatomically, ECCs are subdivided into perihilar and distal ECCs. Perihilar ECCs are proximally separated from the ICC by the second-order bile ducts, and distally separated from distal ECC at the level of the insertion of the cystic duct into the extrahepatic biliary tree [3, 9] (Fig. 6.1). Perihilar ECCs are further classified by their patterns of involvement of the hepatic ducts, utilizing the Bismuth-Corlette classification system [16]: type I tumors exist below the confluence of the left and right hepatic

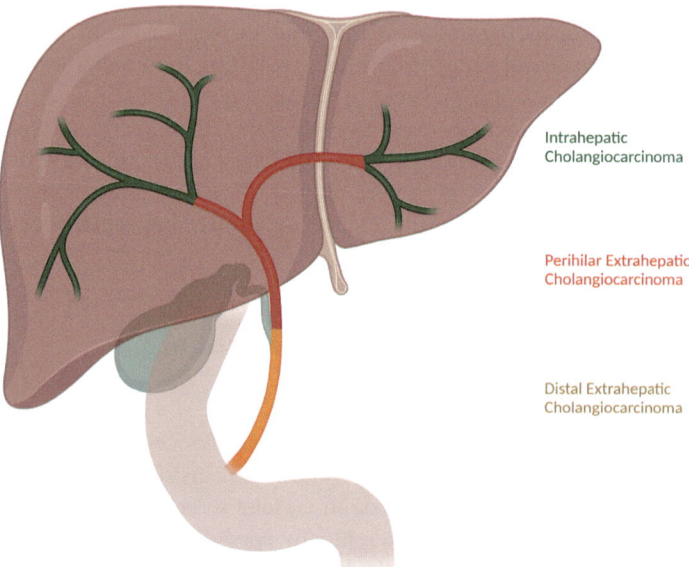

Fig. 6.1 Anatomic definitions of cholangiocarcinoma. Intrahepatic cholangiocarcinomas (ICC) constitute lesions proximal to the level of the confluence of the second-order biliary ducts, whereas extrahepatic cholangiocarcinomas (ECC) are defined by lesions distal to this level. ECCs are further subdivided into perihilar and distal ECCs, at the level of the insertion of the cystic duct into the extrahepatic biliary tree

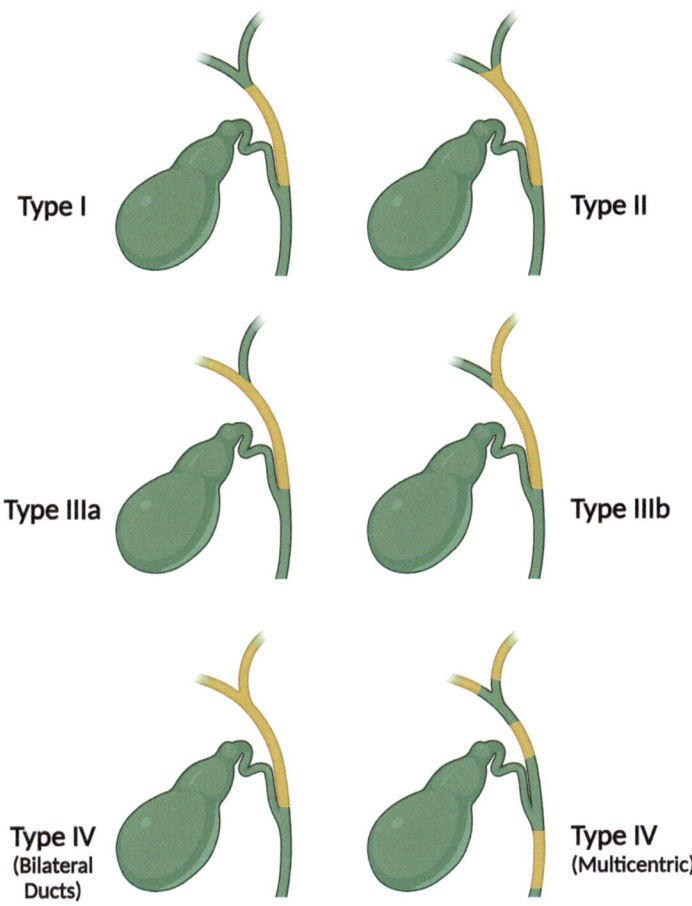

Fig. 6.2 Bismuth-Corlette classification system of perihilar extrahepatic cholangiocarcinoma

ducts, type II tumors reach the confluence of the hepatic ducts, type IIIa and IIIb extend into the right and left hepatic ducts respectively, and type IV involve both hepatic ducts or are multicentric (Fig. 6.2).

Modern staging of extrahepatic cholangiocarcinoma relies on the American Joint Committee on Cancer (AJCC)/Union for

International Cancer Control (UICC) TNM staging system [17], though uniquely, differs between perihilar and distal ECC. For example, T stage is stratified by measured depth of invasion in distal ECC, whereas invasion of specific surrounding structures defines T stage for perihilar ECC. However, similar to most adenocarcinomas, extent of local invasion and lymph node metastasis as a whole appear to be major prognostic factors, regardless of ECC subtype.

Importantly, the AJCC and Bismuth-Corlette staging systems do not accurately assess resectability, which is of paramount importance given that complete resection of perihilar ECCs is a critical determinant of survival. Thus, the Blumgart pre-surgical

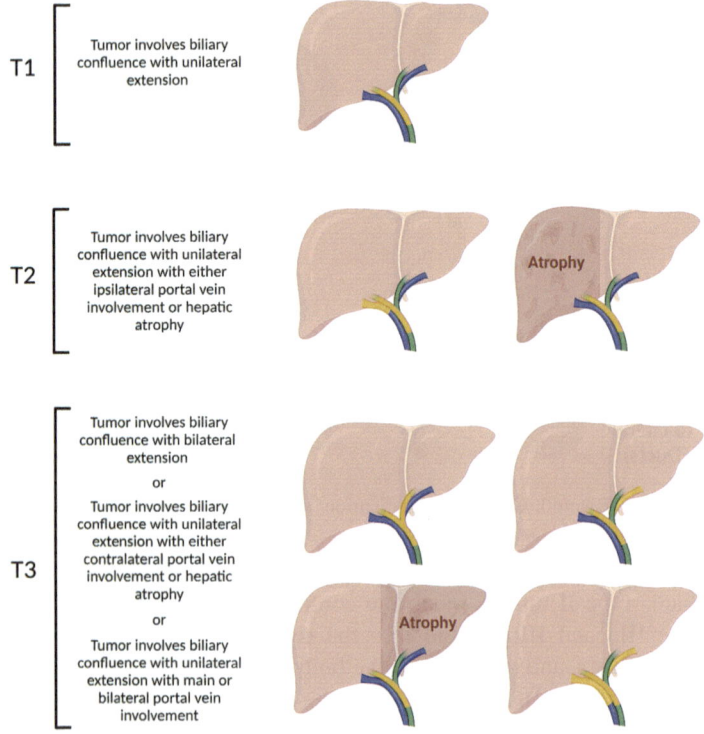

Fig. 6.3 The Blumgart pre-surgical clinical T-staging system for perihilar extrahepatic cholangiocarcinoma

clinical T staging system—defined by biliary tumor extent, the presence or absence of portal vein involvement, and the presence or absence of hepatic lobar atrophy—was devised, in order to better assess surgical resectability (Fig. 6.3). This T staging system has been demonstrated to more accurately predict tumor resectability, R0 resection, and presence of metastatic disease, particularly when compared to the AJCC tumor stage [18].

Diagnostic Workup

Once a clinical suspicion of cholangiocarcinoma has been established, a full diagnostic evaluation should commence. Given that most patients will present with signs and symptoms of biliary obstruction, liver chemistries will typically reveal direct hyperbilirubinemia, and elevated alkaline phosphatase and γ-glutamyl transferase levels. Specific markers of hepatic synthetic function such as prothrombin time and albumin levels may also be affected, though often are normal in earlier stages of disease. Tumor markers such as carcinoembryonic antigen (CEA) and carbonic anhydrase 19–9 (CA 19–9) may also be elevated, though notably, they are both limited by widely variable sensitivities and specificities [19]. These tumor markers are therefore best utilized to track disease response and recurrence, particularly if initially elevated, and are not routinely used as stand-alone diagnostic or screening tests [20].

A number of imaging modalities are utilized when establishing a diagnosis of cholangiocarcinoma. Typically, most patients will initially undergo right upper quadrant ultrasonography, which can generally accurately identify ductal dilatation and the level of obstruction within the biliary tree (Fig. 6.4) though may not consistently identify the extrahepatic cancerous lesions themselves—particularly in the case of the distal bile duct. However, duplex ultrasound may be utilized to better functionally characterize the extent of vascular involvement by tumor. Following an ultrasound evaluation, high-quality cross-sectional imaging is an essential next step in evaluation. Multiphase contrast-enhanced computed tomography (CT) imaging is typically used in order to characterize

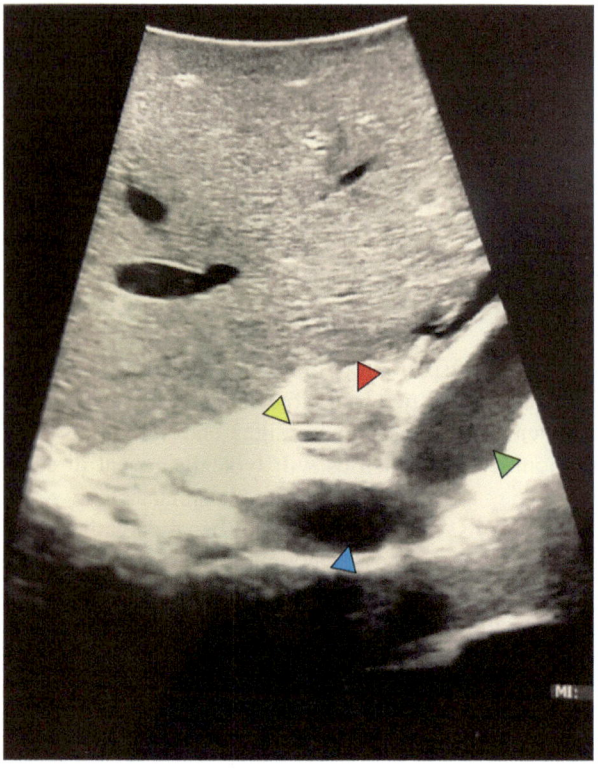

Fig. 6.4 Right upper quadrant ultrasound demonstrating a biliary stent (yellow arrowhead) passing through a perihilar mass (red arrowhead) at the level of the biliary confluence, without clear involvement of the right (blue arrowhead) and left (green arrowhead) portal venous branches

the level and degree of biliary and vascular involvement, as well as to identify hepatic lobar parenchymal atrophy associated with specific perihilar lesions. Additionally, CT imaging provides an opportunity to evaluate for surgical resectability, aberrant vascular anatomy, as well as distant metastatic disease; however, CT imaging may be less sensitive in evaluating for regional lymph node metastasis, and may underestimate the proximal extent of the tumor burden, particularly in the case of perihilar ECC. Given these limitations, most patients will additionally undergo magnetic

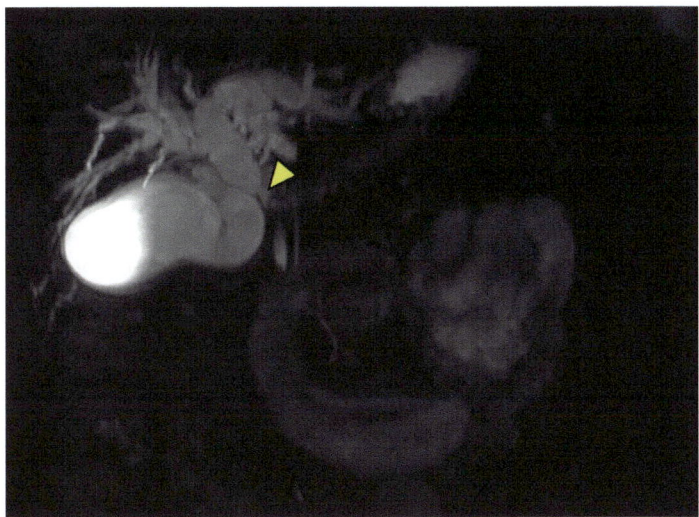

Fig. 6.5 Magnetic resonance cholangiopancreatography (MRCP) imaging demonstrating upstream biliary tree dilatation secondary to malignant obstruction at the level of the proximal common hepatic duct (yellow arrowhead)

resonance imaging (MRI) and magnetic resonance cholangiopancreatography (MRCP), which can provide improved definition of the anatomical extent of tumor burden, through creation of three-dimensional images of the biliary and vascular tree (Fig. 6.5).

Direct cholangiography, through either endoscopic retrograde cholangiopancreatography (ERCP) or percutaneous transhepatic cholangiography (PTC), are frequently utilized, as they provide excellent visualization and evaluation of the biliary tree, and an opportunity to obtain tissue for diagnostic evaluation. However, it is important to note that a tissue diagnosis is not mandatory prior to proceeding with surgical resection for presumed ECC, as accuracy of brush cytology and biopsies can be unreliable, and a negative evaluation does not typically exclude malignant disease [21]. Additionally, modern MRCP techniques have demonstrated similar accuracy in detection of malignant biliary obstructions, with perhaps better anatomical characterization of tumor burden, when compared to ERCP [22, 23]. Thus, in the modern era, MRCP has largely supplanted direct cholangiography. However, direct cholangiography remains an important adjunct in the case of equivocal MRI/MRCP findings, and is used routinely as an interventional tool for biliary drainage.

Preoperative Evaluation

Once a diagnosis or strong clinical suspicion of ECC has been established, preoperative assessment of operative candidacy is assessed. The patient's functional and physiologic state, and ability to tolerate a major abdominal surgery, must be considered prior to moving forth with resection. A number of tumor and anatomic factors must be considered. First, the extent of biliary and vascular involvement, with associated hepatic lobar atrophy, must be assessed; bilateral hepatic arterial or portal venous vascular involvement, bilateral hepatic duct involvement up to the level of the second order biliary ducts, encasement of the main portal vein, and/or encasement of a portal vein branch with associated atrophy of the contralateral hepatic lobe all anatomically preclude safe resection. Secondarily, early identification of metastatic disease including lymph node involvement outside of the hepatoduodenal ligament, as well as metastasis to the liver, lung, peritoneum, or other distant organs, is crucial in classifying patients who do not benefit from surgical resection.

Given that most patients present with biliary obstruction, preoperative biliary decompression plays a role in the management of ECC. The benefits of biliary decompression include addressing hyperbilirubinemia to facilitate systemic chemotherapy administration, amelioration of cholestasis and associated hepatic dysfunction, and to promote liver hypertrophy and regeneration post-surgical resection. It is important to note that the thresholds of preoperative biliary drainage have not been well defined; there are mixed data in regards to survival, clinical benefit, and even quality of life outcomes in those with ECC who undergo biliary decompression. In a systematic review, Liu et al. demonstrated no difference in death rate or postoperative hospital stay in those undergoing preoperative biliary drainage when compared to those without [24], while Robson et al. have prospectively shown that percutaneous biliary drainage did not significantly impact quality of life in patients with malignant biliary obstruction, unless they had associated pruritis [25]. However, Kennedy et al. suggest a survival benefit for preoperative biliary drainage in patients with predicted postoperative future liver remnant (FLR) of <30% [26]. Ultimately, the use of preoperative biliary drainage in ECC varies by center and provider, though generally is utilized when patients experience significant symptoms (pruritis, cholangitis), hyperbilirubinemia, liver dysfunction, need for portal vein embolization, or have planned neoadjuvant therapy with delay to surgical resection. Biliary drainage is largely accomplished with either endoscopic or percutaneous transhepatic techniques. Patients with lower bile duct obstructions are typically treated endoscopically, whereas those with higher obstructions are treated percutaneously. Whether one modality is superior to the other is debated, though limitations to both techniques have been described. Percutaneous drainage has been shown to have a higher overall success rate, though questions regarding tract recurrence and risk of spillage of cancer-containing biliary contents into the peritoneum exist [27, 28]. On the other hand, endoscopic drainage avoids these complications but may not be technically feasible, particularly in the case of proximal perihilar obstruction, and when ineffective, can induce cholangitis [11]. In one randomized multicenter clinical trial, which compared percutaneous and endoscopic biliary drainage in patients with resectable perihilar cholangiocarcinoma, there were similar rates of post-drainage related complications between both modalities, and 56% of those undergoing endoscopic drainage required additional percutaneous drainage; however, this data should be interpreted with caution given a small sample size, and the study being stopped prematurely given higher all-cause mortality rates in the percutaneous biliary drainage cohort [29]. Ultimately, the best approach to biliary drainage involves a careful assessment of anatomic feasibility, and a multidisciplinary assessment of the potential risks/benefits with each technique.

Given that many patients will present with hepatic lobar atrophy and require concomitant hepatic resections, careful calculation of the patient's FLR should be performed with the goal of minimizing risk of postoperative hepatic dysfunction. Preoperative CT imaging allows for volumetric assessment of the liver, which is then utilized to predict future FLR following resection. Patients with a predicted sFLR of <20–40% (depending on the liver characteristics) are considered for preoperative portal vein embolization (PVE) to induce hypertrophy of the future remnant liver [30–33]. PVE is a safe procedure at experienced centers, which has increased the limits of safe hepatic resection and facilitates surgical resection in patients who would otherwise be deemed unresectable.

Operative Strategies

Surgical resection remains the only treatment modality that offers the possibility of cure in ECC. The overall goal is for complete tumor resection with negative histologic (R0) margins, as those with R0 margins have reported 5-year survivals of 54–65%, compared to 0–25% in those with positive (R1) margins [34–37]. Furthermore, it appears that patients with R1 resection margins may have similar survival compared to patients with locally advanced, unresectable disease—thus obtaining R0 margins is of paramount importance in those with ECC [11, 38]. However, achieving an R0 margin can be challenging in ECC, particularly in those proximal hilar tumors with sclerosing histology associated with microscopic radial, subepithelial extension [38]. Reported successful R0 resection rates range from 20% to 40% in perihilar, and 50% in distal tumors [34]. Given that margin-negative resections are of paramount importance, routine frozen sections are sent for pathologic evaluation intraoperatively, in order to improve bile duct margins and optimize survival outcomes for patients undergoing resection. In a recent systematic review by Lenet et al., patients who underwent successful revisions of positive intraoperative bile duct margins had similar overall survival to those with primary negative margin resections, and significantly improved survival when compared to those with R1 resection margins [39].

Despite refinements and improvements in preoperative imaging and staging, a significant number of patients are found to have metastatic disease intraoperatively at the time of surgical resection. Given this, diagnostic laparoscopy is routinely utilized prior to proceeding with a potentially unnecessary, nontherapeutic laparotomy. It is also important to note that true resectability based on vascular involvement is ultimately judged by intraoperative evaluation, as this may not effectively be evident on preoperative staging imaging; however, this is not generally easily clarified by initial diagnostic laparoscopy, thus laparoscopy is best utilized to evaluate for grossly identifiable (most commonly peritoneal) metastatic disease.

Surgical approach is primarily dependent upon the location of the tumor. Patients with distal cholangiocarcinoma are most conventionally managed by a pancreaticoduodenectomy (Whipple procedure), in order to assure negative margins and an adequate lymph node harvest. In patients with perihilar cholangiocarcinoma, the extent of the resection is dependent upon the degree of involvement of the biliary tree. Bismuth type I and II lesions (at or below the level of the hepatic confluence) involve en bloc resection of the bile duct with 5–10 mm negative margins and regional lymphadenectomy. While bile duct resection alone may facilitate appropriate resection margins, most commonly a partial hepatectomy with or without caudate lobectomy is necessary in order to achieve these margins. Bismuth type III lesions generally will require more formal hepatic lobectomy in order to facilitate resection margins and preservation of postoperative hepatic function. Those with Bismuth type IV lesions may be candidates for curative resection, though this may require multiple hepatic segment resections, and may require portal vein resection to achieve negative ductal margins.

Patients with locally advanced, unresectable perihilar disease, without evidence of lymph node or distant metastatic involvement, may achieve R0 resection through orthotopic liver transplantation (OLT). Uniquely, these patients will typically receive preoperative chemoradiation therapy, prior to proceeding with

OLT. This approach is not without controversy, as few patients meet criteria for OLT, and for those who do, the natural limitations of preoperative imaging in ECC may frequently understage these patients, thus incorrectly categorizing patients as appropriate candidates for OLT. However, when appropriately selected, data exist to support the use of transplantation as surgical approach to the management of cholangiocarcinoma, with 5-year survival rates ranging from 39% to 53% [40, 41]. This data must be considered with the context that a significant proportion of patients underwent OLT given history of PSC without confirmed malignancy. Prospective, randomized clinical data are needed to further evaluate OLT as a treatment modality in cholangiocarcinoma.

Systemic Treatment

While surgical resection remains the mainstay management strategy with a clear survival benefit, systemic treatment modalities are often integrated into the therapeutic strategy of patients with ECC, with neoadjuvant, adjuvant, and palliative intent. Neoadjuvant therapy is not considered a standard approach in patients with resectable ECC. However, in patients who are deemed unresectable at the outset, neoadjuvant chemotherapy/chemoradiation may be utilized as a means to downstage initially unresectable disease to resectable disease, in order to facilitate surgical resection. Secondarily, neoadjuvant therapy is generally utilized ahead of OLT, in circumstances when transplantation is the therapeutic strategy to facilitate an R0 resection, as retrospective, pooled systematic review data suggests an improved survival benefit with the integration of neoadjuvant therapy prior to OLT [41]. Specific regimens used in the neoadjuvant setting have historically varied, though most commonly included 5-flurouracil or gemcitabine-based regimens. Based on the results of the ABC-02 trial, gemcitabine/cisplatin-based chemotherapy was considered standard of care for patients with locally advanced or metastatic biliary tract cancers [42]; however, following the results of the TOPAZ-1 trial, combination gemcitabine/cisplatin/durvalumab (GCD) became the new first-line systemic regimen for these patients. It is important to note, however, that the subgroup analysis of those with ECC only within the TOPAZ-1 cohort demonstrated a significant improvement in progression-free survival, but not overall survival, in favor of the GCD cohort [43]. Further investigations into neoadjuvant regimens—even in the setting of upfront resectable disease—are ongoing, to better define the scope and therapeutic strategy for these cytotoxic therapies.

Recurrence remains relatively high following curative resection for cholangiocarcinoma, with rates as high as 76% in patients with perihilar ECC following curative intent surgery [44, 45]. Motivated by this, the integration of adjuvant therapy has been favored following resection of ECC, though until recently, specific regimens and strategies were based off of smaller, retrospective data (Table 6.1). The BCAT phase III trial first evaluated the use of adjuvant gemcitabine against observation alone, in patients with resected ECC, demonstrating no difference in survival outcomes between the two groups, though notably the investigated patient cohort had a relative 50% 5-year survival rate [46]. Similarly, the PRODIGE 12-ACCORD 18-UNICANCER GI phase III trial did not demonstrate a survival benefit in those with cholangiocarcinoma and gallbladder cancer, who received combination gemcitabine/oxaliplatin; though this study was likely underpowered [19, 47]. This was followed by the BILCAP phase III randomized control trial, which recruited 447 patients from 44 centers, comparing adjuvant capecitabine versus observation alone following surgical resection [48]. Within this trial, those receiving adjuvant capecitabine demonstrated a mean overall survival of 53 months compared to 36 months for those treated with observation alone, and an improved recurrence-free survival of 24.4 months versus 17.5 months in favor of the capecitabine group. Given these results, 6 months of adjuvant capecitabine is now considered the current standard of care, though alternate regimens are currently being compared against adjuvant capecitabine in a number of actively recruiting phase III clinical trials. Additionally, based on the results of the SWOG S0809 trial, patients with high-risk features following resection in ECC—such as R1 resection margins, lymph node positivity, advanced T

Table 6.1 Adjuvant therapy clinical trials for resectable biliary tract cancers

Study	Year	Study type	Disease sites	Treatment	No. of patients	Median OS (months)	Median RFS (months)
SWOG 0809	2015	Phase II single-arm	ECC (68%; pECC 51%, dECC 17%) GBC (32%)	Gem/Capecitabine/Radiotherapy	79 patients ($n = 54$ R0 margins, $n = 25$ R1 margins)	35 (34 for R0, 35 for R1) 65% 2-year survival (67% R0 and 60% R1)	26 (26 R0, 23 R1) 52% 2-year survival (54% R0 and 48% R1)
BCAT	2018	Phase III RCT	ECC (pECC 45%, dECC 55%)	Gemcitabine vs. Observation	225 patients ($n = 117$ Gemcitabine vs. $n = 108$ observation)	62.3 vs. 63.8 (HR 1.01, 95% CI 0.70–1.45; $p = 0.964$)	36.0 vs. 39.9 (HR 0.93, 95% CI 0.66–1.32; $p = 0.693$)
PRODIGE 12-ACCORD 18-UNICANCER GI	2019	Phase III RCT	ICC (44%) ECC (36%; pECC 8%, dECC 28%) GBC (20%)	Gem/Ox vs. Observation	196 patients ($n = 95$ Gem/Ox vs. $n = 99$ observation)	75.8 vs. 50.8 (HR 1.08, 95% CI 0.70–1.66; $p = 0.74$)	30.4 vs. 18.5 (HR 0.88, 95% CI 0.62–1.25; $p = 0.48$)
BILCAP	2019	Phase III RCT	ICC (19%) ECC (64%; pECC 29%, dECC 35%) GBC (18%)	Capecitabine vs. Observation	447 patients ($n = 223$ Capecitabine vs. $n = 224$ observation)	53 vs. 36 (HR 0.75, 95% CI 0.58–0.97; $p = 0.028$)	25.9 vs. 17.4 (HR 0.70, 95% CI 0.54–0.92; $p = -0.0093$)

Study	Year	Study type	Disease sites	Treatment	No. of patients	Median OS (months)	Median RFS (months)
ASCOT	2023	Phase III RCT	ICC (13%) ECC (56%) GBC (14%) Ampullary (17%)	S-1 vs. Observation	440 patients ($n = 218$ S-1 vs. $n = 222$ observation)	77.1% vs. 67.6% 3-year survival (HR 0.694, 95% CI 0.514–0.935; $p = 0.008$)	62.4% vs. 50.9% 3-year survival (HR 0.797, 95% CI 0.613–1.035; $p = 0.088$)
STAMP	2023	Phase II RCT	ECC (pECC 45%, dECC 55%)	Gem/Cis vs. Capecitabine	101 patients ($n = 50$ Gem/Cis vs. $n = 51$ capecitabine)	35.7 vs. 35.7 (HR 1.08, 90% CI 0.72–1.64; $p = 0.40$)	14.3 vs. 11.1 (HR 0.96, 90% CI 0.71–1.30; $p = 0.43$)

ECC extrahepatic cholangiocarcinoma, *pECC* perihilar ECC, *dECC* distal ECC, *ICC* intrahepatic cholangiocarcinoma, *GBC* gallbladder carcinoma, *Gem/Cis* gemcitabine/cisplatin, *Gem/Ox* gemcitabine oxaliplatin, *OS* overall survival, *RFS* recurrence free survival, *RCT* randomized control trial stage—are offered concurrent radiation therapy, as a means to decrease recurrence risk and improve survival [49].

Given the rapid adoption and availability of next-generation sequencing, distinct molecular profiles for different biliary tract cancers are being described. Targeted therapies directed toward potentially actionable molecular alterations are now at the forefront of investigation for biliary tract malignancies, and may prove to be an integral component toward improving systemic therapeutic combinations. ERBB2, PI3K/mTOR, KRAS, TP53, and ARID1A are among the notable molecular aberrations that appear to be common and unique to ECCs specifically [50], and development and investigation of therapeutics targeting such aberrations are ongoing.

Palliation

In the majority of patients with ECC, who are technically unresectable or have metastatic disease, management typically focuses on disease control and palliation of symptoms. GCD therapy constitutes the first-line systemic therapy for these patients, and referral for clinical trial participation is key in exposing patients to newer treatment paradigms and modalities which can improve survival and quality of life outcomes. Additionally, given that biliary obstruction remains the major challenge and cause of morbidity in patients with ECC, endoscopic and percutaneous stenting are often incorporated into palliative strategy. Additionally, biliary bypass can be considered to achieve adequate biliary decompression, though this is generally reserved for those who are not candidates for stent-based biliary decompression, as complication and morbidity rates are higher in those undergoing these palliative operations [51].

Summary

Extrahepatic cholangiocarcinoma represents a rare, lethal malignancy with significant diagnostic and therapeutic challenges. While surgical resection offers the best long-term survival outcomes, most patients have advanced disease, precluding them from such intervention. Given this, robust multidisciplinary care is integral to diagnosis, characterizing tumor burden, palliation of symptoms, and ultimately treating or controlling disease. As we enter an exciting era of genomic profiling and learn more about the molecular driver aberrations in ECC, emerging targeted therapies look to meaningfully improve oncologic outcomes, with validation through collaborative multicenter clinical trial efforts.

References

1. Valle JW, Kelley RK, Nervi B, Oh DY, Zhu AX. Biliary tract cancer. Lancet. 2021;397(10272):428–44. https://doi.org/10.1016/s0140-6736(21)00153-7.
2. team TACSmaec. Survival rates for bile duct cancer. 2023.
3. Banales JM, Marin JJG, Lamarca A, Rodrigues PM, Khan SA, Roberts LR, et al. Cholangiocarcinoma 2020: the next horizon in mechanisms and management. Nat Rev Gastroenterol Hepatol. 2020;17(9):557–88. https://doi.org/10.1038/s41575-020-0310-z.
4. Esnaola NF, Meyer JE, Karachristos A, Maranki JL, Camp ER, Denlinger CS. Evaluation and management of intrahepatic and extrahepatic cholangiocarcinoma. Cancer. 2016;122(9):1349–69. https://doi.org/10.1002/cncr.29692.
5. Florio AA, Ferlay J, Znaor A, Ruggieri D, Alvarez CS, Laversanne M, et al. Global trends in intrahepatic and extrahepatic cholangiocarcinoma incidence from 1993 to 2012. Cancer. 2020;126(11):2666–78. https://doi.org/10.1002/cncr.32803.
6. Burak K, Angulo P, Pasha TM, Egan K, Petz J, Lindor KD. Incidence and risk factors for cholangiocarcinoma in primary sclerosing cholangitis. Am J Gastroenterol. 2004;99(3):523–6. https://doi.org/10.1111/j.1572-0241.2004.04067.x.
7. Khan SA, Thomas HC, Davidson BR, Taylor-Robinson SD. Cholangiocarcinoma. Lancet. 2005;366(9493):1303–14. https://doi.org/10.1016/s0140-6736(05)67530-7.

8. Shin HR, Oh JK, Masuyer E, Curado MP, Bouvard V, Fang YY, et al. Epidemiology of cholangiocarcinoma: an update focusing on risk factors. Cancer Sci. 2010;101(3):579–85. https://doi.org/10.1111/j.1349-7006.2009.01458.x.
9. Blechacz B, Komuta M, Roskams T, Gores GJ. Clinical diagnosis and staging of cholangiocarcinoma. Nat Rev Gastroenterol Hepatol. 2011;8(9):512–22. https://doi.org/10.1038/nrgastro.2011.131.
10. Clements O, Eliahoo J, Kim JU, Taylor-Robinson SD, Khan SA. Risk factors for intrahepatic and extrahepatic cholangiocarcinoma: a systematic review and meta-analysis. J Hepatol. 2020;72(1):95–103. https://doi.org/10.1016/j.jhep.2019.09.007.
11. Schoellhammer HF, Fong Y, Singh G. Chapter 51: A extrahepatic bile duct tumors. In: Jarnagin WR, editor. Blumgart's surgery of the liver, biliary tract and pancreas, 2-volume set. 6th ed. Philadelphia: Elsevier; 2017. p. 818–32.e3.
12. Ebata T, Watanabe H, Ajioka Y, Oda K, Nimura Y. Pathological appraisal of lines of resection for bile duct carcinoma. Br J Surg. 2002;89(10):1260–7. https://doi.org/10.1046/j.1365-2168.2002.02211.x.
13. Higuchi R, Ota T, Araida T, Kobayashi M, Furukawa T, Yamamoto M. Prognostic relevance of ductal margins in operative resection of bile duct cancer. Surgery. 2010;148(1):7–14. https://doi.org/10.1016/j.surg.2009.11.018.
14. Castellano-Megías VM, Ibarrola-de Andrés C, Colina-Ruizdelgado F. Pathological aspects of so called "hilar cholangiocarcinoma". World J Gastrointest Oncol. 2013;5(7):159–70. https://doi.org/10.4251/wjgo.v5.i7.159.
15. Nakeeb A, Pitt HA, Sohn TA, Coleman J, Abrams RA, Piantadosi S, et al. Cholangiocarcinoma. A spectrum of intrahepatic, perihilar, and distal tumors. Ann Surg. 1996;224(4):463–73.; discussion 73-5. https://doi.org/10.1097/00000658-199610000-00005.
16. Bismuth H, Nakache R, Diamond T. Management strategies in resection for hilar cholangiocarcinoma. Ann Surg. 1992;215(1):31–8. https://doi.org/10.1097/00000658-199201000-00005.
17. Amin MB, Edge SB, Greene FL, Byrd DR, Brookland RK, Washington MK, et al. AJCC cancer staging manual. Springer; 2017.
18. Matsuo K, Rocha FG, Ito K, D'Angelica MI, Allen PJ, Fong Y, et al. The Blumgart preoperative staging system for hilar cholangiocarcinoma: analysis of resectability and outcomes in 380 patients. J Am Coll Surg. 2012;215(3):343–55. https://doi.org/10.1016/j.jamcollsurg.2012.05.025.
19. Kefas J, Bridgewater J, Vogel A, Stein A, Primrose J. Adjuvant therapy of biliary tract cancers. Ther Adv Med Oncol. 2023;15:17588359231163785. https://doi.org/10.1177/17588359231163785.
20. Chung YJ, Choi DW, Choi SH, Heo JS, Kim DH. Prognostic factors following surgical resection of distal bile duct cancer. J Korean Surg Soc. 2013;85(5):212–8. https://doi.org/10.4174/jkss.2013.85.5.212.

21. Tamada K, Ushio J, Sugano K. Endoscopic diagnosis of extrahepatic bile duct carcinoma: advances and current limitations. World J Clin Oncol. 2011;2(5):203–16. https://doi.org/10.5306/wjco.v2.i5.203.
22. Park HS, Lee JM, Choi JY, Lee MW, Kim HJ, Han JK, et al. Preoperative evaluation of bile duct cancer: MRI combined with MR cholangiopancreatography versus MDCT with direct cholangiography. AJR Am J Roentgenol. 2008;190(2):396–405. https://doi.org/10.2214/ajr.07.2310.
23. Vogl TJ, Schwarz WO, Heller M, Herzog C, Zangos S, Hintze RE, et al. Staging of Klatskin tumours (hilar cholangiocarcinomas): comparison of MR cholangiography, MR imaging, and endoscopic retrograde cholangiography. Eur Radiol. 2006;16(10):2317–25. https://doi.org/10.1007/s00330-005-0139-4.
24. Liu F, Li Y, Wei Y, Li B. Preoperative biliary drainage before resection for hilar cholangiocarcinoma: whether or not? A systematic review. Dig Dis Sci. 2011;56(3):663–72. https://doi.org/10.1007/s10620-010-1338-7.
25. Robson PC, Heffernan N, Gonen M, Thornton R, Brody LA, Holmes R, et al. Prospective study of outcomes after percutaneous biliary drainage for malignant biliary obstruction. Ann Surg Oncol. 2010;17(9):2303–11. https://doi.org/10.1245/s10434-010-1045-9.
26. Kennedy TJ, Yopp A, Qin Y, Zhao B, Guo P, Liu F, et al. Role of preoperative biliary drainage of liver remnant prior to extended liver resection for hilar cholangiocarcinoma. HPB (Oxford). 2009;11(5):445–51. https://doi.org/10.1111/j.1477-2574.2009.00090.x.
27. Hirano S, Tanaka E, Tsuchikawa T, Matsumoto J, Kawakami H, Nakamura T, et al. Oncological benefit of preoperative endoscopic biliary drainage in patients with hilar cholangiocarcinoma. J Hepatobiliary Pancreat Sci. 2014;21(8):533–40. https://doi.org/10.1002/jhbp.76.
28. Takahashi Y, Nagino M, Nishio H, Ebata T, Igami T, Nimura Y. Percutaneous transhepatic biliary drainage catheter tract recurrence in cholangiocarcinoma. Br J Surg. 2010;97(12):1860–6. https://doi.org/10.1002/bjs.7228.
29. Coelen RJS, Roos E, Wiggers JK, Besselink MG, Buis CI, Busch ORC, et al. Endoscopic versus percutaneous biliary drainage in patients with resectable perihilar cholangiocarcinoma: a multicentre, randomised controlled trial. Lancet Gastroenterol Hepatol. 2018;3(10):681–90. https://doi.org/10.1016/s2468-1253(18)30234-6.
30. Abdalla EK, Barnett CC, Doherty D, Curley SA, Vauthey JN. Extended hepatectomy in patients with hepatobiliary malignancies with and without preoperative portal vein embolization. Arch Surg. 2002;137(6):675–80.; discussion 80-1. https://doi.org/10.1001/archsurg.137.6.675.
31. Paik WH, Loganathan N, Hwang JH. Preoperative biliary drainage in hilar cholangiocarcinoma: when and how? World J Gastrointest Endosc. 2014;6(3):68–73. https://doi.org/10.4253/wjge.v6.i3.68.

32. Zorzi D, Laurent A, Pawlik TM, Lauwers GY, Vauthey JN, Abdalla EK. Chemotherapy-associated hepatotoxicity and surgery for colorectal liver metastases. Br J Surg. 2007;94(3):274–86. https://doi.org/10.1002/bjs.5719.
33. Ribero D, Chun YS, Vauthey JN. Standardized liver volumetry for portal vein embolization. Semin Intervent Radiol. 2008;25(2):104–9. https://doi.org/10.1055/s-2008-1076681.
34. Burke EC, Jarnagin WR, Hochwald SN, Pisters PW, Fong Y, Blumgart LH. Hilar Cholangiocarcinoma: patterns of spread, the importance of hepatic resection for curative operation, and a presurgical clinical staging system. Ann Surg. 1998;228(3):385–94. https://doi.org/10.1097/00000658-199809000-00011.
35. Murakami Y, Uemura K, Hayashidani Y, Sudo T, Hashimoto Y, Ohge H, et al. Prognostic significance of lymph node metastasis and surgical margin status for distal cholangiocarcinoma. J Surg Oncol. 2007;95(3):207–12. https://doi.org/10.1002/jso.20668.
36. Nakagohri T, Takahashi S, Ei S, Masuoka Y, Mashiko T, Ogasawara T, et al. Prognostic impact of margin status in distal Cholangiocarcinoma. World J Surg. 2023;47(4):1034–41. https://doi.org/10.1007/s00268-023-06889-7.
37. Wakai T, Shirai Y, Moroda T, Yokoyama N, Hatakeyama K. Impact of ductal resection margin status on long-term survival in patients undergoing resection for extrahepatic cholangiocarcinoma. Cancer. 2005;103(6):1210–6. https://doi.org/10.1002/cncr.20906.
38. Endo I, House MG, Klimstra DS, Gönen M, D'Angelica M, Dematteo RP, et al. Clinical significance of intraoperative bile duct margin assessment for hilar cholangiocarcinoma. Ann Surg Oncol. 2008;15(8):2104–12. https://doi.org/10.1245/s10434-008-0003-2.
39. Lenet T, Gilbert RWD, Smoot R, Tzeng C-WD, Rocha FG, Yohanathan L, et al. Does intraoperative frozen section and revision of margins Lead to improved survival in patients undergoing resection of perihilar cholangiocarcinoma? A systematic review and meta-analysis. Ann Surg Oncol. 2022;29(12):7592–602. https://doi.org/10.1245/s10434-022-12041-x.
40. Darwish Murad S, Kim WR, Harnois DM, Douglas DD, Burton J, Kulik LM, et al. Efficacy of neoadjuvant chemoradiation, followed by liver transplantation, for perihilar cholangiocarcinoma at 12 US centers. Gastroenterology. 2012;143(1):88–98.e3.; quiz e14. https://doi.org/10.1053/j.gastro.2012.04.008.
41. Gu J, Bai J, Shi X, Zhou J, Qiu Y, Wu Y, et al. Efficacy and safety of liver transplantation in patients with cholangiocarcinoma: a systematic review and meta-analysis. Int J Cancer. 2012;130(9):2155–63. https://doi.org/10.1002/ijc.26019.
42. Valle J, Wasan H, Palmer DH, Cunningham D, Anthoney A, Maraveyas A, et al. Cisplatin plus gemcitabine versus gemcitabine for biliary tract

cancer. N Engl J Med. 2010;362(14):1273–81. https://doi.org/10.1056/NEJMoa0908721.
43. Oh D-Y, He AR, Qin S, Chen L-T, Okusaka T, Vogel A, et al. Durvalumab plus gemcitabine and cisplatin in advanced biliary tract cancer. NEJM Evid. 2022;1(8):EVIDoa2200015. https://doi.org/10.1056/EVIDoa2200015.
44. Groot Koerkamp B, Wiggers JK, Allen PJ, Besselink MG, Blumgart LH, Busch OR, et al. Recurrence rate and pattern of perihilar cholangiocarcinoma after curative intent resection. J Am Coll Surg. 2015;221(6):1041–9. https://doi.org/10.1016/j.jamcollsurg.2015.09.005.
45. Shroff RT, Kennedy EB, Bachini M, Bekaii-Saab T, Crane C, Edeline J, et al. Adjuvant therapy for resected biliary tract cancer: ASCO clinical practice guideline. J Clin Oncol. 2019;37(12):1015–27. https://doi.org/10.1200/jco.18.02178.
46. Ebata T, Hirano S, Konishi M, Uesaka K, Tsuchiya Y, Ohtsuka M, et al. Randomized clinical trial of adjuvant gemcitabine chemotherapy versus observation in resected bile duct cancer. Br J Surg. 2018;105(3):192–202. https://doi.org/10.1002/bjs.10776.
47. Edeline J, Benabdelghani M, Bertaut A, Watelet J, Hammel P, Joly JP, et al. Gemcitabine and oxaliplatin chemotherapy or surveillance in resected biliary tract cancer (PRODIGE 12-ACCORD 18-UNICANCER GI): a randomized phase III study. J Clin Oncol. 2019;37(8):658–67. https://doi.org/10.1200/jco.18.00050.
48. Primrose JN, Fox RP, Palmer DH, Malik HZ, Prasad R, Mirza D, et al. Capecitabine compared with observation in resected biliary tract cancer (BILCAP): a randomised, controlled, multicentre, phase 3 study. Lancet Oncol. 2019;20(5):663–73. https://doi.org/10.1016/s1470-2045(18)30915-x.
49. Ben-Josef E, Guthrie KA, El-Khoueiry AB, Corless CL, Zalupski MM, Lowy AM, et al. SWOG S0809: a phase II intergroup trial of adjuvant capecitabine and gemcitabine followed by radiotherapy and concurrent capecitabine in extrahepatic cholangiocarcinoma and gallbladder carcinoma. J Clin Oncol. 2015;33(24):2617–22. https://doi.org/10.1200/jco.2014.60.2219.
50. Bridgewater JA, Goodman KA, Kalyan A, Mulcahy MF. Biliary tract cancer: epidemiology, radiotherapy, and molecular profiling. Am Soc Clin Oncol Educ Book. 2016;35:e194–203. https://doi.org/10.1200/edbk_160831.
51. Singhal D, van Gulik TM, Gouma DJ. Palliative management of hilar cholangiocarcinoma. Surg Oncol. 2005;14(2):59–74. https://doi.org/10.1016/j.suronc.2005.05.004.

Part III

Liver

Hepatic Pre-malignant Lesions

7

Fatima Mustansir and Juan M. Sarmiento

Introduction

Hepatocellular carcinoma (HCC) is the principal type of primary liver cancer, accounting for 73% of liver and intrahepatic bile duct malignancies [1]. The American Cancer Society estimates that 41,260 cases and 30,520 deaths attributable to liver and intrahepatic bile duct cancer will occur in the United States in 2022 [1].

The vast majority of HCCs arise in the background of cirrhosis [2, 3], which starts a cascade of pathologic events beginning with dysplasia and culminating in malignancy. The formative process of HCC, known as hepatocarcinogenesis, follows complex multistep molecular and histological pathways [2, 3], with malignant primary HCC developing either in the absence of identifiable precursor lesions or within existing hepatic nodules.

Advances in molecular, genetic, and clinicopathologic techniques over the years have allowed elucidation of the role of dysplastic lesions in the development of HCC. Evolution of nomenclature, from terms such as hyperplastic nodule, adenoma-

F. Mustansir
Department on Surgery, Washington University, St. Louis, MO, USA

J. M. Sarmiento (✉)
Department of Surgery, Emory University, Atlanta, GA, USA
e-mail: jsarmie@emory.edu

© The Author(s), under exclusive license to Springer Nature Switzerland AG 2025
A. Alseidi et al. (eds.), *The SAGES Manual of Contemporary Indications and Management of Hepatic and Biliary Diseases*, https://doi.org/10.1007/978-3-032-04823-3_7

toid hyperplasia, and multiregenerative nodules to a more standardized format suggested by an international working party (IWP) in 1995 [4], has also been observed. Nomenclature for nodular hepatocellular lesions suggested by this IWP forms the basis for defining many of these lesions. Key premalignant hepatic aberrations discussed in this chapter include dysplastic foci and dysplastic nodules (divided into low-grade and high-grade dysplastic nodules) and hepatic adenomas.

In view of the sizeable healthcare burden attributable to HCC and the significance of precursor lesions in hepatocarcinogenesis, this chapter aims to define the various hepatic premalignant lesions and discuss their histologic, molecular, and radiologic characteristics, and relevant management strategies.

Hepatocarcinogenesis

Molecular (Genetic and Epigenetic) Changes

Hepatocarcinogenesis begins with an underlying disease process with the ability to cause chronic hepatic insult and cirrhosis, such as chronic viral hepatitis (B and C), chronic alcoholic consumption, and aflatoxin-B1 exposure [2, 5]. Cycles of cellular injury and regeneration propagate genomic instability, driving the progression from normal hepatic architecture to a preneoplastic stage, followed by successive escalation of molecular alterations (both genetic and epigenetic) leading to dysplasia and finally, frank HCC.

Genetic alterations refer to changes in genomic or DNA sequences such as chromosomal instability (amplification or loss), or somatic mutations in tumor suppressor genes (most commonly p53 and WNT/B-catenin), while epigenetic changes are modifications like DNA methylation and histone modification that affect gene activation without affecting DNA sequences/structures. These genetic and epigenetic alterations eventually result in deregulation of proto-oncogenes and tumor suppressor genes [2, 6, 7].

Morphologically Distinguishable Hepatocyte Alterations

The presence of identifiable cytoplasmic and/or nuclear changes to form atypical cellular subpopulations that are sufficiently different from normal hepatocytes is characteristic of dysplasia. Small cell change (SCC) and large cell change (LCC), previously known as small cell dysplasia and large cell dysplasia, are two types of morphologic variations in hepatocytes found in dysplastic lesions.

Small Cell Change

SCC results in hepatocytes with decreased cell volume, presence of cytoplasmic basophilia, mild hyperchromasia and nuclear pleomorphism, and an increased nuclear-cytoplasmic ratio. SCC is frequently theorized to play an initial role in hepatocarcinogenesis, with several studies demonstrating the presence of SCC in dysplastic nodules and HCC [8–11]. Evidence of chromosomal changes, interactions with tumor suppressor genes, and histological similarity to HCC support this theory [10, 12–14]. Furthermore, previous investigations revealed that small expansile foci of SCC are more commonly associated with dysplasia/HCC rather than a more widespread diffuse pattern which is indicative of regeneration [15, 16].

Large Cell Change

LCC represents hepatocytes with both nuclear and cytoplasmic enlargement (resulting in preservation of the nuclear-cytoplasmic ratio), nuclear pleomorphism, and abundant nuclear hyperchromasia [4, 15, 17, 18]. In contrast to SCC, LCC is considered to be a consequence of hepatic injury and subsequent regeneration, with uncertain pathogenic and malignant potential. Although several studies have found a statistical association of LCC with HCC [19, 20], debate surrounds whether LCC is an antecedent aberration to HCC via a histologic continuum or an entity coexisting with HCC that has arisen independently through multistep carcinogenesis. Lack of evidence of genetic mutation in LCC linked to HCC further lends credence to the nonmalignant potential of LCC [10].

Currently, though it may be difficult to determine the exact pathologic mechanisms relating LCC and SCC with HCC, it is evident that these aberrations commonly coexist in the hepatocarcinogenesis pathway as potential markers and risk factors for HCC, and thus should be recognized as significant if discovered.

Nomenclature of Hepatic Pre-malignant Lesions

Dysplastic Foci

A dysplastic focus refers to a cluster of hepatocytes measuring less than 1 mm in diameter which possesses dysplastic features (i.e., varying degrees of atypia, nuclear hyperchromasia, and increased proliferative rate) in the absence of obvious malignant characteristics. These foci harbor SCC or LCC, and are frequently detected in cirrhotic livers [14, 21]. Due to their size, dysplastic foci are usually discovered incidentally on microscopic examination of biopsy or resection specimens.

Dysplastic Nodules

Dysplastic nodules are distinctly nodular lesions at least 1 mm in diameter that are visible on radiologic or gross examination, and are dissimilar to the surrounding hepatic parenchyma on the basis of size, color, texture, and degree of protrusion of the cut surface. They are found in 15–25% of cirrhotic livers [22]. They are categorized as low-grade dysplastic nodules (LGDNs) or high-grade dysplastic nodules (HGDNs) based on microscopic morphology. On gross examination, dysplastic nodules usually have a soft texture and bulge above the cut surface of the liver. They may appear more bile-stained or paler than the surrounding liver. Dysplastic nodules contain dysplastic foci with LCC or SCC; some nodules may contain multiple dysplastic foci appearing as subpopulations [4]. HCC may arise in dysplastic nodule, i.e., "nodule in nodule appearance" where the larger outside nodule is dysplastic and the smaller inside nodule is well-differentiated HCC, or in a separate location [13, 17, 23]. Up to 10% of LGDNs [3] may progress to HCC, whereas between 20% and 40% of HGDNs have been observed to transition to HCC [3, 24].

Low-Grade Dysplastic Nodules
Low-grade nodules (LGDNs) lack architectural atypia and demonstrate a mild increase in cellularity compared to surrounding parenchyma. LGDNs may harbor LCC and so are usually classified as nonmalignant nodules. It is challenging to distinguish LGDNs from regenerative nodules [25].

High-Grade Dysplastic Nodules
High-grade dysplastic nodules (HGDNs) display frank cytological and architectural atypia compared to surrounding parenchyma but do not meet the criteria to establish malignancy. SCC is commonly observed within HGDNs [8, 11, 15]. Several prospective research have shown that HGDNs portend a significantly higher risk for progression to HCC than LGDNs [3, 20, 26, 27]. As such, it is difficult to differentiate HGDNs from HCC on histopathological and radiological analysis.

Dysplastic nodules can be differentiated from each other and from HCC on the basis of vascular supply and cytologic appearance. Regenerative nodules, LGDNs, and HGDNs receive vascular supply from portal vessels or from unpaired or nontriadal arteries that have arisen via neoangiogenesis. The presence of nontriadal arteries is suggestive of a malignant process [28, 29]. The greatest density of nontriadal arteries is found in HCC, followed by HGDNs and then LGDNs [15].

As discussed earlier, the presence of SCC is a useful indicator of malignant potential. Cytologic features such as increased nuclear to cytoplasmic ratio have been observed more strongly in HGDNs and HCC[8]. Other features such as clear cell change and fatty change may also be seen in nodules predisposing to malignancy [11]. Additionally, studies of certain immunohistochemical markers (heat-shock protein 70, glutamine synthetase, and glypican-3) have shown that these markers may play a useful role in distinguishing dysplastic lesions from HCC [30, 31].

Hepatocellular Adenoma

Hepatocellular adenomas (HCAs) are principally benign liver lesions; however, they carry a 4–5% risk of malignant transformation. They are monoclonal tumors that can range in size, be monofocal or multifocal, and are typically without a true capsule. Intramural fat lends a yellow appearance on gross examination, while the presence of an extensive arterial supply makes them hypervascular and prone to hemorrhage. Histologically, HCAs appear as sheets of benign hepatocytes without portal venules and bile ductules [32].

Gene sequencing efforts by a team of French researchers allowed subtyping of HCAs into four categories—hepatocyte nuclear factor-1 alpha (HNF1a)-mutated HCA, inflammatory HCA, B-catenin-mutated HCA, and unclassified HCA [33, 34]. In particular, a significant relationship between the B-catenin subtype and HCC has been observed [35, 36], with Zucman-Rossi reporting almost half of B-catenin-mutated HCAs were associated with HCC or borderline malignant lesions [33]. HCAs in men, larger than 5 cm and those that harbor B-catenin mutations portend a greater risk for malignant transformation [35, 37–39]. Between 13% and 19% of HCAs harbor B-catenin mutations and they are more frequently found in men [16, 33].

Management of Hepatic Pre-malignant Lesions

Imaging and Surveillance

The American Association for the Study of Liver Diseases (AASLD) recommends multiphasic CT or MRI as the imaging modalities of choice in high-risk patients with abnormal surveillance results or in whom HCC is strongly suspected [40]. Imaging features on multiphasic scans indicative of HCC are size ≥10 mm, arterial phase hyperenhancement, portal venous washout, interval growth, and an encapsulated appearance. Malignant potential can be roughly assessed by comparing the degree of neoangiogenesis-driven aberrant vascular supply (especially nontriadal arteries and sinusoidal capillarization), which contributes to differences in enhancement between abnormal liver tissue and surrounding normal parenchyma on hepatic, arterial, and portal venous phases. These features are less prominent in HGDNs (which mainly derive vascular supply from portal tracts) and early HCCs due to ongoing neoangiogenesis, therefore resulting in a hypovascular appearance relative to the surrounding tissue. Moreover, size of the lesion also dictates risk of malignancy—lesions smaller than 10 mm have a lesser risk of transformation to HCC[25].

The diagnosis of HCC relative to other solid tumors is unique as it does not necessitate invasive testing such as a biopsy if imaging findings are strongly suggestive of HCC in a cirrhotic liver. Situations which require biopsy to confirm a diagnosis of HCC are when characteristic imaging features are not present but HCC is strongly suspected or when these imaging findings are present in a non-cirrhotic liver.

MRI is the ideal modality to image HCAs, which appear as heterogenous or homogenous hypervascular masses with variable enhancement and washout dependent on the subtype. Although HNF1a-mutated and inflammatory HCAs possess identifying characteristics on imaging such as arterial enhancement, and presence of hemorrhage and intramural fat, B-catenin-mutated HCAs lack these defining features. However, they may show arterial and hepatobiliary phase enhancement and washout in the portal venous phase (mimicking HCC) [32, 40, 41]. Contra-enhanced ultrasound (CEUS) may be a useful adjunct in multiphasic imaging of HCAs, as it is radiation-free, can differentiate HCAs from focal nodular hyperplasia, and potentially help identify certain HCA subtypes such as inflammatory HCA. Characteristic features of HCAs on CEUS include rapid homogenous contrast enhancement in the arterial phase, delayed washout (particularly apparent in inflammatory HCAs), centripetal filling pattern, and hyperenhancement of subcapsular arteries [42, 43].

Surveillance

Patients with cirrhosis and a dysplastic nodule on CT or MRI can be surveilled with follow-up imaging (such as ultrasound at appropriate intervals), alternative imaging (i.e., CT if MRI was used initially), alternative contrast agent, or biopsy. However, the AASLD does not recommend routine biopsy of dysplastic lesions.

The Liver Reporting and Data System (CT/MRI LI-RADS) [44], published by the American College of Radiology (ACR), allows stratification and interpretation of lesions ≥10 mm on multiphase CT or MRI. The LI-RADS categories and associated risk of HCC are shown in Table 7.1. If multiphasic imaging does not identify any lesions or if the identified lesions are LI-RADS 1 or 2, patients should be routinely surveilled using ultrasound. The AASLD suggests that a follow-up CT or MRI in 6 months or less may be considered for LI-RADS 2 observations. If the identified abnormality cannot be categorized, the same diagnostic test can be repeated or an alternative one performed.

Treatment

Curative intent therapies for HCC include surgical resection, ablative therapies (e.g., thermal ablation), and liver transplantation. Although dysplastic nodules, particularly HGDNs, are associated

Table 7.1 CT/MRI LI-RADS 2018 classification

LI-RADS category [45]	Description [45]	Risk of HCC (%) [40]
1	Definitely benign	0
2	Probably benign	11
3	Intermediate probability of malignancy	33
4	Probably HCC	80 (64–87)
5	Definitely HCC	96 (95–99)
M	Probably or definitely malignant but not HCC specific	

HCC hepatocellular carcinoma

with a significant risk of malignant transformation, there is currently no guidance on the management of these lesions beyond aggressive active surveillance.

HCAs, on the other hand, carry risk for malignant transformation and hemorrhage and should be considered for elective surgical resection if they are symptomatic, growing, exceed 5 cm in size, or are found in men or display B-catenin mutations, as these features are highly concerning for malignant potential. For adenomas found in women, and those smaller than 5 cm, cessation of oral contraceptives (if applicable) should be implemented, followed by close surveillance [43].

Summary

- Hepatic premalignant lesions include dysplastic foci, dysplastic nodules, and hepatocellular adenomas.
- High-grade dysplastic nodules have the highest risk for malignant transformation to hepatocellular carcinoma.
- Of the four subtypes of hepatocellular adenoma, the B-catenin-mutated subtype is implicated in conversion to hepatocellular carcinoma.
- It may be challenging to reliably differentiate premalignant dysplastic lesions, such as high-grade dysplastic nodules from hepatocellular carcinoma on histopathology and imaging.
- Premalignant lesions suspicious for malignancy based on features such as degree of atypia and size should be actively surveilled or considered for more definitive management such as resection.

References

1. American Cancer Society. Cancer facts and figures 2022. Published 2022. https://www.cancer.org/research/cancer-facts-statistics/all-cancer-facts-figures/cancer-facts-figures-2022.html. Accessed 18 May 2022.

2. Farazi PA, DePinho RA. Hepatocellular carcinoma pathogenesis: from genes to environment. Nat Rev Cancer. 2006;6(9):674–87. https://doi.org/10.1038/nrc1934.
3. Kobayashi M, Ikeda K, Hosaka T, et al. Dysplastic nodules frequently develop into hepatocellular carcinoma in patients with chronic viral hepatitis and cirrhosis. Cancer. 2006;106(3):636–47. https://doi.org/10.1002/cncr.21607.
4. International Working Party. Terminology of nodular hepatocellular lesions. Hepatology. 1995;22(3):983–93. https://doi.org/10.1016/0270-9139(95)90324-0.
5. Badvie S. Hepatocellular carcinoma. Postgrad Med J. 2000;76(891):4–11. https://doi.org/10.1136/pmj.76.891.4.
6. Niu ZS, Niu XJ, Wang WH, Zhao J. Latest developments in precancerous lesions of hepatocellular carcinoma. World J Gastroenterol. 2016;22(12):3305–14. https://doi.org/10.3748/wjg.v22.i12.3305.
7. Liu M, Jiang L, Guan XY. The genetic and epigenetic alterations in human hepatocellular carcinoma: a recent update. Protein Cell. 2014;5(9):673–91. https://doi.org/10.1007/s13238-014-0065-9.
8. Chang O, Yano Y, Masuzawa A, Fukushima N, Teramura K, Hayashi Y. The cytological characteristics of small cell change of dysplasia in small hepatic nodules. Oncol Rep. 2010;23(5):1229–32. https://doi.org/10.3892/or_00000754.
9. Seki S, Sakaguchi H, Kitada T, et al. Outcomes of dysplastic nodules in human cirrhotic liver: a Clinicopathological study. Clin Cancer Res. 2000;6(9):3469–73.
10. Marchio A, Terris B, Meddeb M, et al. Chromosomal abnormalities in liver cell dysplasia detected by comparative genomic hybridisation. Mol Pathol. 2001;54(4):270–4. https://doi.org/10.1136/mp.54.4.270.
11. Terasaki S, Kaneko S, Kobayashi K, Nonomura A, Nakanuma Y. Histological features predicting malignant transformation of nonmalignant hepatocellular nodules: a prospective study. Gastroenterology. 1998;115(5):1216–22. https://doi.org/10.1016/S0016-5085(98)70093-9.
12. Gong L, Li YH, Su Q, Chu X, Zhang W. Clonality of nodular lesions in liver cirrhosis and chromosomal abnormalities in monoclonal nodules of altered hepatocytes. Histopathology. 2010;56(5):589–99. https://doi.org/10.1111/j.1365-2559.2010.03523.x.
13. Hytiroglou P. Morphological changes of early human hepatocarcinogenesis. Semin Liver Dis. 2004;24(1):65–75. https://doi.org/10.1055/s-2004-823097.
14. Watanabe S, Okita K, Harada T, et al. Morphologic studies of the liver cell dysplasia. Cancer. 1983;51(12):2197–205. https://doi.org/10.1002/1097-0142(19830615)51:12<2197::aid-cncr2820511208>3.0.co;2-5.

15. Park YN. Update on precursor and early lesions of hepatocellular carcinomas. Arch Pathol Lab Med. 2011;135(6):704–15. https://doi.org/10.5858/2010-0524-RA.1.
16. Le Bail B, Bernard PH, Carles J, Balabaud C, Bioulac-Sage P. Prevalence of liver cell dysplasia and association with HCC in a series of 100 cirrhotic liver explants. J Hepatol. 1997;27(5):835–42. https://doi.org/10.1016/s0168-8278(97)80321-2.
17. Hytiroglou P, Park YN, Krinsky G, Theise ND. Hepatic precancerous lesions and small hepatocellular carcinoma. Gastroenterol Clin N Am. 2007;36(4):867–87., vii. https://doi.org/10.1016/j.gtc.2007.08.010.
18. Zimmermann A. Precursor lesions of hepatocellular carcinoma. In: Tumors and tumor-like lesions of the hepatobiliary tract. 1st ed. Cham: Springer; 2016. p. 167–93. https://doi.org/10.1007/978-3-319-26956-6_7.
19. Lee RG, Tsamandas AC, Demetris AJ. Large cell change (liver cell dysplasia) and hepatocellular carcinoma in cirrhosis: matched case-control study, pathological analysis, and pathogenetic hypothesis. Hepatology. 1997;26(6):1415–22. https://doi.org/10.1002/hep.510260607.
20. Borzio M, Fargion S, Borzio F, et al. Impact of large regenerative, low grade and high grade dysplastic nodules in hepatocellular carcinoma development. J Hepatol. 2003;39(2):208–14. https://doi.org/10.1016/s0168-8278(03)00190-9.
21. Cohen C, Berson SD. Liver cell dysplasia in normal, cirrhotic, and hepatocellular carcinoma patients. Cancer. 1986;57(8):1535–8. https://doi.org/10.1002/1097-0142(19860415)57:8<1468::AID-CNCR2820570806>3.0.CO;2-0.
22. Theise ND. Macroregenerative (dysplastic) nodules and hepatocarcinogenesis: theoretical and clinical considerations. Semin Liver Dis. 1995;15(4):360–71. https://doi.org/10.1055/s-2007-1007287.
23. Lee M, Kim K, Kim SY, et al. Genomic structures of dysplastic nodule and concurrent hepatocellular carcinoma. Hum Pathol. 2018;81:37–46. https://doi.org/10.1016/j.humpath.2018.06.026.
24. Di Tommaso L, Sangiovanni A, Borzio M, Park YN, Farinati F, Roncalli M. Advanced precancerous lesions in the liver. Best Pract Res Clin Gastroenterol. 2013;27(2):269–84. https://doi.org/10.1016/j.bpg.2013.03.015.
25. Roncalli M, Terracciano L, Di Tommaso L, David E, Colombo M. Liver precancerous lesions and hepatocellular carcinoma: the histology report. Dig Liver Dis. 2011;43:S361–72. https://doi.org/10.1016/S1590-8658(11)60592-6.
26. Iavarone M, Manini MA, Sangiovanni A, et al. Contrast-enhanced computed tomography and ultrasound-guided liver biopsy to diagnose dysplastic liver nodules in cirrhosis. Dig Liver Dis. 2013;45(1):43–9. https://doi.org/10.1016/j.dld.2012.08.009.

27. Ng CH, Chan SW, Lee WK, et al. Hepatocarcinogenesis of regenerative and dysplastic nodules in Chinese patients. Hong Kong Med J Xianggang Yi Xue Za Zhi. 2011;17(1):11–9.
28. Terada T, Nakanuma Y. Arterial elements and perisinusoidal cells in borderline hepatocellular nodules and small hepatocellular carcinomas. Histopathology. 1995;27(4):333–9. https://doi.org/10.1111/j.1365-2559.1995.tb01523.x.
29. Park YN, Yang CP, Fernandez GJ, Cubukcu O, Thung SN, Theise ND. Neoangiogenesis and sinusoidal "capillarization" in dysplastic nodules of the liver. Am J Surg Pathol. 1998;22(6):656–62. https://doi.org/10.1097/00000478-199806000-00002.
30. Nguyen TB, Roncalli M, Di Tommaso L, Kakar S. Combined use of heat-shock protein 70 and glutamine synthetase is useful in the distinction of typical hepatocellular adenoma from atypical hepatocellular neoplasms and well-differentiated hepatocellular carcinoma. Mod Pathol. 2016;29(3):283–92. https://doi.org/10.1038/modpathol.2015.162.
31. Di Tommaso L, Franchi G, Park YN, et al. Diagnostic value of HSP70, glypican 3, and glutamine synthetase in hepatocellular nodules in cirrhosis. Hepatology. 2007;45(3):725–34. https://doi.org/10.1002/hep.21531.
32. Dharmana H, Saravana-Bawan S, Girgis S, Low G. Hepatocellular adenoma: imaging review of the various molecular subtypes. Clin Radiol. 2017;72(4):276–85. https://doi.org/10.1016/j.crad.2016.12.020.
33. Zucman-Rossi J, Jeannot E, Van NJT, et al. Genotype-phenotype correlation in hepatocellular adenoma: new classification and relationship with HCC. Hepatology. 2006;43(3):515–24. https://doi.org/10.1002/hep.21068.
34. Bioulac-Sage P, Sempoux C, Balabaud C. Hepatocellular adenoma: classification, variants and clinical relevance. Semin Diagn Pathol. 2017;34(2):112–25. https://doi.org/10.1053/j.semdp.2016.12.007.
35. Sempoux C, Balabaud C, Bioulac-Sage P. Malignant transformation of hepatocellular adenoma. Hepatic Oncol. 2014;1(4):421–31. https://doi.org/10.2217/hep.14.14.
36. Farges O, Dokmak S. Malignant transformation of liver adenoma: an analysis of the literature. Dig Surg. 2010;27(1):32–8. https://doi.org/10.1159/000268405.
37. Stoot JHMB, Coelen RJS, De Jong MC, Dejong CHC. Malignant transformation of hepatocellular adenomas into hepatocellular carcinomas: a systematic review including more than 1600 adenoma cases. HPB. 2010;12(8):509–22. https://doi.org/10.1111/j.1477-2574.2010.00222.x.
38. Dokmak S, Paradis V, Vilgrain V, et al. A single-center surgical experience of 122 patients with single and multiple hepatocellular adenomas. Gastroenterology. 2009;137(5):1698–705. https://doi.org/10.1053/j.gastro.2009.07.061.

39. Farges O, Ferreira N, Dokmak S, Belghiti J, Bedossa P, Paradis V. Changing trends in malignant transformation of hepatocellular adenoma. Gut. 2011;60(1):85–9. https://doi.org/10.1136/gut.2010.222109.
40. Marrero JA, Kulik LM, Sirlin CB, et al. Diagnosis, staging, and management of hepatocellular carcinoma: 2018 practice guidance by the American Association for the Study of Liver Diseases. Hepatology. 2018;68(2):723–50. https://doi.org/10.1002/hep.29913.
41. Grazioli L, Olivetti L, Mazza G, Bondioni MP. MR imaging of hepatocellular adenomas and differential diagnosis dilemma. Int J Hepatol. 2013;2013:374170. https://doi.org/10.1155/2013/374170.
42. Laumonier H, Cailliez H, Balabaud C, et al. Role of contrast-enhanced sonography in differentiation of subtypes of hepatocellular adenoma: correlation with MRI findings. Am J Roentgenol. 2012;199(2):341–8. https://doi.org/10.2214/AJR.11.7046.
43. European Association for the Study of the Liver. EASL clinical practice guidelines on the management of benign liver tumours. J Hepatol. 2016;65(2):386–98. https://doi.org/10.1016/j.jhep.2016.04.001.
44. Elsayes KM, Kielar AZ, Chernyak V, et al. LI-RADS: a conceptual and historical review from its beginning to its recent integration into AASLD clinical practice guidance. J Hepatocell Carcinoma. 2019;6:49–69. https://doi.org/10.2147/JHC.S186239.
45. CT/MRI LI-RADS v2018. Accessed from https://www.acr.org/Clinical-Resources/Reporting-and-Data-Systems/LI-RADS/CT-MRI-LI-RADS-v2018.

Hepatocellular Carcinoma

Guido Fiorentini and Sean P. Cleary

Introduction

Hepatocellular carcinoma (HCC) is the third most common cancer worldwide and the most common form of liver cancer, responsible for 90% of the tumors arising from the liver [1–3]. Hepatitis B virus (HBV) infection is the most common risk factor for HCC development worldwide, especially in areas of endemic infection including Asia and sub-Saharan Africa. Hepatitis C virus (HCV) is more evenly distributed globally with high prevalence areas in Eastern and Southern Europe, Japan, Egypt, and central Africa [4]. In the West countries, non-alcoholic steatohepatitis (NASH), associated with metabolic syndrome or diabetes mellitus, is an increasingly important contributor to HCC risk [5, 6].

The management of HCC has markedly improved in the recent decade [7]. Hepatic resection, ablation, and liver transplantation have been the mainstay curative treatments in HCC cases, with outstanding 10-year post-liver transplantation (LT) survival rates

G. Fiorentini
Hepatobiliary and Pancreas Surgery Division, Mayo Clinic, Rochester, MN, USA

S. P. Cleary (✉)
Department of Surgery, University of Toronto, Toronto, CA, USA
e-mail: sean.cleary@uhn.ca

for tumors within the Milan criteria [8]. Additionally, locoregional treatments including transarterial-chemoembolization (TACE), transarterial (bland) embolization (TAE), and radioembolization (TARE), and external beam radiation may be used to treat intermediate-stage HCC [9]. More recently, systemic treatments such as tyrosine kinase inhibitors, immune checkpoint inhibitors, and monoclonal antibodies have become available particularly for the disease's most advanced stages.

The selection of treatment modalities depends not only on the stage and on the extent of tumor, but also on the patient's performance status and underlying liver function. Finally, the Barcelona Clinic Liver Cancer (BCLC) classification stratifies patients according to these factors with treatment recommendations [10].

Risk Factors

The major risk factors [2] for HCC include chronic alcohol consumption, diabetes or obesity-related NASH, and HBV or HCV infection.

Alcohol Chronic sustained alcohol intake causes chronic inflammation leading to liver disease and, eventually, cirrhosis and HCC. Alcohol-related cirrhosis has an annual incidence of 1–2% among patients, and accounts for up to 30% of HCC cases depending on the geographical region.

NASH [5, 11] Non-alcoholic steatohepatitis is the precursor step for HCC in metabolic conditions associated with fat deposition into the liver. Fat infiltration in the liver is associated with chronic inflammation which will eventually progress to fibrosis and cirrhosis throughout the years, with a consequential functional hepatic dysfunction in the most advanced stages. The annual incidence of HCC is lower in NASH-related cirrhosis (1–2% per year) than in viral-mediated cirrhosis (3–5% per year); however, the increasing prevalence of NASH over the viral-mediated cirrhosis are making NASH among the first causes for HCC. In fact, since 2010, the proportion of HCC attributed to NASH has increased up to 15–20% of cases in the West. In addition, NASH-associated HCC cases can occur in the absence of cirrhosis.

Hepatitis Infection

Hepatitis B (HBV) Infection [12] HBV is a double-stranded DNA virus capable of integrating its viral DNA into the host genome inducing insertional mutagenesis, genomic instability, and oncogene activation. The mutagenic potential of HBV can lead to the development of cancer in the absence of cirrhosis, while longstanding infection-related inflammation can result in cancers following the development of cirrhosis. HBV infection is a risk factor for HCC in regions where infection is endemic, particularly in Africa and parts of Asia. The annual incidence of HCC is estimated to be <1% for non-cirrhotic HBV-infected patients and 2–3% for those with cirrhosis, although the annual risk can be even higher depending on some HBV viral subtype and on the geographical distribution. Anti-viral therapy as well as vaccination programs have significantly reduced the burden of HBV-associated HCC in certain regions.

Hepatitis D virus (HDV) is an RNA virus that requires the presence of HBV surface antigens for its replication and, therefore, for infectivity. HBV-HDV co-infection is associated with an increased risk of HCC compared with HBV infection alone.

Hepatitis C (HCV) Infection [13, 14] Chronic HCV infection is the most common underlying viral liver disease among patients with HCC in North America, Europe, and Japan. The use of direct-acting antiviral (DAA) therapy has resulted in a significant reduction in the risk of HCC for this cause over the last decade in developed countries. Otherwise, HCV-related cirrhosis is associated with 1–4% risk of HCC per year.

Diagnosis and Screening

Many patients are diagnosed through surveillance of chronic hepatitis or known cirrhosis. Nevertheless, an incidental diagnosis occurs in up to 50% of cases globally, with patients being diagnosed on cross-sectional imaging performed for other reasons or owing to symptomatic advanced-stage HCC after developing abdominal pain, weight loss, or worsening of liver dysfunction [7].

Serum Markers [15] High serum α-fetoprotein levels (AFP >20 ng/ml) in subjects under surveillance can be an indicator of potential malignancy. While specific, AFP is not a sensitive marker since many tumors do not secrete AFP. Screening with AFP alone has been shown to be inferior to screening with ultrasound with or without AFP. An increase in the AFP associated with an elevated Ca19-9 can be seen in mixed forms of hepatocholangio carcinoma, whose prognosis and natural history are usually worse than HCC.

Screening [15] HCC is largely asymptomatic until it progresses to an advanced stage. This combined with an identifiable at-risk population provides a compelling case for routine screening. Current American Association for the Study of Liver Disease (AASLD) guidelines [16] recommend surveillance with ultrasound +/− AFP every 6 months in patients with cirrhosis from any cause, including patients who have successfully treated with antiviral therapy. In case of an abnormal US, cross-sectional imaging with CT or MRI should be the next step to confirm the diagnosis. HBV-infected individuals at high risk of HCC (Asian and African males >40 years old, Asian women >50, and those with a family history of HCC) should undergo screening even in the absence of cirrhosis.

Imaging [17] In lesions less than 1 cm in diameter detected on ultrasonography, it is difficult to discern cancer vs. precancerous or benign lesions. In the absence of conclusive imaging findings

Table 8.1 Liver imaging reporting and data system (LI-RADS). LR = LI-RADS

Category	Description
LR-1	Definitely benign
LR-2	Probably benign
LR-3	Intermediate probability of HCC
LR-4	High probability of HCC
LR-5	Definitely HCC

for malignancy, lesions <1 cm detected on screening should be assessed with follow-up imaging in 3–6 months. For lesions ≥1 cm in diameter, either quadruple-phase (non-contrast, arterial, portal venous, hepatic venous, and delayed phases) CT or dynamic contrast-enhanced MRI should be performed [18]. The diagnosis of HCC is usually based on non-invasive criteria defined by the AASLD guidelines and Liver Imaging Reporting and Data system (LI-RADS) criteria [19] (Table 8.1). Larger lesions should be interrogated with contrast-enhanced CT or MRI. Arterial phase hyperenhancing lesions are assessed for the presence of washout, the presence of capsular enhancement, and growth on serial imaging. Benign lesions (LI-RADS 1 and 2) can undergo repeat imaging in ≤6 months. Intermediate lesions (LI-RADS 3) should undergo repeat or alternate modality imaging in 3–6 months. LI-RADS 4 lesions are "probable HCC" and should undergo a multidisciplinary assessment that could include additional complementary imaging and possible biopsy. Lesions deemed LI-RADS 5 are considered diagnostic for HCC and do not require biopsy or further diagnostic testing.

Management

Treatment Options

The armamentarium for localized and systemic disease is wide and complex. We provide an overview of the possible treatment strategies, acknowledging that individualized patient management is best achieved through multi-disciplinary decision-making including hepatology, hepatobiliary and transplant surgery, interventional radiology, and medical and radiation oncology. Outcomes for treatment of HCC are best achieved at tertiary referral centers with a full spectrum of specialized physicians. Management of HCC must incorporate both the extent and biology of the tumor as well as the patients' liver function and performance status. The BCLC staging has gained widespread acceptance through its incorporation of liver and tumor factors as well as evidence behind various treatment strategies.

Surgical Resection

Hepatic resection is considered the treatment of choice in patients with HCC without cirrhosis since liver decompensation is less common [20]. In patients with cirrhosis, BCLC criteria have restricted resection to single tumors with a well-preserved liver function and with no clinically relevant portal hypertension or a hepatic venous pressure gradient <10 mmHg, as well as with a good performance status [10]. Surrogates for portal hypertension, including thrombocytopenia <100,000 and radiologic evidence of porto-systemic collaterals including varices, can be used more readily in clinical assessments. In studies where resection has been performed in patients with portal hypertension or Child-Pugh B cirrhosis, 5-year survival was <50% and mortality rate was as high as 4%.

Recurrence rate after resection can be as high as 70% at 5 years [21]. Currently, evidence supporting the use of neoadjuvant treatments (mainly embolization [22]) or adjuvant treatment (such as Sorafenib [23]) to reduce the rate of recurrence is lacking. Early detection and aggressive management of recurrence contribute significantly to improved long-term survival in these patients.

One of the main limitations to surgical resection is related to the amount of functional liver left in place after the resection, referred to as the future remnant liver (FRL) [24]. Adequate FRL should be at least 20% in case of a normal liver parenchyma. However, considering HCC oftentimes arises in the background of liver steatosis/fibrosis/cirrhosis, the FRL cut-off is set up to 40–50% to avoid any post-hepatectomy liver failure. Some techniques of vascular interventional radiology are available to induce a contralateral hypertrophy of the FRL: these are the portal vein embolization [25] (i.e., the embolization of the portal vein of the side of the liver to be harvested), the trans-arterial radioembolization, the association of liver partitioning with portal vein ligation for staged hepatectomy (namely, ALPPS), or the liver vein deprivation (the simultaneous portal vein embolization and occlusion of one or more hepatic veins) [26]. Finally, the implementation of minimally invasive techniques for liver resection has proved to be responsible for a less severe impact on liver function thanks to a decreased biologic insult, with lower rates of morbidity and risks for liver decompensation [27–30].

Liver Transplantation

Patients with cirrhosis and tumor burden within the Milan criteria [31] (single tumor ≤5 cm or up to 3 tumors ≤3 cm, without vascular invasion) can be considered eligible for transplantation in most regions. Outcomes have been very good, with 5- and 10-year survival of 70% and 50% respectively. However, the number of liver grafts available for cadaveric transplantation is limited and many regions have prolonged wait times. Long wait times for cadaveric organs in some regions are a concern as this increases the risk of drop out of patients from the waiting list due to tumor progression. Accessibility to and waiting time for LT are characteristics related to the volume of a transplant center. If the expected waiting time will exceed 6 months, it is recommended to consider treatment as bridge to transplant such as ablation, TAE (bland), TACE or TARE, depending on the case. When neoadjuvant therapies successfully demonstrate a tumor response, the dropout from the waiting list and risk of post-transplant recurrence are reduced. Other strategies to overcome the scarcity of cadaveric organs have consisted in the use of living donors and marginal donors (donors >60 years of age, those with diabetes, BMI >35 kg/m2, or severe graft steatosis). However, some studies have reported a higher recurrence risk in the use of living donors [32]: this is thought to be related to the shorter wait time to transplant, which could assist in selecting out aggressive forms of HCC.

No adjuvant treatment has been shown to prevent recurrence after LT; selection of patients within the Milan criteria is still the best way for the lowest recurrence rates. Over time, other criteria emerged predicting the results of transplantation for HCC, like that proposed by the University of California, San Francisco (UCSF) [33] (single tumor ≤ 6.5 cm or ≤ 3 tumors with the largest tumor diameter ≤ 4.5 cm and total tumor diameter ≤ 8 cm). Both Milan and UCSF criteria have proven equivalent survival rate, thus a greater number of patients might benefit from liver transplant despite the adoption of a less restrictive method.

Tumor Ablation

Image-guided ablation is accepted as a potentially curative therapy for small, early-stage HCC tumors [34, 35]. Ablations and liver resection are alternatively used as a first choice in very early (<2 cm) tumors, providing both excellent results. The choice between the two options relies on tumor location, liver function, presence of cirrhosis, performance status, and possibility to perform the resection in a minimally invasive fashion. Ablation is used to direct injury to the tumor and is achieved via chemical, thermal, or electrical methods. Microwave (MWA) and radiofrequency ablation (RFA) are currently used for tumor ablation. Other non-thermal techniques consist of cryoablation and irreversible electroporation and have particular advantage when tumors are close to main biliary pedicles known to be heat sensitive.

Radiotherapy

In HCC tumors confined to the liver, external beam radiation therapy can achieve radiological responses in HCC across a range of sizes and stages in the liver or can be used for palliation of extrahepatic metastasis [36]. Most studies comparing radiotherapy with other locoregional therapies in HCC are retrospective in nature, supporting a potential role for radiotherapy in selected patients. Modern RT has an increased utility in managing HCC patients, mainly due to two driving forces. First, technological advancement [37] (e.g., stereotactic body radiotherapy and advanced proton-beam therapy) enables delivery of radiation to increase tumor control and reduce collateral effects in the surrounding normal tissue. Second, the boom in developing target therapies and checkpoint-blockade immunotherapy prolongs overall survival in HCC patients, re-emphasizing the importance of local tumor control.

Transarterial Therapies

HCC derives most of its blood supply from arterial flow (hepatic artery or sometimes phrenic arteries for lesions in the liver dome). This provides a selective advantage for hepatic arterial directed therapies, like TAE (bland), TARE and TACE [1].

TAE (bland) as well as TACE has been globally adopted as standard of care for patients with intermediate-stage HCC, with a median survival rate up to 37 months in RCT and a mortality rate inferior to 1%.

During TACE, doxorubicin alone or with cisplatin and/or mitomycin C, mixed with radio-opaque lipiodol are deployed selectively to the tumor area through a trans-arterial access and subsequent angiogram. The most common side effects following TACE are transient abdominal pain, nausea, fever, increased liver enzymes, fatigue, and less commonly worsening liver function, bile duct injury, and abscess. Drug-Eluting-Bead-Chemoembolization refers to the use of doxorubicin loaded bead-based TACE (DEB-TACE) [38], that according to some studies have higher rate of response in comparison to conventional TACE (DEB-TACE 52% versus 35% with classic TACE); however, no survival benefits are proven thus far over TACE. Transarterial embolization (TAE) without chemotherapy is primarily used for the treatment of a ruptured HCC [39]; however, many institutions use this standard instead of TACE for HCC, since TACE or TAE are arguably equally effective. Patients candidate to receive a trans-arterial chemo or bland embolization need to have a well-preserved liver function, since a total bilirubin beyond 2 mg/dl or the presence of ascites are associated with an increased risk of adverse events secondary to liver decompensation.

TARE consists of the trans-arterial deployment of glass microspheres or resin microspheres embedded with yttrium-90 [40, 41]. Use of TARE is usually reserved to intermediate BCLC stage HCC and in advanced stages or in case of vascular invasion such as portal vein neoplastic thrombosis.

Systemic Therapies

First-Line Therapies Associating the anti-PDL1 atezolizumab with the anti-VEGF antibody bevacizumab was the first regimen to improve overall survival compared with sorafenib [42]. The combination of atezolizumab with bevacizumab is currently the first choice for a first-line treatment, with some patients exhibiting durable complete responses. Durvalumab-Tremelimumab [43] is another regimen implemented in the first-line setting. Therefore, immunotherapy has now become a part of the first-line treatment for HCC. Side effects are related to gastrointestinal symptoms (diarrhea) induced from immunotherapy, and an increased risk of variceal bleeding related to the use of bevacizumab. Sorafenib, Lenvatinib, or Durvalumab in monotherapy are used in the first-line setting if none of the previous regimens are feasible.

Tyrosine kinase [44] inhibitors such as regorafenib or carbozantinib or alternate immunotherapy regimens are used as second-line treatment for HCC.

BCLC Staging System

The most recent edition of the BCLC [10] is updated to 2022 (Fig. 8.1). Baseline principle of the BCLC staging system is having resection and transplant for patients with early-stage HCC

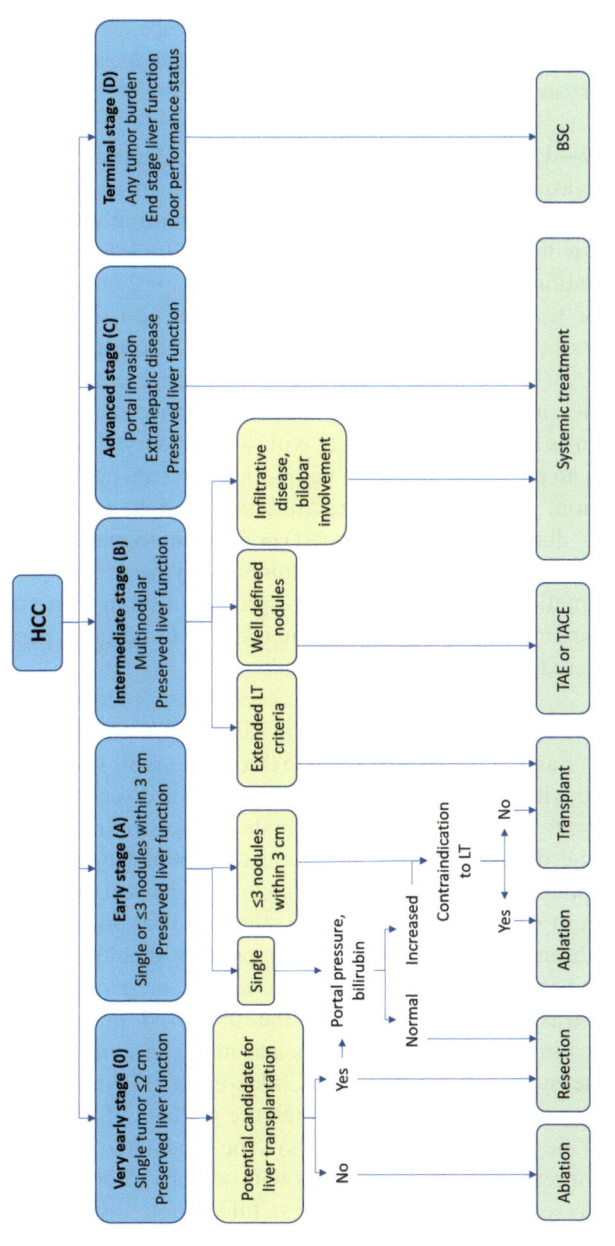

Fig. 8.1 BCLC staging and treatment strategy

tumors, while patients at intermediate stages are candidates for transarterial therapies and patients with advanced disease will first receive systemic treatments.

BCLC 0—Very Early Stage Solitary HCC ≤ 2 cm without vascular invasion or extrahepatic disease is defined as very early stage. Management varies for BCLC-0 according to whether patients with a single HCC < 2 cm are eligible for liver transplant prioritization. In countries/regions where HCC < 2 cm is not eligible for transplant, very early HCC may be best treated with ablation or resection as the first-line therapy. At this time, radiofrequency (RF) or microwave (MW) ablation are both viable modalities associated with similar survival outcomes. Surgical resection is an option in patients with well-preserved liver function and no portal hypertension with lesions that are not amenable to ablation, lesions in peripheral/difficult locations (close to the stomach, diaphragm, GI tract, heart) or adjacent to major intrahepatic vascular structures. BCLC-0 tumors may be considered for transplantation if they can get tumor prioritization in their country/region or if liver function is compromised or portal hypertension precludes ablation or resection.

BCLC A—Early Stage Defined as a solitary HCC irrespective of the size or as a multifocal HCC up to three lesions all smaller than 3 cm and without vascular invasion, extrahepatic disease, and preserved liver function. Liver function should be stratified according to the degree of portal hypertension, defined by a hepatic venous pressure gradient >10 mmHg while many will use a platelet count of <100,000 as a surrogate measure. For solitary nodule and in absence of portal hypertension, patients should be considered for hepatic resection. Preference should be given to minimally invasive resection due to the improved peri-operative outcomes in patients with cirrhosis and may allow patients with moderate synthetic dysfunction (Childs-Pugh B7) or moderate portal hypertension (defined as a pressure gradient of 8–9 mmHg between the portal and hepatic veins) to be considered viable candidate for resection. Within patients with solitary ≥2 cm HCC and moderate-severe liver dysfunction (Childs-Pugh B8 or higher) and/or portal hypertension (a pressure gradient >10 mmHg), LT should be considered the primary treatment modality if the tumor fits transplant eligibility criteria. For solitary HCC not amenable to resection or transplantation, other forms of locoregional treatment may be considered as the next line of treatment. Ablation may also be considered in select circumstances, recognizing that the rate of incomplete ablation and local recurrence rises significantly in lesions >3–5 cm.

For patients with multifocal disease (≤ 3 lesions each ≤ 3 cm) within the Milan criteria, LT should be offered as a first-line therapy, with ablation as a second-line option for patients deemed ineligible for transplantation.

Resection and ablation offer the same survival benefit for HCC ≤ 2 cm. Ablation for size larger than 3 cm is less effective for a higher risk of local recurrence and lower rate of complete response. In these cases, resection is still preferred over ablation. Lobar treatment through transarterial radio embolization (TARE) may increase remnant liver volume and may be considered in some patients as valid alternative to major hepatectomy, which is associated with significant morbidity and mortality in patients with cirrhosis.

Minimally invasive resections are proven to be oncologically equivalent to open procedures, with less morbidity impact and on liver function even in patients with clinically significant portal hypertension. However, the feasibility of these procedures is related to the expertise of a center and to tumor location [29, 30]. It is worth mentioning that the 2022 version of the BCLC staging system does not recommend resection for multinodular HCC within the Milan criteria.

BCLC B—Intermediate Stage Defined as a multifocal disease exceeding BCLC A, but still with well-preserved liver function and no extra-hepatic disease. According to the most recent BCLC guidelines from 2022, BCLC-B is divided into three subgroups. The first subgroup is comprised of patients with well-defined nodules that meet local extended transplant eligibility beyond Milan criteria (e.g., UCSF criteria and others); these patients should be offered LT as a first-line therapy. The second subgroup includes patients who are outside local transplant eligibility criteria but who have defined tumor burden and preserved portal flow; these patients should be considered for transarterial therapies. If patients are downsized to transplant criteria, then re-evaluation for potential transplant listing should be considered. An acceptable post-LT survival may be obtained in a selected group of patients at BCLC stage B beyond the Milan criteria. AFP cut-offs have been used to exclude LT with values beyond 1000 ng/ml widely accepted as a contraindication for LT. Downstaging has emerged as a reliable tool for selecting patients for LT, with the goal of bringing patient disease within the Milan criteria.

In the third subgroup there are patients with diffuse, infiltrative, extensive HCC liver involvement that would not benefit from locoregional therapy and systemic therapy should be the recommended option.

BCLC C—Advanced Stage Includes patients with HCC with vascular invasion or extrahepatic dissemination and who have preserved liver function. If the performance status is adequate, these patients are candidates for systemic therapy.

BCLC D—End Stage Includes patients with major cancer-related symptoms and/or impaired liver function without the option of LT because of tumor burden or patient-related factors (mainly as for consequences of a cirrhosis in an advanced stage). Expected survival is limited to months and these patients should be assessed for clinical trial or supportive care.

Summary

Hepatocellular carcinoma is a common liver cancer, burdened by high mortality. Several complex treatment strategies are best determined by a multidisciplinary team with access to appropriate surgical, hepatology, pathology, interventional radiology, medical and radiation oncology expertise plus supportive and palliative care teams. Most of the background causes for liver cirrhosis can nowadays in western countries be prevented and treated (such as

HBC and HCV), making non-alcoholic fatty liver disease among the most common causes for developing steatohepatitis and, eventually, cirrhosis and/or HCC. Specific surveillance is recommended in patients presenting with risk factors for HCC, aimed at early detection of the disease. The choice of the most appropriate treatment relies on tumor extension, background liver pathology and hepatic function, and the patients' overall functional/performance status. Resection, transplantation, and (in some cases) ablations have potential curative intents, while other treatment strategies such as trans-arterial embolization, systemic therapy, and radiation therapy are used either as primary treatment or bridging to other curative treatments (resection or transplant) or with palliative intent, with the goal of impacting the natural history of HCC.

References

1. Brown ZJ, Tsilimigras DI, Ruff SM, Mohseni A, Kamel IR, Cloyd JM, Pawlik TM. Management of hepatocellular carcinoma: a review. JAMA Surg. 2023;158(4):410–20. https://doi.org/10.1001/jamasurg.2022.7989.
2. Akinyemiju T, Abera S, Ahmed M, Alam N, Alemayohu MA, Allen C, Al-Raddadi R, Alvis-Guzman N, Amoako Y, Artaman A, Ayele TA. The burden of primary liver cancer and underlying etiologies from 1990 to 2015 at the global, regional, and national level. JAMA Oncol. 2017;3:1683.
3. Llovet JM, et al. Hepatocellular carcinoma. Nat Rev Dis Prim. 2016;2:16018.
4. Kanwal F, et al. Risk of hepatocellular cancer in HCV patients treated with direct- acting antiviral agents. Gastroenterology. 2017;153:996–1005.e1.
5. Anstee QM, Reeves HL, Kotsiliti E, Govaere O, Heikenwalder M. From NASH to HCC: current concepts and future challenges. Nat Rev Gastroenterol Hepatol. 2019;16:411–28.
6. Friedman SL, Neuschwander-Tetri BA, Rinella M, Sanyal AJ. Mechanisms of NAFLD development and therapeutic strategies. Nat Med. 2018;24:908–22.
7. Marrero JA, et al. Diagnosis, staging, and management of hepatocellular carcinoma: 2018 practice guidance by the American Association for the Study of Liver Diseases. Hepatology. 2018;68:723–50.

8. Tabrizian P, et al. A US multicenter analysis of 2529 HCC patients undergoing liver transplantation: 10-year outcome assessing the role of downstaging to within Milan criteria [abstract 15]. Hepatology. 2019;70:10–1.
9. Vogel A, et al. Hepatocellular carcinoma: ESMO clinical practice guidelines for diagnosis, treatment and follow- up. Ann Oncol. 2018;29(Suppl 4):iv238–55.
10. Reig M, Forner A, Rimola J, Ferrer-Fàbrega J, Burrel M, Garcia-Criado Á, Kelley RK, Galle PR, Mazzaferro V, Salem R, Sangro B, Singal AG, Vogel A, Fuster J, Ayuso C, Bruix J. BCLC strategy for prognosis prediction and treatment recommendation: The 2022 update. J Hepatol. 2022;76(3):681–93. https://doi.org/10.1016/j.jhep.2021.11.018. Epub 2021 Nov 19. PMID: 34801630; PMCID: PMC8866082
11. Negro F. Natural history of NASH and HCC. Liver Int. 2020;40:72–6.
12. Levrero M, Zucman-Rossi J. Mechanisms of HBV-induced hepatocellular carcinoma. J Hepatol. 2016;64(1 Suppl):S84–S101. https://doi.org/10.1016/j.jhep.2016.02.021.
13. Zhao P, Malik S, Xing S. Epigenetic mechanisms involved in HCV-induced hepatocellular carcinoma (HCC). Front Oncol. 2021;11:677926. https://doi.org/10.3389/fonc.2021.677926. PMID: 34336665; PMCID: PMC8320331
14. Singal AG, et al. Direct-acting antiviral therapy for hepatitis C virus infection is associated with increased survival in patients with a history of hepatocellular carcinoma. Gastroenterology. 2019;157:1253–1263.e2.
15. Poustchi H, et al. Feasibility of conducting a randomized control trial for liver cancer screening: is a randomized controlled trial for liver cancer screening feasible or still needed? Hepatology. 2011;54:1998–2004.
16. Heimbach JK, et al. AASLD guidelines for the treatment of hepatocellular carcinoma. Hepatology. 2018;67:358–80.
17. Tzartzeva K, et al. Surveillance imaging and alpha fetoprotein for early detection of hepatocellular carcinoma in patients with cirrhosis: a meta-analysis. Gastroenterology. 2018;154:1706–1718.e1.
18. Wilson GC, Cannella R, Fiorentini G, Shen C, Borhani A, Furlan A, Tsung A. Texture analysis on preoperative contrast-enhanced magnetic resonance imaging identifies microvascular invasion in hepatocellular carcinoma. HPB (Oxford). 2020;22(11):1622–30. https://doi.org/10.1016/j.hpb.2020.03.001. Epub 2020 Mar 27
19. Centonze L, De Carlis R, Vella I, Carbonaro L, Incarbone N, Palmieri L, Sgrazzutti C, Ficarelli A, Valsecchi MG, Dello Iacono U, Lauterio A, Bernasconi D, Vanzulli A, De Carlis L. From LI-RADS classification to HCC pathology: a retrospective single-institution analysis of clinicopathological features affecting oncological outcomes after curative surgery. Diagnostics (Basel). 2022;12(1):160. https://doi.org/10.3390/diagnostics12010160. PMID: 35054327; PMCID: PMC8775107
20. Roayaie S, et al. The role of hepatic resection in the treatment of hepatocellular cancer. Hepatology. 2015;62:440–51.

21. Tabrizian P, Jibara G, Shrager B, Schwartz M, Roayaie S. Recurrence of hepatocellular cancer after resection: patterns, treatments, and prognosis. Ann Surg. 2015;261:947–55.
22. Gao ZH, Bai DS, Jiang GQ, Jin SJ. Review of preoperative transarterial chemoembolization for resectable hepatocellular carcinoma. World J Hepatol. 2015;7(1):40–3. https://doi.org/10.4254/wjh.v7.i1.40. PMID: 25624995; PMCID: PMC4295192
23. Bruix J, Takayama T, Mazzaferro V, Chau GY, Yang J, Kudo M, Cai J, Poon RT, Han KH, Tak WY, Lee HC, Song T, Roayaie S, Bolondi L, Lee KS, Makuuchi M, Souza F, Berre MA, Meinhardt G, Llovet JM. STORM investigators. Adjuvant sorafenib for hepatocellular carcinoma after resection or ablation (STORM): a phase 3, randomised, double-blind, placebo-controlled trial. Lancet Oncol. 2015;16(13):1344–54. https://doi.org/10.1016/S1470-2045(15)00198-9. Epub 2015 Sep 8
24. Memeo R, Conticchio M, Deshayes E, Nadalin S, Herrero A, Guiu B, Panaro F. Optimization of the future remnant liver: review of the current strategies in Europe. Hepatobiliary Surg Nutr. 2021;10(3):350–63. https://doi.org/10.21037/hbsn-20-394. PMID: 34159162; PMCID: PMC8188135
25. Langella S, Russolillo N, Sijberden J, Fiorentini G, Guglielmo N, Primrose J, Modi S, Massella V, Ettorre GM, Aldrighetti L, Hilal MA, Ferrero A. Safety of laparoscopic compared to open right hepatectomy after portal vein occlusion: results from a multicenter study. Surg Endosc. 2025; https://doi.org/10.1007/s00464-025-11591-x.
26. Fiorentini G, Ratti F, Aldrighetti L. The LiTOS-approach: liver partitioning and total venous occlusion for staged hepatectomy. J Gastrointest Surg. 2022;26(10):2244–7. https://doi.org/10.1007/s11605-022-05402-0. Epub 2022 Jul 11. Erratum in: J Gastrointest Surg; 26(11):2416
27. Fiorentini G, Ratti F, Cipriani F, Cinelli L, Catena M, Paganelli M, Aldrighetti L. Theory of relativity for Posterosuperior segments of the liver. Ann Surg Oncol. 2019;26(4):1149–57. https://doi.org/10.1245/s10434-019-07165-6. Epub 2019 Jan 23
28. Fiorentini G, Ratti F, Cipriani F, Marino R, Cerchione R, Catena M, Paganelli M, Aldrighetti L. Correlation between type of retrieval incision and postoperative outcomes in laparoscopic liver surgery: a critical assessment. J Laparoendosc Adv Surg Tech A. 2021;31(4):423–32. https://doi.org/10.1089/lap.2020.0470. Epub 2020 Aug 20
29. Ratti F, Cipriani F, Fiorentini G, Catena M, Paganelli M, Aldrighetti L. Reappraisal of the advantages of laparoscopic liver resection for intermediate hepatocellular carcinoma within a stage migration perspective: propensity score analysis of the differential benefit. J Hepatobiliary Pancreat Sci. 2020;27(8):510–21. https://doi.org/10.1002/jhbp.736. Epub 2020 Apr 16
30. Cipriani F, Ratti F, Fiorentini G, Catena M, Paganelli M, Aldrighetti L. Pure laparoscopic right hepatectomy: a risk score for conversion for

the paradigm of difficult laparoscopic liver resections. A single Centre case series. Int J Surg. 2020;82:108–15. https://doi.org/10.1016/j.ijsu.2020.08.013. Epub 2020 Aug 27

31. Mazzaferro V, et al. Liver transplantation for the treatment of small hepatocellular carcinomas in patients with cirrhosis. N Engl J Med. 1996;334:693–700.

32. Hwang S, Song GW, Ahn CS, Kim KH, Moon DB, Ha TY, Jung DH, Park GC, Yoon YI, Lee SG. Salvage living donor liver transplantation for hepatocellular carcinoma recurrence after hepatectomy: quantitative prediction using ADV score. J Hepatobiliary Pancreat Sci. 2021;28(11):1000–13. https://doi.org/10.1002/jhbp.863. Epub 2020 Dec 22

33. Unek T, Karademir S, Arslan NC, Egeli T, Atasoy G, Sagol O, Obuz F, Akarsu M, Astarcioglu I. Comparison of Milan and UCSF criteria for liver transplantation to treat hepatocellular carcinoma. World J Gastroenterol. 2011;17(37):4206–12. https://doi.org/10.3748/wjg.v17.i37.4206. PMID: 22072852; PMCID: PMC3208365

34. Ng KKC, et al. Randomized clinical trial of hepatic resection versus radiofrequency ablation for early stage hepatocellular carcinoma. Br J Surg. 2017;104:1775–84.

35. Xu X-L, Liu X-D, Liang M, Luo B-M. Radiofrequency ablation versus hepatic resection for small hepatocellular carcinoma: systematic review of randomized controlled trials with meta- analysis and trial sequential analysis. Radiology. 2018;287:461–72.

36. Wu G, Huang G, Huang J, Lu L, Peng S, Li Y, Zhao W. Comparison of external beam radiation therapy modalities for hepatocellular carcinoma with macrovascular invasion: a meta-analysis and systematic review. Front Oncol. 2022;12:829708. https://doi.org/10.3389/fonc.2022.829708. PMID: 35242713; PMCID: PMC8887617

37. Kimura T, Fujiwara T, Kameoka T, Adachi Y, Kariya S. The current role of stereotactic body radiation therapy (SBRT) in hepatocellular carcinoma (HCC). Cancers (Basel). 2022;14(18):4383. https://doi.org/10.3390/cancers14184383. PMID: 36139545; PMCID: PMC9496682

38. Gao S, Yang Z, Zheng Z, Yao J, Deng M, Xie H, Zheng S, Zhou L. Doxorubicin-eluting bead versus conventional TACE for unresectable hepatocellular carcinoma: a meta-analysis. Hepato-Gastroenterology. 2013;60(124):813–20. https://doi.org/10.5754/hge121025. Epub 2013 Jan 3

39. Sahu SK, Chawla YK, Dhiman RK, Singh V, Duseja A, Taneja S, Kalra N, Gorsi U. Rupture of hepatocellular carcinoma: a review of literature. J Clin Exp Hepatol. 2019;9(2):245–56. https://doi.org/10.1016/j.jceh.2018.04.002. Epub 2018 Apr 26. PMID: 31024207; PMCID: PMC6476943

40. Salem R, et al. Y90 radioembolization significantly prolongs time to progression compared with chemoembolization in patients with hepatocellular carcinoma. Gastroenterology. 2016;151:1155–1163.e2.
41. Hilgard P, et al. Radioembolization with yttrium-90 glass microspheres in hepatocellular carcinoma: European experience on safety and long- term survival. Hepatology. 2010;52:1741–9.
42. Finn RS, et al. Atezolizumab plus bevacizumab in unresectable hepatocellular carcinoma. N Engl J Med. 2020;382:1894–905.
43. Kelley RK, Sangro B, Harris W, Ikeda M, Okusaka T, Kang YK, Qin S, Tai DW, Lim HY, Yau T, Yong WP, Cheng AL, Gasbarrini A, Damian S, Bruix J, Borad M, Bendell J, Kim TY, Standifer N, He P, Makowsky M, Negro A, Kudo M, Abou-Alfa GK. Safety, efficacy, and pharmacodynamics of tremelimumab plus durvalumab for patients with unresectable hepatocellular carcinoma: randomized expansion of a phase I/II study. J Clin Oncol. 2021;39(27):2991–3001. https://doi.org/10.1200/JCO.20.03555. Epub 2021 Jul 22. PMID: 34292792; PMCID: PMC8445563
44. Bruix J, et al. Regorafenib for patients with hepatocellular carcinoma who progressed on sorafenib treatment (RESORCE): a randomised, double- blind, placebo- controlled, phase 3 trial. Lancet. 2017;389:56–66.

Surgical Management of Colorectal Liver Metastases

Gloria Y. Chang, Nicole M. Nevarez, and Georgios Karagkounis

Introduction

Colorectal cancer (CRC) is the third most commonly diagnosed cancer and third highest cause of cancer-related death, affecting women and men equally [1]. Almost 150,000 new CRC cases and over 50,000 deaths occur each year in the United States alone [1, 2]. Despite advances in screening and diagnosis, up to 25% of patients diagnosed with CRC will develop colorectal liver metastases (CRLM), and only 25% of these patients are determined to be resectable [3]. CRLM can be either synchronous, meaning they are diagnosed at the same time as the primary tumor, or metachronous, when they are diagnosed at a later point. Engstrand and colleagues reported that patients with CRC developed synchronous

CRLM in 16.2% of cases, and metachronous in 10.3%. It should be noted, however, that there is no uniform definition of "metachronous", which may refer to "after resection of the primary" or after a set time from diagnosis (typically 6 or 12 months). Regardless of the definition, though, most (>90%) metachronous CRLM develop within 3 years from the original diagnosis [3].

The role of surgery for the management of CRLM has expanded dramatically over the past 3 decades. Once limited to patients with one to two small liver metastases [4], surgical therapy is now offered to an ever-wider group of patients with more extensive disease, without compromising outcomes [5]. Many advances allowed for an expanded role for surgery in the management of CRLM. Modern chemotherapy regimens offer tumor downsizing with possible conversion to resectability and improvement in disease control; imaging techniques offer improved estimates of future liver remnant (FLR) after resection; if insufficient FLR, techniques such as portal vein embolization (PVE) or hepatic vein embolization (HVE) allow liver optimization prior to hepatectomy; and parenchymal preservation techniques offer surgical options for patients with extensive bilobar disease. With these advances, 5-year overall survival (OS) in CRC with liver metastases that undergo resection is now 48–60% [2, 3].

Surgical Evaluation

Imaging

Once a diagnosis of CRC has been made, the next step is staging with a computed tomography (CT) of the chest, abdomen, and pelvis with intravenous contrast. This aims to detect metastasis and evaluate the local extent of disease. In CRLM, CT abdomen and pelvis is helpful for identifying liver metastases >10 millimeters (mm). For smaller liver metastases (<10 mm), CT accuracy is somewhat limited though recent advances with the availability of dual-energy imaging and thin slice scanners have improved the detection of smaller lesions [6]. A multi-phase CT can help: among the arterial, portal venous, and non-contrasted phases, the portal venous phase offers the most information for the mapping of metastatic disease. This phase of the CT has an 85% detection rate and 96% positive predictive value for CRLM [7]. Compared to other liver tumors, the arterial phase benefit is more limited as CRLM are hypovascular; however, it is often very helpful for surgical planning.

While magnetic resonance imaging (MRI) is not part of the standard staging workup of the primary tumor in colon cancer, it is an integral part of defining CRLM. Once hepatic metastases have been identified or if there is a high suspicion that small indeterminate lesions are metastases, an MRI is often an appropriate next step. In general, CRLM are hypointense on T1 phase. Specifically for CRLM, certain gadolinium-based contrast agents are used such as gadoxetate disodium (Eovist, Bayer) and gadobenate dimeglumine (MultiHance, Bracco), which are hepatocyte-specific, meaning they are preferentially absorbed by hepatocytes and excreted via the biliary system. These hepatocyte-specific contrast agents allow for detection of smaller lesions not seen on other imaging modalities and/or other sequences of MRI [8].

The use of positron emission tomography with CT (PET-CT) in the staging of CRLM is controversial. Smaller, indeterminate liver or lung lesions on CT scan are typically below the detection size of PET, limiting the added benefit of this modality. Even though PET-CT can improve detection of extra-hepatic metastases, potentially altering treatment plans, prospective data suggest that it impacts fewer than 10% of cases [9]. It may be useful in patients with renal disease where use of intravenous iodinated contrast may not be optimal.

Determining Resectability

Resectable CRLM are CRLM that can be completely removed or ablated, while preserving at least two contiguous liver segments of adequate volume (FLR) with intact inflow, venous outflow, and biliary drainage. Determining whether a patient is resectable relies on a multidisciplinary approach. Clinicians can not only identify the involved part of the liver and associated vasculature but also estimate the FLR using volumetrics. In patients without underlying liver dysfunction, a minimum FLR of 20–25% has been recommended. In patients with liver dysfunction or cirrhosis, an FLR of at least 30–40% has been recommended to avoid post-operative liver failure, a feared and potentially lethal complication of liver resection [10, 11]. When volumetrics is not sufficient to assess function due to concurrent liver dysfunction, indocyanine green clearance [12, 13] and hepatobiliary scintigraphy can be utilized [11, 14–16].

If a patient is found to have insufficient FLR, there are several options to help mitigate this: PVE (with or without HVE), Associating Liver Partition and Portal vein Ligation for Staged hepatectomy (ALPPS), and two-stage hepatectomy (TSH). PVE is a strategy for inducing liver hypertrophy, most commonly used in the setting of insufficient FLR where the portal vein on the ipsilateral side to the tumor is embolized. The kinetic growth rate (KGR, defined as degree of hypertrophy at initial volume assessment divided by number of weeks elapsed after PVE) is a commonly used predictor of postoperative hepatic insufficiency, with a KGR of at least 2.0% demonstrating protection against hepatic insufficiency and liver-related 90-day mortality [17]. Importantly, PVE does not compromise oncologic outcomes. In a recent retrospective analysis with propensity-score matching by Huiskens and colleagues, the authors found that among 745 patients undergoing major liver resection for CRLM, the disease-free survival and OS were not significantly different between the two groups ($p = 0.776$ and $p = 0.537$) [18]. Additionally, there was no significant difference in 90-day mortality or R0 resections. The only statistically significant difference was a higher complication rate in the PVE group compared to the non-PVE group (48% vs.24%, $p = 0.029$).

When PVE alone does not allow for an adequate FLR, more advanced approaches can be pursued. Classical TSH is performed with or without portal vein embolization or ligation and involves a first stage of resecting or ablating ("clearing") the segments that will form the FLR and returning at a later date after liver hypertrophy for the second stage (resection of remaining disease) [19]. A modification of TSH, ALPPS is an operation where the liver is transected in the planned plane and the portal vein on the side planned for resection is ligated; this is then followed by completion hepatectomy after the contralateral side has hypertrophied [20]. In 2018, a randomized controlled trial from Scandinavia sought to answer whether ALPPS or TSH is superior for increasing FLR [21]. The authors randomized 100 patients with advanced CRLM with FLR <30% to either ALPPS or TSH. 92% of the ALPPS group reached a sufficient FLR of 30% compared to 57% in the TSH group (p < 0.0001). Notably, the ALPPS group reached sufficient FLR faster than the TSH group and time to final intervention was significantly shorter at 11 days in the ALPPS group compared to 43 days in the TSH group (p < 0.0001). No significant differences in complications were observed between the two groups (HR 1.01, 95% CI 0.4–2.6; $p = 0.99$). In a separate retrospective analysis of 189 patients out of Scandinavia, the successful resection rates and degree of upfront ALPPS and PVE with rescue ALPPS were compared. The authors found that upfront ALPPS offered a modestly higher successful resection rate (84.5%) compared to PVE with rescue ALPPS (73.3%) ($p = 0.080$). The combination PVE with ALPPS had a higher overall degree of hypertrophy at 96% (82–113%) compared to upfront ALPPS at 71% (48–97%) ($p = 0.010$) [22].

Prognostic Factors

Clinical Risk Scores

Assessing the prognosis of patients with resectable CRLM is important for guiding therapeutic decisions, including selecting patients for operative management (Table 9.1). While a number of large retrospective studies have identified relevant clinicopathological factors to inform prognostication of patients with CRLMs, the two most widely cited clinical risk scoring systems are by Nordlinger and Fong [23, 24].

Nordlinger et al. proposed a prognostic scoring system based on a large multicenter retrospective study of 1568 patients who underwent resection of CRLM. Seven independent risk factors associated with worse OS were identified: (1) age > 60 years, (2) primary cancer extension into serosa, (3) lymphatic spread of pri-

Table 9.1 Clinical risk score models for patients with CRLM undergoing hepatic resection

Series author	Year	Patients (n)	Outcome	Prognostic factors included	Groups
Nordlinger [23]	1996	1568	OS	Extension of primary tumor into serosa (1 point). Node-positive primary (1 point). Age ≥ 60 years (1 point). Number of CRLM ≥4 (1 point). Disease-free interval < 2 years (1 point). Largest CRLM diameter > 5 cm (1 point). Surgical margin <1 cm (1 point).	Low risk (0–2 points). Intermediate risk (3–4 points). High risk (5–7 points).
Fong (CRS) [24]	1999	1001	RFS	Node-positive primary (1 point). Disease-free interval < 12 months (1 point). Number of CRLM >1 (1 point). Largest CRLM diameter > 5 cm (1 point). CEA > 200 ng/mL (1 point).	Low risk (0–1 point). Intermediate risk (2–3 points). High risk (4–5 points).
Brudvik (m-CRS) [28]	2019	564	OS, RFS	Node-positive primary (1 point). Largest CRLM diameter > 5 cm (1 point). RAS alteration (1 point).	Low risk (0–1 point). Intermediate risk (2 points). High risk (3 points).

(continued)

Table 9.1 (continued)

Series author	Year	Patients (n)	Outcome	Prognostic factors included	Groups
Margonis (GAME) [29]	2018	502	OS	Node-positive primary (1 point). CEA ≥ 20 ng/mL (1 point). Extrahepatic disease (2 points). Tumor burden score[a] 3–8 (1 point) or ≥ 9 (2 points). KRAS-mutation (1 point).	Low risk (0–1 point). Intermediate risk (2–3 points). High risk (4–7 points).
Lang (e-CS) [133]	2019	139	RFS	Node-positive primary (1 point). Largest CRLM diameter > 5 cm (1 point). RAS/RAF alterations (1 point). SMAD alteration (1 point).	Low-intermediate risk (0–2 points). High risk (3–4 points).
Chen (CERR) [134]	2020	787	RFS	Node-positive primary (1 point). CEA > 200 ng/mL or CA 19–9 > 200 u/mL (1 point). KRAS/NRAS/BRAF-mutated tumor (1 point). Extrahepatic disease (1 point). Modified tumor burden score[b] 5–11 (1 point) or ≥ 12 (2 points).	Low risk (0–1 point). Intermediate risk (2 points). High risk (3 points).

[a]Tumor burden score: a prognostic indicator defined by calculating the distance from the origin to a set of coordinates using maximum CRLM size (x-axis) and CRLM number (y-axis) on a Cartesian plane [29]

[b]Modified tumor burden score: a prognostic indicator defined by a mathematical equation incorporating CRLM size, CRLM number, and unilobar or bilobar metastasis [134]

mary cancer, (4) time interval of <2 years from primary tumor to metastases, (5) largest metastasis diameter > 5 cm, (6) number of metastases ≥4, and (7) resection margin <1 cm. In their clinical risk score model, patients could be stratified into one of three risk groups based on how many of the 7 prognostic factors were present: low risk (0–2 factors), intermediate risk (3–4 factors), and high risk (5–7 factors) [23].

Fong et al. proposed a separate clinical risk score model focusing on risk factors available preoperatively in order to predict long-term outcome for patients being considered for resection. In their series, 1001 patients at a single institution undergoing resection for CRLM were examined and five independent risk factors available preoperatively and associated with recurrence free survival were incorporated into the Clinical Risk Score (CRS), often referred to as the "Fong score": (1) node-positive primary, (2) disease-free interval from primary to metastases <12 months, (3) number of hepatic tumors >1, (4) largest CRLM diameter > 5 cm, and (5) carcinoembryonic antigen (CEA) level > 200 ng/ml. A single point is assigned to each parameter, with a sum score of 0–2 having a highly favorable outcome supporting surgical resection, sum of 3 or 4 a more guarded prognosis with surgical resection being considered mostly in the context of adjuvant therapies, and sum score of 5 predictive of poor outcome, discouraging use of resection outside the context of additional adjuvant therapies or trials [24].

These CRS systems provide valuable insight on risk stratification for patients and help with patient selection. Both scoring systems were developed in the 1990s, prior to the more widespread use of neoadjuvant chemotherapy and prior to the recognition of other significant prognostic parameters. Genetic alterations have been increasingly investigated as potential prognostic factors in considering the treatment of CRLM. RAS mutations have been the most widely studied and are associated with a poor prognosis for both RFS and OS after CRLM resection [25, 26]. BRAF V600E alterations (substitution of valine for glutamate in codon 600) have also been demonstrated to be a negative prognostic factor for colorectal cancer with studies reporting worse RFS and OS after CRLM resection compared to those with BRAF V600E wild-type [27] (Table 9.2).

Table 9.2 Prognostic and management impact of genetic biomarkers

Genetic biomarker	Prognostic impact	Management impact
RAS	Negative prognostic biomarker for patients who undergo resection of CRLM [25, 26]. Associated with worse OS compared to WT-RAS after CRLM resection [25, 26]. RAS alteration is a risk factor for recurrence after CRLM resection. Increased risk persists even after 2 years. [25, 26].	RAS testing (KRAS and NRAS) generally recommended prior to use of anti-EGFR systemic therapy as mutation predicts resistance and poor treatment response to these agents [138]. RAS-mutated patients who have undergone CRLM resection may benefit from higher intensity surveillance even after 2 years from resection [136].
BRAF	BRAF V600E makes up 90% of all BRAF mutations. Found in up to 15% of CRC patients but only up to 5.5% of those with resectable CRLM [27]. Marker of aggressive disease and is typically associated with unresectable extrahepatic disease [27]. BRAF mutation correlates with worse OS and RFS after liver resection compared to BRAF-WT patients, but median OS has been reported better than BRAF-mutated patients with metastatic CRC undergoing chemotherapy alone. [27]. Negative impact on prognosis is greater than the negative impact of RAS alteration [135].	Mutation is a predictor of poor response to anti-EGFR therapy as BRAF alteration is associated with resistance to these agents. While BRAF mutation is a negative prognostic marker for those with resectable CRLM, surgery should still be considered, with the caveat that patients are well-selected, and counseled on risk of recurrence. [139].
PIK3CA	Mutation status associated with poor prognosis in the context [140] of co-mutation with APC.	Demonstrated resistance to anti-EGFR therapy [141].

(continued)

Table 9.3 (continued)

Genetic biomarker	Prognostic impact	Management impact
TP53	TP53 alteration is associated with poor prognosis. TP53 mutation with concurrent RAS mutation is associated with worse OS than RAS mutation alone [137].	
SMAD4	SMAD4 alteration is associated with poor prognosis, particularly when co-altered with RAS [142].	

More recent prognostic scoring systems have been proposed that incorporate newer parameters, including the modified-Fong CRS and the Genetic and Morphological Evaluation (GAME) score [28, 29]. The modified-Fong CRS integrates largest CRLM diameter >5 cm, primary lymph node metastases, and RAS alteration while the GAME score includes primary lymph node metastases, preoperative CEA $\geq$ 20, extrahepatic disease, resection margin <1 mm, KRAS alteration, and the "Tumor Burden Score" which takes into consideration primary tumor size as well as number of liver lesions [28, 29].

Adjuncts to Surgical Treatment

Ablation

Surgical resection is the "gold standard" for local control of CRLM but is not always feasible or the most appropriate option. In certain cases, concerns over the morbidity of hepatectomy in patients with borderline overall health may prioritize a less invasive approach. In other cases, an unfavorable tumor location (deep in the parenchyma or adjacent to a major vascular structure) may require the resection of an extensive volume of normal liver parenchyma along with the tumor. In both scenarios, ablative therapies can offer an additional therapeutic option. These include thermal ablative options such as cryotherapy, radiofrequency ablation (RFA), and microwave ablation (MWA) as well as non-thermal therapies such as irreversible electroporation (IRE) and stereotactic body radiotherapy (SBRT) (Table 9.3).

Table 9.3 Advantages and disadvantages of local ablative therapies

Treatment option	Advantages	Disadvantages
Cryoablation	Well-tolerated, less painful procedure. Can visualize ice-ball formation as procedure progresses.	Risk of bleeding and cold shock. Higher complication rate.
Radiofrequency ablation	Widely studied and generally available at most institutions. Good local control for tumors up to 3 cm [35].	Not as effective for tumors >3 cm. Susceptible to the heat sink effect, not great for lesions adjacent to vessels. Risk of thermal injury to important structures [32]. Less predictable ablation zone. Tissue charring resulting in increased impedance.
Microwave ablation	Larger ablation zone with shorter procedural time [38]. Less susceptible to the heat sink effect [39].	Risk of thermal injury to important structures [41].
Irreversible electroporation	Can treat tumors adjacent to critical structures [45]. No heat sink effect.	Limited evidence and not widely available. Requires general anesthesia with muscular relaxation and cardiac monitoring [45].
Stereotactic body radiotherapy	Can treat tumors up to 5 cm in diameter. No heat sink effect. Can treat lesions in close proximity to critical structures [49]. High rates of local control with limited toxicity [48]. Non-invasive; does not require anesthesia.	May not be as widely available due to the need for high level of motion management with imaging. Potentially less effective for lesions adjacent to luminal structures due to the need for reduced dose to avoid toxicity.

Cryoablation

With cryoablation, liquid nitrogen or argon gas is brought into direct contact with a tumor surface and repeated freeze-thaw cycles cause intracellular ice crystal formation, leading to organelle damage and cellular death [30]. Due to more challenging delivery and reports of similar or inferior outcomes, cryoablation has fallen out of favor and has been largely supplanted by radiofrequency and microwave ablation.

Radiofrequency Ablation (RFA)

RFA consists of the placement of a needle electrode into a metastatic lesion and the delivery of high-frequency alternating electrical currents. Frictional heat is generated, resulting in thermocoagulation and cellular necrosis [31]. Consensus guidelines recommend the use of RFA for tumors smaller than 3 cm. A common concern with RFA when used for tumors near major vessels is the potential for the heat sink effect, whereby heat is lost to nearby blood flow, leading to undertreatment of the tumor of interest. RFA is also not recommended for lesions in close proximity to important structures such as major bile ducts, other organs, or large vessels due to risk of heat injury [32]. An ablation margin of at least 1 cm is recommended to minimize local recurrence [33].

The EORTC-CLOCC trial was a randomized Phase II trial comparing 119 patients with unresectable CRLM who underwent either systemic therapy alone or combination treatment with systemic therapy plus RFA with or without additional resection. At 10-year follow-up, the combined treatment group had longer OS compared to the systemic therapy alone group (HR = 0.58, 95% CI = 0.38–0.88, $p = 0.01$), improved OS at 8 years (36% vs.9%), and longer median OS (45.6 months vs.40.5 months). These findings further support the use of aggressive local therapy combined with systemic treatment in select patients with extensive CRLM [34].

The use of RFA in the context of resectable CRLM is being investigated in the ongoing COLLISION trial, a Phase III randomized clinical trial exploring the potential non-inferiority of thermal ablation compared to hepatic resection for resectable CRLM ≤3 cm [35]. Examination of available retrospective series demonstrates improved recurrence rate, 3- and 5-year DFS and OS with hepatic resection over RFA [36]. As such, with the exception of deep-seated CRLM, where RFA can offer benefits of parenchymal preservation, most consensus recommendations favor hepatic resection over RFA for patients with resectable CRLM who are candidates for hepatectomy [37].

Microwave Ablation (MWA)

MWA uses electromagnetic radiation via an antenna to generate heat from the oscillation of polar molecules, resulting in coagulation necrosis of hepatic parenchyma. Compared to RFA, MWA generates heat faster, more homogeneously, and over a larger volume [38]. Because there is no electrical conduction, it is also less susceptible to the heat-sink effect observed with RFA, making MWA a favored approach for CRLMs in close proximity to major vessels [39]. MWA shares many of the same indications and contraindications as RFA [40], while also having reports of similar rates of adverse events [41].

While MWA has not been studied as extensively as RFA and there is no level 1 data comparing the two, MWA has been increasingly used with some reports favoring its use over RFA. A retrospective matched-cohort analysis of 134 patients undergoing MWA or RFA for CRLM at a single institution found that those undergoing MWA had lower ablation-site recurrence rates (6% vs.20%, p < 0.01) suggesting potentially better local control with MWA [42]. A recent systematic review demonstrated decreased 5-year DFS for RFA (RR 0.53, 95%CI 0.28–0.98) and 5-year OS (RR 0.76, 95%CI 0.58–0.98) compared to MWA [41].

Irreversible Electroporation (IRE)

IRE exposes cell membranes to repeated electrical pulses to irreversibly increase the membrane permeability of targeted cells, resulting in cellular apoptosis [43]. Current indications for its use include ablation of tumors that are unresectable and not amenable to thermal ablation. Its efficacy has been described for tumors ≤3 cm in patients with four or fewer lesions [44]. Due to its selectivity and sparing of adjacent structures, IRE's primary role has been in the ablation of lesions too closely associated with critical vessels or biliary anatomy to safely utilize thermal ablation [45]. IRE requires careful cardiac monitoring and general anesthesia with muscular relaxation as the electrical pulses can cause uncontrolled muscle contractions [45]. There is a relative paucity of data for IRE and further investigation is needed regarding its safety and efficacy.

Stereotactic Body Radiotherapy (SBRT)

SBRT is used in conjunction with image-guidance and motion management to deliver a high dose of radiation to a well-defined target [46]. While there are no Phase III randomized clinical trials for SBRT, there are two Phase II trials that have reported on its benefits.

In the SABR-COMET trial, 99 patients with a controlled primary tumor and up to 5 metastatic lesions were randomized to receive standard of care palliative treatment with or without SBRT. The palliative treatment with SBRT arm demonstrated improved PFS (6 months vs.12 months) and OS (28 months vs.41 months). However, this study was limited by heterogeneous primary histologies, with only 18.2% of the 99 patients having colorectal cancer [47].

A separate Phase II trial reported on 42 patients who underwent SBRT for treatment of CRLM. Patients with liver-limited disease who were deemed inoperable and not amenable for RFA were included. All 42 patients received pre-SBRT chemotherapy and 6 patients (14%) received post-SBRT chemotherapy. This study demonstrated complete response in 43% of lesions with a median PFS of 12 months and median OS of 29 months. There were no reports of radiation-induced liver disease or grade ≥ 3 toxicity [48].

SBRT is most efficacious for lesions <5 cm in diameter with particular benefit for lesions in close proximity to large vessels or critical structures [49]. SBRT, either alone or in conjunction with hepatic resection, presents a potentially beneficial therapeutic option when patients are deemed inoperable or are not amenable for other forms of ablation [50].

Hepatic Artery Infusion Therapy

The hepatic artery infusion pump (HAIP) is an implanted catheter device that allows for the direct local infusion of chemotherapy. Because CRLM derive their blood supply primarily from the hepatic artery, intra-arterial chemotherapy allows for the infusion of higher concentrations and a more selective delivery, thereby improving tumor cytotoxic effects while minimizing systemic toxicity [51]. Many initial randomized clinical trials found a significant survival advantage to hepatic artery infusion (HAI) therapy when combined with 5-FU systemic chemotherapy [52]. Since the establishment of modern chemotherapy regimens, no randomized trials exist to prove if HAI still provides this same advantage. In initially unresectable CRLM, HAI therapy can improve survival and offer potential for conversion to resectability. In a study investigating its use in this setting, fluorodeoxyuridine (FUDR) HAI with either oxaliplatin/irinotecan or 5-FU/oxaliplatin/irinotecan was successful in converting 52% of patients to resectable [53].

More recently, studies have focused on HAI with systemic chemotherapy as an adjuvant therapy for CRLM. Groot Koerkamp and colleagues retrospectively studied 1442 patients who underwent perioperative modern systemic chemotherapy with or without HAI [54]. The median OS was statistically improved at 67 months with HAI compared with 47 months in patients who did not receive HAI ($p < 0.001$), and these results persisted even after propensity-matching. Additionally, in 2020, Gholami and colleagues had similar findings. In an analysis of 674 patients who underwent resection CRLM, HAI therapy was associated with 5-year recurrence-free survival and OS advantages compared with no HAI therapy (RFS 33% vs.25%, $p < 0.006$) and OS 70% vs.50%, HR 0.52, $p < 0.0001$) [55]. Most (96%) of these patients underwent systemic chemotherapy as well. Though these retrospective analyses suggest a significant benefit from HAI therapy when combined with systemic chemotherapy, further data from randomized controlled trials, such as the PUMP trial comparing resection alone and resection and adjuvant HAI and systemic therapy, are eagerly awaited [56].

Systemic Chemotherapy

Patients with CRLM are typically offered systemic chemotherapy if their functional status allows it. In patients with resectable disease, this can be offered in either the neoadjuvant or the adjuvant setting; in those with unresectable disease, chemotherapy may be the primary treatment modality. The most commonly prescribed first-line regimen is 5-fluorouracil (5-FU), leucovorin, and oxaliplatin (FOLFOX), though capecitabine with oxaliplatin (XELOX) and 5-FU/leucovorin with irinotecan (FOLFIRI) are also common regimens [57–59]. EGFR blockade such as cetuximab and panitumumab and anti-angiogenic agents such as bevacizumab can be added, especially in unresectable disease where no surgical intervention is intended [60–63].

In patients with initially resectable CRLM, neoadjuvant or perioperative chemotherapy is popular and has been the focus of several studies. With purported benefits of treating micrometastatic disease, improving patient selection by allowing a "test of time" or "biology", and decreasing tumor size to allow for less morbid interventions, neoadjuvant chemotherapy is frequently offered in this setting. However, data on the benefit of this approach remain limited. In the landmark EORTC 40983, patients with resectable CRLM who had never received oxaliplatin based chemotherapy were randomized to either liver resection alone versus FOLFOX followed by liver resection followed by FOLFOX [64, 65]. While progression-free survival was significantly improved in the perioperative chemotherapy group, in an analysis of the long-term results of the study, there was no significant difference in the OS between the two groups. A phase III clinical trial by Kanemitsu and colleagues aimed to determine whether adjuvant FOLFOX was superior to resection alone in patients with resectable CRLM. Similar to the EORTC trial, Kanemitsu and colleagues demonstrated that FOLFOX after resection significantly improved 5-year disease-free survival (49.8% versus 38.7%), though there was no significant difference in 5-year OS [66]. Finally, though not a randomized clinical trial, a meta-analysis by Liu and colleagues confirmed this lack of OS benefit with neoadjuvant chemotherapy in patients with resectable CRLM [67]. As such, the use of neoadjuvant chemotherapy for resectable CRLM remains controversial.

Despite initial enthusiasm, support has waned with regard to neoadjuvant EGFR blockade. In 2014, Primrose and colleagues randomized KRAS wild-type patients with resectable CRLM to perioperative systemic chemotherapy with or without cetuximab [68]. Surprisingly, the addition of cetuximab to standard chemotherapy resulted in poorer progression-free survival.

With regard to patients presenting with initially unresectable disease, the decision to use systemic chemotherapy is more straightforward, as it often is the only treatment available. In addition to improving OS for these patients, systemic chemotherapy can also convert unresectable disease to resectable, allowing curative-intent liver-directed therapy. In this setting, 32–67% of patients with liver-only metastatic disease who were initially unresectable ultimately may be able to undergo surgery [69–71], with FOLFIRINOX offering the highest rate of conversion among systemic chemotherapy regimens [71].

Surgical Therapy

Identification of Lesions in the Operating Room

A combination of visual inspection, manual palpation (in open cases), and the use of intraoperative ultrasound (IOUS) is critical for the intraoperative identification of CRLM. A thorough inspection of the abdomen is also performed to evaluate for extrahepatic disease, confirm findings previously seen on imaging, and locate any radiologically occult superficial lesions.

Thorough palpation and IOUS of the liver are facilitated by dividing the ligamentum Teres and the falciform ligament. A combination of palpation and IOUS can detect CRLM with reports of sensitivity up to 84% [72]. In addition to the detection of CRLM, IOUS is vital for identifying biliary and vascular anatomy and the demarcation of a safe and oncologic plane of transection [73, 74].

While IOUS for hepatic resection has become routine, there has been recent growing interest in the addition of contrast. Though contrast-enhanced IOUS (CE-IOUS) has yet to become widely available or adopted in the United States, its use has been described by a number of groups in Europe and Asia with reports of increased sensitivity and accuracy in detecting CRLM [72, 75–78].

Maximizing Parenchymal Preservation

Anatomic resection (AR), wherein the hepatectomy is performed along the boundaries of hepatic segments defined by their vascular supply and biliary drainage (Couinaud's segments), is a concept developed for the management of primary hepatic malignancies (mainly hepatocellular carcinoma), and its role in the surgical management of CRLM is unclear. In the absence of randomized controlled trials proving the benefits of AR over non-anatomic resection (NAR) (also referred to as parenchymal-sparing resection) in CRLM, retrospective data are useful. One series of 253 patients undergoing wedge or anatomic resection for CRLM found no difference in rate of positive surgical margin, overall recurrence rates, patterns of recurrence, and survival [79]. Subsequent studies have described reduced operation time and blood transfusion requirement while perioperative morbidity and mortality remained similar. No significant differences were found in surgical margins, or rates of intrahepatic recurrence, OS, and DFS, suggesting that NAR is safe for CRLM and does not compromise oncological outcomes, even in the context of more aggressive tumor biology as with RAS mutation [80–84]. A systematic review by Moris and colleagues included 12 studies and 2505 patients who underwent either AR or NAR resections for CRLM [84]. They found no significant difference in R0 resection between NAR (66.7–100%) and AR (71.6–98.6, $p = 0.58$), and the post-operative major morbidity rates were similar (NAR 3.2–27.8% versus AR 6.3–29.3%, $p = 0.218$). Crucially, OS rates in the two groups were nearly identical (5-year OS for NAR 44.7%, for AR 44.6%). Taking into consideration the importance of FLR in both short-term outcomes and potential future need for liver-directed therapy, a parenchymal-sparing approach is often favored for resectable CRLM [81].

Perioperative Management

Minimizing Blood Loss

Because the liver is a highly vascular organ, hepatic resection can result in significant blood loss. Increased perioperative blood loss and need for transfusion have been associated with adverse perioperative events as well as worse oncologic outcomes including long-term survival [85–87]. Accordingly, techniques that limit blood loss are critical during hepatic resection for CRLM.

Hemorrhage can result from either inflow or outflow vessels and different maneuvers can be performed to help address potential blood loss from either source. Hepatic venous bleeding is typically considered more difficult to control but can be minimized by maintaining a low central venous pressure (CVP) of less than 4 cm H2O [88]. Intravenous fluid should be administered judiciously, increased PEEP should be avoided, and a slight Trendelenburg positioning can help improve cardiac preload while decreasing hepatic venous pressure [89], though the latter may interfere with exposure. Raising the liver, either by placing gauze pads behind it or lifting its surface with retraction sutures, can further decrease the pressure in the hepatic vein branches.

For control of blood loss from inflow vessels, the hepatic pedicle can be temporarily occluded, a move known as the Pringle maneuver [90]. In order to mitigate the risk of ischemic and reperfusion injury, the Pringle maneuver is typically performed intermittently, though there is no consensus regarding the optimal duration [91]. Studies examining the impact of the Pringle maneuver in CRLM patients have not found any significant negative impact on recurrence [92], morbidity, or OS [93]. One retrospective study demonstrated lower rates of increased transfusion demand and improved RFS (36 vs.24 months, $p = 0.03$) for patients who underwent the Pringle maneuver during CRLM resection compared to those who did not [94].

Antimicrobial Prophylaxis

A dose of prophylactic antibiotics with adequate biliary coverage should be administered less than 1 hour before skin incision and re-dosed as appropriate [95]. There is no evidence of added benefit from continuing antibiotics postoperatively after hepatic resection [96–97].

Venous Thromboembolism Prophylaxis

Patients undergoing hepatic resection for CRLM are at increased risk of postoperative venous thromboembolism (VTE) and correlates with the magnitude of resection [98, 99]. Sequential compression devices should be placed prior to anesthesia induction [99] while chemical VTE prophylaxis can be administered preoperatively and post-operatively [99, 100]. While the overall clinical picture, any evidence of bleeding, and hemodynamics should be taken into account, patients who have laboratory values including INR less than 1.8, platelet count greater than 100,000/mm^3, and stable hemoglobin should receive chemical VTE prophylaxis [98].

Postoperative Management

Electrolyte Abnormalities

Patients who undergo major liver resection often develop hypokalemia, hypophosphatemia, hyponatremia, and hypoglycemia in the postoperative period as a result of metabolic changes associated with liver regeneration. Electrolytes should be monitored closely and replaced as necessary. Critical electrolyte derangements can potentially be mitigated with the administration of saline-based intravenous fluids supplemented with dextrose and potassium phosphate for the first 24 hours.

Fluid Resuscitation

Balanced fluid resuscitation after hepatic resection is of the utmost importance postoperatively for adequate liver perfusion to avoid postoperative liver failure while keeping in mind the risk of volume-related pulmonary, cardiac, and renal complications. A variety of measures, such as urine output, serum blood urea nitrogen, serum creatinine, invasive measurements of cardiac output and intravascular volume, as well as BNP are valuable tools and markers that can be utilized for goal-directed fluid administration [101].

Liver Function

Liver function tests and coagulation profile should be closely followed post-operatively. Liver transaminase, bilirubin, and INR values should peak and decline in a predictable pattern; failure to do so in the days following surgery may prolong recovery and has the potential to progress to post-operative liver failure.

Surveillance

According to the National Comprehensive Cancer Network (NCCN, Colon Cancer and Rectal Cancer separately), patients with stage IV colon or rectal cancer should undergo surveillance for at least 5 years after treatment. This protocol calls for history and physical examination and CEA every 3–6 months for 2 years then every 6 months for the remaining 3 years. Additionally, a CT chest, abdomen, and pelvis is recommended every 3–6 months for the first 2 years, then 6–12 months for the remaining 3 years and a colonoscopy at 1 year. A colonoscopy is recommended earlier (at 3–6 months) if no pre-operative colonoscopy was performed. As mentioned in a previous section, PET-CT is not routinely recommended [102].

In this surveillance protocol, if there is suspicion for recurrence, then workup proceeds in a similar fashion to the initial diagnosis of CRLM. Once diagnosed with recurrence of CRLM, all the modalities for treating liver lesions enumerated above can be considered again.

Controversies in Surgical Management of CRLM

Importance of Margin
While there is consensus that a microscopically positive (R1) resection margin is a negative prognostic predictor of recurrence, the optimal width of the resection margin in an R0 resection is unclear. Historically, the target resection margin width was 1 centimeter (cm), but several studies have questioned this. A recent study by Hamady and colleagues prospectively compared different resection margins among patients undergoing resection for CRLM [103]. Those with resection margins >1 mm achieved significantly improved 5-year disease-free survival compared to those with <1 mm resection margins. When the >1 mm resection margin group was stratified, there was no difference in disease-free survival between 1–9.9 mm and > 1 cm resection margins. In addition, it remains unclear to what extent the negative prognostic value of an R1 (or close margin) resection is secondary to the risk of residual disease at the margin, or whether it is reflective of disease biology and extent (as a widely negative margin is more challenging in patients with larger tumors, more tumors, or more infiltrative disease).

Role of HAI Therapy
HAI chemotherapy can be beneficial in patients with unresectable liver metastases without extrahepatic disease, in particular those who have progressed on initial therapy. Among these patients, conversion rates to resectability of up to 52% have been reported [55]. In addition, prospective studies in the era prior to the current chemotherapy regimens and recent retrospective studies have shown improvement in recurrence-free and OS in the adjuvant setting (after hepatectomy), when combined with systemic chemotherapy [52, 54]. However, with most available data originating at a single institution, further prospective validation would help solidify the role of HAI therapy for CRLM; upcoming trials in US (HAI Consortium) and in the Netherlands (PUMP trial) will hopefully provide critical information.

Resection Versus Ablation

Ablation is helpful for select patients who are medically unfit to undergo resection. However, for those who are candidates for resection, the decision between resection and ablation can be difficult. Surgical resection offers more consistent disease control, with lower local recurrence rates [42]. However, it can be associated with greater morbidity and decreased rates of parenchymal preservation. For tumors >3 cm and for superficial lesions, resection should be preferred. For smaller lesions, deep in the hepatic parenchyma, the decision to proceed with resection or ablation should be individualized, depending on the patient's disease burden, concurrent procedures, and the surgeon's expertise.

Open Versus Minimally Invasive Approach

Advances in minimally invasive surgery have led to more widespread use of laparoscopic techniques for hepatic resection. Retrospective studies comparing outcomes of laparoscopic vs. open liver resection for CRLM reported laparoscopic resection to be associated with reduced EBL and major morbidity while maintaining comparable oncologic outcomes [104, 105].

Two randomized controlled trials comparing laparoscopic and open hepatic resection for CRLM have been published. OSLO-COMET randomized 280 patients with resectable CRLM to laparoscopic or open liver resections for resectable CRLM. The laparoscopic surgery group had a lower post-operative 30-day complication rate (19% vs. 31%, $p = 0.021$) and gained 0.011 quality-adjusted life years ($p = 0.001$) compared to the open surgery group. There was no difference in EBL, operation time, resection margins, 90-day mortality, or cost comparison at 4 months. Importantly, this trial was able to demonstrate that the laparoscopic liver resection resulted in a lower post-operative complication rate while maintaining comparable resection margins and cost effectiveness compared to open liver resection [106].

In a subsequent single-center prospective randomized controlled trial, LapOpHuva compared clinical and oncological outcomes of laparoscopic vs. open liver resection for CRLM in 193 patients. They confirmed the short-term outcomes reported in OSLO-COMET while also demonstrating lower global morbidity (11.5% vs. 23.7%, $p = 0.025$), similar rates of severe complications (13.4% vs. 6.25%, $p = 0.095$), and similar 5-year OS (49.3% vs. 47.4%, $p = 0.82$) and DFS (22.7% vs. 23.9%, $p = 0.23$) for the laparoscopic compared to open resection group [107].

While the OSLO-COMET and LapOpHuva trials demonstrated that a minimally invasive approach improved short-term outcomes without compromising early oncologic indicators, it remains difficult to make conclusions on long-term outcomes due to relatively short minimum patient follow-up times in the studies. However, recent meta-analyses have reported comparable long-term outcomes [108, 109] with one patient-level meta-analysis reporting a long-term survival benefit of laparoscopic resection over open resection of CRLM [110].

Recent advancements in robotic surgery have resulted in increasing use of the robotic system for major liver resections. While larger studies demonstrating long-term outcomes, specifically for robotic liver resections for CRLM are scarce, a number of retrospective studies have described robotic liver surgery to be associated with shorter ICU and overall hospital length of stay while not compromising oncological margins [111, 112].

Transplantation

For patients with unresectable CRLM without extrahepatic disease, liver transplantation could offer an avenue for an R0 resection. Transplantation for unresectable CRLM remains controversial due to the limited evidence supporting its use and the scarcity of liver grafts in most countries. With advancements in systemic therapy for colorectal cancer and in liver transplantation, there has been a renewed interest in the potential benefit of liver transplant for patients with unresectable CRLM.

SECA-I was the first prospective trial examining liver transplantation for non-resectable CRLM and it reported a 60% 5-year survival [113]. The subsequent SECA-II study employed stricter selection criteria and reported an improved 5-year survival of 83% [114]. It should be noted that this was a highly selected population of 15 patients, and at the time of last report, 8 had experienced recurrent disease. While these recent studies have demonstrated more promising results, they also highlight the need for further studies at high-volume transplant centers with strict selection criteria before liver transplantation can be widely recommended for a highly selected group of patients.

Disappearing Liver Metastases

After initial systemic chemotherapy, CRLM may shrink dramatically in size and sometimes disappear completely on repeat cross-sectional imaging studies. These lesions that demonstrate complete radiographic response are termed disappearing liver metastases (DLM). Though DLMs may vanish radiographically, DLMs may only represent complete pathological response in 17% to 69% of cases [115–120]. For the remainder of cases, the sites of DLMs may harbor persistent residual disease posing the risk of future regrowth if those sites are not resected.

When there is concern over a DLM, additional imaging with higher sensitivity should be performed. MRI with gadoxetate disodium is an excellent preoperative imaging modality for assessing DLMs after chemotherapy [121]. A systematic review and meta-analysis comparing imaging modalities for DLMs after chemotherapy found MRI using gadoxetate disodium and CE-IOUS to have the highest negative predictive values at 0.73 and 0.79, respectively, when compared with IOUS, CT, and PET (0.54, 0.47, and 0.22, respectively) [121]. For tumors not identified preoperatively, careful use of IOUS to attempt identification of DLMs should be performed. CE-IOUS, though not widely used in the United States, has been shown to further improve detection of DLMs [78].

If despite rigorous preoperative imaging, intraoperative US, palpation, and visual inspection the lesion cannot be located, it is deemed a "missing lesion." While missing lesions in areas of the liver that will already be resected do not present an issue, the challenge arises when they are located in a part of the liver that would drastically change the surgical plan or affect the future liver remnant volume. There remains no true consensus for how these lesions are managed. Due to the low rate of true complete response, the typical paradigm has been to recommend complete resection of all original DLM sites when possible [119]. Multiple systematic reviews have reported that resection of DLM sites has been associated with decreased local recurrence risk and longer disease-free survival. However, resection of all sites of DLMs has not been shown to have a clear OS benefit [122, 123].

Postoperatively, close follow-up with repeat MRI every 3 months for the first year and then every 6 months thereafter has been recommended for patients with unresected DLM sites to allow for rigorous monitoring and timely intervention for any detectable recurrence [121]. Interestingly, postoperative FUDR HAIP chemotherapy may also help sustain remission in the setting of multiple missing lesions [117].

Treatment Sequencing for Synchronous Colorectal Cancer and Liver Metastasis

Synchronous CRLM occurs in 15–20% of patients presenting with colorectal cancer [124]. This setting poses the therapeutic dilemma of determining the optimal approach for the sequencing and combinations of treatment modalities. Historically, patients with synchronous disease underwent staged resection with initial resection of the primary tumor followed by hepatic resection for CRLM in a second operation. With improvements in operative experience and technique, as well as in perioperative management, simultaneous resection has become progressively more popular, carrying the purported benefits of shorter time to definitive control of all tumor burden, earlier initiation of adjuvant chemotherapy, decreasing the need for repeat interventions, and reducing the potential costs and complications that may be associated with multiple interventions.

A number of retrospective studies comparing these two approaches have been published with often contradictory results, largely failing to generate a consensus. In an attempt to answer this question, METASYNC, the first prospective randomized controlled trial comparing patients with synchronous colorectal cancer and resectable CRLM who were randomized to either simultaneous ($n = 39$) or delayed ($n = 46$) resection of the metastases was recently published. The primary outcome was the percentage of patients with major postoperative complications at either surgical site, for which they found no significant difference between the two groups. Interestingly, in the secondary outcomes, they found that at 2 years, OS and DFS tended to be improved for the simultaneous-resection group ($p = 0.05$) [125]. While METASYNC provides evidence to support simultaneous resection, it did not address more challenging situations such as scenarios involving a major hepatectomy combined with complex rectal surgery. Ultimately, all presented factors including the degree of metastatic liver disease, the patient's symptomatology, adjuvant therapy, and degree of complexity of each site's surgical resection need to be carefully considered when deciding on the best approach [126, 127].

A third strategy in which a liver-first staged approach is taken has also been described in the context of synchronous CRLM. In the setting of an asymptomatic primary tumor and initially unresectable or borderline metastases, patients can undergo preoperative conversion chemotherapy followed by hepatectomy and further chemotherapy before undergoing resection of the primary tumor. This approach confers the advantage of earlier delivery of systemic chemotherapy to treat micrometastatic disease and, in the current era of rectal cancer care, the potential for non-operative management of the primary tumor if a complete clinical response is achieved (particularly after radiation therapy to the rectum has also been delivered). Studies have demonstrated comparable perioperative morbidity and survival rates between primary-first and liver-first management approaches [128–130], with a relatively low rate of up to 19% for primary tumor-related complications while on chemotherapy [131, 132].

Conclusion

Once considered the terminal, universally lethal manifestation of colorectal cancer, colorectal liver metastases can now be managed with a diverse array of locoregional therapies, offering potential for cure in certain well-selected patients. Strides in imaging have allowed for the earlier detection and more accurate assessment of resectability while advancements in systemic therapy have increased the number of potential patients who may benefit from curative-intent surgical therapy. Thanks to improvements in surgical techniques and perioperative care, hepatic resection can be safely performed in experienced centers. As research continues to expand our understanding of the disease, allowing the development of better diagnostic, prognostic, and therapeutic tools, and as we refine our treatment paradigm to optimize the delivery of local and systemic care, there is reason to hope and anticipate that the prognosis and quality of life of patients with colorectal liver metastases will continue to improve.

References

1. Siegel RL, Miller KD, Fuchs HE, Jemal A, et al. Cancer J Clin. 2021;71(1):7–33. https://doi.org/10.3322/caac.21654. Epub 2021 Jan 12. Erratum in: CA Cancer J Clin. 2021;71(4):359
2. Kow AWC. Hepatic metastasis from colorectal cancer. J Gastrointest Oncol. 2019;10(6):1274–98. https://doi.org/10.21037/jgo.2019.08.06.
3. Engstrand J, Nilsson H, Strömberg C, Jonas E, Freedman J. Colorectal cancer liver metastases—a population-based study on incidence, management and survival. BMC Cancer. 2018;18(1):78. https://doi.org/10.1186/s12885-017-3925-x.
4. Adson MA. Resection of liver metastases—when is it worthwhile? World J Surg. 1987;11(4):511–20. https://doi.org/10.1007/BF01655817.
5. House MG, Ito H, Gönen M, Fong Y, Allen PJ, DeMatteo RP, Brennan MF, Blumgart LH, Jarnagin WR, D'Angelica MI. Survival after hepatic resection for metastatic colorectal cancer: trends in outcomes for 1,600 patients during two decades at a single institution. J Am Coll Surg. 2010;210(5):744–52. https://doi.org/10.1016/j.jamcollsurg.2009.12.040.
6. Sahani DV, Bajwa MA, Andrabi Y, Bajpai S, Cusack JC. Current status of imaging and emerging techniques to evaluate liver metastases from colorectal carcinoma. Ann Surg. 2014;259(5):861–72. https://doi.org/10.1097/SLA.0000000000000525.
7. Soyer P, Poccard M, Boudiaf M, Abitbol M, Hamzi L, Panis Y, Valleur P, Rymer R. Detection of hypovascular hepatic metastases at triple-phase helical CT: sensitivity of phases and comparison with surgical and histopathologic findings. Radiology. 2004;231(2):413–20. https://doi.org/10.1148/radiol.2312021639. Epub 2004 Mar 24
8. Owen JW, Fowler KJ, Doyle MB, Saad NE, Linehan DC, Chapman WC. Colorectal liver metastases: disappearing lesions in the era of

Eovist hepatobiliary magnetic resonance imaging. HPB (Oxford). 2016;18(3):296–303. https://doi.org/10.1016/j.hpb.2015.10.009. Epub 2016 Mar 14
9. Moulton CA, Gu CS, Law CH, Tandan VR, Hart R, Quan D, Fairfull Smith RJ, Jalink DW, Husien M, Serrano PE, Hendler AL, Haider MA, Ruo L, Gulenchyn KY, Finch T, Julian JA, Levine MN, Gallinger S. Effect of PET before liver resection on surgical management for colorectal adenocarcinoma metastases: a randomized clinical trial. JAMA. 2014;311(18):1863–9. https://doi.org/10.1001/jama.2014.3740.
10. Bennink RJ, Dinant S, Erdogan D, Heijnen BH, Straatsburg IH, van Vliet AK, van Gulik TM. Preoperative assessment of postoperative remnant liver function using hepatobiliary scintigraphy. J Nucl Med. 2004;45(6):965–71.
11. Dinant S, de Graaf W, Verwer BJ, Bennink RJ, van Lienden KP, Gouma DJ, van Vliet AK, van Gulik TM. Risk assessment of posthepatectomy liver failure using hepatobiliary scintigraphy and CT volumetry. J Nucl Med. 2007;48(5):685–92. https://doi.org/10.2967/jnumed.106.038430.
12. Wakiya T, Kudo D, Toyoki Y, Ishido K, Kimura N, Narumi S, Kijima H, Hakamada K. Evaluation of the usefulness of the indocyanine green clearance test for chemotherapy-associated liver injury in patients with colorectal cancer liver metastasis. Ann Surg Oncol. 2014;21(1):167–72. https://doi.org/10.1245/s10434-013-3203-3.
13. Yokoyama Y, Nishio H, Ebata T, Igami T, Sugawara G, Nagino M. Value of indocyanine green clearance of the future liver remnant in predicting outcome after resection for biliary cancer. Br J Surg. 2010;97(8):1260–8. https://doi.org/10.1002/bjs.7084.
14. Mizutani Y, Hirai T, Nagamachi S, Nanashima A, Yano K, Kondo K, Hiyoshi M, Imamura N, Terada T. Prediction of posthepatectomy liver failure proposed by the international study group of liver surgery: residual liver function estimation with 99mTc-galactosyl human serum albumin scintigraphy. Clin Nucl Med. 2018;43(2):77–81. https://doi.org/10.1097/RLU.0000000000001913.
15. Rassam F, Olthof PB, Bennink RJ, van Gulik TM. Current modalities for the assessment of future remnant liver function. Visc Med. 2017;33(6):442–8. https://doi.org/10.1159/000480385. Epub 2017 Nov 30
16. de Graaf W, Bennink RJ, Veteläinen R, van Gulik TM. Nuclear imaging techniques for the assessment of hepatic function in liver surgery and transplantation. J Nucl Med. 2010;51(5):742–52. https://doi.org/10.2967/jnumed.109.069435. Epub 2010 Apr 15
17. Shindoh J, Truty MJ, Aloia TA, Curley SA, Zimmitti G, Huang SY, Mahvash A, Gupta S, Wallace MJ, Vauthey JN. Kinetic growth rate after portal vein embolization predicts posthepatectomy outcomes: toward zero liver-related mortality in patients with colorectal liver metastases and small future liver remnant. J Am Coll Surg. 2013;216(2):201–9. https://doi.org/10.1016/j.jamcollsurg.2012.10.018. Epub 2012 Dec 7

18. Huiskens J, Olthof PB, van der Stok EP, Bais T, van Lienden KP, Moelker A, Krumeich J, Roumen RM, Grünhagen DJ, Punt CJA, van Amerongen M, de Wilt JHW, Verhoef C, Van Gulik TM. Does portal vein embolization prior to liver resection influence the oncological outcomes—a propensity score matched comparison. Eur J Surg Oncol. 2018;44(1):108–14. https://doi.org/10.1016/j.ejso.2017.09.017. Epub 2017 Sep 20
19. Adam R, Laurent A, Azoulay D, Castaing D, Bismuth H. Two-stage hepatectomy: a planned strategy to treat irresectable liver tumors. Ann Surg. 2000;232(6):777–85. https://doi.org/10.1097/00000658-200012000-00006.
20. Lang H, Baumgart J, Mittler J. Associated liver partition and portal vein ligation for staged hepatectomy (ALPPS) registry: what have we learned? Gut Liver. 2020;14(6):699–706. https://doi.org/10.5009/gnl19233.
21. Sandström P, Røsok BI, Sparrelid E, Larsen PN, Larsson AL, Lindell G, Schultz NA, Bjørnbeth BA, Isaksson B, Rizell M, Björnsson B. ALPPS improves resectability compared with conventional two-stage hepatectomy in patients with advanced colorectal liver metastasis: results from a scandinavian multicenter randomized controlled trial (LIGRO trial). Ann Surg. 2018;267(5):833–40. https://doi.org/10.1097/SLA.0000000000002511.
22. Sparrelid E, Hasselgren K, Røsok BI, et al. How should liver hypertrophy be stimulated? A comparison of upfront associating liver partition and portal vein ligation for staged hepatectomy (ALPPS) and portal vein embolization (PVE) with rescue possibility. Hepatobiliary Surg Nutr. 2021;10(1):1–8. https://doi.org/10.21037/hbsn.2019.10.36.
23. Nordlinger B, Guiguet M, Vaillant JC, Balladur P, Boudjema K, Bachellier P, Jaeck D. Surgical resection of colorectal carcinoma metastases to the liver. A prognostic scoring system to improve case selection, based on 1568 patients. Cancer. 1996;77(7):1254–62.
24. Fong Y, Fortner J, Sun RL, Brennan MF, Blumgart LH. Clinical score for predicting recurrence after hepatic resection for metastatic colorectal cancer: analysis of 1001 consecutive cases. Ann Surg. 1999;230(3):309–18.; discussion 318–21. https://doi.org/10.1097/00000658-199909000-00004.
25. Karagkounis G, Torbenson MS, Daniel HD, Azad NS, Diaz LA Jr, Donehower RC, Hirose K, Ahuja N, Pawlik TM, Choti MA. Incidence and prognostic impact of KRAS and BRAF mutation in patients undergoing liver surgery for colorectal metastases. Cancer. 2013;119(23):4137–44. https://doi.org/10.1002/cncr.28347. Epub 2013 Sep 19
26. Vauthey JN, Zimmitti G, Kopetz SE, Shindoh J, Chen SS, Andreou A, Curley SA, Aloia TA, Maru DM. RAS mutation status predicts survival and patterns of recurrence in patients undergoing hepatectomy for

colorectal liver metastases. Ann Surg. 2013;258(4):619–26.; discussion 626–7. https://doi.org/10.1097/SLA.0b013e3182a5025a.
27. Margonis GA, Buettner S, Andreatos N, Kim Y, Wagner D, Sasaki K, Beer A, Schwarz C, Løes IM, Smolle M, Kamphues C, He J, Pawlik TM, Kaczirek K, Poultsides G, Lønning PE, Cameron JL, Burkhart RA, Gerger A, Aucejo FN, Kreis ME, Wolfgang CL, Weiss MJ. Association of BRAF mutations with survival and recurrence in surgically treated patients with metastatic colorectal liver cancer. JAMA Surg. 2018;153(7):e180996. https://doi.org/10.1001/jamasurg.2018.0996. Epub 2018 Jul 18
28. Brudvik KW, Jones RP, Giuliante F, Shindoh J, Passot G, Chung MH, Song J, Li L, Dagenborg VJ, Fretland ÅA, Røsok B, De Rose AM, Ardito F, Edwin B, Panettieri E, Larocca LM, Yamashita S, Conrad C, Aloia TA, Poston GJ, Bjørnbeth BA, Vauthey JN. RAS mutation clinical risk score to predict survival after resection of colorectal liver metastases. Ann Surg. 2019;269(1):120–6. https://doi.org/10.1097/SLA.0000000000002319.
29. Margonis GA, Sasaki K, Gholami S, Kim Y, Andreatos N, Rezaee N, Deshwar A, Buettner S, Allen PJ, Kingham TP, Pawlik TM, He J, Cameron JL, Jarnagin WR, Wolfgang CL, D'Angelica MI, Weiss MJ. Genetic and morphological evaluation (GAME) score for patients with colorectal liver metastases. Br J Surg. 2018;105(9):1210–20. https://doi.org/10.1002/bjs.10838. Epub 2018 Apr 25
30. Bryant G. DSC measurement of cell suspensions during successive freezing runs: implications for the mechanisms of intracellular ice formation. Cryobiology. 1995 Apr;32(2):114–28. https://doi.org/10.1006/cryo.1995.1011.
31. McGahan JP, Brock JM, Tesluk H, Gu WZ, Schneider P, Browning PD. Hepatic ablation with use of radio-frequency electrocautery in the animal model. J Vasc Interv Radiol. 1992;3(2):291–7. https://doi.org/10.1016/s1051-0443(92)72028-4.
32. Wood TF, Rose DM, Chung M, Allegra DP, Foshag LJ, Bilchik AJ. Radiofrequency ablation of 231 unresectable hepatic tumors: indications, limitations, and complications. Ann Surg Oncol. 2000;7(8):593–600. https://doi.org/10.1007/BF02725339.
33. Gillams A, Goldberg N, Ahmed M, Bale R, Breen D, Callstrom M, Chen MH, Choi BI, de Baere T, Dupuy D, Gangi A, Gervais D, Helmberger T, Jung EM, Lee F, Lencioni R, Liang P, Livraghi T, Lu D, Meloni F, Pereira P, Piscaglia F, Rhim H, Salem R, Sofocleous C, Solomon SB, Soulen M, Tanaka M, Vogl T, Wood B, Solbiati L. Thermal ablation of colorectal liver metastases: a position paper by an international panel of ablation experts, the interventional oncology sans Frontières meeting 2013. Eur Radiol. 2015;25(12):3438–54. https://doi.org/10.1007/s00330-015-3779-z. Epub 2015 May 22

34. Ruers T, Van Coevorden F, Punt CJ, Pierie JE, Borel-Rinkes I, Ledermann JA, Poston G, Bechstein W, Lentz MA, Mauer M, Folprecht G, Van Cutsem E, Ducreux M, Nordlinger B, European Organisation for Research and Treatment of Cancer (EORTC), Gastro-Intestinal Tract Cancer Group; Arbeitsgruppe Lebermetastasen und tumoren in der Chirurgischen Arbeitsgemeinschaft Onkologie (ALM-CAO), National Cancer Research Institute Colorectal Clinical Study Group (NCRI CCSG). Local treatment of unresectable colorectal liver metastases: Results of a randomized phase II trial. J Natl Cancer Inst. 2017;109(9):djx015. https://doi.org/10.1093/jnci/djx015.
35. Puijk RS, Ruarus AH, Vroomen LGPH, van Tilborg AAJM, Scheffer HJ, Nielsen K, de Jong MC, de Vries JJJ, Zonderhuis BM, Eker HH, Kazemier G, Verheul H, van der Meijs BB, van Dam L, Sorgedrager N, Coupé VMH, van den Tol PMP, Meijerink MR, COLLISION Trial Group. Colorectal liver metastases: surgery versus thermal ablation (COLLISION)—a phase III single-blind prospective randomized controlled trial. BMC Cancer. 2018;18(1):821. https://doi.org/10.1186/s12885-018-4716-8.
36. Gavriilidis P, Roberts KJ, de Angelis N, Aldrighetti L, Sutcliffe RP. Recurrence and survival following microwave, radiofrequency ablation, and hepatic resection of colorectal liver metastases: a systematic review and network meta-analysis. Hepatobiliary Pancreat Dis Int. 2021;20(4):307–14. https://doi.org/10.1016/j.hbpd.2021.05.004. Epub 2021 Jun 4
37. Nieuwenhuizen S, Puijk RS, van den Bemd B, Aldrighetti L, Arntz M, van den Boezem PB, Bruynzeel AME, Burgmans MC, de Cobelli F, Coolsen MME, Dejong CHC, Derks S, Diederik A, van Duijvendijk P, Eker HH, Engelsman AF, Erdmann JI, Fütterer JJ, Geboers B, Groot G, Haasbeek CJA, Janssen JJ, de Jong KP, Kater GM, Kazemier G, Kruimer JWH, Leclercq WKG, van der Leij C, Manusama ER, Meier MAJ, van der Meijs BB, Melenhorst MCAM, Nielsen K, Nijkamp MW, Potters FH, Prevoo W, Rietema FJ, Ruarus AH, Ruiter SJS, Schouten EAC, Serafino GP, Sietses C, Swijnenburg RJ, Timmer FEF, Versteeg KS, Vink T, de Vries JJJ, de Wilt JHW, Zonderhuis BM, Scheffer HJ, van den Tol PMP, Meijerink MR. Resectability and ablatability criteria for the treatment of liver only colorectal metastases: multidisciplinary consensus document from the COLLISION trial group. Cancers (Basel). 2020;12(7):1779. https://doi.org/10.3390/cancers12071779.
38. Jones C, Badger SA, Ellis G. The role of microwave ablation in the management of hepatic colorectal metastases. Surgeon. 2011;9(1):33–7. https://doi.org/10.1016/j.surge.2010.07.009. Epub 2010 Aug 21
39. Shady W, Petre EN, Do KG, Gonen M, Yarmohammadi H, Brown KT, Kemeny NE, D'Angelica M, Kingham PT, Solomon SB, Sofocleous CT. Percutaneous microwave versus radiofrequency ablation of colorectal liver metastases: ablation with clear margins (A0) provides the best

local tumor control. J Vasc Interv Radiol. 2018;29(2):268–275.e1. https://doi.org/10.1016/j.jvir.2017.08.021. Epub 2017 Dec 6
40. Vogl TJ, Farshid P, Naguib NN, Darvishi A, Bazrafshan B, Mbalisike E, Burkhard T, Zangos S. Thermal ablation of liver metastases from colorectal cancer: radiofrequency, microwave and laser ablation therapies. Radiol Med. 2014;119(7):451–61. https://doi.org/10.1007/s11547-014-0415-y. Epub 2014 Jun 4
41. Di Martino M, Rompianesi G, Mora-Guzmán I, Martín-Pérez E, Montalti R, Troisi RI. Systematic review and meta-analysis of local ablative therapies for resectable colorectal liver metastases. Eur J Surg Oncol. 2020;46(5):772–81. https://doi.org/10.1016/j.ejso.2019.12.003. Epub 2019 Dec 4
42. Correa-Gallego C, Fong Y, Gonen M, D'Angelica MI, Allen PJ, DeMatteo RP, Jarnagin WR, Kingham TP. A retrospective comparison of microwave ablation vs. radiofrequency ablation for colorectal cancer hepatic metastases. Ann Surg Oncol. 2014;21(13):4278–83. https://doi.org/10.1245/s10434-014-3817-0. Epub 2014 Jun 3
43. Davalos RV, Mir IL, Rubinsky B. Tissue ablation with irreversible electroporation. Ann Biomed Eng. 2005;33(2):223–31. https://doi.org/10.1007/s10439-005-8981-8.
44. Scheffer HJ, Nielsen K, de Jong MC, van Tilborg AA, Vieveen JM, Bouwman AR, Meijer S, van Kuijk C, van den Tol PM, Meijerink MR. Irreversible electroporation for nonthermal tumor ablation in the clinical setting: a systematic review of safety and efficacy. J Vasc Interv Radiol. 2014;25(7):997–1011. https://doi.org/10.1016/j.jvir.2014.01.028. quiz 1011; Epub 2014 Mar 18
45. Scheffer HJ, Melenhorst MC, Echenique AM, Nielsen K, van Tilborg AA, van den Bos W, Vroomen LG, van den Tol PM, Meijerink MR. Irreversible electroporation for colorectal liver metastases. Tech Vasc Interv Radiol. 2015;18(3):159–69. https://doi.org/10.1053/j.tvir.2015.06.007. Epub 2015 Jun 18
46. Timmerman RD, Herman J, Cho LC. Emergence of stereotactic body radiation therapy and its impact on current and future clinical practice. J Clin Oncol. 2014;32(26):2847–54. https://doi.org/10.1200/JCO.2014.55.4675. Epub 2014 Aug 11
47. Palma DA, Olson R, Harrow S, Gaede S, Louie AV, Haasbeek C, Mulroy L, Lock M, Rodrigues GB, Yaremko BP, Schellenberg D, Ahmad B, Griffioen G, Senthi S, Swaminath A, Kopek N, Liu M, Moore K, Currie S, Bauman GS, Warner A, Senan S. Stereotactic ablative radiotherapy versus standard of care palliative treatment in patients with oligometastatic cancers (SABR-COMET): a randomised, phase 2, open-label trial. Lancet. 2019;393(10185):2051–8. https://doi.org/10.1016/S0140-6736(18)32487-5. Epub 2019 Apr 11
48. Scorsetti M, Comito T, Tozzi A, Navarria P, Fogliata A, Clerici E, Mancosu P, Reggiori G, Rimassa L, Torzilli G, Tomatis S, Santoro A,

Cozzi L. Final results of a phase II trial for stereotactic body radiation therapy for patients with inoperable liver metastases from colorectal cancer. J Cancer Res Clin Oncol. 2015;141(3):543–53. https://doi.org/10.1007/s00432-014-1833-x. Epub 2014 Sep 23
49. McPartlin A, Swaminath A, Wang R, Pintilie M, Brierley J, Kim J, Ringash J, Wong R, Dinniwell R, Craig T, Dawson LA. Long-term outcomes of phase 1 and 2 studies of SBRT for hepatic colorectal metastases. Int J Radiat Oncol Biol Phys. 2017;99(2):388–95. https://doi.org/10.1016/j.ijrobp.2017.04.010. Epub 2017 Apr 13
50. Yoshino T, Arnold D, Taniguchi H, Pentheroudakis G, Yamazaki K, Xu RH, Kim TW, Ismail F, Tan IB, Yeh KH, Grothey A, Zhang S, Ahn JB, Mastura MY, Chong D, Chen LT, Kopetz S, Eguchi-Nakajima T, Ebi H, Ohtsu A, Cervantes A, Muro K, Tabernero J, Minami H, Ciardiello F, Douillard JY. Pan-Asian adapted ESMO consensus guidelines for the management of patients with metastatic colorectal cancer: a JSMO-ESMO initiative endorsed by CSCO, KACO, MOS, SSO and TOS. Ann Oncol. 2018;29(1):44–70. https://doi.org/10.1093/annonc/mdx738.
51. Lewis HL, Bloomston M. Hepatic artery Infusional chemotherapy. Surg Clin North Am. 2016;96(2):341–55. https://doi.org/10.1016/j.suc.2015.11.002. Epub 2016 Feb 16
52. Kemeny N, Huang Y, Cohen AM, Shi W, Conti JA, Brennan MF, Bertino JR, Turnbull AD, Sullivan D, Stockman J, Blumgart LH, Fong Y. Hepatic arterial infusion of chemotherapy after resection of hepatic metastases from colorectal cancer. N Engl J Med. 1999;341(27):2039–48. https://doi.org/10.1056/NEJM199912303412702.
53. Pak LM, Kemeny NE, Capanu M, Chou JF, Boucher T, Cercek A, Balachandran VP, Kingham TP, Allen PJ, DeMatteo RP, Jarnagin WR, D'Angelica MI. Prospective phase II trial of combination hepatic artery infusion and systemic chemotherapy for unresectable colorectal liver metastases: long term results and curative potential. J Surg Oncol. 2018;117(4):634–43. https://doi.org/10.1002/jso.24898. Epub 2017 Nov 22
54. Groot Koerkamp B, Sadot E, Kemeny NE, Gönen M, Leal JN, Allen PJ, Cercek A, DeMatteo RP, Kingham TP, Jarnagin WR, D'Angelica MI. Perioperative hepatic arterial infusion pump chemotherapy is associated with longer survival after resection of colorectal liver metastases: a propensity score analysis. J Clin Oncol. 2017;35(17):1938–44. https://doi.org/10.1200/JCO.2016.71.8346. Epub 2017 Apr 20
55. Gholami S, Kemeny NE, Boucher TM, Gönen M, Cercek A, Kingham TP, Balachandran V, Allen P, DeMatteo R, Drebin J, Jarnagin W, D'Angelica M. Adjuvant hepatic artery infusion chemotherapy is associated with improved survival regardless of KRAS mutation status in patients with resected colorectal liver metastases: a retrospective analysis of 674 patients. Ann Surg. 2020;272(2):352–6. https://doi.org/10.1097/SLA.0000000000003248.

56. Buisman FE, Homs MYV, Grünhagen DJ, Filipe WF, Bennink RJ, Besselink MGH, Borel Rinkes IHM, Bruijnen RCG, Cercek A, D'Angelica MI, van Delden OM, Donswijk ML, van Doorn L, Doornebosch PG, Emmering J, Erdmann JI, NS IJ, Grootscholten C, Hagendoorn J, Kemeny NE, Kingham TP, Klompenhouwer EG, Kok NFM, Koolen S, Kuhlmann KFD, Kuiper MC, Lam MGE, Mathijssen RHJ, Moelker A, Oomen-de Hoop E, Punt CJA, Te Riele WW, Roodhart JML, Swijnenburg RJ, Prevoo W, Tanis PJ, Vermaas M, Versleijen MWJ, Veuger FP, Weterman MJ, Verhoef C, Groot Koerkamp B. Adjuvant hepatic arterial infusion pump chemotherapy and resection versus resection alone in patients with low-risk resectable colorectal liver metastases—the multicenter randomized controlled PUMP trial. BMC Cancer. 2019;19(1):327. https://doi.org/10.1186/s12885-019-5515-6.
57. de Gramont A, Figer A, Seymour M, Homerin M, Hmissi A, Cassidy J, Boni C, Cortes-Funes H, Cervantes A, Freyer G, Papamichael D, Le Bail N, Louvet C, Hendler D, de Braud F, Wilson C, Morvan F, Bonetti A. Leucovorin and fluorouracil with or without oxaliplatin as first-line treatment in advanced colorectal cancer. J Clin Oncol. 2000;18(16):2938–47. https://doi.org/10.1200/JCO.2000.18.16.2938.
58. Giacchetti S, Perpoint B, Zidani R, Le Bail N, Faggiuolo R, Focan C, Chollet P, Llory JF, Letourneau Y, Coudert B, Bertheaut-Cvitkovic F, Larregain-Fournier D, Le Rol A, Walter S, Adam R, Misset JL, Lévi F. Phase III multicenter randomized trial of oxaliplatin added to chronomodulated fluorouracil-leucovorin as first-line treatment of metastatic colorectal cancer. J Clin Oncol. 2000;18(1):136–47. https://doi.org/10.1200/JCO.2000.18.1.136.
59. Douillard JY, Cunningham D, Roth AD, Navarro M, James RD, Karasek P, Jandik P, Iveson T, Carmichael J, Alakl M, Gruia G, Awad L, Rougier P. Irinotecan combined with fluorouracil compared with fluorouracil alone as first-line treatment for metastatic colorectal cancer: a multicentre randomised trial. Lancet. 2000;355(9209):1041–7. https://doi.org/10.1016/s0140-6736(00)02034-1. Erratum in: Lancet 2000 Apr 15;355(9212):1372
60. Petrelli F, Cabiddu M, Barni S. 5-Fluorouracil or capecitabine in the treatment of advanced colorectal cancer: a pooled-analysis of randomized trials. Med Oncol. 2012;29(2):1020–9. https://doi.org/10.1007/s12032-011-9958-0. Epub 2011 Apr 24
61. Hurwitz H, Fehrenbacher L, Novotny W, Cartwright T, Hainsworth J, Heim W, Berlin J, Baron A, Griffing S, Holmgren E, Ferrara N, Fyfe G, Rogers B, Ross R, Kabbinavar F. Bevacizumab plus irinotecan, fluorouracil, and leucovorin for metastatic colorectal cancer. N Engl J Med. 2004;350(23):2335–42. https://doi.org/10.1056/NEJMoa032691.
62. Saltz LB, Clarke S, Díaz-Rubio E, Scheithauer W, Figer A, Wong R, Koski S, Lichinitser M, Yang TS, Rivera F, Couture F, Sirzén F, Cassidy

J. Bevacizumab in combination with oxaliplatin-based chemotherapy as first-line therapy in metastatic colorectal cancer: a randomized phase III study. J Clin Oncol. 2008;26(12):2013–9. https://doi.org/10.1200/JCO.2007.14.9930. Erratum in: J Clin Oncol. 2008 Jun;26(18):3110. Erratum in: J Clin Oncol 2009 Feb 1;27(4):653
63. Macedo LT, da Costa Lima AB, Sasse AD. Addition of bevacizumab to first-line chemotherapy in advanced colorectal cancer: a systematic review and meta-analysis, with emphasis on chemotherapy subgroups. BMC Cancer. 2012;12:89. https://doi.org/10.1186/1471-2407-12-89.
64. Nordlinger B, Sorbye H, Glimelius B, Poston GJ, Schlag PM, Rougier P, Bechstein WO, Primrose JN, Walpole ET, Finch-Jones M, Jaeck D, Mirza D, Parks RW, Collette L, Praet M, Bethe U, Van Cutsem E, Scheithauer W, Gruenberger T, EORTC Gastro-Intestinal Tract Cancer Group, Cancer Research UK, Arbeitsgruppe Lebermetastasen und-tumoren in der Chirurgischen Arbeitsgemeinschaft Onkologie (ALM-CAO), Australasian Gastro-Intestinal Trials Group (AGITG), Fédération Francophone de Cancérologie Digestive (FFCD). Perioperative chemotherapy with FOLFOX4 and surgery versus surgery alone for resectable liver metastases from colorectal cancer (EORTC Intergroup trial 40983): a randomised controlled trial. Lancet. 2008;371(9617):1007–16. https://doi.org/10.1016/S0140-6736(08)60455-9.
65. Nordlinger B, Sorbye H, Glimelius B, Poston GJ, Schlag PM, Rougier P, Bechstein WO, Primrose JN, Walpole ET, Finch-Jones M, Jaeck D, Mirza D, Parks RW, Mauer M, Tanis E, Van Cutsem E, Scheithauer W, Gruenberger T, EORTC Gastro-Intestinal Tract Cancer Group, Cancer Research UK, Arbeitsgruppe Lebermetastasen und–tumoren in der Chirurgischen Arbeitsgemeinschaft Onkologie (ALM-CAO), Australasian Gastro-Intestinal Trials Group (AGITG), Fédération Francophone de Cancérologie Digestive (FFCD). Perioperative FOLFOX4 chemotherapy and surgery versus surgery alone for resectable liver metastases from colorectal cancer (EORTC 40983): long-term results of a randomised, controlled, phase 3 trial. Lancet Oncol. 2013;14(12):1208–15. https://doi.org/10.1016/S1470-2045(13)70447-9. Epub 2013 Oct 11
66. Kanemitsu Y, Shimizu Y, Mizusawa J, Inaba Y, Hamaguchi T, Shida D, Ohue M, Komori K, Shiomi A, Shiozawa M, Watanabe J, Suto T, Kinugasa Y, Takii Y, Bando H, Kobatake T, Inomata M, Shimada Y, Katayama H, Fukuda H, JCOG Colorectal Cancer Study Group. Hepatectomy followed by mFOLFOX6 versus hepatectomy alone for liver-only metastatic colorectal cancer (JCOG0603): a phase II or III randomized controlled trial. J Clin Oncol. 2021;39(34):3789–99. https://doi.org/10.1200/JCO.21.01032. Epub 2021 Sep 14
67. Liu W, Zhou JG, Sun Y, Zhang L, Xing BC. The role of neoadjuvant chemotherapy for resectable colorectal liver metastases: a systematic

review and meta-analysis. Oncotarget. 2016;7(24):37277–87. https://doi.org/10.18632/oncotarget.8671.
68. Primrose J, Falk S, Finch-Jones M, Valle J, O'Reilly D, Siriwardena A, Hornbuckle J, Peterson M, Rees M, Iveson T, Hickish T, Butler R, Stanton L, Dixon E, Little L, Bowers M, Pugh S, Garden OJ, Cunningham D, Maughan T, Bridgewater J. Systemic chemotherapy with or without cetuximab in patients with resectable colorectal liver metastasis: the new EPOC randomised controlled trial. Lancet Oncol. 2014;15(6):601–11. https://doi.org/10.1016/S1470-2045(14)70105-6. Epub 2014 Apr 7. Erratum in: Lancet Oncol. 2014 Jun;15(7):e253
69. Alberts SR, Horvath WL, Sternfeld WC, Goldberg RM, Mahoney MR, Dakhil SR, Levitt R, Rowland K, Nair S, Sargent DJ, Donohue JH. Oxaliplatin, fluorouracil, and leucovorin for patients with unresectable liver-only metastases from colorectal cancer: a north central cancer treatment group phase II study. J Clin Oncol. 2005;23(36):9243–9. https://doi.org/10.1200/JCO.2005.07.740. Epub 2005 Oct 17
70. Pozzo C, Basso M, Cassano A, Quirino M, Schinzari G, Trigila N, Vellone M, Giuliante F, Nuzzo G, Barone C. Neoadjuvant treatment of unresectable liver disease with irinotecan and 5-fluorouracil plus folinic acid in colorectal cancer patients. Ann Oncol. 2004;15(6):933–9. https://doi.org/10.1093/annonc/mdh217.
71. Ychou M, Rivoire M, Thezenas S, Quenet F, Delpero JR, Rebischung C, Letoublon C, Guimbaud R, Francois E, Ducreux M, Desseigne F, Fabre JM, Assenat E. A randomized phase II trial of three intensified chemotherapy regimens in first-line treatment of colorectal cancer patients with initially unresectable or not optimally resectable liver metastases. The METHEP trial. Ann Surg Oncol. 2013;20(13):4289–97. https://doi.org/10.1245/s10434-013-3217-x. Epub 2013 Aug 17
72. Chen JY, Dai HY, Li CY, Jin Y, Zhu LL, Zhang TF, Zhang YX, Mai WH. Improved sensitivity and positive predictive value of contrast-enhanced intraoperative ultrasound in colorectal cancer liver metastasis: a systematic review and meta-analysis. J Gastrointest Oncol. 2022;13(1):221–30. https://doi.org/10.21037/jgo-21-881.
73. Castaing D, Emond J, Kunstlinger F, Bismuth H. Utility of operative ultrasound in the surgical management of liver tumors. Ann Surg. 1986;204(5):600–5. https://doi.org/10.1097/00000658-198611000-00015.
74. Rifkin MD, Rosato FE, Branch HM, Foster J, Yang SL, Barbot DJ, Marks GJ. Intraoperative ultrasound of the liver. An important adjunctive tool for decision making in the operating room. Ann Surg. 1987;205(5):466–72. https://doi.org/10.1097/00000658-198705000-00004.
75. Shah AJ, Callaway M, Thomas MG, Finch-Jones MD. Contrast-enhanced intraoperative ultrasound improves detection of liver metasta-

ses during surgery for primary colorectal cancer. HPB (Oxford). 2010;12(3):181–7. https://doi.org/10.1111/j.1477-2574.2009.00141.x.
76. Fioole B, de Haas RJ, Wicherts DA, Elias SG, Scheffers JM, van Hillegersberg R, van Leeuwen MS, Borel Rinkes IH. Additional value of contrast enhanced intraoperative ultrasound for colorectal liver metastases. Eur J Radiol. 2008;67(1):169–76. https://doi.org/10.1016/j.ejrad.2007.03.017. Epub 2007 Apr 30
77. Stavrou GA, Stang A, Raptis DA, Schadde E, Zeile M, Brüning R, Wagner KC, Huber TM, Oldhafer KJ. Intraoperative (contrast-enhanced) ultrasound has the highest diagnostic accuracy of any imaging modality in resection of colorectal liver metastases. J Gastrointest Surg. 2021;25(12):3160–9. https://doi.org/10.1007/s11605-021-04925-2. Epub 2021 Jun 22
78. Liu W, Zhang ZY, Yin SS, Yan K, Xing BC. Contrast-enhanced intraoperative ultrasound improved sensitivity and positive predictive value in colorectal liver metastasis: a systematic review and meta-analysis. Ann Surg Oncol. 2021;28(7):3763–73. https://doi.org/10.1245/s10434-020-09365-x. Epub 2020 Nov 27
79. Zorzi D, Mullen JT, Abdalla EK, Pawlik TM, Andres A, Muratore A, Curley SA, Mentha G, Capussotti L, Vauthey JN. Comparison between hepatic wedge resection and anatomic resection for colorectal liver metastases. J Gastrointest Surg. 2006;10(1):86–94. https://doi.org/10.1016/j.gassur.2005.07.022.
80. Sui CJ, Cao L, Li B, Yang JM, Wang SJ, Su X, Zhou YM. Anatomical versus nonanatomical resection of colorectal liver metastases: a meta-analysis. Int J Color Dis. 2012;27(7):939–46. https://doi.org/10.1007/s00384-011-1403-5. Epub 2012 Jan 4
81. Mise Y, Aloia TA, Brudvik KW, Schwarz L, Vauthey JN, Conrad C. Parenchymal-sparing hepatectomy in colorectal liver metastasis improves salvageability and survival. Ann Surg. 2016;263(1):146–52. https://doi.org/10.1097/SLA.0000000000001194.
82. Matsumura M, Mise Y, Saiura A, Inoue Y, Ishizawa T, Ichida H, Matsuki R, Tanaka M, Takeda Y, Takahashi Y. Parenchymal-sparing hepatectomy does not increase intrahepatic recurrence in patients with advanced colorectal liver metastases. Ann Surg Oncol. 2016;23(11):3718–26. https://doi.org/10.1245/s10434-016-5278-0. Epub 2016 May 20
83. Joechle K, Vreeland TJ, Vega EA, Okuno M, Newhook TE, Panettieri E, Chun YS, Tzeng CD, Aloia TA, Lee JE, Vauthey JN. Anatomic resection is not required for colorectal liver metastases with RAS mutation. J Gastrointest Surg. 2020;24(5):1033–9. https://doi.org/10.1007/s11605-019-04299-6. Epub 2020 Mar 10
84. Moris D, Ronnekleiv-Kelly S, Rahnemai-Azar AA, Felekouras E, Dillhoff M, Schmidt C, Pawlik TM. Parenchymal-sparing versus anatomic liver resection for colorectal liver metastases: a systematic review.

J Gastrointest Surg. 2017;21(6):1076–85. https://doi.org/10.1007/s11605-017-3397-y. Epub 2017 Mar 31
85. Masatsune S, Kimura K, Kashiwagi S, En W, Okazaki Y, Maeda K, Hirakawa K, Ohira M. Impact of intraoperative blood loss and blood transfusion on the prognosis of colorectal liver metastasis following curative resection. Anticancer Res. 2021;41(11):5617–23. https://doi.org/10.21873/anticanres.15377.
86. Postlewait LM, Squires MH 3rd, Kooby DA, Weber SM, Scoggins CR, Cardona K, Cho CS, Martin RCG, Winslow ER, Maithel SK. The relationship of blood transfusion with peri-operative and long-term outcomes after major hepatectomy for metastatic colorectal cancer: a multi-institutional study of 456 patients. HPB (Oxford). 2016;18(2):192–9. https://doi.org/10.1016/j.hpb.2015.08.003. Epub 2015 Nov 14
87. Margonis GA, Kim Y, Samaha M, Buettner S, Sasaki K, Gani F, Amini N, Pawlik TM. Blood loss and outcomes after resection of colorectal liver metastases. J Surg Res. 2016;202(2):473–80. https://doi.org/10.1016/j.jss.2016.01.020. Epub 2016 Jan 21
88. Melendez JA, Arslan V, Fischer ME, Wuest D, Jarnagin WR, Fong Y, Blumgart LH. Perioperative outcomes of major hepatic resections under low central venous pressure anesthesia: blood loss, blood transfusion, and the risk of postoperative renal dysfunction. J Am Coll Surg. 1998;187(6):620–5. https://doi.org/10.1016/s1072-7515(98)00240-3.
89. Cunningham JD, Fong Y, Shriver C, Melendez J, Marx WL, Blumgart LH. One hundred consecutive hepatic resections. Blood loss, transfusion, and operative technique. Arch Surg. 1994;129(10):1050–6. https://doi.org/10.1001/archsurg.1994.01420340064011.
90. Pringle JH. Notes on the arrest of hepatic Hemorrhage due to trauma. Ann Surg. 1908;48(4):541–9. https://doi.org/10.1097/00000658-190810000-00005.
91. Lesurtel M, Lehmann K, de Rougemont O, Clavien PA. Clamping techniques and protecting strategies in liver surgery. HPB (Oxford). 2009;11(4):290–5. https://doi.org/10.1111/j.1477-2574.2009.00066.x.
92. Matsuda A, Miyashita M, Matsumoto S, Matsutani T, Sakurazawa N, Akagi I, Kishi T, Yokoi K, Uchida E. Hepatic pedicle clamping does not worsen survival after hepatic resection for colorectal liver metastasis: results from a systematic review and meta-analysis. Ann Surg Oncol. 2013;20(12):3771–8. https://doi.org/10.1245/s10434-013-3048-9. Epub 2013 Jun 18
93. Schiergens TS, Stielow C, Schreiber S, Hornuss C, Jauch KW, Rentsch M, Thasler WE. Liver resection in the elderly: significance of comorbidities and blood loss. J Gastrointest Surg. 2014;18(6):1161–70. https://doi.org/10.1007/s11605-014-2516-2. Epub 2014 Apr 9
94. Schiergens TS, Drefs M, Dörsch M, Kühn F, Albertsmeier M, Niess H, Schoenberg MB, Assenmacher M, Küchenhoff H, Thasler WE, Guba

MO, Angele MK, Rentsch M, Werner J, Andrassy J. Prognostic impact of pedicle clamping during liver resection for colorectal metastases. Cancers (Basel). 2020;13(1):72. https://doi.org/10.3390/cancers13010072.

95. Bratzler DW, Dellinger EP, Olsen KM, Perl TM, Auwaerter PG, Bolon MK, Fish DN, Napolitano LM, Sawyer RG, Slain D, Steinberg JP, Weinstein RA, American Society of Health-System Pharmacists (ASHP), Infectious Diseases Society of America (IDSA), Surgical Infection Society (SIS), Society for Healthcare Epidemiology of America (SHEA). Clinical practice guidelines for antimicrobial prophylaxis in surgery. Surg Infect (Larchmt). 2013;14(1):73–156. https://doi.org/10.1089/sur.2013.9999. Epub 2013 Mar 5

96. Hirokawa F, Hayashi M, Miyamoto Y, Asakuma M, Shimizu T, Komeda K, Inoue Y, Uchiyama K, Nishimura Y. Evaluation of postoperative antibiotic prophylaxis after liver resection: a randomized controlled trial. Am J Surg. 2013;206(1):8–15. https://doi.org/10.1016/j.amjsurg.2012.08.016. Epub 2013 May 22

97. Murtha-Lemekhova A, Fuchs J, Teroerde M, Chiriac U, Klotz R, Hornuss D, Larmann J, Weigand MA, Hoffmann K. Routine postoperative antibiotic prophylaxis offers no benefit after hepatectomy-a systematic review and meta-analysis. Antibiotics (Basel). 2022;11(5):649. https://doi.org/10.3390/antibiotics11050649.

98. Tzeng CW, Katz MH, Fleming JB, Pisters PW, Lee JE, Abdalla EK, Curley SA, Vauthey JN, Aloia TA. Risk of venous thromboembolism outweighs post-hepatectomy bleeding complications: analysis of 5651 National Surgical Quality Improvement Program patients. HPB (Oxford). 2012;14(8):506–13. https://doi.org/10.1111/j.1477-2574.2012.00479.x. Epub 2012 May 15

99. Aloia TA, Geerts WH, Clary BM, Day RW, Hemming AW, D'Albuquerque LC, Vollmer CM Jr, Vauthey JN, Toogood GJ. Venous thromboembolism prophylaxis in liver surgery. J Gastrointest Surg. 2016;20(1):221–9. https://doi.org/10.1007/s11605-015-2902-4.

100. Gould MK, Garcia DA, Wren SM, Karanicolas PJ, Arcelus JI, Heit JA, Samama CM. Prevention of VTE in nonorthopedic surgical patients: antithrombotic therapy and prevention of thrombosis, 9th ed: American College of Chest Physicians Evidence-Based Clinical Practice Guidelines. Chest. 2012;141(2 Suppl):e227S–77S. https://doi.org/10.1378/chest.11-2297. Erratum in: Chest 2012 May;141(5):1369

101. Patel SH, Kim BJ, Tzeng CD, Chun YS, Conrad C, Vauthey JN, Aloia TA. Reduction of cardiopulmonary/renal complications with serum BNP-guided volume status management in posthepatectomy patients. J Gastrointest Surg. 2018;22(3):467–76. https://doi.org/10.1007/s11605-017-3600-1. Epub 2017 Oct 11

102. Metcalfe MS, Mullin EJ, Maddern GJ. Choice of surveillance after hepatectomy for colorectal metastases. Arch Surg. 2004;139(7):749–54. https://doi.org/10.1001/archsurg.139.7.749.

103. Hamady ZZ, Lodge JP, Welsh FK, Toogood GJ, White A, John T, Rees M. One-millimeter cancer-free margin is curative for colorectal liver metastases: a propensity score case-match approach. Ann Surg. 2014;259(3):543–8. https://doi.org/10.1097/SLA.0b013e3182902b6e.
104. Hallet J, Beyfuss K, Memeo R, Karanicolas PJ, Marescaux J, Pessaux P. Short and long-term outcomes of laparoscopic compared to open liver resection for colorectal liver metastases. Hepatobiliary Surg Nutr. 2016;5(4):300–10. https://doi.org/10.21037/hbsn.2016.02.01.
105. Karagkounis G, Akyuz M, Guerron AD, Yazici P, Aucejo FN, Quintini C, Miller CM, Vogt DP, Fung JJ, Berber E. Perioperative and oncologic outcomes of minimally invasive liver resection for colorectal metastases: A case-control study of 130 patients. Surgery. 2016;160(4):1097–103. https://doi.org/10.1016/j.surg.2016.04.043. Epub 2016 Jul 30
106. Fretland ÅA, Dagenborg VJ, Bjørnelv GMW, Kazaryan AM, Kristiansen R, Fagerland MW, Hausken J, Tønnessen TI, Abildgaard A, Barkhatov L, Yaqub S, Røsok BI, Bjørnbeth BA, Andersen MH, Flatmark K, Aas E, Edwin B. Laparoscopic versus open resection for colorectal liver metastases: the OSLO-COMET randomized controlled trial. Ann Surg. 2018;267(2):199–207. https://doi.org/10.1097/SLA.0000000000002353.
107. Robles-Campos R, Lopez-Lopez V, Brusadin R, Lopez-Conesa A, Gil-Vazquez PJ, Navarro-Barrios Á, Parrilla P. Open versus minimally invasive liver surgery for colorectal liver metastases (LapOpHuva): a prospective randomized controlled trial. Surg Endosc. 2019;33(12):3926–36. https://doi.org/10.1007/s00464-019-06679-0. Epub 2019 Jan 30
108. Ciria R, Ocaña S, Gomez-Luque I, Cipriani F, Halls M, Fretland ÅA, Okuda Y, Aroori S, Briceño J, Aldrighetti L, Edwin B, Hilal MA. A systematic review and meta-analysis comparing the short- and long-term outcomes for laparoscopic and open liver resections for liver metastases from colorectal cancer. Surg Endosc. 2020;34(1):349–60. https://doi.org/10.1007/s00464-019-06774-2. Epub 2019 Apr 15
109. Taillieu E, De Meyere C, Nuytens F, Verslype C, D'Hondt M. Laparoscopic liver resection for colorectal liver metastases—short- and long-term outcomes: A systematic review. World J Gastrointest Oncol. 2021;13(7):732–57. https://doi.org/10.4251/wjgo.v13.i7.732.
110. Syn NL, Kabir T, Koh YX, Tan HL, Wang LZ, Chin BZ, Wee I, Teo JY, Tai BC, Goh BKP. Survival advantage of laparoscopic versus open resection for colorectal liver metastases: a meta-analysis of individual patient data from randomized trials and propensity-score matched studies. Ann Surg. 2020;272(2):253–65. https://doi.org/10.1097/SLA.0000000000003672.
111. Yang HY, Rho SY, Han DH, Choi JS, Choi GH. Robotic major liver resections: surgical outcomes compared with open major liver resections. Ann Hepatobiliary Pancreat Surg. 2021;25(1):8–17. https://doi.org/10.14701/ahbps.2021.25.1.8.

112. Shapera E, Ross S, Crespo K, Syblis C, Przetocki V, Rosemurgy A, Sucandy I. Analysis of surgical approach and tumor distance to margin after liver resection for colorectal liver metastasis. J Robot Surg. 2022; https://doi.org/10.1007/s11701-022-01387-9. Epub ahead of print

113. Hagness M, Foss A, Line PD, Scholz T, Jørgensen PF, Fosby B, Boberg KM, Mathisen O, Gladhaug IP, Egge TS, Solberg S, Hausken J, Dueland S. Liver transplantation for nonresectable liver metastases from colorectal cancer. Ann Surg. 2013;257(5):800–6. https://doi.org/10.1097/SLA.0b013e3182823957.

114. Dueland S, Syversveen T, Solheim JM, Solberg S, Grut H, Bjørnbeth BA, Hagness M, Line PD. Survival following liver transplantation for patients with nonresectable liver-only colorectal metastases. Ann Surg. 2020;271(2):212–8. https://doi.org/10.1097/SLA.0000000000003404.

115. Benoist S, Brouquet A, Penna C, Julié C, El Hajjam M, Chagnon S, Mitry E, Rougier P, Nordlinger B. Complete response of colorectal liver metastases after chemotherapy: does it mean cure? J Clin Oncol. 2006;24(24):3939–45. https://doi.org/10.1200/JCO.2006.05.8727.

116. Elias D, Goere D, Boige V, Kohneh-Sharhi N, Malka D, Tomasic G, Dromain C, Ducreux M. Outcome of posthepatectomy-missing colorectal liver metastases after complete response to chemotherapy: impact of adjuvant intra-arterial hepatic oxaliplatin. Ann Surg Oncol. 2007;14(11):3188–94. https://doi.org/10.1245/s10434-007-9482-9. Epub 2007 Aug 20

117. Auer RC, White RR, Kemeny NE, Schwartz LH, Shia J, Blumgart LH, Dematteo RP, Fong Y, Jarnagin WR, D'Angelica MI. Predictors of a true complete response among disappearing liver metastases from colorectal cancer after chemotherapy. Cancer. 2010;116(6):1502–9. https://doi.org/10.1002/cncr.24912.

118. Ferrero A, Langella S, Russolillo N, Vigano' L, Lo Tesoriere R, Capussotti L. Intraoperative detection of disappearing colorectal liver metastases as a predictor of residual disease. J Gastrointest Surg. 2012;16(4):806–14. https://doi.org/10.1007/s11605-011-1810-5. Epub 2012 Jan 19

119. van Vledder MG, de Jong MC, Pawlik TM, Schulick RD, Diaz LA, Choti MA. Disappearing colorectal liver metastases after chemotherapy: should we be concerned? J Gastrointest Surg. 2010;14(11):1691–700. https://doi.org/10.1007/s11605-010-1348-y. Epub 2010 Sep 14

120. Tanaka K, Takakura H, Takeda K, Matsuo K, Nagano Y, Endo I. Importance of complete pathologic response to prehepatectomy chemotherapy in treating colorectal cancer metastases. Ann Surg. 2009;250(6):935–42. https://doi.org/10.1097/sla.0b013e3181b0c6e4.

121. Muaddi H, Silva S, Choi WJ, Coburn N, Hallet J, Law C, Cheung H, Karanicolas PJ. When is a ghost really gone? A systematic review and meta-analysis of the accuracy of imaging modalities to predict com-

plete pathological response of colorectal cancer liver metastases after chemotherapy. Ann Surg Oncol. 2021;28(11):6805–13. https://doi.org/10.1245/s10434-021-09824-z. Epub 2021 Mar 26

122. Barimani D, Kauppila JH, Sturesson C, Sparrelid E. Imaging in disappearing colorectal liver metastases and their accuracy: a systematic review. World J Surg Oncol. 2020;18(1):264. https://doi.org/10.1186/s12957-020-02037-w.

123. Tsilimigras DI, Ntanasis-Stathopoulos I, Paredes AZ, Moris D, Gavriatopoulou M, Cloyd JM, Pawlik TM. Disappearing liver metastases: a systematic review of the current evidence. Surg Oncol. 2019;29:7–13. https://doi.org/10.1016/j.suronc.2019.02.005. Epub 2019 Feb 11

124. Manfredi S, Lepage C, Hatem C, Coatmeur O, Faivre J, Bouvier AM. Epidemiology and management of liver metastases from colorectal cancer. Ann Surg. 2006;244(2):254–9. https://doi.org/10.1097/01.sla.0000217629.94941.cf.

125. Boudjema K, Locher C, Sabbagh C, Ortega-Deballon P, Heyd B, Bachellier P, Métairie S, Paye F, Bourlier P, Adam R, Merdrignac A, Tual C, Le Pabic E, Sulpice L, Meunier B, Regimbeau JM, Bellissant E, METASYNC Study Group. Simultaneous versus delayed resection for initially Resectable synchronous colorectal cancer liver metastases: A prospective, open-label, randomized, controlled trial. Ann Surg. 2021;273(1):49–56. https://doi.org/10.1097/SLA.0000000000003848.

126. Adam R, de Gramont A, Figueras J, Kokudo N, Kunstlinger F, Loyer E, Poston G, Rougier P, Rubbia-Brandt L, Sobrero A, Teh C, Tejpar S, Van Cutsem E, Vauthey JN, Påhlman L; of the EGOSLIM (Expert Group on OncoSurgery management of LIver Metastases) Group. Managing synchronous liver metastases from colorectal cancer: a multidisciplinary international consensus. Cancer Treat Rev. 2015;41(9):729–41. https://doi.org/10.1016/j.ctrv.2015.06.006. Epub 2015 Jun 30

127. Tzeng CD. Synchronous colorectal liver metastases with asymptomatic primary tumors: an individualized sequencing approach remains ideal. Surgery. 2021;170(1):319. https://doi.org/10.1016/j.surg.2021.03.052. Epub 2021 May 2

128. Andres A, Toso C, Adam R, Barroso E, Hubert C, Capussotti L, Gerstel E, Roth A, Majno PE, Mentha G. A survival analysis of the liver-first reversed management of advanced simultaneous colorectal liver metastases: a LiverMetSurvey-based study. Ann Surg. 2012;256(5):772–8.; discussion 778–9. https://doi.org/10.1097/SLA.0b013e3182734423.

129. Welsh FK, Chandrakumaran K, John TG, Cresswell AB, Rees M. Propensity score-matched outcomes analysis of the liver-first approach for synchronous colorectal liver metastases. Br J Surg. 2016;103(5):600–6. https://doi.org/10.1002/bjs.10099. Epub 2016 Feb 10

130. Lam VW, Laurence JM, Pang T, Johnston E, Hollands MJ, Pleass HC, Richardson AJ. A systematic review of a liver-first approach in patients with colorectal cancer and synchronous colorectal liver metastases. HPB (Oxford). 2014;16(2):101–8. https://doi.org/10.1111/hpb.12083. Epub 2013 Mar 19
131. McCahill LE, Yothers G, Sharif S, Petrelli NJ, Lai LL, Bechar N, Giguere JK, Dakhil SR, Fehrenbacher L, Lopa SH, Wagman LD, O'Connell MJ, Wolmark N. Primary mFOLFOX6 plus bevacizumab without resection of the primary tumor for patients presenting with surgically unresectable metastatic colon cancer and an intact asymptomatic colon cancer: definitive analysis of NSABP trial C-10. J Clin Oncol. 2012;30(26):3223–8. https://doi.org/10.1200/JCO.2012.42.4044. Epub 2012 Aug 6
132. Karoui M, Roudot-Thoraval F, Mesli F, Mitry E, Aparicio T, Des Guetz G, Louvet C, Landi B, Tiret E, Sobhani I. Primary colectomy in patients with stage IV colon cancer and unresectable distant metastases improves overall survival: results of a multicentric study. Dis Colon Rectum. 2011;54(8):930–8. https://doi.org/10.1097/DCR.0b013e31821cced0. Erratum in: Dis Colon Rectum 2011 Oct;54(10):1338. DesGuetz, Gaetan [corrected to Des Guetz, Gaetan]
133. Lang H, Baumgart J, Heinrich S, Tripke V, Passalaqua M, Maderer A, Galle PR, Roth W, Kloth M, Moehler M. Extended molecular profiling improves stratification and prediction of survival after resection of colorectal liver metastases. Ann Surg. 2019;270(5):799–805. https://doi.org/10.1097/SLA.0000000000003527.
134. Chen Y, Chang W, Ren L, Chen J, Tang W, Liu T, Jian M, Liu Y, Wei Y, Xu J. Comprehensive evaluation of relapse risk (CERR) score for colorectal liver metastases: development and validation. Oncologist. 2020;25(7):e1031–41. https://doi.org/10.1634/theoncologist.2019-0797. Epub 2020 Mar 17
135. Schirripa M, Bergamo F, Cremolini C, Casagrande M, Lonardi S, Aprile G, Yang D, Marmorino F, Pasquini G, Sensi E, Lupi C, De Maglio G, Borrelli N, Pizzolitto S, Fasola G, Bertorelle R, Rugge M, Fontanini G, Zagonel V, Loupakis F, Falcone A. BRAF and RAS mutations as prognostic factors in metastatic colorectal cancer patients undergoing liver resection. Br J Cancer. 2015;112(12):1921–8. https://doi.org/10.1038/bjc.2015.142. Epub 2015 May 5
136. Kawaguchi Y, Kopetz S, Lillemoe HA, Hwang H, Wang X, Tzeng CD, Chun YS, Aloia TA, Vauthey JN. A New surveillance algorithm after resection of colorectal liver metastases based on changes in recurrence risk and RAS mutation status. J Natl Compr Cancer Netw. 2020;18(11):1500–8. https://doi.org/10.6004/jnccn.2020.7596.

137. Kawaguchi Y, Lillemoe HA, Panettieri E, Chun YS, Tzeng CD, Aloia TA, Kopetz S, Vauthey JN. Conditional recurrence-free survival after resection of colorectal liver metastases: persistent deleterious association with RAS and TP53 co-mutation. J Am Coll Surg. 2019;229(3):286–294.e1. https://doi.org/10.1016/j.jamcollsurg.2019.04.027. Epub 2019 May 2
138. Van Cutsem E, Cervantes A, Adam R, Sobrero A, Van Krieken JH, Aderka D, Aranda Aguilar E, Bardelli A, Benson A, Bodoky G, Ciardiello F, D'Hoore A, Diaz-Rubio E, Douillard JY, Ducreux M, Falcone A, Grothey A, Gruenberger T, Haustermans K, Heinemann V, Hoff P, Köhne CH, Labianca R, Laurent-Puig P, Ma B, Maughan T, Muro K, Normanno N, Österlund P, Oyen WJ, Papamichael D, Pentheroudakis G, Pfeiffer P, Price TJ, Punt C, Ricke J, Roth A, Salazar R, Scheithauer W, Schmoll HJ, Tabernero J, Taïeb J, Tejpar S, Wasan H, Yoshino T, Zaanan A, Arnold D. ESMO consensus guidelines for the management of patients with metastatic colorectal cancer. Ann Oncol. 2016;27(8):1386–422. https://doi.org/10.1093/annonc/mdw235. Epub 2016 Jul 5
139. Gau L, Ribeiro M, Pereira B, Poirot K, Dupré A, Pezet D, Gagnière J. Impact of BRAF mutations on clinical outcomes following liver surgery for colorectal liver metastases: an updated meta-analysis. Eur J Surg Oncol. 2021;47(11):2722–33. https://doi.org/10.1016/j.ejso.2021.05.039. Epub 2021 May 31
140. Yamashita S, Chun YS, Kopetz SE, Maru D, Conrad C, Aloia TA, Vauthey JN. APC and PIK3CA mutational cooperativity predicts pathologic response and survival in patients undergoing resection for colorectal liver metastases. Ann Surg. 2020;272(6):1080–5. https://doi.org/10.1097/SLA.0000000000002245.
141. Yang ZY, Wu XY, Huang YF, Di MY, Zheng DY, Chen JZ, Ding H, Mao C, Tang JL. Promising biomarkers for predicting the outcomes of patients with KRAS wild-type metastatic colorectal cancer treated with anti-epidermal growth factor receptor monoclonal antibodies: a systematic review with meta-analysis. Int J Cancer. 2013;133(8):1914–25. https://doi.org/10.1002/ijc.28153. Epub 2013 Jul 13. Erratum in: Int J Cancer. 2014 Jul 15;135(2):E2
142. Kawaguchi Y, Kopetz S, Newhook TE, De Bellis M, Chun YS, Tzeng CD, Aloia TA, Vauthey JN. Mutation status of *RAS*, *TP53*, and *SMAD4* is superior to mutation status of *RAS* alone for predicting prognosis after resection of colorectal liver metastases. Clin Cancer Res. 2019;25(19):5843–51. https://doi.org/10.1158/1078-0432.CCR-19-0863. Epub 2019 Jun 20

10. Neuroendocrine Liver Metastasis

Pranay S. Ajay and David A. Kooby

Introduction

Neuroendocrine tumors (NET) are a heterogenous group of neoplasms capable of emerging in any organ harboring neuroendocrine cells, albeit 60–80% stem from gastroenteropancreatic sites identified as GEP-NET [1]. The overall incidence of NETs is increasing, with a prevalence higher than most gastrointestinal cancers likely due to an indolent disease process, early detection, and stage migration [2–4]. Genetic syndromes, such as multiple endocrine neoplasia type 1, are implicated in 10–20% of these tumors, while the remainder of cases are thought to be sporadic [5–7].

Apart from their categorization as functional and nonfunctional tumors based on their distinct ability to produce neuroactive amines and peptide hormones, neuroendocrine neoplasms are also classified as well-differentiated or poorly differentiated, as per the most recent World Health Organization update in 2017. Those classified as well-differentiated are designated as "neuroendocrine tumors (NET)", and the poorly differentiated as "neu-

P. S. Ajay · D. A. Kooby (✉)
Division of Surgical Oncology, Department of Surgery, Emory University School of Medicine, Atlanta, GA, USA
e-mail: dkooby@emory.edu

roendocrine carcinomas (NEC)". NETs are further graded in three tiers as G1, G2, and G3, corresponding to low-grade, intermediate-grade, and high-grade based on parameters of prognostic relevance including Ki-67 index and mitotic count, whereas NECs are always high grade [8].

GEP-NETs have a proclivity to spread to the liver, seen in 40–85% of patients [9, 10], a critical prognostic factor regardless of primary tumor site [11]. While surgical resection remains the primary treatment option, up to 60% of patients have extensive bilateral liver disease [9] rendering them inoperable for a curative resection favoring a cytoreductive procedure or debulking [12]. Nonsurgical and multimodal treatment strategies including ablation, intra-arterial therapy, and systemic therapy aid in slowing tumor progression and palliating symptoms [13, 14]. Liver transplantation as a treatment option has been reconsidered in patients with extensive disease [15–17] bearing its own limitations.

This chapter reviews the care of patients with neuroendocrine liver metastasis (NELM) and elucidates the multitude of treatment approaches and their role in select patients.

Diagnosis and Staging

Symptoms and Biochemical Characterization

The majority of NETs belong to a sub-group of non-functioning tumors [1], incidentally discovered during imaging studies for other reasons. Patients with symptomatic NETs present with protean clinical manifestations with respect to the type of hormone/peptide amine it produces. Symptoms only present when hepatic metabolism is bypassed, usually seen in patients with NELM, and leading to a cluster of pathognomic symptoms, including episodic flushing, diarrhea, and asthma-like pulmonary complaints [18]. Upon indicatory symptoms or findings, biochemical characterization of NET with specific markers such as Chromogranin A, 5-hydroxy indoleacetic acid, insulin, glucagon, gastrin, vasoactive intestinal peptide, and serotonin aid in facilitating an exact diagnosis and establishing a baseline status [19].

Imaging

The development of new imaging techniques has played a pivotal role in improving localization and defining extent of this disease. Gallium 68-Dotatoc (^{68}Ga) positron emission tomography—computed tomography (PET-CT) is an accepted imaging modality in patients with suspected NETs [20]. Compared to ^{68}Ga Dotatoc, ^{64}Cu-Dotatate is a new PET tracer with a longer half-life (12.7 h vs 68 min), and a scanning window of at least 3 h with improved detection of lesions [21]. In patients with NELM, extent of liver disease is best assessed using a multi-phase contrast CT or gadolinium-based contrast magnetic resonance imaging (MRI), owing to the hypervascular nature of these tumors [22, 23]. ^{18}F-fluorodeoxyglucose (^{18}F-FDG) PET can be considered in patients with high-grade tumors [24]. In addition, an echocardiogram may be essential in looking for serotonin-related valvular disease prior to resection [25].

Endoscopic Assessment in Pursuit of Primary Tumor

In the setting of an unknown primary seen in 11–14% of NETs [26], esophagogastroduodenoscopy and colonoscopy have been effective in diagnosing gastric, colorectal, and ileal lesions. Most of the lesions found intraoperatively are located in the small intestines [27]. Double balloon enteroscopy (DBE) and capsule endoscopy (CE) are useful in the diagnosis of small bowel NETs with similar diagnostic yield [28, 29]. While CE is noninvasive, it can be followed by DBE which has the advantage of interventional capabilities. A biopsy of the metastatic lesion with positive immunohistochemistry may also aid in indicating the primary tumor's most probable location of origin [30].

The extent of pursuit for primary tumor remains controversial as some studies have suggested that an unresected primary does not significantly affect overall survival (OS) [9, 31], while others have advocated the localization and resection of primary even among patients in whom the primary is asymptomatic [32].

Treatment Strategies

Patients with untreated NELM have an overall 5-year survival ranging from 30% to 40% [33, 34]. Initial treatment should be directed at symptomatic management—addressing the consequences of functional tumors. The goals of curative treatment strategies are often hindered by the presence of more extensive disease and a high disease recurrence rate [12], with strategies focusing on increasing survival and palliating symptoms. Surgical resection is the primary treatment option, and patients with resectable disease have a better survival compared to those with unresectable disease [35, 36] (Fig. 10.1). The 5-year survival following resection ranges from 60–85% [12, 37–39], and most disease-specific deaths are usually due to liver failure [40]. NELM are

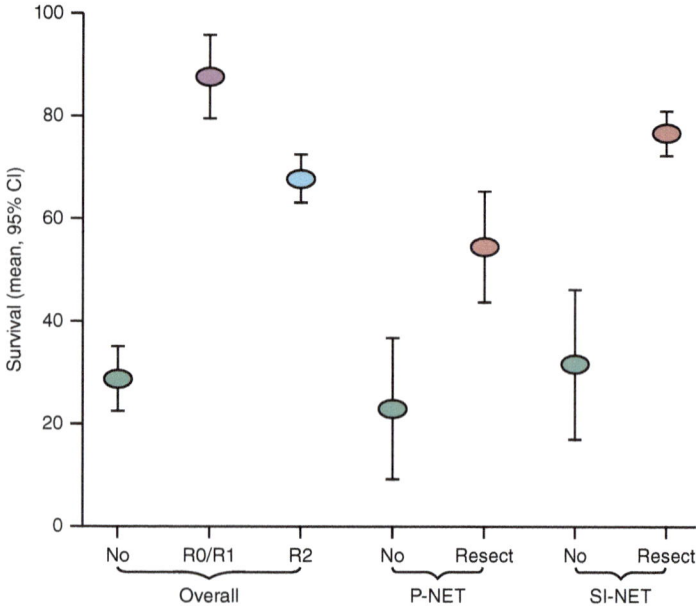

Fig. 10.1 5-year survival after neuroendocrine liver metastases resection. (Reprinted from Frilling et al. [36], Copyright 2014, with permission from Elsevier)

highly vascular and predominantly draw their blood supply from the hepatic artery rather than portal vein [41], forming basis for intra-arterial therapies. While new systemic treatment modalities have shown promise, further studies are warranted before an optimal strategy is promulgated.

Role of Resection and Cytoreductive Approach

Despite recent advances in medicine, surgical resection of primary tumor and hepatic lesions remain the centerpiece of treatment strategies in patients with NELM. Their inherent nature to grow in an expansile rather than infiltrative pattern allows for enucleation of individual metastatic lesions without the need to violate critical adjacent structures. Depending on locational anatomy, wedge resection, lobectomy, and trisegmentectomy are other surgical options with the end goal of removing the majority of the tumor while leaving an adequate hepatic remnant. A cytoreductive procedure remains a viable option in patients with disseminated or bilateral disease.

A multi-institutional study by Mayo et al. in 2010 analyzed 339 patients who underwent surgical management (67% with curative intent) for NELM with resection (78%), ablation (3%), or resection + ablation (19%) [9]. The median OS in all patients was over 10 years while the median survival time for patients with nonfunctional tumors and R2 resections (19%) was in excess of 7 years. A similar study by glazer et al. analyzing 172 patients with NELM (84% R0 resection) showed no difference in OS or progression-free survival (PFS) ($p \geq 0.05$ for both) with respect to margin status (R0 vs R1 vs R2), advocating for an aggressive surgical approach even in the absence of a possibility for complete resection [42].

Evolving Trends in Cytoreductive Surgery

Curative-intent resection may not always be possible as more than half of these patients present with extensive bilateral disease [9, 12, 39] or anatomically challenging locations. Cytoreductive surgery is a viable option for some patients with symptomatic disease not amenable to curative intent resection while asymptomatic patients should be discussed via multidisciplinary tumor board review, and decision making should be based on extent of disease, rate of progression, and patient fitness. Conventional wisdom recommends a debulking procedure when >90% of the tumor can be excised or in functional patients [43, 44] to reduce burden of disease.

Sarmiento and colleagues in 2003 analyzed 170 patients managed with surgical resection for NELM [12]. R0 resection was achieved in less than half of these patients. With a debulking threshold of 90%, almost all patients had partial or complete relief of symptoms, justifying the role of a palliative debulking procedure as long as 90% of disease remains resectable. The 5-year OS rate was 61% with no significant difference in OS between patients who had functional and nonfunctional tumors. In a multi-institutional study of 612 patients by Ejaz et al., 29% of patients underwent cytoreductive surgery with a minimum debulking threshold of 80%. An acceptable 5-year OS rate of 61% was reported in this subset of patients, despite the cohort including higher rates of high-grade tumors (35.0%), lymph node metastasis (72.9%), bilateral liver metastasis (72.6%), and extrahepatic disease (19%) (all $p < 0.001$) compared to patients who underwent a curative intent resection.[39]. Presence of hormonal symptoms did not impact survival in all patients (median survival = 138 months; $p = 0.29$) or in patients who received only a debulking procedure ($p = 0.79$) when compared to asymptomatic patients. Among patients with ≥50% liver involvement (19%), median OS was still almost 5 years.

A study by Graff-Baker et al. in 2014 analyzed 52 patients with neuroendocrine liver metastasis undergoing debulking procedures with a reduced minimum threshold of 70% tumor clearance [40]. The 5-year disease-specific survival was 90% and median PFS was 72 months demonstrating no significant detrimental effects of using this reduced threshold. Progression did not correlate with the percentage of disease debulked as approximately 30% of patients had progression of liver disease regardless of the extent of debulking. Similarly, a study by Maxwell et al. in 2017 analyzed 108 patients with SBNET and PNET who primarily underwent parenchyma-sparing debulking procedures including ablation, enucleation, and wedge resection [45]. The 5-year OS rate was 76% with two-thirds of the patients (69/108) achieving ≥70% cytoreduction, and 60% of these patients (42/69) achieving ≥90% cytoreduction. Greater than 70% cytoreduction was associated with significant improvements in both PFS (3 vs 0.51 years; p < 0.001) and OS (not reached vs 1.7 years; p < 0.001) compared to patients with <70% cytoreduction (Fig. 10.2). While ≥90% cytoreduction (4.4 vs 1.3 years; p = 0.05) is associated with improved PFS compared to <90%, differences in OS remained insignificant (not reached vs 6.1 years; p = 0.14). Consistent with the above-mentioned series, the current trend in literature raises a plea to reassess and reduce the conventional debulking target

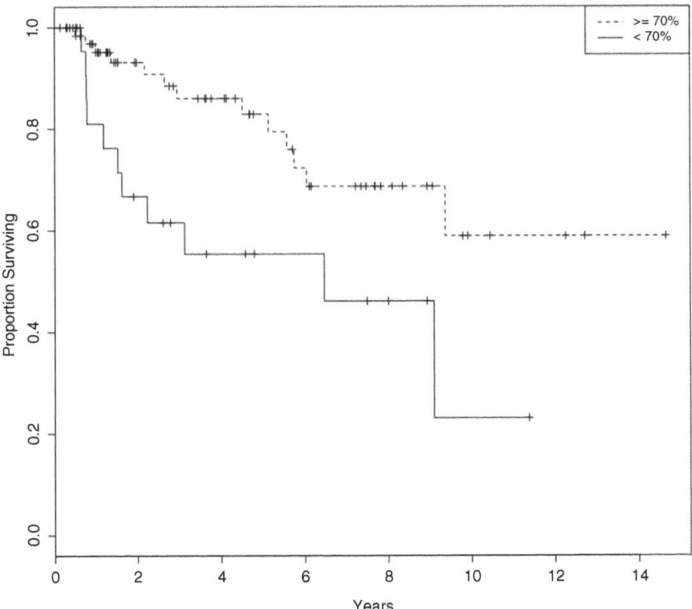

Fig. 10.2 Overall survival in pancreatic and small bowel neuroendocrine tumor by % of liver debulked. (Reprinted from Maxwell et al. [45], Copyright 2016, with permission from Elsevier)

threshold from 90% to increase eligibility and benefit a larger proportion of patients with NELM. Owing to a lack of randomized trials and selection bias in who gets surgery and who achieves higher levels of debulking, patient and disease selection including extent of disease, biology, comorbidities, and response to nonsurgical therapies remain key factors in patient selection for a debulking procedure.

The study by Ejaz et al. showed no difference in OS when stratified by tumor functionality but patients with <50% NELM involvement and those patients with well-differentiated tumors seemed to benefit the most from cytoreductive surgery [39]. A few of the above-mentioned series have also indicated that patients with functional tumors or symptomatic disease benefit the most from a debulking procedure [9, 12].

Tackling Extrahepatic Disease

The presence of extrahepatic disease was noted in most of the above-mentioned series. In the study by Graff-Baker et al., 65% had extrahepatic disease, and 35% continued to have extrahepatic disease after operation [40]. Critically, this did not have an adverse impact on liver progression-free or disease-specific survival as all disease-specific deaths were due to liver failure and not extrahepatic disease. While two other analyses of large series in patients with NELM noted extrahepatic disease to be an adverse prognostic factor, the median OS was still around 85 months [9, 39], justifying resection in a select subset of patients with extrahepatic disease. Counterintuitively, the presence of extrahepatic disease, even when found intraoperatively should not stand as a lone limiting factor to resection.

The Issue of Recurrence and Progression

While patients with NELM have an exceptional long-term survival rate, the rate of PFS remains dismal with recurrence rates ranging from 85% to 94% through the course of the disease [9,

12]. A systematic review by Saxena et al. revealed a median PFS of only 21 months (range, 13–46 months), and well more than half of these patients recur within 5 years [46]. The majority of patients experience recurrent disease confined to the liver, which is associated with better long-term survival outcomes compared to extrahepatic recurrence or a combination of both [47]. Repeat liver resection is deemed safe in patients with NELM and is known to offer reasonable long-term survival outcomes [42, 47].

Ablation—Efficacy and Indications

Radiofrequency ablation (RFA), microwave ablation (MA), and laser ablation (LA) are accepted hyperthermia-based ablative techniques used in the management of NELM, each with its own peculiar benefits and limitations.

RFA is used alone or as an adjunct to surgery in patients receiving debulking procedures due to oligometastatic disease or an inoperable tumor location. Laparoscopic and open techniques are thought to provide better outcomes as compared with percutaneous technique and should be preferred whenever feasible as it provides improved local control [48]. Tumor size is a crucial factor as tumors >2 cm in size are less likely to be effectively treated by RFA [49]. In a study by Akyildiz et al. in 2010, 89 patients with NELM (56% asymptomatic) who failed to respond to other treatments underwent laparoscopic RFA, and symptom relief was achieved in 97% of these patients [50]. Repeat RFA was effective in maintaining a low tumor burden and was performed up to 4 times in this series. Median disease-free survival was 15 months with a 5-year survival rate of 57%, comparable to survival rates in previously mentioned series after cytoreductive surgery. In another study by Taner et al. in 2013, 94 patients underwent hepatic resection and intraoperative ablation of NELM [51]. Rate of 5- and 10-year OS was excellent at 80% and 59%, respectively. Interestingly, tumor grade and need for repeat ablation had no significant association with survival. (Fig. 10.3—Case study of a patient with a 10-year timeline of multiple ablative procedures) Symptom-free survival was 34% at 3 years consistent with exist-

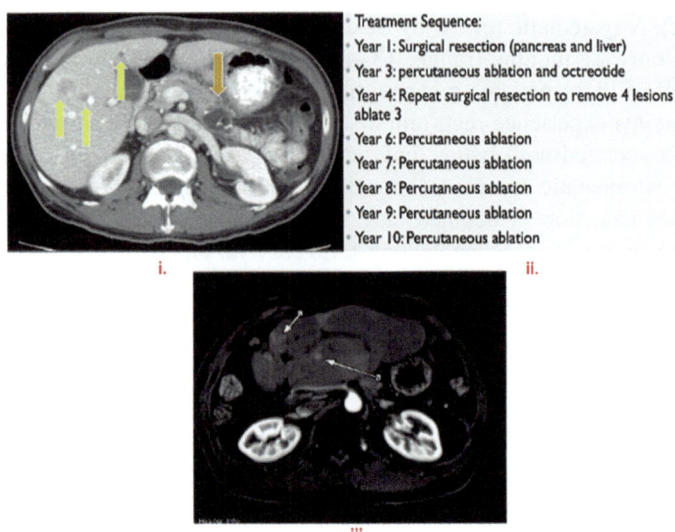

Fig. 10.3 (i) Initial scan showing pancreatic primary with multiple metastatic hepatic lesions; (ii) highlights the sequence of treatment; (iii) denotes a scan after 10 years following a history of multiple percutaneous ablative procedures including resection of the pancreatic primary and right hepatic trisegmentectomy

ing literature regardless of treatment approach [47]. The heat sink effect remains an important limitation leading to increased recurrence in malignant perivascular hepatic lesions after RFA [52].

MA has the added benefit of providing a large ablation zone (up to 6 cm) in a short time and is not impacted as much by the heat sink effect in comparison to RFA [53]. Although majority of studies have reported the use of RFA for NELM, a recent study of 50 patients receiving MA by Pickens et al., in whom 44% underwent concomitant resection, 95% showed symptomatic improvement with 1- and 5- year survival rates of 94% and 70%, respectively [54].

LA has the advantage of smaller diameter needles compared to RFA and MA, a technical characteristic that can be beneficial when the tumors are in at-risk locations [55]. It can also be performed with MRI guidance to optimize needle placement. While data on patients with NELM treated with LA is limited, a recent study in 21 patients with 189 metastatic liver lesion showed promising 1-, 3-, and 5-year survival rates of 95%, 66%, and 40%, respectively, with complete symptom relief in all symptomatic patients [56].

Irreversible electroporation (IRE) is a non-thermal ablative technique ideal in treating central lesions (<3 cm in size) that are unsuitable for thermal ablation as it has the advantage of sparing the collagenous structures preserving the biliary ducts and major hepatic vasculature, thus decreasing the risk of strictures and perforation [57–59]. A recent study in 34 patients including 65 malignant tumors (3 NELM) receiving IRE revealed promising 3-, 6-, and 12-month local recurrence-free survival rates of 87%, 80%, and 75%, respectively [60]. Contraindications to IRE include patients with significant cardiac history as it has the potential of inducing arrhythmias [61].

Intra-arterial Therapy

Less than 15% of patients with NELM are amenable to resection owing primarily to multicentric lesions, bilobar disease, or insufficient liver remnant following resection [10]. In this subset of patients, angiographic liver-directed techniques including transarterial embolization (TAE), transarterial chemoembolization (TACE), selective internal radiotherapy, or radioembolization (RE) with yttrium-90 microspheres can be used to control symptoms, aid in locoregional control by reducing tumor burden, and improve PFS [13, 62, 63].

Eighteen studies (11 TAE or TACE; 7 RE) were reviewed in the NET-Liver-Metastasis conference in 2015 to recommend guidelines for the role of intra-arterial therapies (IAT) (Fig. 10.4—proposed non-surgical treatment approach guidelines) [64]. The study concluded that neither of the treatment modalities can be promulgated as superior compared to the others, while RE may have benefits due to fewer side effects and the requirement of fewer treatments. However, data on long-term toxicity, such as chronic radiation-induced liver disease following TARE, is still

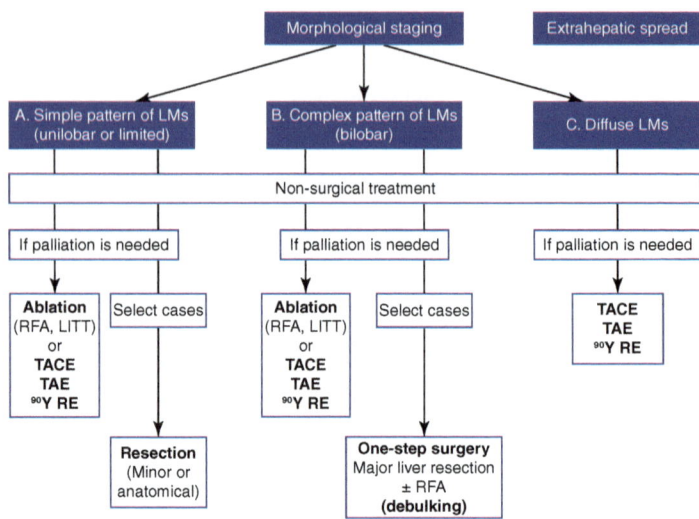

Fig. 10.4 Proposed treatment approach in liver-only metastases from neuroendocrine tumors. *LITT* laser-induced thermotherapy, *LMs* liver metastases, *RE* radioembolization, *RFA* radiofrequency ablation, *TAE* transarterial embolization, *TACE* transarterial chemoembolization, ^{90}Y, yttrium-90. (Reprinted from Kennedy et al. [64], Copyright 2015, with permission from Elsevier)

limited. On the contrary, a study by Minh et al. in 2017 showed an improved association with OS in patients who received conventional TACE compared to drug-eluting beads TACE and RE [65]. While more recently, a multi-institutional analysis of 248 patients by Eggar et al. comparing TACE and RE showed no difference in overall morbidity ($p = 0.17$) [66]. Albeit an improved disease control rate per RECIST in patients who received TACE ($p = <0.01$), no difference in median OS ($p = 0.3$) or PFS ($p = 0.37$) was noted. Randomized trials comparing these treatment strategies on a head-to-head basis are warranted to elucidate the ideal liver-directed IAT.

A propensity-matched analysis comparing surgery vs IAT in 753 patients by Mayo et al. indicated that surgical resection was most beneficial in NELM patients with low volume disease (<25% hepatic tumor burden) or those with symptomatic high volume

(>25%) hepatic burden [67]. No difference was noted between surgery and IAT in patients with asymptomatic, high-volume (25%) liver disease.

Systemic Therapy

An improved understanding of pathogenesis of NET at a molecular level has led to the development of new targeted therapies in this field. The rarity of this disease truncates our ability to effectively compare these treatment strategies leading to a multitude of options with the bane of a lacking consensus in approaching these novel strategies.

Somatostatin analogues (SSA) are primarily used to manage symptoms in NET patients with the added benefit of arresting tumor growth. Octreotide (long-acting repeatable), in the PROMID trial significantly lengthened PFS when compared to placebo (14.3 vs 6 months), with the most favorable effects observed in patients with low hepatic burden and resected primary tumor [68]. The CLARINET trial investigating lanreotide showed similar results in patients with metastatic enteropancreatic neuroendocrine tumors [69]. More recently, in patients with SSA refractory diarrhea, *telotristat ethyl* has been approved in combination with SSA for adults [70].

The use of *mammalian target of rapamycin (mTOR) inhibitor, everolimus*, has been associated with improved PFS in patients with progressive lung or gastrointestinal nonfunctional NETs [71], while a tyrosine kinase inhibitor, sunitib, has been approved for treatment in patients with advanced pancreatic NET [72].

The synergistic chemotherapeutic regimen of *temozolomide-capecitab*ine in a randomized controlled trial has shown to significantly improve PFS and OS in patients with progressive PNETs [73]. Its role in nonpancreatic NET is still to be defined.

Peptide receptor radionuclide therapy (PRRT) is an emerging therapeutic form of targeted radiotherapy, wherein radiolabeled SSAs deliver radioactive isotopes (^{90}Yttrium or ^{177}Lutetium) to somatostatin receptor expressing tumors. The NETTER-1 trial in patients with well-differentiated midgut NETs showed a signifi-

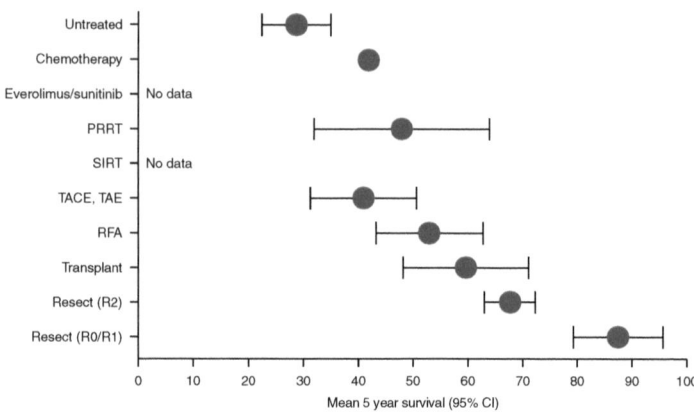

Fig. 10.5 Rates of 5-year survival by treatment method. (Reprinted from Frilling et al. [36], Copyright 2014, with permission from Elsevier)

cantly prolonged PFS in patients receiving ^{177}Lu-Dotatate compared to high-dose octreotide LAR [74]. These results have led to further investigations with PRRT in combination with other treatment strategies such as chemotherapy with capecitabine, and SSAs which have revealed promising results in patients with unresectable GEP-NET [75, 76]. (Fig. 10.5: Rates of 5-year survival by treatment method).

Transplantation

Liver transplantation (LT) has been reconsidered as a treatment option in patients with well-controlled, unresectable NELM and maybe offered to patients with low or intermediate grade tumors (Ki67 < 20%) in the absence of unresectable extrahepatic disease [77]. Guidelines for the selection of NELM patients for LT have been outlined by Mazzaferro et al. in the Milan criteria for NELM which include a low-grade tumor, GEP-NET, <50% liver involvement, stable disease for ≥6 months, and age ≤ 55 years [78].

Indications and Prognostic Factors

A systematic review of literature by Moris et al. in NELM patients with LT—analyzing aggregate single-center reports—demonstrated that the indications for LT were presentation of debilitating or low-grade symptoms related to the underlying NET in 66.1% of patients, and burden of tumor bulk in the rest [79]. Prognostic factors that have been associated with worse OS include resection of primary tumor during LT, >50% liver tumor involvement, high Ki67 index, and PNET compared to gastrointestinal NET, with recurrence rates ranging from 31.3% to 56.8% [16, 79].

Positive Trend in Survival Rates: 1982–2014

A review of the United Network for Organ Sharing (UNOS) database by Gedaly et al. reported 150 LT (0.2% of 87,280) performed for NELM patients (between 1988 and 2008) with a 5-year OS rate of 49%, and 1-, 3-, and 5-year DFS rates of 77%, 50%, and 32% respectively [80]. Patients analyzed in the European Liver Transplant Registry database (1982–2009) revealed a 5-year survival rate of 53% in 213 patients [16]. A similar study, utilizing the UNOS database (1988–2011) with 184 patients, analyzed the impact of model for end-stage liver disease/pediatric model for end-stage liver disease (MELD/PELD) scores and showed an improvement in the 5-year OS rate in the post-MELD/PELD score era (49% vs 58%), with outcomes not significantly different from patients transplanted for HCC [81]. This 5-year OS rate increased to 63% when the database was analyzed from 2002 to 2014 [82].

The interpretation of these results remains tricky due to the inherent selection bias of these large retrospective studies along with disparate patient populations further complicated with a heterogenous disease process.

Conclusion

A multitude of treatment options exist in patients with neuroendocrine liver metastasis depending on the nature, primary site, and extent of disease. Surgical resection is the primary treatment option in patients with resectable disease, and concomitant ablation is an acceptable treatment strategy. As vast majority of patients present with bilateral liver disease, cytoreductive surgery is a favorable option if feasible depending on the location of tumor. In patients with unresectable disease, ablation and liver-directed transarterial therapies are preferred. Peptide receptor radionuclide therapy has shown promise, and results from multiple ongoing randomized trials will help elucidate the optimal therapy sequence in combination with available strategies. Patients with advanced and progressive disease are managed with systemic therapies with or without the use of somatostatin analogues. Liver transplantation has proven to be effective in select patients.

References

1. Modlin IM, et al. Gastroenteropancreatic neuroendocrine tumours. Lancet Oncol. 2008;9(1):61–72.
2. Yao JC, et al. One hundred years after "carcinoid": epidemiology of and prognostic factors for neuroendocrine Tumors in 35,825 cases in the United States. J Clin Oncol. 2008;26(18):3063–72.
3. Lawrence B, et al. The epidemiology of gastroenteropancreatic neuroendocrine Tumors. Endocrinol Metab Clin N Am. 2011;40(1):1–18.
4. Dasari A, et al. Trends in the incidence, prevalence, and survival outcomes in patients with neuroendocrine Tumors in the United States. JAMA Oncol. 2017;3(10):1335–42.
5. Zikusoka MN, et al. The molecular genetics of gastroenteropancreatic neuroendocrine tumors. Cancer. 2005;104(11):2292–309.
6. Marx SJ. Recent topics around multiple endocrine neoplasia type 1. J Clin Endocrinol Metabol. 2018;103(4):1296–301.
7. Wang R, et al. Management of Gastrointestinal Neuroendocrine Tumors. Clin Med Insights Endocrinol Diab. 2019;12:1179551419884058.
8. Rindi G, et al. A common classification framework for neuroendocrine neoplasms: an International Agency for Research on Cancer (IARC) and

World Health Organization (WHO) expert consensus proposal. Mod Pathol. 2018;31(12):1770–86.
9. Mayo SC, et al. Surgical management of hepatic neuroendocrine tumor metastasis: results from an international multi-institutional analysis. Ann Surg Oncol. 2010;17(12):3129–36.
10. John BJ, Davidson BR. Treatment options for unresectable neuroendocrine liver metastases. Expert Rev Gastroenterol Hepatol. 2012;6(3):357–69.
11. Rindi G, et al. Prognostic factors in gastrointestinal endocrine tumors. Endocr Pathol. 2007;18(3):145–9.
12. Sarmiento JM, et al. Surgical treatment of neuroendocrine metastases to the liver: a plea for resection to increase survival. J Am Coll Surg. 2003;197(1):29–37.
13. Gupta S, et al. Hepatic artery embolization and chemoembolization for treatment of patients with metastatic carcinoid tumors: the M.D. Anderson experience. Cancer J. 2003;9(4):261–7.
14. Forrer F, et al. Peptide receptor radionuclide therapy. Best Pract Res Clin Endocrinol Metab. 2007;21(1):111–29.
15. Pavel M, et al. ENETS consensus guidelines for the management of patients with liver and other distant metastases from neuroendocrine neoplasms of foregut, midgut, hindgut, and unknown primary. Neuroendocrinology. 2012;95(2):157–76.
16. Le Treut YP, et al. Liver transplantation for neuroendocrine tumors in Europe—results and trends in patient selection: a 213-case European liver transplant registry study. Ann Surg. 2013;257(5).
17. Olausson M, et al. Orthotopic liver or multivisceral transplantation as treatment of metastatic neuroendocrine tumors. Liver Transpl. 2007;13(3):327–33.
18. Warner RRP. Carcinoid case presentation and discussion: the American perspective. Endocr Relat Cancer. 2003;10(4):489–96.
19. Miękus N, Bączek T. Non-invasive screening for neuroendocrine tumors—biogenic amines as neoplasm biomarkers and the potential improvement of "gold standards". J Pharm Biomed Anal. 2016;130:194–201.
20. Frilling A, et al. The impact of 68Ga-DOTATOC positron emission tomography/computed tomography on the multimodal management of patients with neuroendocrine tumors. Ann Surg. 2010;252(5).
21. Johnbeck CB, et al. Head-to-head comparison of (64)Cu-DOTATATE and (68)Ga-DOTATOC PET/CT: a prospective study of 59 patients with neuroendocrine Tumors. J Nucl Med. 2017;58(3):451–7.
22. Tan EH, Tan CH. Imaging of gastroenteropancreatic neuroendocrine tumors. World J Clin Oncol. 2011;2(1):28–43.
23. Dromain C, et al. MR imaging of hepatic metastases caused by neuroendocrine tumors: comparing four techniques. Am J Roentgenol. 2003;180(1):121–8.

24. Deroose CM, et al. Molecular imaging of gastroenteropancreatic neuroendocrine tumors: current status and future directions. J Nucl Med. 2016;57(12):1949–56.
25. Luis SA, Pellikka PA. Carcinoid heart disease: diagnosis and management. Best Pract Res Clin Endocrinol Metab. 2016;30(1):149–58.
26. Hauso O, et al. Neuroendocrine tumor epidemiology: contrasting Norway and North America. Cancer. 2008;113(10):2655–64.
27. Wang SC, et al. Identification of unknown primary tumors in patients with neuroendocrine liver metastases. Arch Surg. 2010;145(3):276–80.
28. Rossi RE, et al. Endoscopic techniques to detect small-bowel neuroendocrine tumors: a literature review. United European Gastroenterol J. 2017;5(1):5–12.
29. Pasha SF, et al. Double-balloon enteroscopy and capsule endoscopy have comparable diagnostic yield in small-bowel disease: a meta-analysis. Clin Gastroenterol Hepatol. 2008;6(6):671–6.
30. Chan ES, et al. PDX-1, CDX-2, TTF-1, and CK7: a reliable immunohistochemical panel for pancreatic neuroendocrine neoplasms. Am J Surg Pathol. 2012;36(5):737–43.
31. Ho AS, et al. Long-term outcome after chemoembolization and embolization of hepatic metastatic lesions from neuroendocrine tumors. AJR Am J Roentgenol. 2007;188(5):1201–7.
32. Givi B, et al. Operative resection of primary carcinoid neoplasms in patients with liver metastases yields significantly better survival. Surgery. 2006;140(6):891–7. discussion 897–8
33. Thompson GB, et al. Islet cell carcinomas of the pancreas: a twenty-year experience. Surgery. 1988;104(6):1011–7.
34. Chen H, et al. Isolated liver metastases from neuroendocrine tumors: does resection prolong survival? J Am Coll Surg. 1998;187(1):88–92. discussion 92–3
35. Frilling A, et al. Treatment of liver metastases from neuroendocrine tumours in relation to the extent of hepatic disease. J Br Surg. 2009;96(2):175–84.
36. Frilling A, et al. Recommendations for management of patients with neuroendocrine liver metastases. Lancet Oncol. 2014;15(1):e8–e21.
37. Chamberlain RS, et al. Hepatic neuroendocrine metastases: does intervention alter outcomes? J Am Coll Surg. 2000;190(4):432–45.
38. Scigliano S, et al. Clinical and imaging follow-up after exhaustive liver resection of endocrine metastases: a 15-year monocentric experience. Endocr Relat Cancer. 2009;16(3):977–90.
39. Ejaz A, et al. Cytoreductive debulking surgery among patients with neuroendocrine liver metastasis: a multi-institutional analysis. HPB (Oxford). 2018;20(3):277–84.
40. Graff-Baker AN, et al. Expanded criteria for carcinoid liver debulking: maintaining survival and increasing the number of eligible patients. Surgery. 2014;156(6):1369–77.

41. Vogl TJ, et al. Liver metastases of neuroendocrine carcinomas: interventional treatment via transarterial embolization, chemoembolization and thermal ablation. Eur J Radiol. 2009;72(3):517–28.
42. Glazer ES, et al. Long-term survival after surgical management of neuroendocrine hepatic metastases. HPB (Oxford). 2010;12(6):427–33.
43. Que FG, et al. Hepatic resection for metastatic neuroendocrine carcinomas. Am J Surg. 1995;169(1):36–42. discussion 42–3
44. McEntee GP, et al. Cytoreductive hepatic surgery for neuroendocrine tumors. Surgery. 1990.
45. Maxwell JE, et al. Liver-directed surgery of neuroendocrine metastases: what is the optimal strategy? Surgery. 2016;159(1):320–33.
46. Saxena A, et al. Surgical resection of hepatic metastases from neuroendocrine neoplasms: a systematic review. Surg Oncol. 2012;21(3):e131–41.
47. Spolverato G, et al. Management and outcomes of patients with recurrent neuroendocrine liver metastasis after curative surgery: an international multi-institutional analysis. J Surg Oncol. 2017;116(3):298–306.
48. Eisele RM, et al. Open surgical is superior to percutaneous access for radiofrequency ablation of hepatic metastases. World J Surg. 2009;33(4):804–11.
49. Elvin A, Skogseid B, Hellman P. Radiofrequency ablation of neuroendocrine liver metastases. Abdom Imaging. 2005;30(4):427–34.
50. Akyildiz HY, et al. Laparoscopic radiofrequency thermal ablation of neuroendocrine hepatic metastases: long-term follow-up. Surgery. 2010;148(6):1288–93. discussion 1293
51. Taner T, et al. Adjunctive radiofrequency ablation of metastatic neuroendocrine cancer to the liver complements surgical resection. HPB. 2013;15(3):190–5.
52. Lin ZY, et al. Effect of heat sink on the recurrence of small malignant hepatic tumors after radiofrequency ablation. J Cancer Res Ther. 2016;12(Supplement):C153–c158.
53. Vogl TJ, et al. Microwave ablation (MWA): basics, technique and results in primary and metastatic liver neoplasms—review article. Rofo. 2017;189(11):1055–66.
54. Pickens RC, et al. Operative microwave ablation for the multimodal treatment of neuroendocrine liver metastases. J Laparoendosc Adv Surg Tech. 2020;31(8):917–25.
55. Sartori S, et al. Laser ablation of liver tumors: an ancillary technique, or an alternative to radiofrequency and microwave? World J Radiol. 2017;9(3):91–6.
56. Sartori S, et al. Percutaneous laser ablation of liver metastases from neuroendocrine neoplasm. A retrospective study for safety and effectiveness. Cardiovasc Intervent Radiol. 2019;42(11):1571–8.
57. Silk M, et al. The state of irreversible electroporation in interventional oncology. Semin Intervent Radiol. 2014;31(2):111–7.

58. Ruarus AH, et al. Irreversible electroporation for hepatic tumors: protocol standardization using the modified Delphi technique. J Vasc Interv Radiol. 2020;31(11):1765–1771.e15.
59. Din ATU, et al. Irreversible electroporation for liver tumors: a review of literature. Cureus. 2019;11(6).
60. Niessen C, et al. Percutaneous ablation of hepatic Tumors using irreversible electroporation: a prospective safety and midterm efficacy study in 34 patients. J Vasc Interv Radiol. 2016;27(4):480–6.
61. O'Neill CH, Martin RCG 2nd. Cardiac synchronization and arrhythmia during irreversible electroporation. J Surg Oncol. 2020;122(3):407–11.
62. Roche A, et al. Trans-catheter arterial chemoembolization as first-line treatment for hepatic metastases from endocrine tumors. Eur Radiol. 2003;13(1):136–40.
63. Gupta S, et al. Hepatic arterial embolization and chemoembolization for the treatment of patients with metastatic neuroendocrine tumors: variables affecting response rates and survival. Cancer. 2005;104(8):1590–602.
64. Kennedy A, et al. Role of hepatic intra-arterial therapies in metastatic neuroendocrine tumours (NET): guidelines from the NET-liver-metastases consensus conference. HPB. 2015;17(1):29–37.
65. Do Minh D, et al. Intra-arterial therapy of neuroendocrine tumour liver metastases: comparing conventional TACE, drug-eluting beads TACE and yttrium-90 radioembolisation as treatment options using a propensity score analysis model. Eur Radiol. 2017;27(12):4995–5005.
66. Egger ME, et al. Transarterial chemoembolization vs Radioembolization for neuroendocrine liver metastases: a multi-institutional analysis. J Am Coll Surg. 2020;230(4):363–70.
67. Mayo SC, et al. Surgery versus intra-arterial therapy for neuroendocrine liver metastasis: a multicenter international analysis. Ann Surg Oncol. 2011;18(13):3657–65.
68. Rinke A, et al. Placebo-controlled, double-blind, prospective, randomized study on the effect of octreotide LAR in the control of tumor growth in patients with metastatic neuroendocrine midgut tumors: a report from the PROMID study group. J Clin Oncol. 2009;27(28):4656–63.
69. Caplin ME, et al. Lanreotide in metastatic enteropancreatic neuroendocrine tumors. N Engl J Med. 2014;371(3):224–33.
70. Pavel M, et al. Telotristat ethyl in carcinoid syndrome: safety and efficacy in the TELECAST phase 3 trial. Endocr Relat Cancer. 2018;25(3):309–22.
71. Yao JC, et al. Everolimus for the treatment of advanced, non-functional neuroendocrine tumours of the lung or gastrointestinal tract (RADIANT-4): a randomised, placebo-controlled, phase 3 study. Lancet. 2016;387(10022):968–77.

72. Raymond E, et al. Sunitinib malate for the treatment of pancreatic neuroendocrine tumors. N Engl J Med. 2011;364(6):501–13.
73. Kunz PL, et al. A randomized study of temozolomide or temozolomide and capecitabine in patients with advanced pancreatic neuroendocrine tumors: a trial of the ECOG-ACRIN cancer research group (E2211). Am Soc Clin Oncol; 2018.
74. Strosberg J, et al. Phase 3 trial of (177)Lu-dotatate for midgut neuroendocrine tumors. N Engl J Med. 2017;376(2):125–35.
75. Ballal S, et al. Concomitant 177Lu-DOTATATE and capecitabine therapy in patients with advanced neuroendocrine tumors: a long-term-outcome, toxicity, survival, and quality-of-life study. Clin Nucl Med. 2017;42(11):e457–66.
76. Yordanova A, et al. The role of adding somatostatin analogues to peptide receptor radionuclide therapy as a combination and maintenance therapy. Clin Cancer Res. 2018;24(19):4672–9.
77. Frilling A, Clift AK. Therapeutic strategies for neuroendocrine liver metastases. Cancer. 2015;121(8):1172–86.
78. Mazzaferro V, Pulvirenti A, Coppa J. Neuroendocrine tumors metastatic to the liver: how to select patients for liver transplantation? J Hepatol. 2007;47(4):460–6.
79. Moris D, et al. Liver transplantation in patients with liver metastases from neuroendocrine tumors: a systematic review. Surgery. 2017;162(3):525–36.
80. Gedaly R, et al. Liver transplantation for the treatment of liver metastases from neuroendocrine tumors: an analysis of the UNOS database. Arch Surg. 2011;146(8):953–8.
81. Nguyen NT, et al. Neuroendocrine liver metastases and Orthotopic liver transplantation: the US experience. Int J Hepatol. 2011;2011:742890.
82. Nobel YR, Goldberg DS. Variable use of model for end-stage liver disease exception points in patients with neuroendocrine tumors metastatic to the liver and its impact on patient outcomes. Transplantation. 2015;99(11):2341–6.

Non-CR, Non-NE Liver Metastases

David Henault, Hala Muaddi, and Chaya Shwaartz

Introduction

Colorectal cancer (CRC) is the second cause of cancer-related mortality in North America [1, 2]. Colorectal liver metastases (CRLM) occur in 30% of patients and are responsible for two-thirds of CRC-related deaths. At presentation, up to 50% of patients with CRC have liver metastases; however, the majority of these liver metastases are unresectable [3].

Liver resection is considered standard of care in CRLM and is the only treatment to offer potential long-term survival. Modern surgical advances have led to a significant decrease in morbidity and mortality to less than 20% and 5% respectively associated with major hepatectomies [4, 5]. Patients previously deemed palliative can nowadays achieve better long-term outcome. Recent analyses have in fact shown 5- and 10-year survival rates as high

D. Henault · C. Shwaartz (✉)
HPB Surgical Oncology, University Health Network, University of Toronto, Toronto, ON, Canada
e-mail: David.Henault@uhn.ca; Chaya.Shwaartz@uhn.ca

H. Muaddi
Department of General Surgery, University of Toronto, Toronto, Canada
e-mail: Hala.Muaddi@mail.utoronto.ca

as 40–58% and 12–36%, respectively, when eradication of all disease was achieved [6–10].

In parallel to the increasingly aggressive surgical approach to CRLM, neuroendocrine liver metastases (NELM) have also gained interest. While liver metastases from neuroendocrine tumor (NET) generally portend a poor prognosis, resection with either debulking or curative intent has shown favorable long-term outcome [11–13]. Resection of NELM is associated with 5-year overall survival rates of 61–74% [5, 11, 14, 15]. Many of the first studies evaluating outcome of resected non-CRLM included metastases from both neuroendocrine and non-neuroendocrine origin. Early analyses have then shown patients with NELM to be a group with better prognosis [16–32].

Advances in surgical techniques and the promising results observed for CRLM and NELM have generated renewed enthusiasm in the role of hepatectomy for non-colorectal non-endocrine liver metastases (NCRNNELMs). The benefit of resection is still under debate for NCRNNELMs and the indications for surgery must be redefined in line with these developments. Not only are liver metastases from non-CRC and non-NET primaries less frequent, but liver involvement in these cases more often reflects widespread disease and an impossibility to achieve R0 resection.

Only a minority of patients with NCRNNELMs are candidate for R0 resection, giving rise to paucity of data in the literature. Moreover, NCRNNELMs are a heterogenous group of tumors with drastically different outcomes. Small case series, grouping together metastases behaving differently due to their biologically distinct origin, complicates outcome analyses. The retrospective nature of these series, obliged by the rarity of cases, also gives rise to a serious selection bias concern.

Epidemiology

In 2006, Adam et al. published a milestone series of 1452 NCRNNELMs resected patients in 41 centers, hence assisting with patient selection for surgery [33]. In this study, they have established a prognostic score based on predictors of poor survival outcome such as patient age >60 years, tumor origin non-breast/squamous histology/choroid melanoma, disease-free interval <12 months, extrahepatic metastases, R2 resection, and major hepatectomy. For a long time, this study has remained the largest one published in the literature and these factors have been used to help in surgical decision making.

A 2022 systematic review by Bauschke et al. found a slim total of 13 studies including >100 patients with NCRNNELM since 2005 [34]. The time span of patient inclusion in these studies is 1983–2017, with only 6 studies being multicentric and 3 studies including patients treated in 2015 or after. The 5-year and median overall survival for the whole cohort were 18% and 16 months. Drastic differences however were seen based on the primary tumor origin, with 5-year survival as good as 75% for GISTs or 29% for breast cancer, and as disappointing as 8% for lung cancer or 0% of pancreatic adenocarcinoma. The encouraging outcomes for some cancers must be disentangled from the poor outcomes seen in others.

Only one series larger than the one by Adam et al. has been published on the surgical treatment of NCRNNELMs in 2018 by Sano et al. [35]. In this Japanese series of 1539 patients treated in 124 institutions, the 5 most frequent primary tumor types were gastric carcinoma (540 patients [35%]), gastrointestinal stromal tumor (GIST) (204 patients [13%]), biliary carcinoma (150 patients [10%]), ovarian cancer (107 patients [7%]), and pancreatic carcinoma (77 patients [5%]). Breast primary represented 31% of cases in the study by Adam et al. vs. 5% of cases in the study by Sano et al. Following hepatic resection, these patients experienced 5-year survivals of 41% vs. 50%, with a median survival of 45 vs. 62 months, respectively. As for gastric cancer, these patients represented 4% of the cohort by Adam et al. with a 5-year survival of 27% and a median survival of 15 months compared to 32% and 30 months in the cohort by Sano et al. The difference in incidence of cancer by country highlights the complexity in generalizing outcomes of available evidence. Whether results from Eastern studies can be applied to Western population remains to be determined.

Serious advances in targeted therapy, immunomodulation, and loco-regional treatment have occurred in the recent years and have yet to be reflected in the outcomes of modern studies in NCRNNELMs. Surgeons face an increase of patients responding to some form of therapy and with now technically resectable disease by modern surgical standards. It remains unclear however which patient truly benefits from an aggressive surgical approach due to the poorly defined and varying tumor biology. The treatment algorithm varies increasingly as the therapeutic options multiply and patients are treated differently based on local expertise and reference pattern. This only adds to the difficulty in creating comparative studies and ultimately leads to clinical conundrum and absence of consensus and guidelines.

In this chapter, we aim to review the management and outcome of liver resection based on primary tumor type of NCRNNELMs. Each individual surgeon will have very limited opportunities to treat every one of these rare cases of liver metastases. It is our hope that this work will help guide state-of-the-art clinical decision-making.

Biology

Initial Hypotheses

The liver is a prime target for metastases. Cancer cells develop in such a way that they acquire survival and invasion capabilities through their evolution, but intrinsic features of the liver contribute to its qualities as a pro-metastatic niche.

The liver is the most common site of metastatic disease after lymph nodes [36]. In 1858, Virchow published his most outstanding scientific contribution stating that metastases can be explained by the lodgment of tumor-cell emboli in the vasculature [37]. This theory was later backed by James Ewing in 1929 who proposed that the anatomical structure of the vascular system was the pure mechanical contributor to the metastatic dissemination process [38].

A different school of thought was put forward early on by Paget in 1889, the "seed and soil" hypothesis. He stated the following principle: "When a plant goes to seed, its seeds are carried in all directions; but they can only live and grow if they fall on congenial soil". Paget's seminal paper was virtually unknown outside the metastasis community and was not accorded serious consideration during his lifetime [39]. It was only later in the 1970s where studies have shown the importance of organ selectivity to the metastatic spread, confirming the importance of cross-talk between 'seed' and 'soil' [40].

Achieving cure requires the complete eradication of all tumor cells. If the latter of the two hypotheses is correct (and which is now widely accepted), then and only then does local therapy—i.e., surgery—offer a logical treatment to a systemic disease. Surgical excision is the cornerstone of treatment of metastatic disease because it is site-specific. Nonetheless, micrometastatic disease explains the high rate of recurrence despite complete macroscopic excision. This is often treated with (neo)adjuvant systemic therapy.

As will be described below, many key features make the liver prone to developing metastatic disease and it is difficult to single out one specific characteristic as they are likely inter-related and influence one another. They all, however, carry part of the key in understanding and treating hepatic metastases.

Mechanical and Hemodynamic Properties of the Liver

Early observations gave rise to the concept that the peculiar vascular architecture of the liver (i.e., sinusoids), as well as its hemodynamic properties make it a prime target for metastatic seeding [41]. The liver is the largest internal organ in human beings, receiving approximately 25% of the total cardiac output at any moment, and the arterial to portal blood supply ratio is approximately 1:3 [42]. The important blood flow reaching the liver after draining other organs gives an increased statistical probability that circulating cells will reach this organ more often than others. Moreover, the hepatic microcirculation is rich in adhesion molecules and gives an opportunity to tumor cells to obstruct sinusoids, adhere to endothelial walls, and extravasate into the liver [43]. The transient ischemia resulting from tumor emboli causes an inflammatory response mediated by the release of nitrous oxide (NO), reactive oxygen species (ROS), tumor necrosis factor (TNF)-α, and interferon (IFN)-γ [44]. The local inflammation acts as a signal for endothelial cells to upregulate adhesion molecules and direct leukocyte homing. Unfortunately, this also opens the door to tumor cells to infiltrate the liver parenchyma [45, 46].

The liver vascular architecture can also easily supply metastases in nutrients and oxygen. Most tumors flip on the 'angiogenic switch', which refers to the tipping moment when tumors start to stimulate existing vessels to sprout toward them through hormonal regulation of pro-angiogenic factors [47]. Tumors can however also resort to alternative methods of gathering the required nutrients by hijacking liver sinusoids. This vascular feature of the liver easily allows tumors to acquire the necessary blood supply by resorting to vessel co-option [48]. This process was found to be a non-angiogenic mechanism for tumors to acquire blood supply and may be an explanation to the anti-angiogenic therapy resistance seen in some cancers [49].

Pathophysiology and Molecular Basis

The clonal selection model of the metastatic process suggests that heterogeneity develops within a population of cancer cells through mutational events, allowing a subpopulation to randomly acquire the necessary traits to disseminate successfully [39]. Alternatively, it has been argued that within cancers of the same pathological type, i.e., breast cancer, some tumors are a priori more likely to develop metastases than others. This is supported by gene expression data where specific molecular signatures have been found to accurately predict prognosis in breast cancer [50, 51], ovarian cancer [52], and melanoma [53]. Similarly, in CRC the genotype of microsatellite instability correlates with a decreased likelihood of metastatic spread [54].

Immunology

Every cancer has a type-specific pattern of cytokine expression that appears to direct both malignant and non-malignant cells to specific distant organs. The influx and clustering of bone-marrow-derived hematopoietic cells is one of the earliest events in the development of a metastatic deposit. This is closely followed by local inflammation and the release of matrix metalloproteinases. These local events appear to mediate remodeling of the extracellular matrix, creating a more permissive microenvironment for the eventual deposition and growth of malignant cells [55].

A recent study by Lee et al. brings a more sophisticated and detailed insight from an immunological standpoint as to why the liver is so commonly affected by metastases of various solid organ cancers [56]. In short, in a pancreatic cancer model, they explain that interleukin 6 (IL-6) secreted by the primary tumor stimulates the STAT3-signaling cascade in hepatocytes, ultimately resulting in liver fibrosis and myeloid cell accumulation in the liver. This finding was consistently found in humans as well, altogether suggesting that IL-6 production by the primary tumor might be a systemic way through which the nascent cancer prepares its distant metastatic site. Blockade of this axis in animal model ultimately leads to reduction of metastatic burden in pancreatic cancer.

Indications and Management of Liver Metastases by Primary Tumor

Adrenal

Adrenocortical carcinoma (ACC) is a poor-prognosis endocrine neoplasm with a worldwide incidence of approximately 0.5–2 per million population [57]. Because of the limited efficacy of systemic treatment, loco-regional therapies, or surgical resection, the 5-year survival rate for patients with stage IV disease is as low as 0–24%, with a median survival between 6 and 20 months [58–61]. Approximately one-third of patients present with synchronous metastases, the most common sites being the liver (40–90%), lungs (40–80%), and bones (5–20%) [62, 63].

Currently, the main treatment modality for synchronous metastatic ACC is mitotane plus chemotherapy regimen based on the First International Randomized Trial in Locally Advanced and Metastatic Adrenocortical Carcinoma Treatment study [64]. However, the survival remains dismal, and the cytotoxicity and narrow therapeutic range of this regimen limits its efficacity. For patients who are surgical candidates and who can potentially achieve total tumor burden eradication, resection is recommended and remains the only potential curative treatment [59, 60].

The literature on the management of this disease is rare, even more so regarding liver metastases. Case series have reported long-term survivors following aggressive treatment of ACC liver metastases [65]. However, factors relating to survival outcomes have failed to be consistent across studies, making patient selection difficult.

A series on liver resection for ACC metastases published by Gaujoux et al. in 2012 reported a median overall survival of 31.5 months and a 5-year survival of 39% following aggressive surgical resection [60]. After hepatectomy, all patients recurred. Dy et al. have studied a pure cohort of synchronous metastatic ACC undergoing surgery with intent of cure [66]. Patients achieving R0 vs. R2 resection had improved 1- and 2-year overall survival (69.9%, 46.9% vs. 53.0%, 22.1%; $p = 0.02$). They also noted a trend in improved disease-free survival for patients treated with perioperative therapy, which unfortunately did not translate to overall survival. Baur et al. reported median OS of 76 months in patients following liver resection compared to patients who did not undergo resection (10 months). However, disease-free survival after liver resection was only 9 months. Of note, patients with a time interval to the first metastasis/recurrence >12 months or solitary liver metastases showed significantly prolonged survival [67]. In 2020, Ayabe et al. published the largest series to date on ACC liver metastases treated with resection/ablation. In this cohort of 62 patients, they found 44 survivors >24 months. Longer disease-free interval and non-functioning tumors were associated with longer overall survival [68].

To this date, there is limited evidence supporting the use of locoregional treatment for metastatic ACC, but recent guidelines still support its use [69]. They offer the advantage of better tolerability for patient, but the outcome report related to these techniques is even more rare than for surgical resection. Veltri et al. reported their experience in 32 ACC metastases (4 lung and 28 liver) from 16 patients and were able to achieve a liver disease-free survival of 25 months and a median overall survival of

48.6 months, speaking to the benefits of RFA/MWA as a treatment option for ACC liver metastases [70]. As expected, larger tumors (mean 20 mm vs. 34.5 mm) were significantly more prone to local progression. Hormonal secretion was also an independent predictor of poor overall survival.

Finally, even in patients in whom curative intent surgery is not possible, aggressive debulking of 80–90% of the tumor when hormonal secretion is not achievable otherwise can significantly improve the quality of life of patients.

In conclusion, ACC is an aggressive disease with little effective treatment. The ability to achieve R0 resection, a longer disease-free interval and the non-secretory status of tumors are all related to better prognosis following liver resection. Surgery is not precluded in select cases of synchronous disease. Metachronous disease resection may be superior in patients with at least 12 months of disease-free interval. Promising advances in locoregional and ablative therapy may benefit patients with ACC liver metastases.

Breast

Breast cancer spreads systemically, and the liver represents the third most common site of metastases after the lungs and bones [71]. Breast cancer patients rarely present with isolated liver metastasis. Therefore, the role of liver resection in breast cancer liver metastasis (BCLM) remains controversial and the primary treatment remains systemic therapy and palliative local regimens [72]. If left untreated, survival of patients with BCLM is poor and does not exceed 8 months [73–75].

Breast cancer is heterogenous with respect to histology and molecular profiling. The majority of breast cancer are invasive ductal carcinomas, and approximately 10% are lobular ductal carcinomas [76]. Furthermore, the different hormonal subtypes have a different propensity to metastasize to the liver and respond to different treatment combinations. It is also common to see a discrepancy between the hormonal status of breast cancer primary tumors and BCLM.

Breast cancer with hormonal status ER−/PR−/HER2+ has the highest incidence of liver metastasis. This profile is found in 4.6% of all breast cancer cases but accounts for 32.7–46.5% of liver metastases [75, 77–79]. Patients with ER+/PR+/HER2+ breast cancer also have a high probability of liver metastasis, and represent 20.3% of all BCLM [77]. The most common primary tumor hormonal profile is ER+/PR+/HER2− and the incidence of BCLM in these patients is fourfold lower than patients with HER2+ disease [80].

Multiple retrospective studies examined patient outcomes after liver resection of BCLM. The outcomes reported vary widely, with a 5-year survival rate from 9% to 78%. This is likely attributable to the inconsistent inclusion criteria for hepatic resection across studies [81–83]. No consensus has been reached on the benefit of liver resection for BCLM. The 5th European School of Oncology–European Society of Medical Oncology (ESO–ESMO) International Consensus Guidelines for Advanced Breast Cancer (ABC 5) suggest that liver resection for BCLM can be considered in carefully select patients with good performance status and limited tumor burden [84]. Yet, the National Comprehensive Cancer Network (NCCN) guidelines do not discuss liver resection as a treatment option for patients with BCLM [85].

Adam et al. in a study of 454 patients undergoing hepatic resection for BCLM succeeded in showing a 10-year survival rate of 22% after liver resection [33]. A propensity score matching analysis found superior overall survival after liver resection in 384 patients with BCLM, with a median and 5-year OS of 61.8 vs. 38.6 months and 54.7% vs. 21.9%, respectively, when compared to systemic therapy alone [86]. Carefully selected patients with BCLM have been found to have a median OS as high as 116 months [87]. A recent systematic review endeavored to describe the factors that can identify patients with BCLM with superior 5-year OS survival. In an analysis of 35 series, patients with axillary lymph node positivity at the time of primary resection were found to have a significantly worst survival following liver resection [88, 89]. In addition, hormonal status of the primary tumor was significantly related to survival outcomes, with ER+ primaries having better overall survival than ER− primary tumors [90–92]. This shifts the focus on making the decision to resect the liver disease based on the primary disease receptor status rather than the BCLM receptor status [93, 94]. Of note 1/3 of BCLM are triple negative, however the receptor status of the liver metastases does not correlate with survival after resection. Good prognostic factors related to the BCLM include size <30 mm, solitary metastases or unilobar distribution, minor hepatectomy, and longer disease-free interval [87, 93–98]. Response to systemic therapy also appears to be an important predictor of survival. In one study, patients who progressed during pre-hepatectomy chemotherapy had a 5-year survival rate of 0% compared to 11% in responders [99].

Other locoregional treatment modalities may include TACE, TARE, and radiofrequency ablation [100, 101]. These are offered to a selected group of patients and can be combined with other surgical or nonsurgical treatments. The evidence for those modalities is still limited and in its early stages. Patients treated with RFA have achieved a median overall survival between 30 and 60 months. However, it is still thought that liver resection, when applicable, can lead to superior outcomes in comparable patients [102–105]. Therefore, these modalities are reserved for patients who are poor surgical candidates.

Endometrial

Uterine cancer is the most common gynecologic cancer in the United States. Most patients are diagnosed at an early stage of the disease with 10–15% of patients having advanced disease at the time of diagnosis. Metastatic endometrial cancer is usually multifocal and rarely managed operatively. Around 4% of patients develop metastatic disease and 0.9% of all metastatic endometrial cancer have liver involvement [105].

There is limited evidence on patient outcomes after endometrial liver metastases resection. Over a period of 10 years, one center reported five women in whom liver metastases developed between 11 months and 10 years following endometrial cancer resection. These patients underwent hepatic resection with disease-free survival of 8–66 months post-resection [106]. Based on limited data, it appears that complete cytoreduction of visible disease is associated with improved overall survival as well as progression-free survival [107–109]. Complete cytoreduction and adjuvant radiation were both positively associated with survival, whereas adjuvant chemotherapy alone was associated with decreased survival [110]. Furthermore, for each 10% increase in the proportion of patients undergoing complete cytoreduction, survival improved by 9.3 months.

Esophagus

Esophageal cancer is the sixth cause of cancer-related mortality worldwide and half of patients have metastatic disease on presentation [2, 111]. Metastatic esophageal cancer is usually widely disseminated and is associated with a 5-year survival of 3–5% when multiple sites of disease are present and 7–8% when disease is limited to the liver [112]. The liver is the most common site of metastases and is involved in isolation in approximately 35% of patients [113]. Compared to hepatic metastases from adenocarcinoma of other gastrointestinal origin, patients with esophageal cancer liver metastases fare worse.

Most of the evidence on liver resection is anecdotal, with small series reporting adequate survival from 14 to 22 months, often with recurrence [114–116]. One patient from this series with metachronous metastases was alive 92 months after liver resection. Oligometastatic esophageal cancer may represent an entity with more favorable biology and is generally defined as spread to 1 organ with ≤3 metastases or 1 extra-regional lymph node station [117].

Adam et al. reported a 3-year median overall survival following hepatic resection of 32% and 16 months in 20 patients with esophageal cancer metastases [33]. Sano et al. reported 51 patients that underwent liver resection for esophageal cancer liver metastases with a median survival of 15 months and 5-year overall survival of 15% [35]. A recent meta-analysis aimed at determining the survival benefit associated with local directed treatment of oligometastatic esophageal cancer. The overall survival data was available on 740 patients from 16 non-randomized studies. Compared to systemic therapy alone, the addition of local therapy (metastasectomy or SBRT) was associated with improved survival for all-sites metastases (pooled aHR 0.47, 95% CI: 0.30–0.74) and for liver oligometastases (pooled aHR 0.39, 95% CI: 0.22–0.59) [117].

In conclusion, patients with esophageal cancer liver metastases are rarely candidates for surgery because of disseminated disease, but there are favorable reports published on the benefit of radical surgery in well-selected patients with oligometastatic disease.

Gastric

Gastric cancer currently ranks as the fifth most frequently diagnosed cancer worldwide and the third leading cause of cancer death [2]. The incidence of gastric cancer varies by geographic region, with half of the cases worldwide occurring in Eastern Asia. Gastric cancer is notoriously aggressive with approximately 35% of patients with metastatic disease at presentation [118]. The liver is a common site of spread in 9–40% of patients although patients with gastric cancer liver metastases (GCLM) often present with bilobar disease, peritoneal dissemination, or lymph node invasion [119–121]. Hepatic metastases are diagnosed synchronously in 3–14% of patients, and metachronously in up to 37% of patients [122]. Most cases of GCLM are considered incurable and liver resection in these patients has historically been contraindicated.

Overall, 5-year survival in patients with GCLM ranges from 0% to 10% and the median survival with systemic chemotherapy is 7–14 months [123, 124]. However, encouraging results were put forward recently with 5-year survival rates as high as 10–40% in carefully selected patients for liver resection [122, 125, 126]. The two largest series published on NCRNNELMs found that following resection of GCLM, patients had 5-year overall survival of 27–32% and a median OS of 15–30 months [33, 35].

There is a lack of consensus guideline on patients who can potentially benefit from liver resection due to absence of prospective studies or randomized data. Many retrospective studies and meta-analyses have consistently reported similar outcomes and prognostic factors. These reviews often included patients from overlapping studies, sometimes with extra-hepatic disease or evaluating non-surgical ablative treatment [122, 126, 127]. In an effort to rigorously address these pitfalls, Granieri et al. published a systematic review of 29 studies from year 2000 and onward [128]. They identified 1132 patients undergoing hepatectomy for GCLM. More than one liver metastases and T3–4 primary tumor were non-significantly related to worst survival. These two factors, as well as lymphatic invasion, have been shown in multiple prior studies to significantly predict outcome [129–132]. Significant prognostic predictors also included bilobar disease (HR: 2.46; $p < 0.001$) and metastasis greatest dimension ≥ 5 cm (HR: 1.77; $p < 0.001$). Synchronous liver metastases resulted in an increased risk of death (HR: 1.08; $p = 0.001$) with 23.5% 5-year overall survival compared to 29.2% 5-year overall survival for patients with metachronous metastases.

Resection vs. No Resection

Markar et al. reported improved OS for liver resection and a median of 1-year, 3-year, and 5-year survival of 68%, 31%, and 27% respectively in an analysis of 9 studies with 679 patients: 235 in the resection group and 444 in the non-resected group (HR = 0.50; 95% CI 0.41–0.61; $p < 0.001$) [122].

A systematic review by Gavriilidis et al. aimed at evaluating the benefits of hepatectomy and gastrectomy (349 patients) compared to gastrectomy alone (512 patients) in 11 studies. Six hundred and seven (62%) patients underwent resection for synchronous metastases and 376 (38%) for metachronous metastases. Significantly better 5-year overall survival was demonstrated for patients who underwent gastrectomy plus hepatic resection compared to gastrectomy alone (HR = 0.83 (0.78, 0.90), $P < 0.001$) [122].

Loco-Regional Modalities

A 2021 meta-analysis of Sun et al. reviewed 23 studies, involving 5472 GCLM patients, comparing survival outcomes of patients treated with gastrectomy alone, gastrectomy and hepatectomy, RFA and gastrectomy, TACE and gastrectomy, palliative chemotherapy. Overall survival was significantly better for hepatic resection or RFA plus gastrectomy compared to gastrectomy alone or palliative chemotherapy.

In conclusion, metastasectomy for gastric cancer is feasible and safe in both metachronous and synchronous scenarios. In well-selected patients, it appears to offer a survival benefit. Patients with a high burden of liver disease, synchronous metastases, and locally advanced primary tumors or lymphatic spread are less likely to benefit from aggressive surgical management. The currently undergoing RENNAISSANCE TRIAL will hopefully provide further guidance by evaluating in a randomized prospective fashion the benefit of systemic therapy with or without radical surgery in oligometastatic gastric and gastroesophageal junction cancer [133]. Emerging evidence are showing benefits to local ablative therapies compared with resection, but more data is required before drawing definitive conclusions.

Gastrointestinal Stromal Tumors (GIST)

Gastrointestinal stromal tumors (GISTs) are mesenchymal neoplasms of the gastrointestinal tract. They arise from the interstitial cells of cajal in the muscularis propria layer of the GI tract. GISTs account for 1–2% of all neoplasms of the digestive track and most frequently occur in the stomach (50–70%), small intestine (25–35%), the colon and rectum (5–10%), and the esophagus (<5%) [134, 135].

The majority of GISTs (75–80%) have a gain-of-function KIT mutation. The most common mutation in KIT gene is exon 11 (65%). In-frame deletions in exon 11, particularly in codons 557 and 558, are associated with worse prognosis compared to kit exon 11 point mutations [136]. Other KIT mutations can occur in exon 9 (8–10%) which is often found in small or large bowel tumors, and less commonly in exons 13, 17, 18. Other mutations include platelet-derived growth factor receptor alpha (PDGFRA) mutants which is the second most common molecular subtype found in 10% of GISTs and more frequently in GISTs that arise in the stomach [137]. Exon 18 of PDGFRA is the most commonly mutated region and it's found in 8% of GISTs. GISTs associated with *PDGFRA* mutation due to Asp842Val substitution in exon18 is resistant to tyrosine kinase inhibitor (TKI) imatinib. Less common mutations are found in exon 12 or 14 of PDGFRA. The remainder 10–15% of GISTs do not have detectable *KIT* or *PDGFRA* gene mutation and are so-called "wild-type" GISTs. Often these GISTs harbor a gain-of-function mutation in RAS or BRAF, loss-of-function neurofibromatosis type 1 (NF1) mutations, or succinate dehydrogenase deficiency [137]. The introduction of molecular targeting therapy with tyrosine kinase inhibitors such as imatinib has revolutionized the clinical management of GISTs, but treatment needs to be tailored to mutation sensitivity. KIT and PDGFRA wild-type GIST have no standard/effective therapeutic alternative.

The primary GIST tumor can be classified into four prognostic categories, ranging from very low risk to high risk, according to site of the primary lesion, size of the primary lesion, and the number of mitotic figures identified on histology. The liver is the most common site of metastasis (90%) [138]. Metastatic GIST disease is seen in up to 50% of patients at primary presentation and up to 80% may experience liver metastasis within the first 2 years [139–141]. For GIST liver metastases, the therapeutic modalities include systemic therapies such as chemotherapy and targeted therapy, tumor ablation and trans-arterial embolization, and resection.

Surgical resection with or without TKI is the standard of care for resectable primary GIST. However, in the presence of liver metastases, tyrosine kinase inhibitors (TKI) such as imatinib are the first-line treatment of choice [142, 143]. GIST metastatic to the liver is usually unresponsive to cytotoxic agents with response rate as low as 5% [144]. Treatment with imatinib can achieve very high survival rates, unfortunately, initial or acquired resistance to

TKI usually appears years after its use. Nearly 50% of patients will develop resistance within 18 months of its administration [145, 146]. Second- (e.g., sunitinib) and third-line agents (e.g., nilotinib and masitinib) have shown promise in patients resistant to imatinib [147].

Complete response of metastatic disease after TKI is uncommon [148]. Surgery after TKI is thought to prolong the disease control time by resecting remaining disease resistant to TKI and through decreasing the risk of secondary resistance by reducing the tumor volume reaching 5-year survival rates as high as 91% [149–152]. Overall, surgery is recommended after 6–9 months from the initiation of imatinib for maximal treatment response and is usually appropriate for patients with response to preoperative imatinib treatment. Therefore, the decision on whether to perform surgery is based on radiologic findings and strict parameters to guide this decision are lacking. A randomized controlled trials evaluated liver resections with neoadjuvant and adjuvant imatinib therapy compared to imatinib alone. After a median follow-up of 36 months, the OS was significantly better in the surgical arm compared with the non-operative arm (1- and 3-year OS; 100% and 89% versus 85% and 60%, respectively, $p = 0.03$) [153]. Another study evaluated 48 patients who underwent liver resection for GIST metastases, 36 of whom received TKI therapy either pre- or postoperatively. Median survival was 7.5 years and 5-year overall survival was 76%. Multivariate analysis demonstrated that R0 resection of the liver metastasis was the only significant predictor of survival [154].

One prospective phase III study explored the role of surgery in GIST-LM. No difference was found in DFS, but there was a significantly longer median OS achieved in the surgery group (median not reached) vs. 49 months in the non-surgery group [155]. Most of the data comes from retrospective studies which suggest that, in order to achieve good outcomes, adequate patient selection based on the response to TKI is essential [148, 149, 152, 156–159]. Therefore, resection may drastically improve survival in the case of good response (OS of 100% and DFS >60% at two years) and is not recommended in cases of widespread progression (OS of 0%–60% and DFS of 0% at two years) [140, 156, 160, 161].

Patients could receive upfront surgical resection followed by TKI treatment. A multicenter European study retrospectively evaluated 239 patients undergoing hepatic metastectomy, all of whom received adjuvant imatinib. R0/R1 resection was found to be a significant predictor of survival and median survival in this group was 8.7 years and 5.3 years in patients with R2 resection ($p < 0.0001$) [148]. Other significant predictors of survival were female gender and metastases confined to the liver.

Disease progression is managed by imatinib dose escalation followed by second- and third-line agents. In the event of tumor rupture or hemorrhage, surgery or hepatic artery embolization may be performed in an emergency setting. Six to twelve months of imatinib therapy is recommended for patients with unresectable hepatic metastases and if the tumor responds, resection can be considered if an R0 resection can be anticipated [162].

Percutaneous ablation, embolization, and intra-arterial therapies are reserved for palliative purposes or combined with resection. The data on their efficacy for the treatment of liver metastases from GIST is scarce [163–168]. All of these procedures seem to be equivalent and their use depends on local availability.

In the case of unresectable LM, liver transplantation (LT), the last and most radical option for locoregional management, remains in its early stages with limited evidence supporting its use [169].

Lung

Lung cancer is the leading cause of cancer-related mortality worldwide [170]. Overall survival for all types at 5 years is 19% [171]. Importantly, 70% of patients present with advanced-stage disease at diagnosis [172]. Specifically, patients with liver metastasis have the worst prognosis with a median OS of 3–12 months and often have multiple metastatic sites involved [173–177].

The management of lung cancer liver metastases mainly consists of chemotherapy and radiation. Most of the surgical experience with this disease comes from the broader context of studies reporting on NCRNNELM. Adam et al. found a 5-year survival of

8% in 32 resected patients, whereas Sano et al. reported a 23% 5-year overall survival in 25 resected patients. Of interest, these studies were published more than 10 years apart and improvement in adjunct therapies may play a role in the improved outcomes of the latter series [33, 35]. Long-term survival following hepatectomy has been reported in selected patients with few metastases, but the evidence remains anecdotal [178–180].

A recent retrospective study from 2014 to 2019 on 58 patients with liver metastases from lung cancer undergoing RFA found acceptable local tumor control especially in tumors ≤3 cm. The overall survival (OS) rate at 5 years after RFA was 14.4% and the median OS was 14.0 ± 1.6 months.

In conclusion, the presence of liver metastases in the context of lung cancer represents a worst prognosis. Nevertheless, the role of surgery as well as other treatment modalities (RFA, TAE/TACE) may be beneficial, but cannot be definitively determined with current evidence. Recent advances in targeted therapy and immunotherapy may guide future decision-making [181].

Melanoma

Malignant melanoma can arise from a uveal, cutaneous, or a mucosal origin, and each has a different clinical course. Cutaneous melanoma is most common and spreads to lungs, lymph nodes, and soft tissue with fewer patients developing liver metastasis (10–20%) [182, 183]. Uveal melanoma is rare and spreads hematogenously most commonly to the liver (89%) and 45% of patients will develop liver metastasis at 10 years [184, 185]. Mucosal melanoma is most rare and 36% of the patients will develop liver metastases [186, 187].

Surgical resection has not been accepted as a therapeutic option as most patients will have several sites of involvement with a limited median survival of 4–6 months without therapy [188]. There is scarce information on outcomes following resection in patients with disease limited to the liver, however its judicial use in a selected group of patients can be appropriate. Of note, there are currently no randomized controlled studies to define the role of surgery in the treatment of hepatic metastases from melanoma.

Six studies compared surgical to nonsurgical resection of melanoma liver metastases. The overall survival in all studies was longer after liver resection [189–193]. In patients with ocular melanoma, a median survival 14–24 months was observed after liver resection compared to 3–12 months for patients who were treated with chemotherapy or non-operatively [189–192]. Similar trends were observed in patients with cutaneous melanoma that metastasized to the liver such that the median survival for resected patients was 28 months compared to 6 months for non-surgical patients [193]. Other single-arm retrospective studies reporting the outcomes of patients after liver resection show a similar trend of improved median survival at 19–39 months [33, 194–198].

Recurrence rate after liver resection is high (72–75%) [193, 195, 196]. Studies that examined prognostic factors showed a significant impact of R0 vs. R2 resection on survival [192]. Other favorable prognostic factors include fewer number of lesions, long disease-free interval, and localized metastatic disease [33, 190, 191, 194].

Liver resection is offered to 2–7% of patients with metastatic melanoma. Palliative cytotoxic systemic therapy or radiation therapy is resorted to as the mainstay of therapy for most patients with stage IV melanoma [191–193, 198]. Palliative radiotherapy and systemic cytotoxic chemotherapy are not effective in conferring a survival advantage. Biological agents such as interferon-α and interleukin-2 have yielded modest response rates but are associated with significant toxicity [199].

New molecular therapies have become standard of care in treatment of metastatic melanoma. BRAF and MEK inhibitors are used for patients with tumor mutations in the *BRAF* gene. These demonstrated superior survival and proved most effective when combined [200–203]. Immunomodulators targeting CTLA-4 (e.g., ipilimumab) and PD-1 (e.g., nivolumab, pembrolizumab) are used increasingly in all patients with advanced melanoma. These agents collectively have improved overall survival for patients with advanced melanoma compared to prior therapies [204].

Large-scale randomized controlled trials on advanced metastatic cutaneous melanoma demonstrated that pembrolizumab had less toxicity and is superior to ipilimumab in with respect to PFS and OS [203, 205]. The widespread use of these agents may lead to an increased number of patients referred for consideration for resection of isolated hepatic metastases. It is difficult to estimate the impact that liver resection will have on these patients, but it seems reasonable to adopt a resectional approach in highly selected patients, i.e., those with a long disease-free interval from treatment of the primary tumor to development of metastases, and patients who can be rendered disease-free following surgery. However, it is imperative to understand the molecular drivers for melanoma as they differ between ocular and cutaneous melanoma. Ocular melanoma has a lower response to targeted agents because BRAF, RAS, and KIT mutations are rare [206–208]. Recent evidence supports the use of immunotherapy in metastatic ocular melanoma.

Regional therapies include hepatic arterial infusions, chemoembolization, and isolated or percutaneous hepatic perfusions, TACE and RFA, but limited data on their efficacy is available, and rates of response vary greatly across studies [192, 209–218].

Ovarian

Epithelial ovarian cancer represents the most common malignancy of the ovary and the liver is the most common site of metastasis followed by the lungs, bones, and brain [219, 220]. Historically, these patients were considered to not be suitable for surgical treatment. Nowadays, cytoreductive surgery and platinum-based chemotherapy are key to the treatment of ovarian cancer liver metastases.

Ovarian cancer can metastasize to the liver through different modes: peritoneal dissemination, hematogenous metastases, and lymph node metastases [221]. Different treatment modalities can be used based on the metastasis approach. Peritoneal dissemination (PD), as the most common pattern, usually leads to tumor implantation in the liver capsule without invasion of the liver parenchyma (Stage III). Hematogenous metastasis can lead to intraparenchymal metastases (stage 4) and has a worse prognosis [222]. Lymph node metastasis results in liver seeding through the portal venous system. Peritoneal metastases that invade the liver parenchyma may be difficult to distinguish from parenchymal metastases. These two entities reflect different biology, response to therapy, and have different survival outcomes [223, 224]. If this distinction can be made preoperatively, patients with parenchymal lesions are considered to have more advanced disease and are generally treated with systemic therapy rather than surgery [223, 224].

Numerous studies have shown that surgical treatment for patients with ovarian cancer liver metastases is safe, effective, and can improve prognosis [223–225]. The National Comprehensive Cancer Network (NCCN) guidelines recommend that part of the liver, gallbladder, tail of pancreas, and diaphragm can be resected if needed to achieve satisfactory cytoreduction [226]. Achieving complete resection of primary and metastatic disease (R0) is the most favorable determinant of patient prognosis. Previous studies have shown a median survival of 50.1 months in patients with stage IV ovarian cancer who underwent hepatic cytoreduction for liver metastasis [227]. Interestingly, optimal hepatic cytoreduction was only achieved in 16% of patients, and nearly 30% of patients achieved suboptimal hepatic disease resection, resulting in a median survival of 27 months. Additionally, the parenchymal liver lesions correlated with survival such that every additional 10% cytoreduction increased the survival rate by 5.5% [227].

Patients not surgical candidates because of extent of disease or poor performance status can receive platinum-based chemotherapy combined with paclitaxel. These treatments can also be utilized in the neoadjuvant setting to reduce perioperative mortality, complications, and improve the possibility of R0 resection [228]. Intraperitoneal chemotherapy also offers survival benefits in stage III disease compared to intravenous therapy alone. However, it requires optimal debulking in order to be the most effective [229–231]. Therefore, successful cytoreduction is a crucial step in the management of advanced ovarian cancer.

TACE and RFA offer potential alternative therapeutic options in achieving local control in patients with contraindications to resection or as adjuncts to systemic therapy [223, 232, 233].

Pancreatic Adenocarcinoma

Pancreatic ductal adenocarcinoma (PDAC) accounts for 90% of all histological subtypes of pancreatic cancer [234]. It is the fourth leading cause of cancer-related death in Europe and the United States [235]. Less than 20% of patients are candidates for curative-intent resection and approximately half of patients have stage IV disease at presentation, the liver being a frequent site of metastases [236]. The average 5-year overall survival for unresectable PDAC is 5%, with a median survival of 8–11 months for patients with metastatic disease receiving chemotherapy [237–239].

Complete surgical resection remains the only potential cure for PDAC, but the role for surgery in the setting of metastatic disease has not been well investigated, especially in the era of modern chemotherapy. Most data are derived from older retrospective analyses. The struggle for the surgeon is even more apparent when complete excision of the metastatic disease is technically feasible, especially considering the recent success of metastasectomies in the setting of other solid organ liver metastases. However, many patients with liver metastases also carry additional systemic disease. As a result, most will not be surgical candidates and chemotherapy represents the backbone of treatment.

An accrued interest in this topic can be seen as the number of publications on hepatectomies for oligometastatic PDAC has increased in the recent years. Experts have put forward an effort in identifying characteristics of patients likely to benefit from such an aggressive approach. One must consider two different scenarios when analyzing the literature; the case of synchronous metastases, which has been traditionally a contraindication to surgery due to lack of benefit when compared to palliative bypass, and the case of metachronous metastases, which is more controversial, especially in the setting of long disease-free interval.

Synchronous

The first study assessing the survival benefit of simultaneous pancreas and liver resection for Stage IV PDAC found no improvement in overall survival in 33 patients compared to palliative bypass (4 vs. 6 months, respectively) [240]. A subsequent study by Gleisner et al. also found an abysmal median overall survival of 5.9 months in 17 patients treated with simultaneous pancreatic and hepatic resection, again no different when compared to patients undergoing palliative bypass [241]. Many more small series around the same period consistently found this lack of survival advantage and increased peri-operative morbidity and mortality [242–244].

In the modern era, these studies are hardly generalizable as little to no chemotherapy was given or documented in these earlier series. Series on synchronous liver resection of stage IV PDAC have since shown the crucial role of chemotherapy in the treatment of these patients and have encouragingly found carefully selected long-term survivors.

In a 2016 study of 69 patients from six European centers with synchronous pancreas and liver resections for PDAC and isolated hepatic metastases, outcomes were compared to 69 matched patients who did not undergo resection. Median survival was greater in the resection group (14.5 months vs 7.5 months) and four resected patients were alive longer than 5 years. However, data on chemotherapy was incomplete and of these, less than 80% of resected patients received adjuvant therapy. It was mainly administered in the form of single-agent gemcitabine in 70% of resected patients and a minority (7%) received post-operative FOLFIRINOX [245].

Andreou et al. found 1-, 3-, and 5-year OS rates of 41%, 13%, and 7%, respectively, following resection of synchronous PDAC liver metastases in 76 patients. Preoperative and postoperative chemotherapy were only administered to 5% and 72% of patients, respectively, and were not standardized due to the long period of time covered by this study. In their multivariate analysis, R1 status and absence of pre- or post-operative chemotherapy were all significantly associated with worst DFS and OS [246].

Since the 2011 landmark publication by Conroy et al., FOLFIRINOX has become the standard chemotherapy regimen for PDAC [237]. Following recent studies in resected patients, the trend even points at superior outcomes following a neoadjuvant strategy, across all stages of PDAC.

Highlighting the importance of neoadjuvant therapy in the context of synchronous resection of PDAC liver metastases, Crippa et al. reported the highest median survival at 39 months in 127 patients treated with primary chemotherapy before resection [247]. As a control group, 116 patients had chemotherapy only and their median OS was only 11 months. Frigerio et al. found that in 24/535 patients with metastatic PDAC and disappearing liver metastases following chemotherapy, pancreatic resection without associated liver resection resulted in OS and DFS was 56 and 27 months, respectively [248].

To separate the early, grim, and chemotherapy-free literature from the more encouraging recent one, a 2020 systematic review focused strictly on series published after 2011 [249]. In 204 patients issued from 6 studies with synchronous resection of PDAC liver metastases, 63% underwent upfront resection and 35% had surgery after primary chemotherapy. Median OS range was significantly improved in patients treated with neoadjuvant chemotherapy (34–56 months) vs. upfront resection (7.6–14.5 months).

In aggregate, the level of data on synchronous resection of PDAC liver metastases is poor and based on small series. Traditionally, it was recommended to avoid resection in these patients due to their poor prognosis. Recent data, mostly owing to the advances in systemic therapy, suggest that provided careful selection, some patients could benefit from an aggressive surgical approach. However, this should only be performed under a well-designed prospective clinical trial. When unsuspected synchronous liver metastases are discovered at the time of surgery, resection of the primary tumor with concomitant resection of the liver lesions should also be strongly discouraged. Moreover, avoiding a bypass procedure (unless indicated) may decrease recovery time and allow earlier initiation of chemotherapy.

A stage III randomized controlled trial is under way (Chinese Study Group for Pancreatic Cancer (CSPAC)–1) in order to establish a strategy for selecting PDAC patients with liver oligometastases who may benefit from synchronous resection after conversion chemotherapy. Complete accrual is expected by 2023 [250].

Metachronous

It has been agreed upon for a longer time that resection in well-selected patients with metachronous disease may provide a survival benefit.

For example, Dünschede et al. reported on 23 patients with pancreatic liver metastases (14 synchronous and 9 metachronous disease). Surgery in synchronous liver disease did not provide a survival benefit when compared to gemcitabine-based chemotherapy (8 vs. 11 months), but it was associated with a longer median survival (31 months) in patients with metachronous disease [251]. In the famous 2006 series by Adam et al., long before the current chemotherapeutic standards were adopted, a subgroup of 40 resected patients with metachronous pancreatic adenocarcinoma liver metastasis had an estimated 5-year survival of 20%—better than anticipated for patients with stage IV disease [33].

In the largest series published to date, Hackert et al. reported on 85 patients after pancreatic and synchronous or metachronous liver resection [252]. The median overall survival after resection was 12.3 months and there were no differences observed between synchronous and metachronous patients. Gemcitabine was the most commonly used agent in adjuvant therapy and 86% of patients completed their course. As previously discussed, FOLFIRINOX might further improve the survival.

While patient selection clearly plays a very important part in explaining the survival benefit associated with surgery, the data suggest that liver resection may be beneficial in a select subset of patients with metachronous disease. The most relevant prognostic factors appear to be response to preoperative chemotherapy, oligometastatic disease, and R0 resection [253]. Molecular stratification biomarkers may prove useful in this rare setting [254].

Renal Cancer

Renal cell carcinoma (RCC) accounts for 3% of all malignancies. Approximately 20–30% of patients with RCC present with synchronous metastatic disease and 20–40% develop metachronous recurrence after primary resection. Hepatic spread is usually an indicator of poor prognosis due to widespread disease and is present in approximately 20% of metastatic kidney cancers [255]. Only 10–15% of patients with metastases have disease confined to the liver. About 10% of metastatic patients present with synchronous disease and the rate of metastases is known to correlate with the size of the primary tumor [256]. Less than 5% of patients with primary renal cell carcinoma <4 cm have metastatic disease at presentation [257, 258].

Systemic therapy options for RCC are limited. The prognosis for metastatic RCC is poor with a 5-year OS of 5–10% [259]. Liver metastases portend a poor prognosis of 7–12 months median survival [260, 261]. Without treatment, patients with metastatic renal cell cancer die within 4 months following diagnosis and have a 1-year survival of 10%.

Interleukin-2 and interferon-α were previously used as first-line therapy for metastatic RCC and were not found to be active against liver metastases [261, 262]. Current regimens employ tyrosine kinase inhibitors like sunitinib, which is associated with an improved progression-free survival in phase III trials, and emerging data suggest that immune checkpoint inhibitors are effective in metastatic RCC [262, 263]. Although this paradigm shift is recent, radical resection of metastatic RCC, when feasible, and in combination with new systemic agents, is likely to improve survival outcome in well-selected patients.

A review by Dabestani et al. found in six studies that complete surgical resection in metastatic RCC was associated with longer OS compared to non-radical treatment (40.8 vs. 14.8 months) [264]. Zaid et al. evaluated eight retrospective studies in a population of 958 patients who underwent metastasectomy compared to 1309 who had not undergone metastasectomy or only partial resection. Completely resected patients had a significantly better

OS (36.4–142 months) compared to the latter group (8.4–27 months) [265].

Specifically, regarding liver resection, it is performed in approximately 1% of patients with liver metastases, consequently there is little literature on this topic and data is limited to retrospective reviews.

A study from the Netherlands examined 33 patients who underwent resection or ablative therapy for RCC hepatic metastases. The study documented no operative mortality, with 5-year disease-free and overall survival of 11% and 43%, respectively. The median overall survival was 33 months [266]. A second retrospective study compared 68 patients who underwent surgery to a cohort of 20 patients who were eligible but refused an operation. Disease in these patients was mostly confined to the liver. Overall survival at 5 years in the treatment arm was 62% in comparison to 29% in the control group [267]. A review of 13 articles and 378 patients who underwent liver resection for RCC metastases showed a median survival after resection that ranged from 15 to 142 months with a 1-, 3-, and 5-year OS that ranged from 69–100%, 26–83.3%, and 0–62% respectively. The median disease-free survival ranged from 7.2 to 27 months [268]. Factors associated with better survival included metachronous metastases, R0 metastasectomy, and non-sarcomatoid histology [261, 266, 267, 269].

More contemporary series have examined liver resection for RCC metastases in the context of TKI use. In one series of 39 patients undergoing liver resection (37 patients) or ablation (2 patients), the overall median survival was 42 months. During a median follow-up period of 2.2 years, 74% of patients who received no targeted therapy recurred, compared to 40% of patients maintained on postoperative treatment. Multivariate analysis identified postoperative TKI therapy as a predictor of survival [270]. Preoperative TKI therapy has also been shown to downsize unresectable RCC liver metastases in order to facilitate safe liver resection [271]. In a cohort of patients with metachronous RCC metastases treated with targeted therapies, Yu et al. reported a median OS of 52 months for patients who underwent complete metastasectomy compared to 16 months for targeted therapy only and 22 months for incomplete resection.

Several new immunotherapies are becoming important in the treatment of kidney cancer and are likely to influence surgical approach to RCC liver metastases [272–274].

Conclusion

Metastatic RCC has a poor survival and liver involvement portends even worst prognosis as it often is accompanied by widespread disease. Nevertheless, there is accumulating evidence that radical resection of all disease, when feasible, improves patient outcomes. A high number of oncological therapies have become available in the recent years and although the results are encouraging, they are still early. Liver surgery in selected patients represents a potential curative option for metastatic kidney cancer. Such undertakings should be done only following accurate patient selection and the multidisciplinary approach is essential.

Sarcomas

Soft-tissue sarcomas (STSs) are rare malignant tumors with an incidence of approximately 1% of all malignancies [275]. Although the lung is the most common site of metastases, the potential for liver metastases is also well recognized. Gastrointestinal organ sarcomas such as gastrointestinal stromal tumors (GISTs) and leiomyosarcomas (LMS) commonly metastasize to the liver, with a reported incidence of 55–72% in patients who underwent a curative resection of the primary tumor [140, 276, 277].

Retroperitoneal and abdominal visceral sarcomas are known to metastasize to the liver through the abdominal lymphatic system, by dissemination through the portal vein or through direct invasion. The liver is a prime target of STS as well, but its mechanism of spread is less well understood [278]. GISTs are the most common STS. Unfortunately, 61% of patients have metastases at the time of diagnosis [279].

There is limited data available on the oncological outcomes following liver resection for sarcoma metastases, mostly owing to their rarity and heterogeneity. Moreover, most studies consist of small case series, and do not differentiate between gastrointestinal stromal tumor (GIST) and non-GIST sarcoma metastases, creating a significant bias in oncological outcomes [280].

Systemic chemotherapy does not prolong survival remarkably and therefore hepatic metastasis is generally associated with a poor prognosis [281]. Liver resection is the curative treatment of choice in well-selected patients.

In order to more properly assess outcomes of non-GIST sarcomas, one must look at the few published studies making the distinction. Tirotta et al. described their experience on 24 patients from 2 European centers [280]. Retroperitoneal leiomyosarcoma was the most common type of sarcoma and metastases were most commonly metachronous (79%), with the median disease-free interval being 33 months. The median OS was 35 months, and 1, 3-, and 5-year OS were 94%, 36%, and 18%, respectively. Patients with extra-hepatic metastases resected at the time of liver resection were found to have a significantly shorter OS, compared to those who had only liver metastases, with median survivals of 27 vs. 36 months ($p = 0.016$). In the largest series reported to date, Goumard et al. reported on 126 patients, half of whom had leiomyosarcoma, undergoing liver resection for non-GIST sarcoma liver metastases [282]. In the entire cohort, 5-year OS and RFS were 49.3% and 14.9%, respectively, and median OS and RFS were 58.0 months and 12.5 months, respectively. Presence of extra-hepatic disease at the time of liver resection was again significantly associated with lower survival outcomes. In the 83 (66%) patients with metachronous liver metastases, disease-free interval > 6 months was associated with improved OS (median 67.3 months vs. 34.1 months, $p = 0.027$) and RFS (median 13 months and 5.1 months, $p = 0.003$). Other smaller studies have suggested better survival trends associated with R0 resection compared to R1/2, but this fails to be consistently significant between studies. Lang et al. showed a tendency toward shorter OS in the incomplete resection group, with a median OS of 12 vs. 32 months ($p = 0.31$) in 24 patients [283]. Chen et al. reported the same association with median OS of 24 vs. 53 months ($p = 0.03$) in favor of complete resection in 11 patients [284].

Chemotherapy is generally viewed as having limited efficacy in the treatment of STS. Whether patients with liver metastases specifically should receive chemotherapy, and if so in what sequence, remains to be answered. In the above-mentioned series, patients did not consistently receive chemotherapy, and fewer even got neoadjuvant treatment [285]. An interesting recent trial on first-line chemotherapy compared doxorubicin alone to combination with ifosfamide or dacarbazine in locally advanced or metastatic leiomyosarcoma. They found an unadjusted median OS survival ranging from 21 to 35 months. A matched analysis found the combination of doxorubicin and dacarbazine to be associated with significantly longer OS. The relatively favorable survival from their study highlights whether patients undergoing liver resection could have an added benefit from systemic therapy and if there is a superior treatment strategy between upfront resection or first-line chemotherapy.

Conclusion

Patients undergoing liver resection for sarcoma liver metastases are more likely to benefit from surgery in the absence of extra-hepatic spread. Based on the limited data available, patients with co-existing extra-hepatic metastases would be most appropriately managed with palliative chemotherapy or best supportive care.

Small Bowel

Primary small bowel malignancy accounts for less than 3% of all gastrointestinal cancers [286]. Adenocarcinoma is the second most common histology after neuro-endocrine [287]. The low prevalence of small-bowel adenocarcinoma limits our understanding of the natural history of tumor spread, restricting the development of clear treatment guidelines. The prognosis of metastatic small bowel adenocarcinoma is less than 6 months without systemic therapy [288, 289].

Liver metastasis is a poor prognostic factor. Risk factors for developing hepatic disease include distal and larger primary tumor, poorer histological grade or signet-ring subtype, nodal spread, and extra-hepatic site of metastases [290, 291].

Although viewed as an incurable disease, long-term favorable outcomes following resection of oligometastatic disease have been reported [32]. In a series of 34 patients with locally advanced or metastatic small bowel cancer treated with first-line chemotherapy, Li et al. reported a disappointing overall survival of 13.8 months [292]. They however found 3 long-term survivors after combined modality systemic chemotherapy and local treatment with survival of 52–96 months, speaking to the potential advantage of an aggressive surgical approach. Adam et al. reported 5-year survival of 49% and a median OS of 58 months in 28 patients with metastatic small bowel adenocarcinoma following hepatectomy compared to 5-year and median OS of 21% and 34 months in 12 patients with non-ampullary duodenal cancer [33]. Rompteaux et al. evaluated 34 patients who underwent curative intent resection of metastatic small bowel adenocarcinoma, from which 9 had isolated liver metastases. The median OS was 28.6 months. Worst prognosis was observed after resection in patients with poor differentiation, R1 margins, or lymphatic invasion [293].

As seen in other types of liver metastases from aggressive primaries, the addition of systemic chemotherapy to radical surgery seems to be the cornerstone of success. In a large SEER database analysis of 2010–2015, 2457 patients with small bowel adenocarcinoma were identified, from which 506 had liver metastases. They found that patients with adenocarcinoma could benefit from chemotherapy alone (HR = 0.35, 95% CI [0.27–0.44], $P < 0.001$) or surgery plus chemotherapy (HR = 0.27, 95% CI [0.18–0.42], $P < 0.001$) when compared with no treatment. Surgery plus chemotherapy was the best therapeutic option compared to surgery alone (HR = 0.37, 95% CI [0.22–0.65], $P < 0.001$) [291].

In conclusion, certain patients with small bowel adenocarcinoma and limited visceral metastases may benefit from radical surgery [294]. The addition of chemotherapy is likely to improve patient outcome.

Testicular

Testicular cancer is a relatively rare but diverse set of tumors that reaches a peak incidence in young adult males between the ages of 25 and 35 years old [295]. They are divided into seminomas and nonseminoma tumors. Thankfully, even in advanced stages, modern systemic therapies have achieved a cure rate as high as 80–95% [296].

Patients with "poor-risk" nonseminomas (defined as those with non-pulmonary metastases, arising from the mediastinum, or associated with marked elevation of tumor markers) have a 5-year overall survival of 48% compared to 80–92% for other nonseminomas. Similarly, seminomas with non-pulmonary metastases carry a 5-year overall survival of 72% when compared to over 86% for those without such metastases [297].

Aggressive surgical management of residual disease following response to systemic therapy is well accepted, but the role of hepatectomy itself remains poorly defined as isolated hepatic metastases are rare [298]. Patients being evaluated for liver resection already represent a subgroup with poor prognosis, but even in these patients, lower tumor marker, significant decline in tumor marker following orchiectomy, and the absence of pulmonary metastases all represent favorable prognostic characteristics [299].

One retrospective series of 15 patients reported an overall 10-year survival of 62% after resection of hepatic metastases [300]. The largest report to date comes from the study by Adam et al. who found 78 patients with a 51% 5-year post-resection survival compared to the cohort average of 36% 5-year overall survival in 1452 patients with NCRNNELMs [33].

Given the paucity of data, it is difficult to develop a cohesive set of prognostic factors for liver surgery candidates. Regarding the size of the liver metastases, resected lesions <1 cm were found to only contain non-viable necrotic tissues, whereas tumors >3 cm were associated with overall worst prognosis [301–303]. Longer disease-free interval and R0 resection also represent favorable attributes.

In a SEER database review of 2010–2016, 1661 patients with metastatic testicular cancer were studied, from which 15.2% had liver metastases at diagnosis. As expected, patients with lung, liver, or bone metastases had poorer overall survival compared to lymph node only metastases. In patients with only one metastatic site, patients with bone or liver involvement represented the worst two groups in terms of survival [304].

In conclusion, patients with liver metastases from testicular cancer may benefit from aggressive surgical resection following response to systemic therapy and when complete surgical excision is possible. Overall, they represent a group with unfavorable outcome compared to all cases of metastatic testicular cancer.

Thyroid Cancer

Thyroid carcinomas represent less than 1% of cancer cases in humans. Liver metastases are especially rare in well-differentiated thyroid cancer with an incidence of less than 1%, but more common in medullary thyroid cancer in up to 21% of patients [305, 306]. Cases of metastatic disease are often widespread and isolated liver metastases are reported with a frequency of less than 0.5% [307]. The mainstay of treatment for metastatic thyroid disease is generally one of radioactive iodine (I^{131}) therapy, with or without loco-regional ablative therapy such as RFA [308]. Surgery is rarely indicated. In the last 30 years, a handful of case series have reported outcomes on hepatic metastases management using combinations of systemic therapy, loco-regional therapies such as RFA and TACE and surgery [309–317]. Patients with metastatic thyroid cancer generally have considerable life expectancy and cases of isolated liver metastases are rare. Drawing conclusions on a superior treatment strategy is therefore impossible with the current literature. It is reasonable to aim for local control of disease with minimally invasive approaches and well-tolerated systemic treatments.

A recent systematic review of the literature evaluated the role of surgery in thyroid cancer liver metastases. They identified 5 patients with a mean time of follow-up after hepatectomy of 22.2 ± 19.9 months. All patients were alive at last follow-up whereas no recurrence of disease was reported [318].

Surgical resection of thyroid cancer liver metastases appears safe and feasible, but there is insufficient data to comment on the survival benefit, especially in the era of effective loco-regional therapies.

Urothelial

Urothelial cancers are the fourth most common tumors in North America [319]. The most common metastatic locations are lymph nodes, lung, liver, and bone [320, 321]. About 20% of the patients will have liver metastasis with liver only metastases in about 9% [322]. Ninety percent of the patients with liver metastases have multiple lesions [320].

Cumulative experience with liver resection for metastatic bladder cancer is limited. Liver involvement is a poor prognostic indicator for metastasectomy, but some authors suggest radical resection in patients with solitary metastases and major response to systemic therapy [323–325].

Abe et al. investigated the effect of metastasectomy in 48 patients with urothelial cancer. Resection of metastases and the absence of liver or bone metastases and local recurrence were some of the independent predictors of prolonged survival. The median survivals of patients with and without metastasis to the liver, bone, or local recurrence were 7 months (5–12) and 28 months (19–40), respectively. Patients undergoing resection of metastases had longer median survival at 42 months (19–92) vs. 10 months (6–17). In a multi-institutional German study, 44 patients who underwent resection for metastatic urothelial carcinoma were included. They reported a median time to recurrence of 9 months (2–42) and a 5-year overall survival of 28% following resection of lung, brain, adrenal, small bowel, or lymph node metastases [326].

Specifically, the experience with liver resection for metastatic bladder cancer is extremely limited. In a SEER database study, Dong et al. found in 337 patients with metastatic urothelial cancer undergoing resection that both liver (HR = 1.507, 95% CI 1.017–2.233, p = 0.041) or brain (HR = 2.435, 95% CI 1.161–5.109, p = 0.019) involvement were unfavorable predictors of overall survival.

Liver resection should only be considered following the opinion of expert urology oncologists and ideal candidates would include patients with good performance status, liver-only and limited burden of disease, and following an objective response to systemic therapy. There is currently too little data to recommend this as a routine surgical practice. The encouraging advances seen in immunotherapy are likely to be a game changer in modern practice [327].

Conclusion

NCRNNELM treatment has changed significantly in the modern era. What was considered unresectable once is now considered for resection in select patients. Available studies are biased, with retrospective studies focusing on rare survivors who exhibit favorable tumor biology.

The most recent advances in modern medicine in terms of advanced chemotherapy, immunomodulation, and targeted therapy have given the highest progress in terms of patient survival.

The most recent studies unfortunately do not account for these improvements, and it will take several years before we can appreciate the progress resulting from research efforts in that field.

Positive prognostic factors of recurrence include low burden of disease, long disease-free interval, achievable R0 resection, and response to preoperative therapy.

When facing a patient who seems to meet criteria favoring resection, a multidisciplinary discussion should take place. Patients with extensive metastatic disease are unlikely to benefit from therapy.

Data is scarce in NCRNNELM and although these pathologies appear worse than other, long-term survivors have been identified. Studies must be directed at identifying long-term potential survivors.

References

1. Yamashita S, et al. Biomarkers in colorectal liver metastases. Br J Surg. 2018;105(6):618–27.
2. Bray F, et al. Global cancer statistics 2018: GLOBOCAN estimates of incidence and mortality worldwide for 36 cancers in 185 countries. CA Cancer J Clin. 2018;68(6):394–424.
3. Siegel R, Naishadham D, Jemal A. Cancer statistics, 2012. CA Cancer J Clin. 2012;62(1):10–29.
4. Kishi Y, et al. Three hundred and one consecutive extended right hepatectomies: evaluation of outcome based on systematic liver volumetry. Ann Surg. 2009;250(4):540–8.
5. Glazer ES, et al. Long-term survival after surgical management of neuroendocrine hepatic metastases. HPB (Oxford). 2010;12(6):427–33.
6. Creasy JM, et al. Actual 10-year survival after hepatic resection of colorectal liver metastases: what factors preclude cure? Surgery. 2018;163(6):1238–44.
7. Engstrand J, et al. Colorectal cancer liver metastases - a population-based study on incidence, management and survival. BMC Cancer. 2018;18(1):78.
8. Hackl C, et al. Treatment of colorectal liver metastases in Germany: a ten-year population-based analysis of 5772 cases of primary colorectal adenocarcinoma. BMC Cancer. 2014;14:810.
9. Dorr NM, Bartels M, Morgul MH. Current treatment of colorectal liver metastasis as a chronic disease. Anticancer Res. 2020;40(1):1–7.
10. Petrowsky H, et al. Modern therapeutic approaches for the treatment of malignant liver tumours. Nat Rev Gastroenterol Hepatol. 2020;17(12):755–72.
11. Frilling A, Clift AK. Therapeutic strategies for neuroendocrine liver metastases. Cancer. 2015;121(8):1172–86.
12. Mayo SC, et al. Surgical management of hepatic neuroendocrine tumor metastasis: results from an international multi-institutional analysis. Ann Surg Oncol. 2010;17(12):3129–36.
13. Fairweather M, et al. Management of Neuroendocrine Tumor Liver Metastases: Long-term outcomes and prognostic factors from a large prospective database. Ann Surg Oncol. 2017;24(8):2319–25.

14. Tran CG, et al. Surgical Management of Neuroendocrine Tumor Liver Metastases. Surg Oncol Clin N Am. 2021;30(1):39–55.
15. Chan MY, Ma KW, Chan A. Surgical management of neuroendocrine tumor-associated liver metastases: a review. Gland Surg. 2018;7(1):28–35.
16. Paineau J, et al. Resection of hepatic metastases from non colorectal cancers. Our experience apropos of 20 cases. J Chir (Paris). 1995;132(1):1–6.
17. Berney T, et al. Results of surgical resection of liver metastases from non-colorectal primaries. Br J Surg. 1998;85(10):1423–7.
18. Lindell G, et al. Liver resection of noncolorectal secondaries. J Surg Oncol. 1998;69(2):66–70.
19. Le Treut YP, Sebag F, Hardwigsen J. Surgery of liver metastases of non-colorectal origin. Ann Chir. 1998;52(1):88–91.
20. Elias D, et al. Resection of liver metastases from a noncolorectal primary: indications and results based on 147 monocentric patients. J Am Coll Surg. 1998;187(5):487–93.
21. Benevento A, et al. Result of liver resection as treatment for metastases from noncolorectal cancer. J Surg Oncol. 2000;74(1):24–9.
22. Hamy AP, et al. Hepatic resections for non-colorectal metastases: forty resections in 35 patients. Hepato-Gastroenterology. 2000;47(34):1090–4.
23. Buell JF, et al. Hepatic resection: effective treatment for primary and secondary tumors. Surgery. 2000;128(4):686–93.
24. van Ruth S, et al. Metastasectomy for liver metastases of non-colorectal primaries. Eur J Surg Oncol. 2001;27(7):662–7.
25. Goering JD, et al. Cryoablation and liver resection for noncolorectal liver metastases. Am J Surg. 2002;183(4):384–9.
26. Harrison LE, et al. Hepatic resection for noncolorectal, nonneuroendocrine metastases: a fifteen-year experience with ninety-six patients. Surgery. 1997;121(6):625–32.
27. Hemming AW, et al. Hepatic resection of noncolorectal nonneuroendocrine metastases. Liver Transpl. 2000;6(1):97–101.
28. Yamada H, et al. Hepatectomy for metastases from non-colorectal and non-neuroendocrine tumor. Anticancer Res. 2001;21(6A):4159–62.
29. Takada Y, et al. Hepatic resection for metastatic tumors from non-colorectal carcinoma. Hepato-Gastroenterology. 2001;48(37):83–6.
30. Karavias DD, et al. Liver resection for metastatic non-colorectal non-neuroendocrine hepatic neoplasms. Eur J Surg Oncol. 2002;28(2):135–9.
31. Weitz J, et al. Partial hepatectomy for metastases from noncolorectal, nonneuroendocrine carcinoma. Ann Surg. 2005;241(2):269–76.
32. Ercolani G, et al. The role of liver resections for noncolorectal, nonneuroendocrine metastases: experience with 142 observed cases. Ann Surg Oncol. 2005;12(6):459–66.

33. Adam R, et al. Hepatic resection for noncolorectal nonendocrine liver metastases: analysis of 1,452 patients and development of a prognostic model. Ann Surg. 2006;244(4):524–35.
34. Bauschke A, et al. Surgical treatment of liver metastases from non-colorectal non-neuroendocrine carcinomas. J Cancer Res Clin Oncol. 2022;148(2):503–15.
35. Sano K, et al. Outcomes of 1,639 hepatectomies for non-colorectal non-neuroendocrine liver metastases: a multicenter analysis. J Hepatobiliary Pancreat Sci. 2018;25(11):465–75.
36. Hidalgo M. Pancreatic cancer. N Engl J Med. 2010;362(17):1605–17.
37. Virchow R. Die Cellularpathologie in ihrer Begründung auf physiologische und pathologische Gewebelehre. Berlin: August Hirschwald; 1858.
38. Hewing J. Neoplastic diseases. 6th ed. Philadelphia: PA:WB Saunders; 1928.
39. Fidler IJ, Poste G. The "seed and soil" hypothesis revisited. Lancet Oncol. 2008;9(8):808.
40. Hart IR, Fidler IJ. Role of organ selectivity in the determination of metastatic patterns of B16 melanoma. Cancer Res. 1980;40(7):2281–7.
41. Clark AM, et al. Liver metastases: microenvironments and ex-vivo models. Exp Biol Med (Maywood). 2016;241(15):1639–52.
42. Adelmann D, Kronish K, Ramsay MA. Anesthesia for liver transplantation. Anesthesiol Clin. 2017;35(3):491–508.
43. Vidal-Vanaclocha F. The prometastatic microenvironment of the liver. Cancer Microenviron. 2008;1(1):113–29.
44. Braet F, et al. The hepatic sinusoidal endothelial lining and colorectal liver metastases. World J Gastroenterol. 2007;13(6):821–5.
45. Laferriere J, et al. Transendothelial migration of colon carcinoma cells requires expression of E-selectin by endothelial cells and activation of stress-activated protein kinase-2 (SAPK2/p38) in the tumor cells. J Biol Chem. 2001;276(36):33762–72.
46. Auguste P, et al. The host inflammatory response promotes liver metastasis by increasing tumor cell arrest and extravasation. Am J Pathol. 2007;170(5):1781–92.
47. Bergers G, Benjamin LE. Tumorigenesis and the angiogenic switch. Nat Rev Cancer. 2003;3(6):401–10.
48. Kuczynski EA, et al. Vessel co-option in cancer. Nat Rev Clin Oncol. 2019.
49. Frentzas S, et al. Vessel co-option mediates resistance to anti-angiogenic therapy in liver metastases. Nat Med. 2016;22(11):1294–302.
50. van 't Veer LJ, et al. Gene expression profiling predicts clinical outcome of breast cancer. Nature. 2002;415(6871):530–6.
51. Patsialou A, et al. Selective gene-expression profiling of migratory tumor cells in vivo predicts clinical outcome in breast cancer patients. Breast Cancer Res. 2012;14(5):R139.

52. Spentzos D, et al. Gene expression signature with independent prognostic significance in epithelial ovarian cancer. J Clin Oncol. 2004;22(23):4700–10.
53. Winnepenninckx V, et al. Gene expression profiling of primary cutaneous melanoma and clinical outcome. J Natl Cancer Inst. 2006;98(7):472–82.
54. Gryfe R, et al. Tumor microsatellite instability and clinical outcome in young patients with colorectal cancer. N Engl J Med. 2000;342(2):69–77.
55. Kaplan RN, et al. VEGFR1-positive haematopoietic bone marrow progenitors initiate the pre-metastatic niche. Nature. 2005;438(7069):820–7.
56. Lee JW, et al. Hepatocytes direct the formation of a pro-metastatic niche in the liver. Nature. 2019;567(7747):249–52.
57. Golden SH, et al. Clinical review: prevalence and incidence of endocrine and metabolic disorders in the United States: a comprehensive review. J Clin Endocrinol Metab. 2009;94(6):1853–78.
58. Assie G, et al. Prognostic parameters of metastatic adrenocortical carcinoma. J Clin Endocrinol Metab. 2007;92(1):148–54.
59. Berruti A, et al. Adrenal cancer: ESMO clinical practice guidelines for diagnosis, treatment and follow-up. Ann Oncol. 2012;23(Suppl 7):vii131–8.
60. Gaujoux S, et al. Resection of adrenocortical carcinoma liver metastasis: is it justified? Ann Surg Oncol. 2012;19(8):2643–51.
61. Icard P, et al. Adrenocortical carcinomas: surgical trends and results of a 253-patient series from the French Association of Endocrine Surgeons study group. World J Surg. 2001;25(7):891–7.
62. Terzolo M, et al. Management of adrenal cancer: a 2013 update. J Endocrinol Investig. 2014;37(3):207–17.
63. Fassnacht M, et al. Adrenocortical carcinoma: a clinician's update. Nat Rev Endocrinol. 2011;7(6):323–35.
64. Fassnacht M, et al. Combination chemotherapy in advanced adrenocortical carcinoma. N Engl J Med. 2012;366(23):2189–97.
65. Di Carlo I, et al. Liver resection for hepatic metastases from adrenocortical carcinoma. HPB (Oxford). 2006;8(2):106–9.
66. Dy BM, et al. Surgical resection of synchronously metastatic adrenocortical cancer. Ann Surg Oncol. 2015;22(1):146–51.
67. Baur J, et al. Outcome after resection of adrenocortical carcinoma liver metastases: a retrospective study. BMC Cancer. 2017;17(1):522.
68. Ayabe RI, et al. Disease-free interval and tumor functional status can be used to select patients for resection/ablation of liver metastases from adrenocortical carcinoma: insights from a multi-institutional study. HPB (Oxford). 2020;22(1):169–75.

69. Fassnacht M, et al. European Society of Endocrinology Clinical Practice Guidelines on the management of adrenocortical carcinoma in adults, in collaboration with the European network for the study of adrenal Tumors. Eur J Endocrinol. 2018;179(4):G1–G46.
70. Veltri A, et al. Oligometastatic adrenocortical carcinoma: the role of image-guided thermal ablation. Eur Radiol. 2020;30(12):6958–64.
71. Charalampoudis P, et al. Surgery for liver metastases from breast cancer. Future Oncol. 2015;11(10):1519–30.
72. Gradishar WJ, et al. Breast cancer, version 3.2020, NCCN clinical practice guidelines in oncology. J Natl Compr Cancer Netw. 2020;18(4):452–78.
73. Crump M, et al. Randomized trial of high-dose chemotherapy with autologous peripheral-blood stem-cell support compared with standard-dose chemotherapy in women with metastatic breast cancer: NCIC MA.16. J Clin Oncol. 2008;26(1):37–43.
74. Horn SR, et al. Epidemiology of liver metastases. Cancer Epidemiol. 2020;67:101760.
75. Zhao HY, et al. Incidence and prognostic factors of patients with synchronous liver metastases upon initial diagnosis of breast cancer: a population-based study. Cancer Manag Res. 2018;10:5937–50.
76. St Romain P, et al. Organotropism and prognostic marker discordance in distant metastases of breast carcinoma: fact or fiction? A clinicopathologic analysis. Hum Pathol. 2012;43(3):398–404.
77. Gong Y, et al. Impact of molecular subtypes on metastatic breast cancer patients: a SEER population-based study. Sci Rep. 2017;7:45411.
78. Wang S, et al. Incidence and prognosis of liver metastasis at diagnosis: a pan-cancer population-based study. Am J Cancer Res. 2020;10(5):1477–517.
79. Liu D, et al. Breast subtypes and prognosis of breast cancer patients with initial bone metastasis: a population-based study. Front Oncol. 2020;10:580112.
80. Harrell JC, et al. Genomic analysis identifies unique signatures predictive of brain, lung, and liver relapse. Breast Cancer Res Treat. 2012;132(2):523–35.
81. Kobryn E, et al. Is there a rationale for aggressive breast cancer liver metastases resections in polish female patients? Analysis of overall survival following hepatic resection at a single Centre in Poland. Ann Agric Environ Med. 2016;23(4):683–7.
82. Vertriest C, et al. Resection of single metachronous liver metastases from breast cancer stage I-II yield excellent overall and disease-free survival. Single center experience and review of the literature. Dig Surg. 2015;32(1):52–9.

83. Rivera K, Jeyarajah DR, Washington K. Hepatectomy, RFA, and other liver directed therapies for treatment of breast cancer liver metastasis: a systematic review. Front Oncol. 2021;11:643383.
84. Cardoso F, et al. 5th ESO-ESMO international consensus guidelines for advanced breast cancer (ABC 5). Ann Oncol. 2020;31(12):1623–49.
85. Gradishar WJ, et al. NCCN guidelines(R) insights: breast cancer, version 4.2021. J Natl Compr Cancer Netw. 2021;19(5):484–93.
86. Feng Y, et al. Comparison of hepatic resection and systemic treatment of breast cancer liver metastases: a propensity score matching study. Am J Surg. 2020;220(4):945–51.
87. Tasleem S, et al. The role of liver resection in patients with metastatic breast cancer: a systematic review examining the survival impact. Ir J Med Sci. 2018;187(4):1009–20.
88. Sunden M, et al. Surgical treatment of breast cancer liver metastases—a nationwide registry-based case control study. Eur J Surg Oncol. 2020;46(6):1006–12.
89. Sadot E, et al. Hepatic resection or ablation for isolated breast cancer liver metastasis: a case-control study with comparison to medically treated patients. Ann Surg. 2016;264(1):147–54.
90. Zegarac M, et al. Prognostic factors for longer disease free survival and overall survival after surgical resection of isolated liver metastasis from breast cancer. J BUON. 2013;18(4):859–65.
91. Koo JS, Jung W, Jeong J. Metastatic breast cancer shows different immunohistochemical phenotype according to metastatic site. Tumori. 2010;96(3):424–32.
92. Hoefnagel LD, et al. Receptor conversion in distant breast cancer metastases. Breast Cancer Res. 2010;12(5):R75.
93. Abbas H, et al. Breast cancer liver metastases in a UK tertiary Centre: outcomes following referral to tumour board meeting. Int J Surg. 2017;44:152–9.
94. Ercolani G, et al. Ten-year survival after liver resection for breast metastases: a single-Center experience. Dig Surg. 2018;35(4):372–80.
95. Galiandro F, et al. Prognostic factors in patients with breast cancer liver metastases undergoing liver resection: systematic review and meta-analysis. Cancers (Basel). 2022;14(7).
96. Golse N, Adam R. Liver metastases from breast cancer: what role for surgery? Indications and results. Clin Breast Cancer. 2017;17(4):256–65.
97. Bale R, Putzer D, Schullian P. Local treatment of breast cancer liver metastasis. Cancers (Basel). 2019;11(9).
98. Cheung TT, et al. Survival analysis of breast cancer liver metastasis treated by hepatectomy: a propensity score analysis for Chinese women in Hong Kong. Hepatobiliary Pancreat Dis Int. 2019;18(5):452–7.

99. Lermite E, et al. Surgical resection of liver metastases from breast cancer. Surg Oncol. 2010;19(4):e79–84.
100. Vlastos G, et al. Long-term survival after an aggressive surgical approach in patients with breast cancer hepatic metastases. Ann Surg Oncol. 2004;11(9):869–74.
101. Schneebaum S, et al. The regional treatment of liver metastases from breast cancer. J Surg Oncol. 1994;55(1):26–31. discussion 32
102. Sofocleous CT, et al. Radiofrequency ablation in the management of liver metastases from breast cancer. AJR Am J Roentgenol. 2007;189(4):883–9.
103. Meloni MF, et al. Breast cancer liver metastases: US-guided percutaneous radiofrequency ablation—intermediate and long-term survival rates. Radiology. 2009;253(3):861–9.
104. Xiao YB, Zhang B, Wu YL. Radiofrequency ablation versus hepatic resection for breast cancer liver metastasis: a systematic review and meta-analysis. J Zhejiang Univ Sci B. 2018;19(11):829–43.
105. Mao W, et al. Clinicopathological study of organ metastasis in endometrial cancer. Future Oncol. 2020;16(10):525–40.
106. Knowles B, et al. Hepatic resection for metastatic endometrioid carcinoma. HPB (Oxford). 2010;12(6):412–7.
107. Chi DS, et al. The role of surgical cytoreduction in stage IV endometrial carcinoma. Gynecol Oncol. 1997;67(1):56–60.
108. Bristow RE, Duska LR, Montz FJ. The role of cytoreductive surgery in the management of stage IV uterine papillary serous carcinoma. Gynecol Oncol. 2001;81(1):92–9.
109. Memarzadeh S, et al. FIGO stage III and IV uterine papillary serous carcinoma: impact of residual disease on survival. Int J Gynecol Cancer. 2002;12(5):454–8.
110. Barlin JN, Ueda SM, Bristow RE. Cytoreductive surgery for advanced and recurrent endometrial cancer: a review of the literature. Womens Health (Lond). 2009;5(4):403–11.
111. Wu SG, et al. Sites of metastasis and overall survival in esophageal cancer: a population-based study. Cancer Manag Res. 2017;9:781–8.
112. Daly JM, Karnell LH, Menck HR. National cancer data base report on esophageal carcinoma. Cancer. 1996;78(8):1820–8.
113. Zhang S, et al. Metastasis pattern and prognosis in men with esophageal cancer patients: a SEER-based study. Medicine (Baltimore). 2021;100(25):e26496.
114. Yamamoto T, et al. Esophagectomy and hepatic arterial chemotherapy following hepatic resection for esophageal cancer with liver metastasis. J Gastroenterol. 2001;36(8):560–3.
115. Hanazaki K, et al. Hepatic metastasis from esophageal cancer treated by surgical resection and hepatic arterial infusion chemotherapy. Hepato-Gastroenterology. 1998;45(19):201–5.

116. Huddy JR, et al. Liver metastases from esophageal carcinoma: is there a role for surgical resection? Dis Esophagus. 2015;28(5):483–7.
117. Kroese TE, et al. Definition of oligometastatic esophagogastric cancer and impact of local oligometastasis-directed treatment: a systematic review and meta-analysis. Eur J Cancer. 2022;166:254–69.
118. Sun Z, et al. Liver metastases in newly diagnosed gastric cancer: a population-based study from SEER. J Cancer. 2019;10(13):2991–3005.
119. Dittmar Y, et al. Resection of liver metastases is beneficial in patients with gastric cancer: report on 15 cases and review of literature. Gastric Cancer. 2012;15(2):131–6.
120. Tiberio GA, et al. Factors influencing survival after hepatectomy for metastases from gastric cancer. Eur J Surg Oncol. 2016;42(8):1229–35.
121. Ueda K, et al. Analysis of the prognostic factors and evaluation of surgical treatment for synchronous liver metastases from gastric cancer. Langenbeck's Arch Surg. 2009;394(4):647–53.
122. Markar SR, et al. Influence of surgical resection of hepatic metastases from gastric adenocarcinoma on Long-term survival: systematic review and pooled analysis. Ann Surg. 2016;263(6):1092–101.
123. Bang YJ, et al. Trastuzumab in combination with chemotherapy versus chemotherapy alone for treatment of HER2-positive advanced gastric or gastro-oesophageal junction cancer (ToGA): a phase 3, open-label, randomised controlled trial. Lancet. 2010;376(9742):687–97.
124. Kang YK, et al. Nivolumab in patients with advanced gastric or gastro-oesophageal junction cancer refractory to, or intolerant of, at least two previous chemotherapy regimens (ONO-4538-12, ATTRACTION-2): a randomised, double-blind, placebo-controlled, phase 3 trial. Lancet. 2017;390(10111):2461–71.
125. Gavriilidis P, et al. Gastrectomy alone or in combination with hepatic resection in the Management of Liver Metastases from Gastric Cancer: a systematic review using an updated and cumulative meta-analysis. J Clin Med Res. 2019;11(8):600–8.
126. Montagnani F, et al. Long-term survival after liver metastasectomy in gastric cancer: systematic review and meta-analysis of prognostic factors. Cancer Treat Rev. 2018;69:11–20.
127. Petrelli F, et al. Hepatic resection for gastric cancer liver metastases: a systematic review and meta-analysis. J Surg Oncol. 2015;111(8):1021–7.
128. Granieri S, et al. Surgical treatment of gastric cancer liver metastases: systematic review and meta-analysis of long-term outcomes and prognostic factors. Crit Rev Oncol Hematol. 2021;163:103313.
129. Ochiai T, et al. Hepatic resection for metastatic tumours from gastric cancer: analysis of prognostic factors. Br J Surg. 1994;81(8):1175–8.

130. Koga R, et al. Liver resection for metastatic gastric cancer: experience with 42 patients including eight long-term survivors. Jpn J Clin Oncol. 2007;37(11):836–42.
131. Shirabe K, et al. Analysis of the prognostic factors for liver metastasis of gastric cancer after hepatic resection: a multi-institutional study of the indications for resection. Hepato-Gastroenterology. 2003;50(53):1560–3.
132. Takemura N, et al. Long-term outcomes after surgical resection for gastric cancer liver metastasis: an analysis of 64 macroscopically complete resections. Langenbeck's Arch Surg. 2012;397(6):951–7.
133. Al-Batran SE, et al. The RENAISSANCE (AIO-FLOT5) trial: effect of chemotherapy alone vs. chemotherapy followed by surgical resection on survival and quality of life in patients with limited-metastatic adenocarcinoma of the stomach or esophagogastric junction—a phase III trial of the German AIO/CAO-V/CAOGI. BMC Cancer. 2017;17(1):893.
134. Chandrasekhara V, Ginsberg GG. Endoscopic management of gastrointestinal stromal tumors. Curr Gastroenterol Rep. 2011;13(6):532–9.
135. Soreide K, et al. Global epidemiology of gastrointestinal stromal tumours (GIST): a systematic review of population-based cohort studies. Cancer Epidemiol. 2016;40:39–46.
136. Martin J, et al. Deletions affecting codons 557-558 of the c-KIT gene indicate a poor prognosis in patients with completely resected gastrointestinal stromal tumors: a study by the Spanish Group for Sarcoma Research (GEIS). J Clin Oncol. 2005;23(25):6190–8.
137. Bannon AE, et al. Using molecular diagnostic testing to personalize the treatment of patients with gastrointestinal stromal tumors. Expert Rev Mol Diagn. 2017;17(5):445–57.
138. Yang DY, et al. Metastatic pattern and prognosis of gastrointestinal stromal tumor (GIST): a SEER-based analysis. Clin Transl Oncol. 2019;21(12):1654–62.
139. Gold JS, Dematteo RP. Combined surgical and molecular therapy: the gastrointestinal stromal tumor model. Ann Surg. 2006;244(2):176–84.
140. DeMatteo RP, et al. Two hundred gastrointestinal stromal tumors: recurrence patterns and prognostic factors for survival. Ann Surg. 2000;231(1):51–8.
141. Ng EH, et al. Prognostic factors influencing survival in gastrointestinal leiomyosarcomas. Implications for surgical management and staging. Ann Surg. 1992;215(1):68–77.
142. von Mehren M, et al. Gastrointestinal stromal tumors, version 2.2014. J Natl Compr Cancer Netw. 2014;12(6):853–62.
143. Blay JY, et al. Consensus meeting for the management of gastrointestinal stromal tumors. Report of the GIST Consensus Conference of 20–21 March 2004, Under the auspices of ESMO. Ann Oncol. 2005;16(4):566–78.

144. Dematteo RP, et al. Clinical management of gastrointestinal stromal tumors: before and after STI-571. Hum Pathol. 2002;33(5):466–77.
145. Demetri GD, et al. Efficacy and safety of sunitinib in patients with advanced gastrointestinal stromal tumour after failure of imatinib: a randomised controlled trial. Lancet. 2006;368(9544):1329–38.
146. van der Zwan SM, DeMatteo RP. Gastrointestinal stromal tumor: 5 years later. Cancer. 2005;104(9):1781–8.
147. Kim EJ, Zalupski MM. Systemic therapy for advanced gastrointestinal stromal tumors: beyond imatinib. J Surg Oncol. 2011;104(8):901–6.
148. Bauer S, et al. Long-term follow-up of patients with GIST undergoing metastasectomy in the era of imatinib—analysis of prognostic factors (EORTC-STBSG collaborative study). Eur J Surg Oncol. 2014;40(4):412–9.
149. Gronchi A, et al. Surgery of residual disease following molecular-targeted therapy with imatinib mesylate in advanced/metastatic GIST. Ann Surg. 2007;245(3):341–6.
150. Mussi C, et al. Post-imatinib surgery in advanced/metastatic GIST: is it worthwhile in all patients? Ann Oncol. 2010;21(2):403–8.
151. Fairweather M, et al. Cytoreductive surgery for metastatic gastrointestinal stromal Tumors treated with tyrosine kinase inhibitors: a 2-institutional analysis. Ann Surg. 2018;268(2):296–302.
152. DeMatteo RP, et al. Results of tyrosine kinase inhibitor therapy followed by surgical resection for metastatic gastrointestinal stromal tumor. Ann Surg. 2007;245(3):347–52.
153. Xia L, et al. Resection combined with imatinib therapy for liver metastases of gastrointestinal stromal tumors. Surg Today. 2010;40(10):936–42.
154. Seesing MF, et al. Resection of liver metastases in patients with gastrointestinal stromal tumors in the imatinib era: a nationwide retrospective study. Eur J Surg Oncol. 2016;42(9):1407–13.
155. Du CY, et al. Is there a role of surgery in patients with recurrent or metastatic gastrointestinal stromal tumours responding to imatinib: a prospective randomised trial in China. Eur J Cancer. 2014;50(10):1772–8.
156. Bonvalot S, et al. Impact of surgery on advanced gastrointestinal stromal tumors (GIST) in the imatinib era. Ann Surg Oncol. 2006;13(12):1596–603.
157. Andtbacka RH, et al. Surgical resection of gastrointestinal stromal tumors after treatment with imatinib. Ann Surg Oncol. 2007;14(1):14–24.
158. Rutkowski P, et al. Surgical treatment of patients with initially inoperable and/or metastatic gastrointestinal stromal tumors (GIST) during therapy with imatinib mesylate. J Surg Oncol. 2006;93(4):304–11.

159. Ecker BL, et al. Surgical Management of Sarcoma Metastatic to liver. Surg Oncol Clin N Am. 2021;30(1):57–67.
160. Raut CP, et al. Surgical management of advanced gastrointestinal stromal tumors after treatment with targeted systemic therapy using kinase inhibitors. J Clin Oncol. 2006;24(15):2325–31.
161. Bauer S, et al. Resection of residual disease in patients with metastatic gastrointestinal stromal tumors responding to treatment with imatinib. Int J Cancer. 2005;117(2):316–25.
162. Mastoraki A, et al. Metastatic liver disease associated with gastrointestinal stromal Tumors: controversies in diagnostic and therapeutic approach. J Gastrointest Cancer. 2015;46(3):237–42.
163. Hakime A, et al. A role for adjuvant RFA in managing hepatic metastases from gastrointestinal stromal tumors (GIST) after treatment with targeted systemic therapy using kinase inhibitors. Cardiovasc Intervent Radiol. 2014;37(1):132–9.
164. Takaki H, et al. Hepatic artery embolization for liver metastasis of gastrointestinal stromal tumor following imatinib and sunitinib therapy. J Gastrointest Cancer. 2014;45(4):494–9.
165. Rajan DK, et al. Sarcomas metastatic to the liver: response and survival after cisplatin, doxorubicin, mitomycin-C, Ethiodol, and polyvinyl alcohol chemoembolization. J Vasc Interv Radiol. 2001;12(2):187–93.
166. Pierce DB, et al. Safety and efficacy outcomes of embolization in hepatic sarcomas. AJR Am J Roentgenol. 2018;210(1):175–82.
167. Rathmann N, et al. Radioembolization in patients with progressive gastrointestinal stromal tumor liver metastases undergoing treatment with tyrosine kinase inhibitors. J Vasc Interv Radiol. 2015;26(2):231–8.
168. Chapiro J, et al. Transarterial chemoembolization in soft-tissue sarcoma metastases to the liver—the use of imaging biomarkers as predictors of patient survival. Eur J Radiol. 2015;84(3):424–30.
169. Fernandez JA, et al. Unresectable GIST liver metastases and liver transplantation: a review and theoretical basis for a new indication. Int J Surg. 2021;94:106126.
170. Sung H, et al. Global cancer statistics 2020: GLOBOCAN estimates of incidence and mortality worldwide for 36 cancers in 185 countries. CA Cancer J Clin. 2021;71(3):209–49.
171. Groome PA, et al. The IASLC lung cancer staging project: validation of the proposals for revision of the T, N, and M descriptors and consequent stage groupings in the forthcoming (seventh) edition of the TNM classification of malignant tumours. J Thorac Oncol. 2007;2(8):694–705.
172. Travis WD, Brambilla E, Riely GJ. New pathologic classification of lung cancer: relevance for clinical practice and clinical trials. J Clin Oncol. 2013;31(8):992–1001.

173. Ren Y, et al. Prognostic effect of liver metastasis in lung cancer patients with distant metastasis. Oncotarget. 2016;7(33):53245–53.
174. Riihimaki M, et al. Metastatic sites and survival in lung cancer. Lung Cancer. 2014;86(1):78–84.
175. Tamura T, et al. Specific organ metastases and survival in metastatic non-small-cell lung cancer. Mol Clin Oncol. 2015;3(1):217–21.
176. Liao Y, Fan X, Wang X. Effects of different metastasis patterns, surgery and other factors on the prognosis of patients with stage IV non-small cell lung cancer: a surveillance, epidemiology, and end results (SEER) linked database analysis. Oncol Lett. 2019;18(1):581–92.
177. Campos-Balea B, et al. Prognostic factors for survival in patients with metastatic lung adenocarcinoma: an analysis of the SEER database. Thorac Cancer. 2020;11(11):3357–64.
178. Nagashima A, et al. Long-term survival after surgical resection of liver metastasis from lung cancer. Jpn J Thorac Cardiovasc Surg. 2004;52(6):311–3.
179. Ileana E, et al. Surgical resection of liver non-small cell lung cancer metastasis: a dual weapon? Lung Cancer. 2010;70(2):221–2.
180. Ercolani G, et al. The role of liver resections for metastases from lung carcinoma. HPB (Oxford). 2006;8(2):114–5.
181. Bansal P, et al. Recent advances in immunotherapy in metastatic NSCLC. Front Oncol. 2016;6:239.
182. Leiter U, et al. The natural course of cutaneous melanoma. J Surg Oncol. 2004;86(4):172–8.
183. Tas F, Erturk K. Recurrence behavior in early-stage cutaneous melanoma: pattern, timing, survival, and influencing factors. Melanoma Res. 2017;27(2):134–9.
184. Diener-West M, et al. Development of metastatic disease after enrollment in the COMS trials for treatment of choroidal melanoma: collaborative ocular melanoma study group report no. 26. Arch Ophthalmol. 2005;123(12):1639–43.
185. Lane AM, Kim IK, Gragoudas ES. Survival rates in patients after treatment for metastasis from uveal melanoma. JAMA Ophthalmol. 2018;136(9):981–6.
186. Lian B, et al. The natural history and patterns of metastases from mucosal melanoma: an analysis of 706 prospectively-followed patients. Ann Oncol. 2017;28(4):868–73.
187. Heppt MV, et al. Prognostic factors and treatment outcomes in 444 patients with mucosal melanoma. Eur J Cancer. 2017;81:36–44.
188. Barth A, Wanek LA, Morton DL. Prognostic factors in 1,521 melanoma patients with distant metastases. J Am Coll Surg. 1995;181(3):193–201.
189. Marshall E, et al. MRI in the detection of hepatic metastases from high-risk uveal melanoma: a prospective study in 188 patients. Br J Ophthalmol. 2013;97(2):159–63.

190. Frenkel S, et al. Long-term survival of uveal melanoma patients after surgery for liver metastases. Br J Ophthalmol. 2009;93(8):1042–6.
191. Mariani P, et al. Surgical management of liver metastases from uveal melanoma: 16 years' experience at the Institut curie. Eur J Surg Oncol. 2009;35(11):1192–7.
192. Rivoire M, et al. Treatment of liver metastases from uveal melanoma. Ann Surg Oncol. 2005;12(6):422–8.
193. Rose DM, et al. Surgical resection for metastatic melanoma to the liver: the John Wayne cancer institute and Sydney melanoma unit experience. Arch Surg. 2001;136(8):950–5.
194. de Ridder J, et al. Hepatic resection for metastatic melanoma in The Netherlands: survival and prognostic factors. Melanoma Res. 2013;23(1):27–32.
195. Groeschl RT, et al. Hepatectomy for noncolorectal non-neuroendocrine metastatic cancer: a multi-institutional analysis. J Am Coll Surg. 2012;214(5):769–77.
196. Pawlik TM, et al. Hepatic resection for metastatic melanoma: distinct patterns of recurrence and prognosis for ocular versus cutaneous disease. Ann Surg Oncol. 2006;13(5):712–20.
197. Ripley RT, et al. Liver resection for metastatic melanoma with postoperative tumor-infiltrating lymphocyte therapy. Ann Surg Oncol. 2010;17(1):163–70.
198. Ryu SW, et al. Liver resection for metastatic melanoma: equivalent survival for cutaneous and ocular primaries. J Surg Oncol. 2013;108(2):129–35.
199. Becker JC, et al. Treatment of disseminated ocular melanoma with sequential fotemustine, interferon alpha, and interleukin 2. Br J Cancer. 2002;87(8):840–5.
200. Dummer R, et al. Encorafenib plus binimetinib versus vemurafenib or encorafenib in patients with BRAF-mutant melanoma (COLUMBUS): a multicentre, open-label, randomised phase 3 trial. Lancet Oncol. 2018;19(5):603–15.
201. Larkin J, et al. Combined vemurafenib and cobimetinib in BRAF-mutated melanoma. N Engl J Med. 2014;371(20):1867–76.
202. Long GV, et al. Combined BRAF and MEK inhibition versus BRAF inhibition alone in melanoma. N Engl J Med. 2014;371(20):1877–88.
203. Robert C, et al. Improved overall survival in melanoma with combined dabrafenib and trametinib. N Engl J Med. 2015;372(1):30–9.
204. Singh BP, Salama AK. Updates in therapy for advanced melanoma. Cancers (Basel). 2016;8(1).
205. Larkin J, Hodi FS, Wolchok JD. Combined Nivolumab and Ipilimumab or monotherapy in untreated melanoma. N Engl J Med. 2015;373(13):1270–1.

206. Hofmann UB, et al. Overexpression of the KIT/SCF in uveal melanoma does not translate into clinical efficacy of imatinib mesylate. Clin Cancer Res. 2009;15(1):324–9.
207. Rimoldi D, et al. Lack of BRAF mutations in uveal melanoma. Cancer Res. 2003;63(18):5712–5.
208. Zuidervaart W, et al. Activation of the MAPK pathway is a common event in uveal melanomas although it rarely occurs through mutation of BRAF or RAS. Br J Cancer. 2005;92(11):2032–8.
209. Leyvraz S, et al. Hepatic intra-arterial versus intravenous fotemustine in patients with liver metastases from uveal melanoma (EORTC 18021): a multicentric randomized trial. Ann Oncol. 2014;25(3):742–6.
210. Agarwala SS, Panikkar R, Kirkwood JM. Phase I/II randomized trial of intrahepatic arterial infusion chemotherapy with cisplatin and chemoembolization with cisplatin and polyvinyl sponge in patients with ocular melanoma metastatic to the liver. Melanoma Res. 2004;14(3):217–22.
211. Farolfi A, et al. Liver metastases from melanoma: hepatic intra-arterial chemotherapy. A retrospective study. J Chemother. 2011;23(5):300–5.
212. Heusner TA, et al. Transarterial hepatic chemoperfusion of uveal melanoma metastases: survival and response to treatment. Rofo. 2011;183(12):1151–60.
213. Peters S, et al. Intra-arterial hepatic fotemustine for the treatment of liver metastases from uveal melanoma: experience in 101 patients. Ann Oncol. 2006;17(4):578–83.
214. Ahrar J, et al. Response, survival, and prognostic factors after hepatic arterial chemoembolization in patients with liver metastases from cutaneous melanoma. Cancer Investig. 2011;29(1):49–55.
215. Gupta S, et al. Hepatic artery chemoembolization in patients with ocular melanoma metastatic to the liver: response, survival, and prognostic factors. Am J Clin Oncol. 2010;33(5):474–80.
216. Patel K, et al. Chemoembolization of the hepatic artery with BCNU for metastatic uveal melanoma: results of a phase II study. Melanoma Res. 2005;15(4):297–304.
217. Schuster R, et al. Transarterial chemoembolization of liver metastases from uveal melanoma after failure of systemic therapy: toxicity and outcome. Melanoma Res. 2010;20(3):191–6.
218. Sharma KV, et al. Hepatic arterial chemoembolization for management of metastatic melanoma. AJR Am J Roentgenol. 2008;190(1):99–104.
219. Gardner AB, et al. Ovarian, uterine, and cervical cancer patients with distant metastases at diagnosis: most common locations and outcomes. Clin Exp Metastasis. 2020;37(1):107–13.
220. Chang SJ, et al. Survival impact of complete cytoreduction to no gross residual disease for advanced-stage ovarian cancer: a meta-analysis. Gynecol Oncol. 2013;130(3):493–8.

221. Nakayama K, et al. Mechanisms of ovarian cancer metastasis: biochemical pathways. Int J Mol Sci. 2012;13(9):11705–17.
222. Prat J, F.C.o.G. Oncology. FIGO'S staging classification for cancer of the ovary, fallopian tube, and peritoneum: abridged republication. J Gynecol Oncol. 2015;26(2):87–9.
223. Gasparri ML, et al. Hepatic resection during cytoreductive surgery for primary or recurrent epithelial ovarian cancer. J Cancer Res Clin Oncol. 2016;142(7):1509–20.
224. Bacalbasa N, et al. Liver resection for ovarian cancer liver metastases as part of cytoreductive surgery is safe and may bring survival benefit. World J Surg Oncol. 2015;13:235.
225. Neumann UP, et al. Clinical outcome of patients with advanced ovarian cancer after resection of liver metastases. Anticancer Res. 2012;32(10):4517–21.
226. Armstrong DK, et al. Ovarian cancer, version 2.2020, NCCN clinical practice guidelines in oncology. J Natl Compr Cancer Netw. 2021;19(2):191–226.
227. Bristow RE, et al. Survival effect of maximal cytoreductive surgery for advanced ovarian carcinoma during the platinum era: a meta-analysis. J Clin Oncol. 2002;20(5):1248–59.
228. Elies A, et al. The role of neoadjuvant chemotherapy in ovarian cancer. Expert Rev Anticancer Ther. 2018;18(6):555–66.
229. Armstrong DK, et al. Intraperitoneal cisplatin and paclitaxel in ovarian cancer. N Engl J Med. 2006;354(1):34–43.
230. van Driel WJ, et al. Hyperthermic intraperitoneal chemotherapy in ovarian cancer. N Engl J Med. 2018;378(3):230–40.
231. Spiliotis J, et al. Cytoreductive surgery and HIPEC in recurrent epithelial ovarian cancer: a prospective randomized phase III study. Ann Surg Oncol. 2015;22(5):1570–5.
232. Mateo R, et al. Optimal cytoreduction after combined resection and radiofrequency ablation of hepatic metastases from recurrent malignant ovarian tumors. Gynecol Oncol. 2005;97(1):266–70.
233. Liu B, et al. Ultrasound-guided percutaneous radiofrequency ablation of liver metastasis from ovarian cancer: a single-Center initial experience. Int J Gynecol Cancer. 2017;27(6):1261–7.
234. Samuel N, Hudson TJ. The molecular and cellular heterogeneity of pancreatic ductal adenocarcinoma. Nat Rev Gastroenterol Hepatol. 2011;9(2):77–87.
235. Malvezzi M, et al. European cancer mortality predictions for the year 2013. Ann Oncol. 2013;24(3):792–800.
236. Iacobuzio-Donahue CA, et al. DPC4 gene status of the primary carcinoma correlates with patterns of failure in patients with pancreatic cancer. J Clin Oncol. 2009;27(11):1806–13.

237. Conroy T, et al. FOLFIRINOX versus gemcitabine for metastatic pancreatic cancer. N Engl J Med. 2011;364(19):1817–25.
238. Ay S, et al. FOLFIRINOX versus gemcitabine plus nab-paclitaxel as the first-line chemotherapy in metastatic pancreatic cancer. J Chemother. 2022:1–7.
239. Kneuertz PJ, et al. Palliative surgical management of patients with unresectable pancreatic adenocarcinoma: trends and lessons learned from a large, single institution experience. J Gastrointest Surg. 2011;15(11):1917–27.
240. Takada T, et al. Simultaneous hepatic resection with pancreato-duodenectomy for metastatic pancreatic head carcinoma: does it improve survival? Hepato-Gastroenterology. 1997;44(14):567–73.
241. Gleisner AL, et al. Is resection of periampullary or pancreatic adenocarcinoma with synchronous hepatic metastasis justified? Cancer. 2007;110(11):2484–92.
242. Shrikhande SV, et al. Pancreatic resection for M1 pancreatic ductal adenocarcinoma. Ann Surg Oncol. 2007;14(1):118–27.
243. Klein F, et al. The impact of simultaneous liver resection for occult liver metastases of pancreatic adenocarcinoma. Gastroenterol Res Pract. 2012;2012:939350.
244. Yamada H, et al. Surgical treatment of liver metastases from pancreatic cancer. HPB (Oxford). 2006;8(2):85–8.
245. Tachezy M, et al. Synchronous resections of hepatic oligometastatic pancreatic cancer: disputing a principle in a time of safe pancreatic operations in a retrospective multicenter analysis. Surgery. 2016;160(1):136–44.
246. Andreou A, et al. The role of hepatectomy for synchronous liver metastases from pancreatic adenocarcinoma. Surg Oncol. 2018;27(4):688–94.
247. Crippa S, et al. Is there a role for surgical resection in patients with pancreatic cancer with liver metastases responding to chemotherapy? Eur J Surg Oncol. 2016;42(10):1533–9.
248. Frigerio I, et al. Downstaging in stage IV pancreatic cancer: a new population eligible for surgery? Ann Surg Oncol. 2017;24(8):2397–403.
249. Crippa S, et al. A systematic review of surgical resection of liver-only synchronous metastases from pancreatic cancer in the era of multiagent chemotherapy. Updat Surg. 2020;72(1):39–45.
250. Wei M, et al. Simultaneous resection of the primary tumour and liver metastases after conversion chemotherapy versus standard therapy in pancreatic cancer with liver oligometastasis: protocol of a multicentre, prospective, randomised phase III control trial (CSPAC-1). BMJ Open. 2019;9(12):e033452.
251. Dunschede F, et al. Treatment of metachronous and simultaneous liver metastases of pancreatic cancer. Eur Surg Res. 2010;44(3–4):209–13.
252. Hackert T, et al. Radical surgery of oligometastatic pancreatic cancer. Eur J Surg Oncol. 2017;43(2):358–63.

253. Kirchweger P, et al. Circulating tumor DNA correlates with tumor burden and predicts outcome in pancreatic cancer irrespective of tumor stage. Eur J Surg Oncol. 2022;48(5):1046–53.
254. Moffitt RA, et al. Virtual microdissection identifies distinct tumor- and stroma-specific subtypes of pancreatic ductal adenocarcinoma. Nat Genet. 2015;47(10):1168–78.
255. Bianchi M, et al. Distribution of metastatic sites in renal cell carcinoma: a population-based analysis. Ann Oncol. 2012;23(4):973–80.
256. Janzen NK, et al. Surveillance after radical or partial nephrectomy for localized renal cell carcinoma and management of recurrent disease. Urol Clin North Am. 2003;30(4):843–52.
257. Kunkle DA, et al. Tumor size predicts synchronous metastatic renal cell carcinoma: implications for surveillance of small renal masses. J Urol. 2007;177(5):1692–6. discussion 1697
258. Thompson RH, et al. Metastatic renal cell carcinoma risk according to tumor size. J Urol. 2009;182(1):41–5.
259. Gupta K, et al. Epidemiologic and socioeconomic burden of metastatic renal cell carcinoma (mRCC): a literature review. Cancer Treat Rev. 2008;34(3):193–205.
260. Dekernion JB, Ramming KP, Smith RB. The natural history of metastatic renal cell carcinoma: a computer analysis. J Urol. 1978;120(2):148–52.
261. Hamada S, et al. Clinical characteristics and prognosis of patients with renal cell carcinoma and liver metastasis. Mol Clin Oncol. 2015;3(1):63–8.
262. Motzer RJ, et al. Sunitinib versus interferon alfa in metastatic renal-cell carcinoma. N Engl J Med. 2007;356(2):115–24.
263. Rini BI, et al. The society for immunotherapy of cancer consensus statement on immunotherapy for the treatment of advanced renal cell carcinoma (RCC). J Immunother Cancer. 2019;7(1):354.
264. Dabestani S, et al. Local treatments for metastases of renal cell carcinoma: a systematic review. Lancet Oncol. 2014;15(12):e549–61.
265. Zaid HB, et al. Outcomes following complete surgical Metastasectomy for patients with metastatic renal cell carcinoma: a systematic review and meta-analysis. J Urol. 2017;197(1):44–9.
266. Ruys AT, et al. Surgical treatment of renal cell cancer liver metastases: a population-based study. Ann Surg Oncol. 2011;18(7):1932–8.
267. Staehler MD, et al. Liver resection for metastatic disease prolongs survival in renal cell carcinoma: 12-year results from a retrospective comparative analysis. World J Urol. 2010;28(4):543–7.
268. Pinotti E, et al. Surgical treatment of liver metastases from kidney cancer: a systematic review. ANZ J Surg. 2019;89(1–2):32–7.
269. Grimes NG, et al. A systematic review of the role of hepatectomy in the management of metastatic renal cell carcinoma. Eur J Surg Oncol. 2014;40(12):1622–8.

270. Hau HM, et al. The value of hepatic resection in metastasic renal cancer in the era of Tyrosinkinase inhibitor therapy. BMC Surg. 2016;16(1):49.
271. Mitomo S, et al. Sunitinib treatment enabling resection of massive liver metastasis: a case report. J Med Case Rep. 2013;7:234.
272. Drake CG, Lipson EJ, Brahmer JR. Breathing new life into immunotherapy: review of melanoma, lung and kidney cancer. Nat Rev Clin Oncol. 2014;11(1):24–37.
273. Hammers H. Immunotherapy in kidney cancer: the past, present, and future. Curr Opin Urol. 2016;26(6):543–7.
274. Nazzani S, Bazinet A, Karakiewicz PI. Role of immunotherapy in kidney cancer. Curr Opin Support Palliat Care. 2018;12(3):325–33.
275. Rehders A, et al. Hepatic metastasectomy for soft-tissue sarcomas: is it justified? World J Surg. 2009;33(1):111–7.
276. Deneve JL, et al. Chemosaturation with percutaneous hepatic perfusion for unresectable isolated hepatic metastases from sarcoma. Cardiovasc Intervent Radiol. 2012;35(6):1480–7.
277. Mudan SS, et al. Salvage surgery for patients with recurrent gastrointestinal sarcoma: prognostic factors to guide patient selection. Cancer. 2000;88(1):66–74.
278. Chua TC, Chu F, Morris DL. Outcomes of single-Centre experience of hepatic resection and cryoablation of sarcoma liver metastases. Am J Clin Oncol. 2011;34(3):317–20.
279. Burkill GJ, et al. Malignant gastrointestinal stromal tumor: distribution, imaging features, and pattern of metastatic spread. Radiology. 2003;226(2):527–32.
280. Tirotta F, et al. Liver resection for sarcoma metastases: a systematic review and experience from two European centres. Eur J Surg Oncol. 2020;46(10 Pt A):1807–13.
281. Le Cesne A, et al. Randomized phase III study comparing conventional-dose doxorubicin plus ifosfamide versus high-dose doxorubicin plus ifosfamide plus recombinant human granulocyte-macrophage colony-stimulating factor in advanced soft tissue sarcomas: a trial of the European Organization for Research and Treatment of cancer/soft tissue and bone sarcoma group. J Clin Oncol. 2000;18(14):2676–84.
282. Goumard C, et al. Long-term survival according to histology and radiologic response to preoperative chemotherapy in 126 patients undergoing resection of non-GIST sarcoma liver metastases. Ann Surg Oncol. 2018;25(1):107–16.
283. Lang H, et al. Hepatic metastases from leiomyosarcoma: a single-center experience with 34 liver resections during a 15-year period. Ann Surg. 2000;231(4):500–5.
284. Chen H, et al. Complete hepatic resection of metastases from leiomyosarcoma prolongs survival. J Gastrointest Surg. 1998;2(2):151–5.

285. D'Ambrosio L, et al. Doxorubicin plus dacarbazine, doxorubicin plus ifosfamide, or doxorubicin alone as a first-line treatment for advanced leiomyosarcoma: a propensity score matching analysis from the European Organization for Research and Treatment of cancer soft tissue and bone sarcoma group. Cancer. 2020;126(11):2637–47.
286. Siegel RL, Miller KD, Jemal A. Cancer statistics, 2016. CA Cancer J Clin. 2016;66(1):7–30.
287. Qubaiah O, et al. Small intestinal cancer: a population-based study of incidence and survival patterns in the United States, 1992 to 2006. Cancer Epidemiol Biomarkers Prev. 2010;19(8):1908–18.
288. Dabaja BS, et al. Adenocarcinoma of the small bowel: presentation, prognostic factors, and outcome of 217 patients. Cancer. 2004;101(3):518–26.
289. Halfdanarson TR, et al. A single-institution experience with 491 cases of small bowel adenocarcinoma. Am J Surg. 2010;199(6):797–803.
290. Ye X, et al. Frequency, prognosis and treatment modalities of newly diagnosed small bowel cancer with liver metastases. BMC Gastroenterol. 2020;20(1):342.
291. Zhou YW, et al. Clinical features, treatment, and prognosis of different histological types of primary small bowel adenocarcinoma: a propensity score matching analysis based on the SEER database. Eur J Surg Oncol. 2021;47(8):2108–18.
292. Li X, et al. Clinicopathological features and treatment outcomes of metastatic or locally unresectable small bowel adenocarcinoma. J BUON. 2019;24(6):2539–45.
293. Rompteaux P, et al. Resection of small bowel adenocarcinoma metastases: results of the ARCAD-NADEGE cohort study. Eur J Surg Oncol. 2019;45(3):331–5.
294. Benson AB, et al. Small bowel adenocarcinoma, version 1.2020, NCCN clinical practice guidelines in oncology. J Natl Compr Cancer Netw. 2019;17(9):1109–33.
295. Shelley MD, Burgon K, Mason MD. Treatment of testicular germ-cell cancer: a cochrane evidence-based systematic review. Cancer Treat Rev. 2002;28(5):237–53.
296. Dearnaley D, Huddart R, Horwich A. Regular review: managing testicular cancer. BMJ. 2001;322(7302):1583–8.
297. Mead GM, Stenning SP, Cook P, Fossa SD, Horwich A, Kaye SB, Oliver RT, de Mulder PH, de Wit R, Stoter G, Sylvester RJ. International germ cell consensus classification: a prognostic factor-based staging system for metastatic germ cell cancers. International germ cell cancer collaborative group. J Clin Oncol. 1997;15(2):594–603.
298. Tonyali S, Yazici S. Does solitary- and organ-confined metastasectomy really improve survival in advanced urologic malignancies? Int Urol Nephrol. 2016;48(5):671–80.

299. Gilligan T, et al. Testicular cancer, version 2.2020, NCCN clinical practice guidelines in oncology. J Natl Compr Cancer Netw. 2019;17(12):1529–54.
300. You YN, Leibovitch BC, Que FG. Hepatic metastasectomy for testicular germ cell tumors: is it worth it? J Gastrointest Surg. 2009;13(4):595–601.
301. Copson E, et al. Liver metastases in germ cell cancer: defining a role for surgery after chemotherapy. BJU Int. 2004;94(4):552–8.
302. Rivoire M, et al. Multimodality treatment of patients with liver metastases from germ cell tumors: the role of surgery. Cancer. 2001;92(3):578–87.
303. Hahn TL, et al. Hepatic resection of metastatic testicular carcinoma: a further update. Ann Surg Oncol. 1999;6(7):640–4.
304. Xu P, et al. Prognosis of patients with testicular carcinoma is dependent on metastatic site. Front Oncol. 2019;9:1495.
305. Song HJ, et al. Rare metastases of differentiated thyroid carcinoma: pictorial review. Endocr Relat Cancer. 2011;18(5):R165–74.
306. Machens A, Dralle H. Prognostic impact of N staging in 715 medullary thyroid cancer patients: proposal for a revised staging system. Ann Surg. 2013;257(2):323–9.
307. Song HJ, et al. Uncommon metastases from differentiated thyroid carcinoma. Hell J Nucl Med. 2012;15(3):233–40.
308. American Thyroid Association Guidelines Taskforce on Thyroid, N, et al. Revised American Thyroid Association management guidelines for patients with thyroid nodules and differentiated thyroid cancer. Thyroid. 2009;19(11):1167–214.
309. Salvatori M, et al. Solitary liver metastasis from Hurthle cell thyroid cancer: a case report and review of the literature. J Endocrinol Investig. 2004;27(1):52–6.
310. Lorenz K, et al. Selective arterial chemoembolization for hepatic metastases from medullary thyroid carcinoma. Surgery. 2005;138(6):986–93. discussion 993
311. Fromigue J, et al. Chemoembolization for liver metastases from medullary thyroid carcinoma. J Clin Endocrinol Metab. 2006;91(7):2496–9.
312. Brown AP, et al. Radioiodine treatment of metastatic thyroid carcinoma: the Royal Marsden Hospital experience. Br J Radiol. 1984;57(676):323–7.
313. Kouso H, et al. Liver metastasis from thyroid carcinoma 32 years after resection of the primary tumor: report of a case. Surg Today. 2005;35(6):480–2.
314. Zhang H, et al. Successful treatment of Hurthle cell thyroid carcinoma with lung and liver metastasis using docetaxel and cisplatin. Jpn J Clin Oncol. 2012;42(11):1086–90.

315. Machens A, Behrmann C, Dralle H. Chemoembolization of liver metastases from medullary thyroid carcinoma. Ann Intern Med. 2000;132(7):596–7.
316. Wertenbroek MW, et al. Radiofrequency ablation of hepatic metastases from thyroid carcinoma. Thyroid. 2008;18(10):1105–10.
317. Waters KM, et al. Smoldering medullary thyroid carcinoma liver metastasis 37 years after resection of an organ-confined tumor. Diagn Cytopathol. 2015;43(1):45–8.
318. Paspala A, et al. Long-term outcomes after hepatic and pancreatic resections for metastases from thyroid cancer: a systematic review of the literature. J Gastrointest Cancer. 2019;50(1):9–15.
319. Roupret M, et al. European guidelines on upper tract urothelial carcinomas: 2013 update. Eur Urol. 2013;63(6):1059–71.
320. Shinagare AB, et al. Metastatic pattern of bladder cancer: correlation with the characteristics of the primary tumor. AJR Am J Roentgenol. 2011;196(1):117–22.
321. Wallmeroth A, et al. Patterns of metastasis in muscle-invasive bladder cancer (pT2-4): an autopsy study on 367 patients. Urol Int. 1999;62(2):69–75.
322. Dong F, et al. Prognostic value of site-specific metastases and therapeutic roles of surgery for patients with metastatic bladder cancer: a population-based study. Cancer Manag Res. 2017;9:611–26.
323. Witjes JA, et al. EAU guidelines on muscle-invasive and metastatic bladder cancer: summary of the 2013 guidelines. Eur Urol. 2014;65(4):778–92.
324. Yafi FA, Kassouf W. Management of patients with advanced bladder cancer following major response to systemic chemotherapy. Expert Rev Anticancer Ther. 2009;9(12):1757–64.
325. Abe T, et al. Impact of multimodal treatment on survival in patients with metastatic urothelial cancer. Eur Urol. 2007;52(4):1106–13.
326. Lehmann J, et al. Surgery for metastatic urothelial carcinoma with curative intent: the German experience (AUO AB 30/05). Eur Urol. 2009;55(6):1293–9.
327. Shimizu T, et al. Organ-specific and mixed responses to pembrolizumab in patients with unresectable or metastatic urothelial carcinoma: a multicenter retrospective study. Cancers (Basel). 2022;14(7).

Part IV

Basic Procedures

Positions and Access

12

Fabio Giannone, Oronzo Ligurgo, and Patrick Pessaux

Open Approach

The open approach is the conventional laparotomic technique. The laparotomic approach has been used for decades and is well established in the surgical field. Moreover, it offers the greatest exposure of the entire abdominal cavity. Depending on the target, it is possible to choose different types of incisions and calibrate their size gaining great visibility and accessibility. The advantages of open surgery are the shortest preparation and operating times and the lowest costs in terms of the materials used. Nevertheless, it is burdened by some major disadvantages such as a higher risk of infection of the operating site directly linked to the dimension of the incision, more intense post-operative pain, and the major risk of development of incisional hernias. We will further discuss about the techniques of patient positioning, the different types of incision used to access the abdominal cavity as well as about specific materials to increase exposure of the surgical field as retractors.

F. Giannone (✉) · O. Ligurgo · P. Pessaux
Department of Visceral and Digestive Surgery, University Hospital of Strasbourg, Strasbourg, France
e-mail: fabio.giannone@ospedale.al.it

Patient Positioning

The first phase of a surgical intervention is the positioning of the patient. In the laparotomic approach, the position of the patient is crucial because it is intended to enable the surgeon to be in the most ergonomic position. Secondly, the changing of the operating bed position during the intervention allows naturally retraction of the different organs thanks to the gravity and finally a better exposition. In open liver surgery, the most used position is undoubtedly the supine decubitus. Patient's arms are generally spread on the armrests at 90 degrees, even if that on the operator side may be positioned alongside the body according surgeon's preference. Is it advisable, however, to spread the left arm to enable vascular access for anesthetists? Lower limbs are closed and parallel. Left lateral decubitus position is rarely used and described for posterior segments allowing a better access to the right posterior lateral sector and to the inferior vena cava.

During the various surgical phases, the available positions may change to facilitate specific maneuvers, including Trendelenburg, reverse-Trendelenburg, and rotation of the operating table to the left or to the right. The Trendelenburg position consists in raising patient's feet higher than his head. It can be recommended during liver resection in order to decrease the risk of venous air embolism even though rare in open surgery. The disadvantage is that this position raises the central venous pressure and may increase blood loss during the parenchymal transection. On the contrary, the reverse-Trendelenburg position (feet lower than the head) effectively lowers the central venous pressure during liver surgery and it is recommended to liver surgeons and anesthetists who have difficulties in maintaining low pressures with the supine or Trendelenburg positions in the presence of bleeding that cannot be controlled by the Pringle maneuver [1]. As concerns lateral tilting, a rotation to the left side allows a better maneuverability and a more precise control of the right posterior segments and the inferior cava vein. The rotation in this sense is often used during right liver complete mobilization, in the dissection of the right hepatic vein, during the dissection of the posterior face of the liver and of the inferior vena cava, and especially if inferior hepatic veins should be controlled. During pedicle dissection, a left-tilt could be used to isolate the portal trunk and the right portal vein. Rotation to the right is not useful a priori in liver surgery while it is frequently used to access the spleen and the pancreas.

Access

Three different surgical times compose the access: preparation of the surgical field, incision, and exposure. At the end, the preparation of the patient is ready and the operation can begin. All these phases have the purpose of allowing the surgeon to work with the best exposition, in the safest position ant in the most ergonomic way.

Surgical Field

During surgical field preparation, skin disinfection of the entire abdomen is always necessary. Furthermore, in some cases, it is possible to widen the disinfection to the chest and/or to the Scarpa triangle. Indeed, surgical field should include the thorax, if a thoracotomy or sternotomy is expected, and it should include triangle of Scarpa in case of vascular reconstruction with the need of a vascular graft or when an extracorporeal circulation could be installed.

Incision

Correct choice of incision plays a pivotal role in the safe performance and success of the surgical intervention. The key points which govern this choice are: optimal exposure of the anticipated organs, ergonomics of dissection at depth, ergonomics of retraction, ease of extension, body habitus, previous surgical scars, rapidity of entry, security of closure, abdominal wall integrity, post-operative pain, surgical site infection, and cosmesis [2].

In open liver surgery, wide ranges of incisions are commonly used:

- The right subcostal incision (Kocher incision). In this case, the skin incision is traced two fingers below the right costal margin. This facilitates closure so that the incision line is not on or over the costal margin. The advantage of this incision is that it is versatile and can easily be extended. It is usually made for cholecystectomy or common bile duct exploration. It permits the exploration of the sole anterior segments.
- The bilateral subcostal incision (Chevron incision) is used to access the liver for transplantation and major liver resections. In addition, most pancreas resections are performed with this incision. The advantage is that a wide and comprehensive view of the upper quadrants is guaranteed.
- Bilateral subcostal incision with midline cephalad extension (Mercedes incision). It theoretically increases liver exposure, especially in supra-elevated and intrathoracic livers. Furthermore, it ensures a better visualization of the suprahepatic inferior vena cava, useful in case of total vascular exclusion or cava resections. Both Chevron and Mercedes incision are described to be associated with a higher risk of postoperative pulmonary complications [3].
- Midline incision is used in liver surgery generally for left-sided resections. The advantage is that it is the only incision that prevents the transversal resection of the rectus abdominis muscles. Nevertheless, in overweight patients and those whose anteroposterior distance is increased, the midline incision does not allow an adequate exposure [4].
- The J-shaped incision (Makuuchi incision) is used most frequently for surgery on the right liver. This incision provides a particularly good access to the area between the inferior vena cava and the right hepatic vein. The J-shaped incision can be extended laterally to a thoracotomy for better exposure.

Retractors

Retractors are useful instruments that help the surgeon to expose the surgical site. They can be divided into standard retractors and self-retractors. Retractors of Leriche, the malleable valve, the valve of Mickulitz, and others belong to the first group. The assistant is supposed to gently pull the different organs during the intervention using these kinds of valves. The latter group of the self-retaining retractors has the important advantage to make traction independently by pivoting on the operating bed:

- The Rochard retractor is composed by two large semicircular blades, which retract the abdominal wall and are attached to a fixed arm at the operating table. The main disadvantage is the unidirectional tension.
- Japanese retractor of Tagasako or Ulrich retractor (Fig. 12.1) is made up by a fixed semicircular arm (frame) that is fixed to the operating table and four semicircular blades. The semicircular blades retract the abdominal wall, and are attached to the fixed arm thanks to a reel that can be used for adjusting traction.

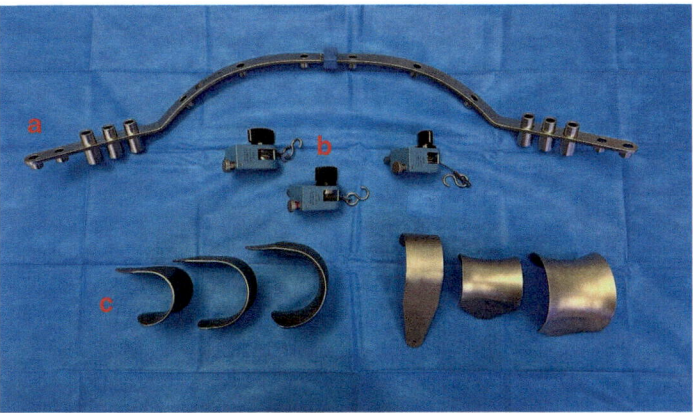

Fig. 12.1 Ulrich retractor. A semicircular frame (**a**) is fixed to the operating table and through 2–4 winch systems (**b**) different blades (**c**) can be used to retract the abdominal wall

- Thompson is a very stable and versatile retractor. The basic components are the rail arm, the two rods, and the different retracting paddles that are attached to a retaining arm. The Thompson retractor is favored for uni- and bilateral subcostal incisions. The exposure of the lower abdominal parts is limited. There is a wide range of blades and paddles available as accessories.
- Omnitract is a newer self-retractor. Although this retractor system needs careful installation, it offers excellent access for most incisions. The open frame system can be utilized as easily as a closed ring where several paddles can be attached.

Laparoscopic Approach

The spread of the minimally invasive approach has undoubtedly affected liver surgery and the indications for diseases of the hepatobiliary sphere. Initially limited to specific indications, as small lesions in anterior segments, it has gained over the past few decades increasing prominence and acceptance in complex cases, hostile locations, and impaired underlying parenchyma. The last consensus guidelines confirmed that laparoscopic liver resections can be safely performed, especially in experts' hands, even in case of major or complex hepatectomies [5]. This approach offers numerous advantages over traditional open surgery, including significantly reduced surgical trauma, minimized blood loss, shorter hospital stays, and faster patient recovery. Proper patient positioning and precise trocar placement are fundamental aspects of this surgical technique, ensuring safety and efficiency throughout the procedure. This chapter provides an in-depth exploration of these critical elements, with detailed tips according to type or resection or specific locations.

Patient Positioning

Supine Position

A well-established patient positioning for laparoscopic liver surgery involves the combination of a two-axis tilt, cranio-caudal and latero-lateral, which allows for optimal access to the liver and the surgical field by utilizing gravity to displace abdominal contents. The most frequently adopted position is the supine split-leg one, with the surgeon standing between the lower limbs of the patient. This approach allows a global visualization of the whole liver parenchyma and the biliary tree. Supine split-leg position is undoubtedly the one of choice in anterior segments resections, right or left hepatectomies, or biliary tree surgery, allowing a direct, frontal view of the target as well as of the liver section slice. Supine approach with a right-left tilt and/or chest lifting has been largely described for posterior segment resections with excellent results [6–8]. In the supine configuration, arms are spread apart or placed along the body as needed by anesthesiologists for arterial or venous access. The pelvis is placed as low as possible, at the edge of the operating bed, to allow more efficient leg opening with a consequent increase in movement space for the first operator. Before preparing the operating field, the surgeon checks whether the patient's position is appropriate. Adequate patient fixation is crucial to prevent unintended movement during surgery or tilting. Techniques such as padded positioning devices, straps, gel mattress, and cushions help maintain the patient's stability and ensure safety throughout the laparoscopic procedure. Straps placement just above the knee or at ankle height avoids patient slipping in reverse Trendelenburg position. After ensuring proper positioning and fixation of the patient, a "crash test" can be done to simulate operative movements. In detail, the table is tilt laterally and cranio-caudally in extreme positions to check for possible body displacement. Once the operative field is done and pneumoperitoneum is created, a 10–30 degrees reverse Trendelenburg position is adopted. This is characterized by elevating the patient's head higher than the feet, causing the abdominal organs, including the liver, to shift away from the diaphragm and expose the hilum. Furthermore, it decreases hepatic venous pressure by reducing venous return. An exclusive lowering of the legs without modifying the cranio-caudal axis of the rest of the body could be useful for avoiding conflicts between surgical instrumentations and lower limbs. Additionally, a lateral tilt, generally left, of approximately 10–15 degrees redirects the liver laterally, facilitating the access to the desired segment. Alternatively, as it happens in our unit, an inflatable pillow can be positioned under the right shoulder to rotate the chest and the right upper quadrant up to 30 degrees in case of postero-lateral resections (Fig. 12.1b). Mainly in this latter case, but also with the patient fully supine, some authors have described lateral resections (both left or right) [9, 10] with surgeon standing on the opposite side of the target throughout the procedure or at particular steps of the operation. While this can be helpful and comfortable in certain circumstances, evident drawbacks are the lack of a global vision during certain maneuvers, difficult access to the hilum in the emergency setting or the need to shift positioning of the screen or instrumentations during surgery.

Lateral Decubitus

Mainly for tumors located in the posterior segments, lateral position of the patient has been largely described in the literature [11–14]. Different variants are reported, as a semi-left lateral position, a vertical or full lateral position [11], and the semi-prone position [12, 15]. All these approaches allow transthoracic trocars placement as well as a better exposure of the poster-lateral surface of the parenchyma. Furthermore, it elevates the right hepatic vein higher than the vena cava, which reduces hepatic venous bleeding. In case of lateral decubitus, legs are normally united and the surgeon is on the left side of the patient. An exception is the case of a semi-lateral decubitus where a 30–45 degrees rotation is considered with split legs and surgeon between. Different steps and much attention are required when choosing this approach, for the risk of joint or muscular damages. A pillow is normally placed between the legs, with the right one slightly rotated forward, especially in the semi-prone decubitus, to maintain a correct axis with the spine and the pelvis. Left arm generally lies perpendicular to the body, while the right one is bent upward, raised by an armrest. Another advice is to correctly place the patient so that the lumbar region could be elevated and exposed after angling the table up to 120° [16], as performed in a right adrenectomy. This allows the extension of the distance between the right costal margin and the right anterior superior iliac spine and the anteriorization of the posterior segments. Pillows, soft gel protections and straps are extensively used to protect surfaces and avoid displacements during surgery. Several series reported the feasibility as well as the advantages of this decubitus over the supine one in some aspects. However, some weaknesses should be reported. First of all, the necessity of repositioning the patient in case of conversion, especially in case of major bleeding, which takes time. In addition, the lateral decubitus position does not allow for a complete and effective visualization of the left-sided segments and it is not replicable in cases of large tumors compressing the diaphragm and the inferior vena cava.

Trocars Placement

The selection of trocar sites in laparoscopic liver surgery is highly dynamic, depending on the specific procedure and patient anatomy [17]. Normally, four to six trocars can be used in a normal setting, while single-site liver resections are rarely reported [18]. Adding a small incision for tape or thread exteriorization is sometimes necessary when opting for an extracorporeal pringle maneuver or in case of round ligament traction. A mix of both 5 mm and 10/12 mm trocars has to be used, planning accurately the exact location for larger trocars due to the greater number of 10-mm instruments in laparoscopic liver resections (ultrasound probe, ultrasonic dissector, clips appliers, etc.). Less frequently, a 15-mm trocar must be used for wider instruments, such as particular staplers. The first port is normally placed after a para-umbilical incision (usually supra-umbilical) for endoscope insertion. A veress technique could be alternatively performed, especially when para-umbilical access is not used. A paramedian or pararectal incision is the alternative, frequently used in right-sided resections. Para-umbilical incisions could be replaced by another type of access in specific situation, like in cirrhotic patients with a preoperative CT-scan identification of umbilical vein recanalization or large collateral veins. Other potential examples in which first trocar placement may be modified are in case of reoperation, with patients having a history of a median incision, or hepatomegaly and obese patients, where trocars should be placed respectively lower and higher than usual. A 30–45° endoscope is suggested to increase visibility during certain maneuvers as liver mobilization. Placement of operative trocars always needs the localization of some internal landmarks, such as the inferior border of the liver. This step is extremely important and should be accurately planned after the first trocar insertion. In patients with high body mass index or intra-thoracic liver for example, ports should be placed from 5 to 10 cm higher, to avoid an excessive distance from the farthest target, theoretically the hepatic-caval confluence, and thus a discomfort for the surgeon. In addition, the general principles of laparoscopic surgery have to be respected, such as the frontal view of the target (i.e., the transection plane), triangulation, and the minimum distance between trocars to avoid a collision between the various instruments. To deal with this issue of unconventional anatomy and misplaced ports, our team described an augmented-reality-based strategy in which a virtual image of the liver parenchyma is projected on the skin surface in relation to some external landmarks allowing targeting of the lesion and liver structures at the beginning of the operation for ports placement [19]. This results in an improved manageability of the operator, above all for posterior segment approach, which can lead to fewer operative times and lower intraoperative complications [20].

Although some general rules can be mentioned, there is currently no standard of care in port placement for laparoscopic and robotic hepatectomies and the main cause of this variability is site of tumor location and thus type of planned surgery [21]. For this reason, a typical setting of laparoscopic accesses will be described specifically for different liver location.

Left-Sided Segments

For left liver resections, the para-umbilical access is commonly employed, providing a central and clear view of the liver. The transection line is normally included between the Cantlie line, as in left hepatectomies, and the left lobe, in case of atypical resections of Sg 2 or 3. The transection plane is therefore very close and not too angled from the line of sight the surgeon has in this setting. A right pararectal trocar could be alternatively used in left hepatectomies or Sg 4 resections, especially in cirrhotic livers with umbilical vessel recanalization or left liver hypertrophy. After identifying some internal landmarks, such as the transection line, exact tumor location (if subcapsular), and liver borders, operative trocars can be accurately placed. In left lateral sectionectomies, the first two ports can be placed to the right and left of the optic access, at least 10 cm apart, at a height that varies according to patient anatomy and liver position. Trocars can be placed at the same level, keeping an exact triangulation with the middle line, or at a different height in specific situation, as in the case when the surgeon stands laterally. It is recommended to use 10/12-mm trocars for these two operative ports, as they should be alternatively used for dissectors, large clip appliers, and staplers according to the best angle. Although some authors describe left lateral sectionectomies using exclusively three ports [22], a fourth 5-mm port is usually added for irrigation/suction or to spread transected parenchyma. This is placed under the xyphoid or laterally, in the left or right hypochondriac/lumbar region in relation to the presence of a second assistant. Single-port laparoscopic approach is also feasible in this kind of operation with similar operative outcomes [23]. In resections located at Sg 4 and in left hepatectomies the same outline can be used for operative trocars, with a possible rightward shift for some trocars. An assistant port is almost always necessary while single-port resections are less described in the literature.

Right-Sided Segments

Right hepatectomies and Sg 5–6 resections are generally performed in a supine position, with a possible left-tilt or a pillow beneath the hemithorax, although some authors prefer a left lateral decubitus position [15]. In the first case, a 5–6 trocars setting is used with the endoscopic port usually placed in a right paramedian or pararectal position. Operative trocars are generally placed on the same axis whose angle varies from the horizontal transumbilical plane to the 45-degree subcostal border. Patient anatomy, the type of resection, and the liver position can modify the exact position of the chosen axis both in the latero-lateral and craniocaudal direction. Using this configuration, the optics are aligned with the main Cantlie line and the two operative trocars follow the triangulation principle of a laparoscopic approach. The use of 12 mm trocars, beyond allowing the universal and ubiquitous use of all the instruments, enables shifting endoscope placement during specific maneuvers. Assistant trocars can be aligned with this main axis or placed under the xyphoid [24]. Alternatively, the classic setting already described for left-sided resection can be used [25]. In left lateral decubitus the same principle of a single-axis port placement can be followed, generally located a couple of centimeters under the costal margin, from the right linea axillaris media to the midline [15]. The laparoscopic port in inserted by an open technique in the pararectal space, on the transumbilical plane or just above.

Posterior Segments

Segments 7 and 8 are undoubtedly the most challenging in minimally invasive liver surgery. The posterior and deep location, difficult exposure, uncomfortable transection plane, and proximity to large hepatic veins are definitely some of the issues encountered in this kind of resection. Several solutions have been proposed with a multitude of approaches used in literature, from supine to semi-prone position, from an exclusive abdominal access to the use of intercostal trocars with a hybrid approach [7, 26–29]. Trocar placement is therefore highly variable depending on surgeon preference, with a difficulty in drawing solid and always applicable tips. A general statement usually reported is the necessity of an experienced surgeon and always being prepared for a possible conversion. Totally abdominal postero-lateral resections can be performed in a semi-lateral position, with a 15–30 degrees left tilt and the surgeon between the legs [6], in a vertical left-lateral decubitus [11] or in the semi-prone position [12]. In the semi-lateral decubitus, a trocars setting similar to that described for left-sided resection has been described, with a multicentric report and good outcomes [6]. As already reported in the previous paragraph, when instead a full left-lateral decubitus is preferred trocars are placed following the costal margin, a few cm lower. Placing the main working ports as close as possible to the subcostal area results in maintaining the distance between the ports and operation field as short as possible. For a patient with a huge body cavity or who is obese, some devices could in fact not reach to the dome of the liver [9]. Even in this case pneumoperitoneum can be created through a right open pararectal access or, alternatively, 2–3 cm cm below the right costal arch in the right anterior axillary line [11]. Similarly, a pararectal access for the endoscopic port and three subcostal trocars were described for the technique in the semi-prone position [12]. The addition of an intercostal trocar is largely described in the literature for postero-lateral segments with encouraging results [27, 28, 30]. The postero-superior view obtained by this access allows a clearer and safer visualization of tumors located in the dome and of the right hepatic vein confluence in the inferior vena cava. One or two ports are usually inserted, of 5 or 10 mm size, normally after placing the abdominal trocars. Although they can be positioned between the ribs below the diaphragm, thus avoiding the perforation of this structure, the anatomical location of posterior segments normally requires a transdiaphragmatic access. Single-lung ventilation is necessary in these cases. Intercostal trocars are described both in the semi-lateral and in the left-lateral decubitus. The exact location of the intercostal port location is chosen after checking the posterior landmarks of the liver, the site of the lesion and of the major vascular structures and, not least, the transection planes. Balloon-tipped trocars are usually used, in order to push the diaphragm against the chest wall, minimizing therefore intra-operative pneumothorax formation. At the end of the liver resection, it is important to close the diaphragmatic incision to avoid organ herniation. Total transthoracic hepatectomies, also called "thoracoscopic", are also described, through case reports or small series [14, 31–33]. In this case, after the intercostal port insertion, a transdiaphragmatic ultrasound is performed to check tumor location and create the transdiaphragmatic access.

Robotic Approach

Robotic-assisted surgery has revolutionized the field of liver surgery, offering enhanced precision and dexterity to surgeons. Indications for robotic liver resection have been enormously expanded since its first application, being currently used even in donor hepatectomies and complex liver resections [34]. Central to the success of robotic liver procedures is the precise positioning of the patient and trocars. These steps are in fact crucial for a good exposure throughout the surgical resection and to avoid conflicts between the arms. This chapter provides a comprehensive overview of patient positioning and trocar placement employed in the literature in robotic hepatectomies, with a specific description based on the type of resection.

Patient Positioning and Operating Room Configuration

Unlike traditional laparoscopic liver surgery, robotic liver surgery almost exclusively employs a supine position for the patient without therefore the large variability seen in the last paragraph [35, 36]. This position offers several advantages in robotic liver resections, including improved patient comfort, better access to the entire abdomen, and ergonomic positioning of the robotic arms for the surgeon. General principles and precautions already described in the analogous paragraph for laparoscopic resections are applicable also in robotic hepatectomies. Patient's arms are normally extended on arm boards or alongside the body and legs are spread apart, leaving space for the first tableside assistant. The rotating overhead boom available in the latest model allows the

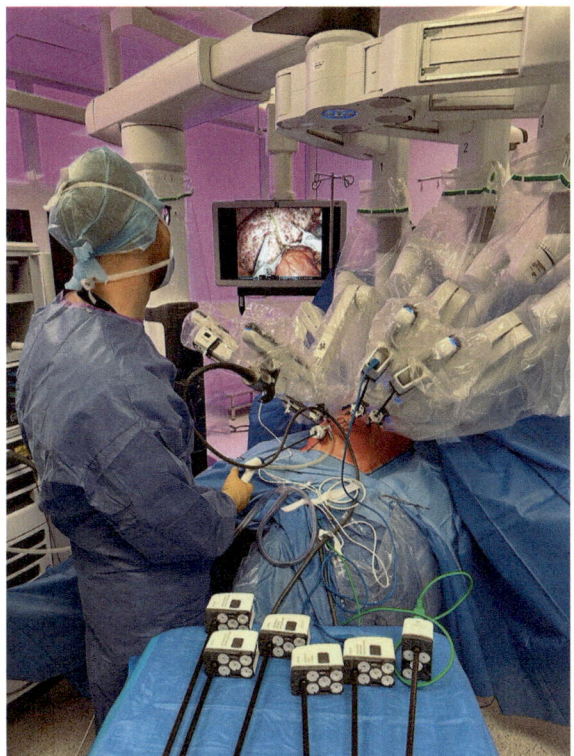

Fig. 12.2 Cart position in a typical liver resection scenario. Cart comes from the right position and the assistant stays between the inferior limbs of the patients

positioning of the patient cart on any side of the operating bed. A right or left positioning is advisable in order to free up enough room for the anesthetists (Fig. 12.2). The operating table is then tilted into a 15–30 degrees reverse Trendelenburg position, with the head of the patient's bed elevated. This positioning aids in providing better visualization and access to the upper abdomen, particularly when working on the liver's superior segments. A light left tilt could be helpful, especially for right-sided resections. These steps as well as all table's movements have to be done before docking the robot, to avoid any dangerous trocars or instrument displacements, unless an integrated table motion is available. In this case, the surgeon can safely dock the arms and move the table immediately before or during the surgical procedure. As in a laparoscopic approach, a semi-lateral or left-lateral decubitus is described by some authors for postero-superior resections [36, 37]. First reports on robotic transthoracic approach have also been published, defining the feasibility of this technique even with the robotic platform [14].

Trocars Placement

Port placement in robotic liver resections only partially follows the principles described in the laparoscopic approach. This is due to the features of the recent platforms and the need to establish a full-movement field for all the robotic arms without any conflicts. Abdominal access and port placement are in fact a crucial point to start robotic liver activity. Pneumoperitoneum can be created following surgeon's preference. If an open technique is chosen, a 12 mm trocar can be inserted in a peri-umbilical position, on the midline or laterally. This will be used as an assistant port and it should be therefore inserted slightly lower than the plane identified for the robotic trocars. In case of a veress technique, the 8 mm robotic ports can be directly placed. General rules of robotic platform include a distance between the target and the camera port (and ideally all the robotic ports) of about 20 cm, as well as a minimum distance of 8 cm between trocars. One or two assistant ports can be added, paying attention to their positioning and a possible conflict with the robotic arms. Generally, they are placed between two robotic ports, 4 cm lower, with a 10–12 mm access to allow for dissector or stapler insertion. All robotic ports should ideally be placed on the same axis, whose angle depends on the type of resection. This axis normally corresponds to the transumbilical plane but it could be higher in patients with an elevated BMI. Four 8 mm trocars should be used or, alternatively, one 12 mm port could be inserted instead for robotic stapling. Specific settings of port placements will be described in detail below.

Left-Sided Segments

In left-sided resections, trocars are usually placed on the horizontal transverse umbilical axis, or slightly higher in obese patients or in supra-elevated livers (Fig. 12.3a, b). The endoscopic port (port 2) should be inserted in front of the transection plane, which means on a right paramedian position in left hepatectomies or supraumbilical in left lateral segmentectomies. Both configurations can be, however, indistinctly used for all left-sided resections [38]. Port 1 and 3 are placed laterally, respectively on the right and on the left side of port 2, respecting the 8 cm distance and with a possible insertion of a 12 mm trocar for stapling in port 3. This setting respects the principle of triangulation already described for laparoscopic resections, with a central view and two

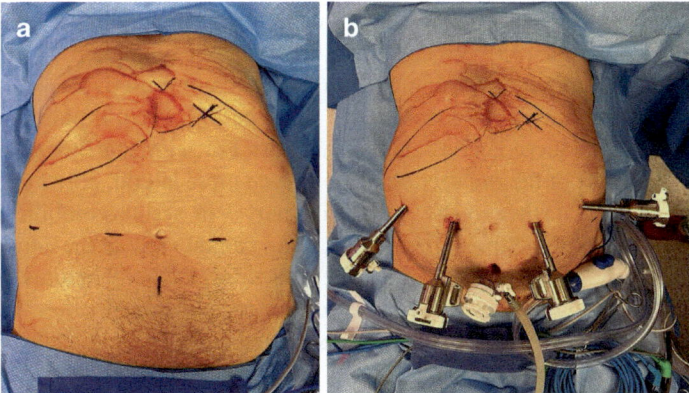

Fig. 12.3 Trocars placement in a robotic atypical liver resection between Sg2 and 3. (**a**) Localization of the lesion (and therefore of the transection axis) is slightly lateralized to the left compared to a classic left lateral sectionectomy, where this plane lies exactly on the midline. The setting used involves the use of port 3 for the camera, which will be placed on a left paramedian position. All trocars are conceptually placed on the same horizontal axis. A subumbilical incision is used for the open access and, later, as assistant trocar. (**b**) After the 12 mm trocar placement and pneumoperitoneum creation, liver exact position is checked before confirming trocars exact placement. In this case, all trocars are placed 2 cm higher than the planned point, whereas port 4 is even higher, following the oblique anterior liver margin

lateral operative arms. The last robotic trocar is finally placed on the left side, approximately on the midclavicular line or more laterally in case of midline endoscopic port insertion. Alternatively, in few cases, it may be moved on the far right to allow for more space for the operative arms on the left [35]. One or two assistant ports can be placed 4 cm inferiorly and triangulated between port 2 and 3 and between port 1 and 2. Assistant trocars can be used for suction or irrigation by the tableside assistant and for ultrasonic dissectors in case of a hybrid approach. This setting has been also described in case of major hepatectomies with the need of biliary reconstructions [39].

Right-Sided Segments

A six trocars configuration is similarly used in resection of the right segments. Optical robotic port always corresponds to the arm 2 of the platform and it is normally placed on a right paramedian position [35]. When pneumoperitoneum is created by an open technique, a median 12 mm trocar may be used, above or under the umbilicus according to the type of resection planned, which will serve later as an assistant port. For segments 5 or 6, in which part of the transection place is even more lateral, port 2 can be shifted further to the right, with port 3 in a supra-umbilical position. This setting allows a direct and frontal view of the entire target. As in all minimally invasive resections, the body habitus of each patient needs to be assessed since adjustments may be needed in order to avoid arm collision and achieve optimal exposure. Other ports are placed following the same axis, as described earlier, whose angle can be tilted up to 15–20 degrees from the transverse umbilical line (Fig. 12.4a, b) [40]. This inclination can be helpful to reach the postero-lateral area of the liver, as during right hepatic vein dissection next to its confluence. Alternatively, ports 1, 2, and 3 can be placed in a totally horizontal axis with or without the last port shifted upwards [39]. A 12 mm access should be used in port 3 or 4 for stapling, especially in right hepatectomies. Assistant trocars are generally placed as described in the previous paragraph.

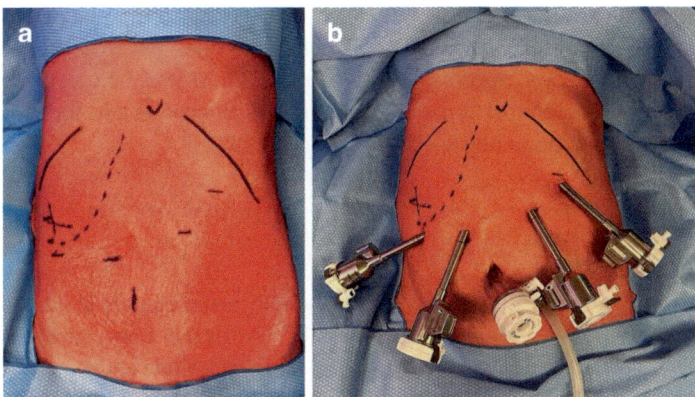

Fig. 12.4 Trocars placement in a robotic liver Sg 6 resection with lymphadenectomy for an intrahepatic cholangiocarcinoma. (**a**) In this patient, given the habitus (20 BMI) and tumor location (Sg 6 with an elevated rib cage and a subcostal right liver), a 12 mm port is placed under the umbilicus for pneumoperitoneum which will be further used by an assistant. The "x" indicates the probable position of the liver and the tumor. Ports will be therefore placed on a tilted axis. (**b**) After insufflation, tumor site is confirmed and four 8 mm robotic ports are placed. The choice of trocar placement is also dictated by the hepatic lymphadenectomy, for which port 1 is placed higher than the axis drawn and port 4 lower

Posterior Segments

The large variability seen in trocar placement for laparoscopic approach could be theoretically reproduced with the robotic platform. However, robotic hepatectomies through a partial transthoracic access (intercostal trocars) are scarcely reported [14] while the semi-prone decubitus has not been reported in literature to the best of our knowledge. In the supine position trocar configuration is similar to that seen for right-sided resections, with patient in a left tilt and port 2 placed laterally on the right anterior axillary line or on the pararectal space after [41]. When a semi-lateral position is chosen, the endoscopic port is placed on a pararectal line or a few cm to the right. Port 1 is placed laterally on the right on the same horizontal axis while ports 3 and 4 follow the right costal border up to the epigastric region, keeping the 20 cm distance from the target as in all robotic procedures [37, 42]. One 12 mm assistant trocar is placed between port 1 and 2. Port placement configuration used in left-lateral decubitus does not differ from the laparoscopic approach, with a first 12 mm assistant port for creating pneumoperitoneum on the right axillary line and three or four robotic ports below the costal borders [36].

Conclusions

This paragraph aims to review the main principles of patient's positioning and type of access in all the different approaches of liver surgery. Standardization of a specific technique is difficult to achieve, being some variations are necessary according to patient's habitus, type of resection, and surgical complexity. However, we describe in detail the most important settings found, with specific applications in relation to tumor location and planned hepatectomy as well as some tips currently used during the different phases of the operation.

References

1. Soonawalla ZF, Stratopoulos C, Stoneham M, Wilkinson D, Britton BJ, Friend PJ. Role of the reverse-Trendelenberg patient position in maintaining low-CVP anaesthesia during liver resections. Langenbeck's Arch Surg. 2008;393(2):195–8. https://doi.org/10.1007/s00423-007-0222-1.
2. Pandit N, Awale L, Adhikary S, et al. Modified Makuuchi incision for major upper abdominal surgeries. Pol Przegl Chir. 2019;91(6):15–9. https://doi.org/10.5604/01.3001.0013.5382.
3. Nobili C, Marzano E, Oussoultzoglou E, et al. Multivariate analysis of risk factors for pulmonary complications after hepatic resection. Ann Surg. 2012;255(3):540–50. https://doi.org/10.1097/SLA.0b013e3182485857.
4. Takei D, Kuroda S, Matsubara K, et al. Usefulness and safety of midline incision for right-sided hepatectomy: cohort study. Ann Med Surg. 2012;2021(67):102498. https://doi.org/10.1016/j.amsu.2021.102498.
5. Abu Hilal M, Aldrighetti L, Dagher I, et al. The Southampton consensus guidelines for laparoscopic liver surgery: from indication to implementation. Ann Surg. 2018;268(1):11–8. https://doi.org/10.1097/SLA.0000000000002524.

6. Giuliani A, Aldrighetti L, Di Benedetto F, et al. Total abdominal approach for postero-superior segments (7, 8) in laparoscopic liver surgery: a multicentric experience. Updat Surg. 2015;67(2):169–75. https://doi.org/10.1007/s13304-015-0305-4.
7. Fuks D, Gayet B. Laparoscopic surgery of postero-lateral segments: a comparison between transthoracic and abdominal approach. Updat Surg. 2015;67(2):141–5. https://doi.org/10.1007/s13304-015-0320-5.
8. Kose E, Kahramangil B, Aydin H, et al. Minimally invasive resection of posterosuperior liver tumors in the supine position using intra-abdominal trocars. Surg Endosc. 2020;34(2):536–43. https://doi.org/10.1007/s00464-019-06789-9.
9. Han HS, Cho JY, Yoon YS. Techniques for performing laparoscopic liver resection in various hepatic locations. J Hepato-Biliary-Pancreat Surg. 2009;16(4):427–32. https://doi.org/10.1007/s00534-009-0118-2.
10. Goh BKP, Chan CY, Lee SY, et al. Laparoscopic liver resection for tumors in the left lateral liver section. JSLS. 2016;20(1):e2015.00112. https://doi.org/10.4293/JSLS.2015.00112.
11. Xiao M, Wang D, Lin GL, Lin X, Tao LY, Li QY. Safely modified laparoscopic liver resection for segment VI and/or VII hepatic lesions using the left lateral decubitus position. Int J Gen Med. 2022;15:6691–9. https://doi.org/10.2147/IJGM.S376919.
12. Ikeda T, Toshima T, Harimoto N, et al. Laparoscopic liver resection in the semiprone position for tumors in the anterosuperior and posterior segments, using a novel dual-handling technique and bipolar irrigation system. Surg Endosc. 2014;28(8):2484–92. https://doi.org/10.1007/s00464-014-3469-y.
13. Anselmo A, Sensi B, Bacchiocchi G, Siragusa L, Tisone G. All the routes for laparoscopic liver segment VIII resection: a comprehensive review of surgical techniques. Front Oncol. 2022;12:864867. https://doi.org/10.3389/fonc.2022.864867.
14. Vega EA, Salehi O, Panettieri E, et al. Subsegmental approaches to S7: anatomic laparoscopic transdiaphragmatic and nonanatomic robotic transthoracic. Surg Endosc. 2023;37(10):8154–5. https://doi.org/10.1007/s00464-023-10310-8.
15. Ikeda T, Yonemura Y, Ueda N, et al. Pure laparoscopic right hepatectomy in the semi-prone position using the intrahepatic Glissonian approach and a modified hanging maneuver to minimize intraoperative bleeding. Surg Today. 2011;41(12):1592–8. https://doi.org/10.1007/s00595-010-4479-6.
16. Chen JC, Zhang RX, Chen MS, et al. Left jackknife position: a novel position for laparoscopic hepatectomy. Chin J Cancer. 2017;36(1):31. https://doi.org/10.1186/s40880-017-0190-y.
17. Patient and port positioning in laparoscopic liver resections. Hepatoma Res. 2021;7(0):null-null. https://doi.org/10.20517/2394-5079.2020.144.

18. Chuang SH, Chuang SC. Single-incision laparoscopic surgery to treat hepatopancreatobiliary cancer: a technical review. World J Gastroenterol. 2022;28(27):3359–69. https://doi.org/10.3748/wjg.v28.i27.3359.
19. Pessaux P, Diana M, Soler L, Piardi T, Mutter D, Marescaux J. Towards cybernetic surgery: robotic and augmented reality-assisted liver segmentectomy. Langenbeck's Arch Surg. 2015;400(3):381–5. https://doi.org/10.1007/s00423-014-1256-9.
20. Giannone F, Felli E, Cherkaoui Z, Mascagni P, Pessaux P. Augmented reality and image-guided robotic liver surgery. Cancer. 2021;13(24):6268. https://doi.org/10.3390/cancers13246268.
21. Goumard C, Farges O, Laurent A, et al. An update on laparoscopic liver resection: the French Hepato-Bilio-pancreatic surgery association statement. J Visc Surg. 2015;152(2):107–12. https://doi.org/10.1016/j.jviscsurg.2015.02.003.
22. Sugawara T, Hashimoto M, Shindoh J. Laparoscopic left lateral sectionectomy: a three-port method. J Minimal Access Surg. 2020;16(3):220. https://doi.org/10.4103/jmas.JMAS_233_17.
23. Wang JC, Pan Y, Chen J, et al. Single versus multiple port laparoscopic left lateral sectionectomy for hepatocellular carcinoma: a retrospective comparative study. Int J Surg Lond Engl. 2020;77:15–21. https://doi.org/10.1016/j.ijsu.2020.03.003.
24. Tsai TJ, Chouillard EK, Gumbs AA. Laparoscopic right hepatectomy with intrahepatic transection of the right bile duct. Ann Surg Oncol. 2012;19(2):467–8. https://doi.org/10.1245/s10434-011-1927-5.
25. Soubrane O, Kwon CHD. Tips for pure laparoscopic right hepatectomy in the live donor. J Hepato-Biliary-Pancreat Sci. 2017;24(2):E1–5. https://doi.org/10.1002/jhbp.425.
26. Hayashi A, Misumi K, Shibahara J, et al. Distinct clinicopathologic and genetic features of 2 histologic subtypes of intrahepatic cholangiocarcinoma. Am J Surg Pathol. 2016;40(8):1021–30. https://doi.org/10.1097/PAS.0000000000000670.
27. Ichida H, Ishizawa T, Tanaka M, et al. Use of intercostal trocars for laparoscopic resection of subphrenic hepatic tumors. Surg Endosc. 2017;31(3):1280–6. https://doi.org/10.1007/s00464-016-5107-3.
28. Schwarz L, Aloia TA, Eng C, Chang GJ, Vauthey JN, Conrad C. Transthoracic port placement increases safety of total laparoscopic posterior sectionectomy. Ann Surg Oncol. 2016;23(7):2167. https://doi.org/10.1245/s10434-016-5126-2.
29. Takagi K, Kuise T, Umeda Y, et al. Laparoscopic liver resection of segment seven: a case report and review of surgical techniques. Int J Surg Case Rep. 2020;73:168–71. https://doi.org/10.1016/j.ijscr.2020.06.107.
30. Hayashi H, Yamashita YI, Okabe H, et al. Varied application of intercostal trans-diaphragmatic ports for laparoscopic hepatectomy. PLoS One. 2020;15(6):e0234919. https://doi.org/10.1371/journal.pone.0234919.

31. Hallet J, Soler L, Diana M, et al. Trans-thoracic minimally invasive liver resection guided by augmented reality. J Am Coll Surg. 2015;220(5):e55–60. https://doi.org/10.1016/j.jamcollsurg.2014.12.053.
32. Yamashita S, Loyer E, Kang HC, et al. Total transthoracic approach facilitates laparoscopic hepatic resection in patients with significant prior abdominal surgery. Ann Surg Oncol. 2017;24(5):1376–7. https://doi.org/10.1245/s10434-016-5685-2.
33. Aikawa M, Miyazawa M, Okamoto K, et al. Thoracoscopic hepatectomy for malignant liver tumor. Surg Endosc. 2014;28(1):314. https://doi.org/10.1007/s00464-013-3128-8.
34. Liu R, Abu Hilal M, Wakabayashi G, et al. International experts consensus guidelines on robotic liver resection in 2023. World J Gastroenterol. 2023;29(32):4815–30. https://doi.org/10.3748/wjg.v29.i32.4815.
35. Giulianotti PC, Bianco FM, Daskalaki D, Gonzalez-Ciccarelli LF, Kim J, Benedetti E. Robotic liver surgery: technical aspects and review of the literature. Hepatobiliary Surg Nutr. 2016;5(4):31121–321. https://doi.org/10.21037/hbsn.2015.10.05.
36. Nota CL, Rinkes IHB, Hagendoorn J. Setting up a robotic hepatectomy program: a Western-European experience and perspective. Hepatobiliary Surg Nutr. 2017;6(4):239–45. https://doi.org/10.21037/hbsn.2016.12.05.
37. Wu CY, Chen PD, Lee CY, Liang JT, Wu YM. Robotic-assisted right posterior segmentectomies for liver lesions: single-center experience of an evolutional method in left semi-lateral position. J Robot Surg. 2019;13(2):231–7. https://doi.org/10.1007/s11701-018-0842-1.
38. Durán M, Briceño J, Padial A, et al. Short-term outcomes of robotic liver resection: an initial single-institution experience. World J Hepatol. 2022;14(1):224–33. https://doi.org/10.4254/wjh.v14.i1.224.
39. D'Hondt M, Wicherts DA. Pure robotic major hepatectomy with biliary reconstruction for hepatobiliary malignancies: first European results. Surg Endosc. 2023;37(6):4396–402. https://doi.org/10.1007/s00464-023-09863-5.
40. Giulianotti PC, Sbrana F, Coratti A, et al. Totally robotic right hepatectomy: surgical technique and outcomes. Arch Surg 1960. 2011;146(7):844–50. https://doi.org/10.1001/archsurg.2011.145.
41. Denglos P, Truant S, El Amrani M, Millet G. Robotic liver resection in the posterosuperior segments as a way to extent the mini-invasive arsenal: a comparison with transthoracic laparoscopic approach. Surg Endosc. 2023;37(6):4478–85. https://doi.org/10.1007/s00464-023-09919-6.
42. Kato Y, Sugioka A, Uyama I. Robotic liver resection for hepatocellular carcinoma: a focus on anatomic resection. Hepatoma Res. 2021;7:10. https://doi.org/10.20517/2394-5079.2020.129.

Instrumentation and Approaches for Parenchymal Transection

13

Ana Luiza Mandelli Gleisner and Sumaya Abdul Ghaffar

Parenchymal transection is a pivotal phase in liver resection procedures. One of the main goals during this part is to minimize blood loss while also reducing the risk of injury to the remnant liver. Failure to achieve this can lead to higher postoperative complications, including liver failure and death. In addition, in patients undergoing liver resection for malignancies, increased blood loss and need for blood transfusion may impact long-term oncologic outcomes. Thus, a comprehensive and multidisciplinary planning is essential when a major liver resection is being contemplated. The preoperative evaluation includes an assessment of the volume of the remnant liver to gauge its functional capacity after surgery. If necessary, portal vein embolization is performed beforehand. A meticulous examination of the liver vasculature is also imperative for the surgical team's preparedness. The anesthesia team should be well-versed in blood loss minimizing techniques, including maintaining a low central venous pressure, controlled hypoventilation, and acute normovolemic hemodilution. Autologous blood transfusion is also employed whenever possible, and its preparation is also initiated in the preoperative setting.

A. L. M. Gleisner (✉) · S. A. Ghaffar
Department of Surgery, University of Colorado, Aurora, CO, USA
e-mail: ana.gleisner@cuanschutz.edu

© The Author(s), under exclusive license to Springer Nature Switzerland AG 2025
A. Alseidi et al. (eds.), *The SAGES Manual of Contemporary Indications and Management of Hepatic and Biliary Diseases*, https://doi.org/10.1007/978-3-032-04823-3_13

Preparation does not conclude once the incision is made. Intraoperative ultrasound has emerged as the primary tool for identifying not only the precise location of the target lesions but also major vascular and biliary structures. New technologies for intraoperative navigation are also on the horizon, such as the use of indocyanine green for biliary duct identification, 3D navigation techniques in laparoscopic and robotic surgery, among others.

As transection techniques have advanced over the years and minimally invasive surgery has gained prominence, other methods for minimizing blood loss have evolved, particularly through the introduction of new devices in electrosurgery. The utilization of vascular occlusion, primarily through the Pringle maneuver, has also been subject to scrutiny over the years, and intermittent occlusion is still frequently employed. The decision regarding whether to use the Pringle maneuver can sometimes be challenging. However, the selection of a device for transection has become increasingly complex with the array of options now available. The use of devices has been extensively debated, with their efficacy, costs, and associated complications undergoing thorough evaluation and comparison. A similar discourse has taken place regarding hemostatic agents used to seal the transection plane at the conclusion of the procedure, with a multitude of choices available, each with its own set of advantages and disadvantages.

In this chapter, all these topics will be comprehensively explored, providing a detailed presentation and evaluation of the devices available for parenchymal transection and the hemostatic agents used for the care of the transected surface of the remnant liver.

Preoperative Preparation Pearls

Preoperative Imaging

Review of preoperative imaging, typically high-quality computer tomography (CT) imaging, is a crucial step in the preoperative evaluation for liver resections. Imaging technology has seen remarkable advancements over the years, resulting in high-speed and high-resolution imaging that is acquired quickly and with reduced motion artifacts. Imaging review aims at determination of the extent of the disease and the volume of the future liver remnant. Disease resectability involves achieving negative margins when indicated and leaving sufficient liver remnant to ensure adequate hepatic function with preserved vascular inflow, outflow, and biliary drainage. Thus, a comprehensive understanding of the general liver anatomy and the relationship of the disease to vital structures is paramount. Magnetic resonance imaging (MRI) can be particularly useful for a thorough evaluation of the biliary ducts. Regardless of the method, it is imperative that images are obtained through thin slices, and contrast-enhanced arterial, venous, and portal phases.

When the volumetric evaluation of the liver suggests that resection would compromise function, two-stage procedures can be considered, such as portal vein embolization (PVE) and associating liver partition and portal vein ligation for staged hepatectomy (ALPPS). These procedures focus on inducing hypertrophy of the future remnant liver beforehand to ensure adequate function after surgery.

Body composition can also be assessed through CT-scan imaging. Recent studies have established a potential relationship between sarcopenia and short-term outcomes after liver surgery for hepatocellular carcinoma, with higher rates of postoperative mortality and morbidity. Visceral adiposity is also of particular interest, as it can pose challenges for laparoscopic techniques, but it has also been associated with increased morbidity in the postoperative period.

Furthermore, CT scans play an indispensable role in the assessment of anatomical variants within the vascular system of the liver. These variants can significantly impact surgical planning and execution. Moreover, with advancements in technology, CT scans allow for the creation of three-dimensional reconstructions, providing surgeons with a comprehensive view of the liver's vascular architecture.

Anatomical Variants

The blood perfusion of the liver is exceptionally intricate, characterized by a dual system. The portal vein supplies 70% of the hepatic blood flow, while the hepatic artery accounts for the remaining 30%. Changes in hepatic inflow can be identified in a CT scan; even if the portal vein remains intact, compromised arterial flow typically does not result in parenchymal infarction. In cases where it is present, a wedge-shaped area of low attenuation can be observed in the periphery of the liver. Vascular inflow complications are more commonly encountered in liver transplantation, with thrombosis and stenosis being of particular concern as they can lead to irreversible loss of the liver graft. In other liver resections, inflow injury can compromise liver regeneration, potentially leading to hepatic failure postoperatively.

The portal vein is formed by the confluence of the superior mesenteric vein and the splenic veins. Upon reaching the porta hepatis, it bifurcates into right and left hepatic branches, alongside branches of the hepatic artery, lymphatic vessels, and the hepatic nerve plexus. The right branch provides portal flow to segments V, VI, VII, and VIII, while the left branch serves segments I, II, III, and IV via the left obliterated umbilical vein, passing through the ligamentum teres. Anatomic variations within the portal system may increase the risk of postoperative complications. Such variations can occur in up to 30% of the population. Common variations to be aware of during a formal hepatectomy in which inflow control will be obtained in the hilum are the portal vein "trifurcation", the main portal vein divides into three branches (left portal vein, right anterior portal vein, right posterior portal vein) and an early take off of the right posterior portal vein.

The proper hepatic artery is a branch of the common hepatic artery, originating separately from the celiac trunk. Upon reaching the porta hepatis, it further divides into the right and left hepatic arteries. A CT scan can identify arteries up to their 3rd or 4th branching, contingent on their caliber, and also pinpoint their anatomical variations. Michel's classification of hepatic artery anatomy (Table 13.1) is widely recognized, with the classical

Table 13.1 Michel's classification of the hepatic arterial anatomy

Type	Frequency	Description
I	55.0%	RHA, MHA, and LHA arise from the common hepatic artery
II	10.0%	RHA, MHA, and LHA arise from common hepatic artery; replaced LHA arises from left gastric artery
III	1.0%	Replaced RHA and LHA
V	8.0%	RHA, MHA, and LHA arise from common hepatic artery; accessory LHA arises from left gastric artery
VI	7.0%	RHA, MHA, and LHA arise from common hepatic artery; accessory RHA
VII	1.0%	Accessory RHA and LHA
VIII	4.0%	Replaced RHA and accessory LHA or replaced LHA and accessory RHA
IX	4.5%	Entire hepatic trunk arises from superior mesenteric artery
X	0.5%	Entire hepatic trunk arises from left gastric artery

RHA right hepatic artery
MHA middle hepatic artery
LHA left hepatic artery

branching pattern (type I) occurring in 76% of the population. Knowledge of these variations streamlines any liver resection and heightens the likelihood of technical success. Particular attention is given to collaterals, as they can serve as a significant source of bleeding after ligation of the main arteries.

Venous drainage of the liver occurs through three primary hepatic veins: the right hepatic vein (RHV), left hepatic vein (LHV), and middle hepatic vein (MHV). All of these converge and drain into the suprahepatic portion of the superior vena cava, with the MHV and the LHV often forming a short common trunk. The RHV typically drains segments V-VII (40% of the liver), the MHV drains segments IV, V, VIII (30% of liver), and the LHV drains segments II and III (20%). Compromising venous drainage can have catastrophic consequences, resulting in parenchymal necrosis and compromising liver function in the remnant as well as its capacity for regeneration, since these regions can only achieve approximately 40% of their normal function. The MHV is often the most critical vein in the liver, running along the mid-plane in the Rex-Cantlie line and draining both sides of the liver. A CT scan can identify early branching, bifurcation, and common variants, which may alter the transection plane of hemihepatectomies. Variants are observed in up to 30% of patients undergoing living donor resection. The most common variants are:

- Accessory RHV.
- Two accessory hepatic veins.
- Accessory vein draining the caudate lobe (MRHV).
- Accessory inferior RHV (IRHV).
- Early branching of the vein that drains the segment VIII into the MHV.

Recent studies have delved into the tributaries of the major veins. The middle right hepatic vein (MRHV) and the inferior right hepatic vein (IRHV), when present, may allow parenchymal preservation when the main hepatic veins need to be resected. Two other tributaries of notable interest in surgical procedures are the left superficial vein (LSV), which drains into the LHV, and the right superficial vein (RSV), which frequently runs immediately inferior to the caval ligament. The LSV may communicate with the left inferior phrenic vein and directly drain into the inferior vena cava. Its visibility on CT scans is often limited, as it runs immediately below the left diaphragm, and the beating heart can interfere with visualization. The RSV should be handled with care, properly ligated, or sealed during the mobilization of the right hemiliver. Finally, the MHV tributaries that drain segments 8 (V8) and 5 (V5). During a hemihepatectomy in which the transection plane is just lateral to MHV, careful identification and ligation of V5 and V8 branches is crucial. This is especially true when V8 is closer to the inferior vena cava, as injury to this branch can result in severe bleeding. V8 is closer to the inferior vena cava compared to other MHV branches, and ultrasound identification has proven highly effective in preventing such injuries.

3D Reconstruction

The emergence of software-powered 3D reconstruction (3DR) of the liver using CT scans offers comprehensive information not only about the complex internal anatomy of the liver but also its external relationship with other organs. 3D reconstruction can also be achieved by combining MRI venous phase and CT venous phase through fusion imaging. Images should be multiphase, with plain, arterial, portal venous, and delayed phases, and ideally thinly sliced (preferably <1 mm). Intrahepatic vascular branches can be identified up to the 3rd or 4th tributary levels. The morphology of the biliary system may be presented in detail. Classification systems are available for each system (arterial, hepatic venous, portal venous) for 3DR, along with consensus recommendations for imaging acquisition and reconstruction. The evaluation of lesions with 3DR can lead to increased surgical eligibility of borderline lesions, enhance the safety of these resections, avoid excessive parenchyma removal, and ultimately assess the adequacy of oncologic margins.

3D models can offer information for liver volume calculation and variations of the intrahepatic blood vessels. They can also enable virtual simulation of the procedure and aid in surgical navigation. In the management of hepatocellular carcinoma, 3D visualization has improved perioperative results, reducing intraoperative blood loss, postoperative complications, operative time, hospital stay, and recurrence rate of liver cancer in short-term follow-up. For laparoscopic surgery, 3DR altered surgical planning preoperatively in up to a third of cases and may help spare patients from unnecessary surgery.

The lack of reliable markers on the liver surface and morphological changes during surgery due to traction and respiratory movement can make the transition from 2D images to an abstract 3D model mentally challenging. High-precision 3D printing has emerged in this context, enabling real-time navigation to assist clinical decision-making in the operating room. Additionally, 3DR has facilitated the development of augmented reality software for real-time surgical navigation, superimposing virtual reconstructions onto the surgical field and adapting to the patient's and surgeon's movements during the procedure. Such navigation tools are especially useful during the transection of the parenchyma during minimally invasive liver resections.

Key Steps

Principles for Parenchymal Transection

Parenchymal transection remains the most crucial aspect of the liver resection procedure. It can be approached either through segmentation or non-anatomically. Transection is the phase where massive blood loss can occur, and it's also when operative times may be prolonged. The primary principles for parenchymal transection involve executing it with minimal blood loss and ensuring the proper sealing of vessels and biliary structures in the remnant liver. Massive bleeding is associated with increased postoperative morbidity and mortality, as well as poorer long-term outcomes. Additionally, timely completion of the transection is crucial, as prolonged operative times are also linked to increased complications and higher healthcare costs.

The key steps in parenchymal transection are consistent for both open and laparoscopic surgery:

1. Defining the transection plane with ultrasound-guided intraoperative assessment of the lesion(s) and intraparenchymal structures to define the transection plane for a resection with appropriate oncologic margins; in anatomic resections, demarcation of the transection plane can be obtained with selective inflow occlusion or injection of different dyes.
2. Intermittent inflow occlusion to decrease blood loss.
3. Execution of parenchymal transection with ligation of vessels and biliary structures.
4. Thorough revision for hemostasis and biliostasis.

Defining the Transection Plane

Intraoperative Ultrasound

Despite advances in preoperative imaging and 3D reconstruction, intraoperative ultrasound remains the gold standard for liver examination and surgical guidance. Prior to the availability of ultrasound, assessing liver tumors and anatomical structures during surgery was restricted to palpation and visual inspection. Offering critical real-time information, ultrasound allows for the identification of vascular anatomy, precise lesion localization, and assessment of their extent, aiding surgeons in accurate dissection. Current technology can detect lesions larger than 2 mm, with reported sensitivity rates ranging from 90% to 95%. Additionally, it exhibits superior discrimination of lesions in cirrhotic livers, and its use correlates with improved surgical outcomes and enhanced procedural safety. In the context of laparoscopic surgery, palpation is not feasible, making intraoperative ultrasound evaluation assessment indispensable. It ensures precise knowledge of the tumor's location, along with its associated vascular and biliary structures, and verifies the absence of additional lesions.

Methods for vascular identification have significantly reduced massive bleeding rates over time, and intraoperative ultrasound assessment has been a key contributor.

After transection, color-Doppler ultrasound can be employed to assess the remnant liver's vascular anatomy, blood flow volume, and velocity, particularly after vessel reconstruction. Identifying any alterations early on can lead to timely intervention, ultimately improving surgical outcomes.

Ultrasound can be further enhanced with microbubble contrast and elastography. With contrast enhancement, intraoperative ultrasound becomes more sensitive in detecting new lesions and influencing surgical decision-making. The significance of contrast-enhanced ultrasound (CE-U) has grown, particularly in cases of disappearing liver metastasis, owing to modern and effective chemotherapy regimens. CE-U surpasses the sensitivity of intraoperative ultrasound alone in identifying DLM, and when combined with previously acquired gadoxetic acid-enhanced MRI (EOB-MRI), the detection rate of such metastasis exceeds 90%, with up to 77% of these lesions exhibiting viable disease. Intraoperative ultrasound can be integrated with 3DR for an enhanced real-time navigation system. Techniques for intraoperative ultrasound evaluation in liver resection will be addressed in a separate chapter.

Parenchymal Demarcation

Traditionally, parenchymal vascular demarcation has been observed during anatomic liver resections as the inflow is selectively ligated. This is easily accomplished for right or left hemi liver resections, when the extrahepatic dissection and ligation of the inflow is routine. However, the selective ligation of the pedicles to the different sectors of the liver (right anterior, right posterior, and left lateral) or even to different segments of the liver, such as segments 2, 3, and 7, is often possible, resulting in a discoloration that will aid the definition of the transection plane so that lesions can be resected with appropriate oncologic margin while leaving minimal devascularized parenchyma behind.

Demarcation of the anatomic hemilivers, sectors, and segments can be enhanced with the use of dyes such as methylene blue and Indocyanine green (ICG). Staining can be positive or negative. Positive staining occurs when the dye is injected into the portal branch of interest under ultrasound guidance. The corresponding segments slated for removal have an obvious discoloration with methylene blue and will enhance through fluorescence with ICG. Using this approach, an anatomic resection is possible even for subsegmental lesions. In the method described by Makuuchi, the portal vein supplying the subsegment where the tumor is located is identified and punctured under ultrasound guidance, followed by injection of the dye. In another method described by Castaing, a balloon catheter is positioned in the feeding vessel and dye is injected as the vessel is occluded.

Although highly effective in delineating the appropriate transection plane, injection of dye into the different branches of the portal system is technically challenging, especially during minimally invasive surgery. As a result, negative staining has emerged as an alternative approach, when dye is injected intravenously after the corresponding portal pedicle is either closed or divided. The area of interest is then identified as it does not stain. Demarcation remains evident even in the deeper parenchyma, aiding in the transection process. Neither method is considered superior, but some hypothesize that negative staining offers a more robust approach for liver segmentation than positive staining, aside from being technically easier to perform.

The utilization of ICG in hepatic resection has demonstrated safety. It promotes a higher R0 resection rate and assists in minimizing blood loss. Importantly, it does not lead to prolonged operative times or extended hospital stays, and it is not associated with increased postoperative complications.

Inflow Occlusion

There are three major techniques for vascular occlusion: selective, complete inflow occlusion (Pringle maneuver), and total hepatic isolation. Selective vascular occlusion is commonly employed in anatomic resections such as left or right hepatectomy as described above. For the Pringle maneuver, the hilar structures are occluded with a vascular clamp, an umbilical tape, or a vessel loop. This maneuver is typically performed intermittently, with a short duration usually around 15 min, followed by a rest period of at least 5 min between occlusions, for a total of 60 min. While the Pringle maneuver has been previously associated with higher mortality rates due to liver ischemia and reperfusion injury, when executed correctly, it effectively reduces blood loss and the need for transfusion. In addition, it allows better visualization of vascular and biliary structures during parenchymal transection. Aside from ischemia-and-reperfusion injury, more rare complications include portal vein emboli and spontaneous rupture of the spleen. Concerns about the Pringle maneuver potentially decreasing the time for tumor recurrence have been refuted in recent studies.

In the total hepatic isolation (THI), inflow occlusion is combined to occlusion of the inferior vena cava and either the superior vena cava or the hepatic veins, therefore eliminating the back-bleeding from branches of the hepatic veins. However, THI presents several challenges. Reduction in cardiac output can lead to rapid hemodynamic instability and injuries to the retrohepatic vascular structures can result in rapid exsanguination. Consequently, this technique is mostly reserved for traumatic injuries or situations where controlled access to vena cava is an intended part of the procedure, such as the resection of tumors with invasion into the retrohepatic vena cava. Veno-veno bypass should be considered in these cases to avoid hemodynamic instability. In most cases, reduced bleeding from the hepatic veins can be achieved with a low central venous pressure and low positive airway pressure using low tidal volumes.

Parenchymal Transection

Techniques for Parenchymal Transection

Several techniques have been described for the transection of the liver parenchyma, with or without the use of numerous devices. Despite various randomized controlled trials (RCT), no particular technique has demonstrated clear superiority in terms of blood loss, surgical outcomes, or oncologic outcomes.

Regardless of the technique, the surgical field should be developed in a peripheral to central fashion. The rationale behind this approach lies in the fact that the peripheral area (up to 2 cm deep) of the parenchyma has fewer thick tributaries and lacks major vessels, resulting in a lower risk of vascular injury. As a result, transection begins in this peripheral region, progressing in a cranial-to-caudal fashion until the transection plane takes on a convex shape, revealing the central area. Within the central area of the parenchyma lie the major structures and thickest tributaries, which are carefully identified and subsequently ligated.

The distinct characteristics of the peripheral and central areas of the parenchyma allow for the tailored use of various electrosurgery devices to address specific needs during this stage. The capsule and the first centimeter of superficial parenchyma can be effectively divided using monopolar cautery or ultrasonic vibration devices. This approach is swift and delivers a bloodless field, facilitating the management of the central parenchyma. The management of the central parenchyma can be accomplished using various electrosurgical devices. Glissonean branches and hepatic veins are carefully exposed and subsequently ligated.

Digitoclasy Technique

Digitoclasy, also known as the "finger-fracture technique", is one of the earliest and most basic methods devised for parenchymal transection. In this approach, after inflow occlusion, the liver parenchyma is compressed between the thumb and the finger. This action isolates structures like vessels and bile ducts, which are then ligated and divided.

Sharp Dissection

Sharp dissection, though seldom employed, involves the use of a scalpel to dissect through a pre-determined plane in the liver. This method necessitates complete vascular occlusion of the liver, which can be achieved through either total hepatic isolation or selective hepatic vascular exclusion. While there are relatively few studies directly comparing sharp dissection to other techniques, the largest study to date, which compared it to clamp-crushing, demonstrated its comparable safety profile in terms of blood loss and morbidity.

Clamp-Crushing Technique

The original clamp crushing technique, as initially described, involved the use of surgical instruments such as small Kelly or Pean clamps to grip and subsequently crush the parenchyma. In contemporary practice, a combination of techniques is often utilized. The surgeon gently divides the liver tissue either using their finger or clamps upon entering the capsule. Vessels and ducts are then identified and ligated, a step that can be accomplished with sutures, clips, or various electrosurgical devices.

In experienced hands, the clamp-crushing approach is associated with decreased blood loss, faster transection times, and lower costs, being the most cost-effective strategy for parenchymal transection.

Stapling Technique

Vascular staplers have played a crucial role in minimizing blood loss and reducing the need for inflow occlusion during hepatectomy. Over time, the development of GIA vascular staplers has further enhanced their utility in parenchymal transection. The technique typically involves initial division of the liver capsule with cautery, followed by parenchyma fracturing using a vascular clamp, and ultimately, transection and division with the vascular stapler.

The use of staplers has been shown to be safe, leading to reduced reliance on the Pringle maneuver in some series and generally faster transection speeds. Moreover, surgical and oncologic outcomes with staplers have been comparable to those achieved with clamp-crushing, CUSA, and LigaSure techniques. Notably, a study examining the postoperative inflammatory response revealed that stapler usage, likely due to its swifter transection process, was associated with lower levels of interleukin-6 compared to CUSA.

Device-Assisted Techniques

The devices specifically developed for parenchymal transection can be broadly categorized into ultrasonic, bipolar sealing, and radiofrequency devices. Some newer devices combine multiple technologies for improved results. Although some surgeons may prefer to use one device for parenchymal transection, most surgeons will use a combination of devices.

Ultrasonic Devices

Ultrasonic devices convert electrical energy into mechanical energy, facilitating cutting and coagulation effects. They generate powerful vibrations at the instrument tip, exerting mechanical forces that rupture tissue and form clots. Examples of devices using this technology include the Harmonic Scalpel, Thunderbeat, and CUSA, among others.

Ultrasonic devices offer several advantages, including minimal thermal spread, reduced tissue charring and smoke formation, and no risk of electrical injury, as there is no electrical current passing through the patient. They are versatile, serving functions in dissection, cutting, and coagulation.

Harmonic Scalpel (Harmonic® Open Shears—Ethicon)

The Harmonic Scalpel (HS) is an ultrasonic device renowned for its ability to provide hemostatic dissection with minimal thermal spread to adjacent tissues. It is proficient at dividing vessels up to 4 mm, and a newer version, the Harmonic ACE, may extend this capability to vessels up to 7 mm. One consideration in its use is that surgeons must adapt their technique and be mindful of the tension applied to tissue, as excessive tension on a vascular pedicle can lead to premature tissue separation and bleeding.

The HS has undergone evaluation in several studies for liver resection. When compared to LigaSure, it demonstrated similar surgical and major outcomes. In contrast to clamp-crushing alone, HS exhibited the lowest rates of overall transfusion, overall complications, and major complications. No significant differences were noted in terms of bile leakage and surgical site infection. In a study comparing clamp-crushing with Pringle maneuver to HS without Pringle maneuver, the latter facilitated an earlier recovery of the liver function. A recent meta-analysis of parenchymal transection techniques indicated that combining HS with clamp-crushing resulted in lower blood loss compared to other devices, with only TissueLink and LigaSure outperforming it. No significant disparities in operative time were observed, but transection times were shorter with the HS, trailing only behind staplers and TissueLink.

Thunderbeat (Olympus Medical Systems)

The Thunderbeat (TB) represents a recent advancement that integrates both ultrasonic and bipolar energy. This dual functionality allows for the simultaneous sealing and cutting of vessels, resulting in swifter tissue division. The device is capable of effectively sealing vessels up to 7 mm in diameter, while maintaining minimal thermal dispersion. It can be employed in two primary modes: the "Seal and Cut" mode, or solely the "Seal" mode, functioning as a pure bipolar device.

In a recent study focused on laparoscopic hepatic parenchymal transection, TB was compared with HS, both with and without the CUSA device. The study reported no significant disparities in terms of intraoperative blood loss, operative time, or postoperative outcomes. Consequently, TB was deemed a safe and proficient tool, though it did not emerge as a markedly superior alternative in this particular evaluation.

Cavitron Ultrasound Surgical Aspirator (CUSA; Tyco Healthcare)

The CUSA is an ultrasonic device designed for fragmenting, rapidly irrigating, and aspirating tissue from the dissection field. Its primary application is in liver resection, where it facilitates the controlled disintegration of liver parenchyma, while preserving larger vessels for appropriate management. As mentioned earlier, CUSA has become the favored device among hepatobiliary surgeons, likely due to the precise and controlled dissection it offers in the delicate central parenchyma.

Despite its popularity, CUSA has been subjected to numerous comparative trials, none of which have conclusively established its superiority over other techniques. When compared to clamp-crushing, it exhibited higher blood loss, increased blood transfusion requirements, and longer operative times. In a study comparing CUSA, clamp-crushing, and LigaSure, all three techniques were found to be equally safe for non-cirrhotic liver resection, yielding similar outcomes. In comparison to staplers, one study reported no discernible differences, while another indicated that CUSA was associated with higher blood loss and longer operative times. Additionally, in one study, CUSA proved to be the most expensive technique, though the cost was offset for high-volume centers.

Bipolar Sealing Devices

Advanced bipolar devices integrate bipolar current energy with tissue superposition and compression for sealing purposes. They can effectively manage blood vessels contained within other tissue, such as the omentum or mesentery, or vessels that have been dissected. These devices can seal vessels up to 7 mm in diameter.

LigaSure (Valleylab)
LigaSure (LS) is a bipolar sealing device that applies precise energy and pressure to bind collagen and elastin within vessel walls, resulting in a permanent seal for vessels up to 7 mm. Concerns regarding an increased risk of bile leakage have been raised as a potential drawback of LS; however, recent studies have not substantiated this claim. One of the primary disadvantages of LS is its relatively high cost, as each device is disposable.

Studies comparing LS to clump-crushing and CUSA have consistently demonstrated safety and effectiveness. Findings regarding liver resection time have been somewhat contradictory, with some studies indicating a clear improvement in transection time, while others have shown no significant difference.

Radiofrequency Devices

Radiofrequency devices (RFD) produce a high-frequency alternating current transmitted through an electrode placed into the tissue under ultrasound guidance. Activation of the device leads to focal tissue destruction. In liver resection, RFD is positioned to target segmental vessels prior to resection, creating coagulated areas that are then resected in a relatively bloodless field.

While few studies on RFD in liver resection are available, they have not shown significant differences in blood loss or blood transfusion. However, some studies have reported an increased incidence of complications like abscesses and biliary fistulas associated with RFD use. The theory is that the necrotic remnant on the resection surface may foster bacterial growth, leading to abscess formation, and subsequent detachment of the necrotic tissue may result in biliary leakage. Currently, RFD technology is predominantly used in conjunction with other technologies (such as ultrasonic or bipolar).

RFD and microwave ablation devices that are typically used for ablation of liver lesions have also been used to pre-coagulate the liver parenchyma at its transection site, generating a zone of coagulative necrosis to minimize bleeding.

TissueLink™ (DS 3.0®; Tissue Link Medical)

TissueLink (TL) is a radiofrequency device that generates heat through a metal probe in conjunction with saline irrigation. It effectively coagulates tissue without causing charring and can seal small vascular and biliary structures by inducing collagen shrinkage. Additionally, it can be utilized as a dissector. It is important to note that TL comes with certain drawbacks, such as the potential risk of biliary injury due to the high temperature of the saline, which can flow into the extrahepatic biliary tree. There is also a risk of scalding the liver parenchyma for the same reason. Therefore, it is advised not to use TL at the porta hepatis, and when preservation of structures is essential, cool wet gauze should be placed over them.

Although there have been a limited number of studies evaluating TL's performance in liver surgery, it has generally been deemed safe with outcomes comparable to other techniques. In an RCT comparing TL to the clamp-crushing technique, TL did not demonstrate significant advantages in reducing blood loss. However, prior studies involving a similar device to DS 3.0 from TissueLink, known as the Floating Ball®, showed significantly reduced blood loss compared to clamp-crushing. A meta-analysis identified higher blood loss with CUSA when compared to TL but noted a shorter transection time compared to RFD.

In terms of cost, TL utilizes the electrosurgical generator for conventional electrocautery, while each handpiece is disposable, potentially leading to higher costs.

Aquamantys™ (Medtronic)

Aquamantys, also classified as a bipolar sealing device, harnesses the power of radiofrequency energy and saline to achieve hemostatic sealing of soft tissues. Notably, it offers the advantage of producing no associated smoke or char. While Aquamantys is not employed for transection in isolation, it is primarily used in conjunction with other devices for achieving hemostasis during the transection process. Its rounded tip allows for coagulation without puncturing the parenchyma.

Initially prominent in orthopedic surgery, Aquamantys has found application in abdominal surgery. However, there is limited trial data available to comprehensively assess its efficacy in liver resection. One study, comparing CUSA with Aquamantys to CUSA with standard bipolar cautery, demonstrated that using Aquamantys instead of the standard bipolar method was associated with reduced blood loss during transection, quicker transection speeds, and no increased morbidity. Another study compared Aquamantys with VIO (Integra LifeSciences Co), a soft coagulation device, both in conjunction with CUSA as the primary parenchymal transection device. It found no disparities in blood loss but noted a higher parenchymal transection speed with Aquamantys, along with similar postoperative complications.

Other Devices

Hydro-Jet® (ERBE)

High-pressure water-jet dissection, originally developed for industrial applications, has recently been adapted for surgical dissection. The Hydro-Jet (HJ) enables precise, controllable, and tissue-selective dissection through a thin, laminar, water jet. Reports suggest minimal trauma to surrounding structures, and one study described it as highly precise, showing reduced perceived "oozing" and a lower need for inflow occlusion.

While HydroJet has not been extensively studied and compared with other devices, it is generally considered safe and on par with devices like CUSA and TissueLink. Studies have reported similar blood loss, transection speed, and overall outcomes. One study even noted that all surgeons in their study transitioned from using CUSA to HJ after becoming proficient with it. Nevertheless, further research is warranted to establish if HJ holds superiority in any specific aspect.

Hotspots for Injury along the Middle Hepatic Vein

Injury to the middle hepatic vein (MHV) is a common cause of major intraoperative bleeding. In addition, the MHV can be used as a crucial guide for parenchymal transection in a right, left, or central hepatectomy. A comprehensive understanding of the MHV anatomy is, therefore, imperative and a "roadmap", indicating the hotspots where injuries are more likely to occur, has been previously described. Typically, the MHV exhibits a consistent branching pattern, with an average of three significant tributaries (each with a diameter of ≥ 2 mm). These three tributaries have a diameter of approximately 4 mm and are typically found within 15 mm of the MHV. Using CT imaging, two notable hotspots where vascular injury is more prone to occur have been identified:

- V8 hotspot: up to 4 but most commonly 2 tributaries drain segment 8 between 9 and 35 mm from the MHV termination.
- V5 hotspot: up to 3 but most commonly 1 tributary draining segment 5 is found between 45 and 90 mm from the MHV termination. It is often the first encountered tributary and close to the portal trunk.

During the transection for a right hepatectomy, the tributary draining liver segment 5 (V5) serves as a guide leading toward the MHV. Once the MHV is located, the transection plane follows along its right side and aligns with the Rex-Cantlie line. Dissection for surgical field development during right hepatectomy should proceed in a peripheral-to-central direction, as described below.

Hemostasis and Biliostasis

After removing the specimen, it is imperative to thoroughly inspect the remnant hepatic liver surface. Any vessels should be meticulously ligated or clipped. Bleeding from the raw surface without an identifiable vessel can be managed using different devices such as an argon beam coagulator, the Aquamantys or Plasmajet. Furthermore, topical hemostatic agents may be applied to the cut surface of the liver. These can be categorized into matrix-based types (made from materials like collagen, cellulose, or gelatine) and those based on fibrin and/or thrombin. Some newer products in the market combine features of both categories, referred to as "carrier-bound fibrine sealants". Use of hemostatic agents may lead to reduced time required for achieving hemostasis, lower transfusion rates, decreased postoperative bleeding, fewer complications, and shorter hospital stays. In addition, use of hemostatic agents has not been shown to increase postoperative collections or intra-abdominal infections.

Residual bile leaks must also be addressed and subsequently ligated. Cholangiography can be effectively employed to identify any persistent bile leaks. Additionally, a Doppler ultrasound should be performed in the remnant liver to confirm adequate flow in the vascular structures.

A falciform ligament flap or an omental pedicle flap can be employed to ensure optimal protection of the raw surface of the liver. Drains can be positioned suprahepatic, infrahepatic, or retrohepatic, but should not be placed in direct contact with the raw surface of the liver. Routine use of drains is not indicated. Randomized controlled trials in the late 1990s and early 2000s have shown that routine abdominal drainage after liver resection does not decrease bile collections nor increase the detection of leaks or hemorrhages. Moreover, routine drainage was associated with prolonged hospital stays and higher postoperative morbidity rates, particularly in patients with chronic liver disease. Drains may be considered in cases at high risk for biliary leakage such as when a bilioenteric anastomosis is performed.

Some hemostatic devices and agents commonly used in liver resections are described below.

Hemostatic Devices

PlasmaJet® (Plasma Surgical)

Employing a distinct technology that utilizes a high-energy flow of ionized gas to seal small vessels, the PlasmaJet swiftly gained prominence in cytoreductive and endometriosis surgeries. By combining this approach with ultrasonic energy, it transforms into a versatile tool capable of dissection, vaporization, coagulation, and surface sealing functions. In the context of liver surgery, PlasmaJet has recently been introduced as a tool for managing hemostasis on the raw surface of the liver.

In the sole available RCT, PlasmaJet was compared to the application of fibrin glue. Though blood transfusion rates and postoperative mortality did not exhibit significant differences, a noteworthy reduction in postoperative complications necessitating percutaneous drainage was observed with PlasmaJet. Further studies are imperative to comprehensively evaluate the role of PlasmaJet in liver resection.

Argon Beam

The argon beam coagulator (ABC) system employs a jet of argon gas to generate a finely dispersed plasma of electrical current, ensuring consistent coagulation of tissue surfaces. This technique effectively clears blood and other debris, thereby reducing oxygen availability at the dissection site. Importantly, it results in minimal carbonization and smoke production. The primary risk associated with ABC use is the potential for argon gas embolism. Its application is somewhat restricted during laparoscopic surgery due to the high-flow infusion of argon gas, which can elevate abdominal pressure.

In liver resection procedures, the argon beam is utilized on the raw surfaces remaining after resection, thereby enhancing hemostasis. Previous comparative studies examining ABC and bipolar cautery for parenchymal transection, both in conjunction with CUSA, demonstrated reduced blood loss and shorter resection times with ABC. Its efficacy is on par with fibrin sealant methods.

Hemostatic Agents

Collagen-Based Topical Hemostatic Agents

Microfibrillar collagen (MC) sourced from bovine collagen serves as a scaffold for clot formation and activates platelets. It can be directly applied in powder form to the raw surface of the liver. Alternatively, a foam sheet variant (Avitene Ultrafoam) is also available.

Key products in the market include Avitene™ (Bard); CollaStat™ (Integra LifeSciences), and Helistat™ (Integra LifeSciences) in sponge form; as well as Instat MCH™ (Johnson & Johnson Company), available in patch form.

Purified Plant Starch Topical Hemostatic Agents

Derived from potato starch, these agents consist of microporous polysaccharide spheres that expedite clot formation. They accomplish this by locally absorbing water, which allows platelets and blood proteins to concentrate. Prior to application, the surface should be adequately dried. The powder is then applied liberally, followed by gentle pressure. This method is considered safe, as is not associated with foreign body reactions and does not serve as a growth media for pathogens. The primary product available in this category is Arista™ (Medafor), which is provided in spray form.

Oxidized Cellulose Topical Hemostatic Agents

Oxidized regenerated cellulose, presented in a dry sterile mesh form, is particularly effective for minor bleeding. It can be applied directly to the area of interest. Due to its mesh structure, it is easy to handle, making it a popular choice for minimally invasive surgeries. However, its use comes with some risks, notably infection and the potential formation of adhesions. Despite being absorbable, there have been instances where the mesh was discovered more than a year after placement.

The primary product available in this category is Surgicel™ (Johnson & Johnson Company). Additionally, there is a combination with polyethylene glycol known as Veriset™ (Covidien Inc.), both available in patch form.

Gelatin Matrix Topical Hemostatic Agents

Gelatin, derived from porcine collagen, is a hydrocolloid known for its high absorption capacity—up to 40 times its weight—and it can expand up to 200% in sponge form. While gelatin is not considered antigenic, its use carries an increased risk of infection, as well as the potential formation of granulomas and fibrosis.

The main products in this category are Gelfoam™ (Pfizer/Pharmacia) and Surgifoam™ (Johnson & Johnson Company), both available in sponge and powder form.

Fibrin Sealants

Fibrin sealants (FS) are composed of fibrinogen, thrombin, and other constituents like ionized calcium, factor XIII, fibronectin, and occasionally an antifibrinolytic agent such as aprotinin. Fibrinogen and factor XII are packaged together in one syringe, while thrombin and calcium are in the other. They function as a type of adhesive, applied using a two-syringe technique. When combined, a fibrin clot forms rapidly at the application site. They can also be used laparoscopically with a dual-lumen applicator.

Risks associated with FS include air or gas embolism, hypotension, potential impacts on wound healing, the theoretical risk of blood-borne disease since they are mostly derived from pooled human sources, and the potential for immune-mediated coagulopathy. FS should be avoided in patients with a history of anaphylactic reactions to plasma products or those with IgA deficiency.

Key products in this category include CryoSeal Fibrin Selant System™ (ThermoGenesis), Tisseel™ (Baxter Healthcare Corporation), and Evicel™ (Johnson & Johnson; OMRIX Biopharmaceuticals).

Thrombin Sealants

Topical thrombin (TT) is also sourced from pooled human blood, although recombinant and bovine thrombin varieties are also available. It is typically applied in spray form, particularly useful for managing diffuse bleeding. Additionally, it can be directly administered to the specific area using a syringe. TT can be combined with gelatin to create an immediate scaffold for clot formation, facilitating faster bleeding control.

Major products in this category include Recothrom™ (ZymoGenetics) recombinant thrombin; Surgiflo™ (Johnson & Johnson Company) which pairs porcine gelatin with thrombin, and FloSeal Hemostatic Matrix™ (Baxter Healthcare Corporation), comprising bovine gelatin and thrombin.

Laparoscopic Liver Resection

Laparoscopic liver resection was initially introduced for minor hepatectomies. However, with the increasing experience gained in minimally invasive surgery over the years, it is now also utilized for major hepatectomies. Nevertheless, this practice is primarily limited to surgeons with the appropriate expertise, often in high-volume institutions. Mastering laparoscopic liver surgery presents significant challenges, with a learning curve estimated at around 50 cases.

While various aspects of laparoscopic surgery, including techniques, patient selection, positioning, peritoneal access, and trocar positioning, will be discussed separately, the core steps of the procedure generally align with those of the state-of-the-art open procedure. Robotic surgery will also be addressed independently.

Laparoscopic surgery has substantially enhanced the understanding of liver anatomy, both internally and externally, owing to its magnified view and unique perspectives from caudal and dorsal angles. The pneumoperitoneum also exerts a tamponade effect, reducing intraoperative bleeding. In terms of outcomes, minimally invasive liver resection surpasses open surgery in various aspects, particularly with regard to blood loss and postoperative complications. Incidence rates of bile leaks and wound infections remain comparable. For malignancies, numerous large series have demonstrated equivalent oncologic outcomes.

However, laparoscopic liver resections usually are associated with prolonged operative times and prolonged time to bleeding control compared to open surgery.

Parenchymal transection during laparoscopic liver resection should follow the same principles as open surgery. Unique aspects related to the laparoscopic approach are described below.

Defining the Transection Plane

Ensuring the transection plane is aligned with the optical trocar adheres to the optimal triangulation rule. Additionally, proper retraction, adjusting the operating table, and evaluating camera positioning are all crucial for achieving optimal exposure. Intraoperative ultrasound is crucial for the determination of the transection line as in the open approach. Selective inflow occlusion and dye injection for the delineation of segments can also be performed but are technically more challenging.

Inflow Occlusion

The intermittent Pringle maneuver can be applied in laparoscopic procedures, and it stands as the most commonly used vascular occlusion technique in minimally invasive surgery. It enhances the visualization of hepatic veins and Glissonean pedicles, providing a nearly bloodless field. This maneuver effectively reduces blood loss and facilitates prompt bleeding control in the event of a conversion to an open procedure. It can be executed using either an intra- or extracorporeal approach, with several variants described.

To initiate the maneuver, a vascular tape is positioned around the hepatoduodenal ligament after opening the lesser omentum and threading it through the foramen of Winslow. In the intracorporeal method, this tape is exteriorized, and a tourniquet is affixed to it, then reinserted into the cavity. The maneuver is performed under direct visual guidance. When necessary, the tourniquet is pushed toward the pedicle and secured fastened with a clip. The clip is later removed, and the tourniquet is released when the maneuver is no longer required.

The extracorporeal technique has been described with some variations. It can be executed using a specialized vascular clamp passed directly through the trocar to clamp the pedicle, or by utilizing the same tourniquet technique, but with clamping control exerted through an instrument outside the patient. Extracorporeal techniques have the advantage of expediting bleeding control and are practical. When utilizing the tourniquet, they also prove to be the most cost-effective option. However, both methods yield comparable outcomes.

While highly effective, implementing the Pringle maneuver in the minimally invasive setting demands a degree of experience, as achieving complete clamping and subsequent unclamping can be technically challenging.

Parenchymal Transection

In minimally invasive surgery, the same peripheral-to-central technique is applied. Handling the liver capsule and the superficial layer is typically accomplished using ultrasonic shears, often without pre-coagulation. For superficial tumors undergoing wedge resection, ultrasonic shears alone can be employed.

Managing the central parenchyma, however, is more challenging. It necessitates the exposure of Glissonean branches and hepatic veins. Tactile techniques like clamp-crushing are not viable for transecting the deeper parenchyma in minimally invasive surgery, making electrosurgery the preferred method. The choice of device is primarily based on the surgeon's preference. The Cavitron Ultrasonic Surgical Aspirator (CUSA) is the most frequently utilized tool. The CUSA's pulsatile mode (TissueSelect®) is especially effective for dissecting major hepatic veins, as it allows for a slowed-down parenchymal transection, minimizing the risk of injury. Laparoscopic bipolar cautery is used in conjunction. Other devices will be discussed in detail below.

Small vessels (≤ 2 mm) can be sealed and then divided. Larger vessels (3–7 mm) may also be managed with sealing devices depending on the specific type, but they can also be clipped. Significant hepatic veins or Glissonean pedicles are dissected, and if necessary, taped for traction which facilitates the positioning of clips, typically the Hem-o-lock® type. The division is carried out with scissors, and vascular staplers are employed for managing major hepatic veins in cases of major hepatectomy.

Hemostasis and Biliostasis

Addressing bleeding during laparoscopy presents unique challenges, in addition to considerations regarding anesthesia, the maintenance of a low central venous pressure, and vascular occlusion.

For minor bleeding, a simple technique involves applying gentle pressure with a small gauze pad for several minutes, followed by direct clipping of the vessel. If bleeding is nonspecified, cautery can be used with caution. Larger vessels may be temporarily controlled using a clip or a grasper, followed by an attempt at direct suturing. For experienced surgeons, attempting sutures can be effective, as converting to an open approach can be time-consuming. It is advised not to increase the pneumoperitoneum for bleeding management, even in cases of massive hemorrhage, due to the high risk of gas embolism.

The use of hemostatic agents is less extensively studied in laparoscopic liver surgery, and proper placement in the transection plane can be technically challenging. The type of hemostatic agent largely depends on the surgeon's preference and experience. In cases of hand-assisted minimally invasive surgery, direct manual pressure on the cut surface with a warm sponge for 5–10 min can be applied. Hemostatic devices (e.g., Aquamantys) are also available for laparoscopic surgery. At the completion of the procedure, the pneumoperitoneum should be slowly released for several minutes and then re-insufflated to examine the cut surface one last time.

References

1. Moggia E, Rouse B, Simillis C, et al. Methods to decrease blood loss during liver resection: a network meta-analysis. Cochrane Database Syst Rev. 2016;2016(10) https://doi.org/10.1002/14651858.cd010683.pub3.
2. Curley SA, Glazer ES. Overview of hepatic resection. In UpToDate, Post TW (Ed). Wolters Kluwer. https://www.uptodate.com. Accessed on 9 Oct 2023.
3. Curley SA, Glazer ES. Open hepatic resection techniques. In UpToDate, Post TW (Ed). Wolters Kluwer. https://www.uptodate.com Accessed on 9 Oct 2023.
4. Pawlik TM, Schmidt C, Lewis HL. Minimally invasive liver resection (MILR). In UpToDate, Post TW (Ed). Wolters Kluwer. https://www.uptodate.com. Accessed on 9 Oct 2023.
5. Firat A, Abbasoglu TT, Karcaaltincaba M, Balaban YH. Clinical anatomy of hepatic vessels by computed tomography angiography: a minireview. World J Radiol. 2023;15(1):1–9. (In eng). https://doi.org/10.4329/wjr.v15.i1.1.
6. Alirr OI, Rahni AAA. Survey on liver tumour resection planning system: steps, techniques, and parameters. J Digit Imaging. 2020;33(2):304–23. https://doi.org/10.1007/s10278-019-00262-8.
7. Guilbaud T, Scemama U, Sarran A, et al. Predictive ability of preoperative CT scan for the intraoperative difficulty and postoperative outcomes of laparoscopic liver resection. Surg Endosc. 2021;35(6):2942–52. https://doi.org/10.1007/s00464-020-07734-x.
8. Tani K, Shindoh J, Akamatsu N, et al. Venous drainage map of the liver for complex hepatobiliary surgery and liver transplantation. HPB (Oxford). 2016;18(12):1031–8. (In eng). https://doi.org/10.1016/j.hpb.2016.08.007.

9. Kamel IR, Kruskal JB, Pomfret EA, Keogan MT, Warmbrand G, Raptopoulos V. Impact of multidetector CT on donor selection and surgical planning before living adult right lobe liver transplantation. AJR Am J Roentgenol. 2001;176(1):193–200. (In eng). DOI: 10.2214/ajr.176.1.1760193
10. Kawaguchi Y, Ishizawa T, Miyata Y, et al. Portal uptake function in veno-occlusive regions evaluated by real-time fluorescent imaging using indocyanine green. J Hepatol. 2013;58(2):247–53. (In eng). https://doi.org/10.1016/j.jhep.2012.09.028.
11. Ito K, Akamatsu N, Tani K, et al. Reconstruction of hepatic venous tributary in right liver living donor liver transplantation: the importance of the inferior right hepatic vein. Liver Transpl. 2016;22(4):410–9. (In eng). https://doi.org/10.1002/lt.24386.
12. Sugawara Y, Makuuchi M, Akamatsu N, et al. Refinement of venous reconstruction using cryopreserved veins in right liver grafts. Liver Transpl. 2004;10(4):541–7. (In eng). https://doi.org/10.1002/lt.20129.
13. Fang C, An J, Bruno A, et al. Consensus recommendations of three-dimensional visualization for diagnosis and management of liver diseases. Hepatol Int. 2020;14(4):437–53. https://doi.org/10.1007/s12072-020-10052-y.
14. Zhang WQ, Fang CH. Meta-analysis of efficacy comparison between diagnosis and treatment of primary hepatocellular carcinoma treated by 3D visualization technology and 2D imaging technology. Chin J Pract Surg. 2019;39:44–50.
15. Montalti R, Rompianesi G, Cassese G, et al. Role of preoperative 3D rendering for minimally invasive parenchyma sparing liver resections. HPB (Oxford). 2023;25(8):915–23. (In eng). https://doi.org/10.1016/j.hpb.2023.04.008.
16. Sheng W, Yuan C, Wu L, Yan J, Ge J, Lei J. Clinical application of a three-dimensional reconstruction technique for complex liver cancer resection. Surg Endosc. 2021:1–8.
17. Montalti R, Rompianesi G, Cassese G, et al. Role of preoperative 3D rendering for minimally invasive parenchyma sparing liver resections. HPB (Oxford). 2023;25(8):915–23. https://doi.org/10.1016/j.hpb.2023.04.008.
18. Huber T, Tripke V, Baumgart J, et al. Computer-assisted intraoperative 3D-navigation for liver surgery: a prospective randomized-controlled pilot study. Ann Transl Med. 2023;11(10):346. https://doi.org/10.21037/atm-22-5489.
19. Yang T, Lin S, Xie Q, et al. Impact of 3D printing technology on the comprehension of surgical liver anatomy. Surg Endosc. 2019;33(2):411–7. https://doi.org/10.1007/s00464-018-6308-8.
20. Kamiyama T, Kakisaka T, Orimo T. Current role of intraoperative ultrasonography in hepatectomy. Surg Today. 2021;51(12):1887–96. https://doi.org/10.1007/s00595-020-02219-9.

21. Lubner MG, Mankowski Gettle L, Kim DH, Ziemlewicz TJ, Dahiya N, Pickhardt P. Diagnostic and procedural intraoperative ultrasound: technique, tips and tricks for optimizing results. Br J Radiol. 2021;94(1121):20201406. https://doi.org/10.1259/bjr.20201406.
22. Wagnetz U, Atri M, Massey C, Wei AC, Metser U. Intraoperative ultrasound of the liver in primary and secondary hepatic malignancies: comparison with preoperative 1.5-T MRI and 64-MDCT. AJR Am J Roentgenol. 2011;196(3):562–8. https://doi.org/10.2214/AJR.10.4729.
23. Makuuchi M, Hasegawa H, Yamazaki S. Ultrasonically guided subsegmentectomy. Surg Gynecol Obstet. 1985;161(4):346–50.
24. Castaing D, Garden OJ, Bismuth H. Segmental liver resection using ultrasound-guided selective portal venous occlusion. Ann Surg. 1989;210(1):20–3.
25. Ishizawa T, Saiura A, Kokudo N. Clinical application of indocyanine green-fluorescence imaging during hepatectomy. Hepatobiliary Surg Nutr. 2016;5(4):322–8. https://doi.org/10.21037/hbsn.2015.10.01.
26. Alomari MAM, Wakabayashi T, Colella M, et al. Comparing the accuracy of positive and negative indocyanine green staining in guiding laparoscopic anatomical liver resection: protocol for a randomised controlled trial. BMJ Open. 2023;13(9):e072926. https://doi.org/10.1136/bmjopen-2023-072926.
27. Wang J, Xu Y, Zhang Y, Tian H. Safety and effectiveness of fluorescence laparoscopy in precise hepatectomy: a meta-analysis. Photodiagn Photodyn Ther. 2023;42:103599. https://doi.org/10.1016/j.pdpdt.2023.103599.
28. Aoki T, Yasuda D, Shimizu Y, et al. Image-guided liver mapping using fluorescence navigation system with Indocyanine green for anatomical hepatic resection. World J Surg. 2008;32(8):1763–7. https://doi.org/10.1007/s00268-008-9620-y.
29. Ogiso S, Okuno M, Shindoh J, et al. Conceptual framework of middle hepatic vein anatomy as a roadmap for safe right hepatectomy. HPB (Oxford). 2019;21(1):43–50. https://doi.org/10.1016/j.hpb.2018.01.002.
30. Hoekstra LT, van Trigt JD, Reiniers MJ, Busch OR, Gouma DJ, van Gulik TM. Vascular occlusion or not during liver resection: the continuing story. Dig Surg. 2012;29(1):35–42. https://doi.org/10.1159/000335724.
31. MacKenzie S, Dixon E, Bathe O, Sutherland F. Intermittent hepatic vein—total vascular exclusion during liver resection: anatomic and clinical studies. J Gastrointest Surg. 2005;9(5):658–66. https://doi.org/10.1016/j.gassur.2004.12.003.
32. Smyrniotis V, Arkadopoulos N, Kostopanagiotou G, et al. Sharp liver transection versus clamp crushing technique in liver resections: a prospective study. Surgery. 2005;137(3):306–11. https://doi.org/10.1016/j.surg.2004.09.012.
33. de Rougemont O, Dutkowski P, Weber M, Clavien PA. Abdominal drains in liver transplantation: useful tool or useless dogma? A matched case-

control study. Liver Transpl. 2009;15(1):96–101. https://doi.org/10.1002/lt.21676.
34. Aldameh A, McCall JL, Koea JB. Is routine placement of surgical drains necessary after elective hepatectomy? Results from a single institution. J Gastrointest Surg. 2005;9(5):667–71. https://doi.org/10.1016/j.gassur.2004.12.006.
35. Yoh T, Cauchy F, Soubrane O. Techniques for laparoscopic liver parenchymal transection. Hepatobiliary Surg Nutr. 2019;8(6):572–81. https://doi.org/10.21037/hbsn.2019.04.16.
36. Chua D, Syn N, Koh YX, Goh BKP. Learning curves in minimally invasive hepatectomy: systematic review and meta-regression analysis. Br J Surg. 2021;108(4):351–8. https://doi.org/10.1093/bjs/znaa118.
37. Piardi T, Lhuaire M, Memeo R, Pessaux P, Kianmanesh R, Sommacale D. Laparoscopic Pringle maneuver: how we do it? HepatoBiliary Surg Nutr. 2016;5(4):345–9. https://doi.org/10.21037/hbsn.2015.11.01.
38. Lim C, Osseis M, Lahat E, Azoulay D, Salloum C. Extracorporeal Pringle Maneuver during laparoscopic and robotic hepatectomy: detailed technique and first comparison with Intracorporeal Maneuver. J Am Coll Surg. 2018;226(5):e19–25. https://doi.org/10.1016/j.jamcollsurg.2018.02.003.
39. Kamarajah SK, Wilson CH, Bundred JR, et al. A systematic review and network meta-analysis of parenchymal transection techniques during hepatectomy: an appraisal of current randomised controlled trials. HPB (Oxford). 2020;22(2):204–14. https://doi.org/10.1016/j.hpb.2019.09.014.
40. Lupo L, Gallerani A, Panzera P, Tandoi F, Di Palma G, Memeo V. Randomized clinical trial of radiofrequency-assisted versus clamp-crushing liver resection. Br J Surg. 2007;94(3):287–91. https://doi.org/10.1002/bjs.5674.
41. Francone E, Muzio E, D'Ambra L, et al. Precoagulation-assisted parenchyma-sparing laparoscopic liver surgery: rationale and surgical technique. Surg Endosc. 2017;31(3):1354–60. https://doi.org/10.1007/s00464-016-5120-6.
42. Lesurtel M, Selzner M, Petrowsky H, McCormack L, Clavien PA. How should transection of the liver be performed?: a prospective randomized study in 100 consecutive patients: comparing four different transection strategies. Ann Surg. 2005;242(6):814–22., discussion 822-3. https://doi.org/10.1097/01.sla.0000189121.35617.d7.
43. Campagnacci R, De Sanctis A, Baldarelli M, et al. Hepatic resections by means of electrothermal bipolar vessel device (EBVS) LigaSure V: early experience. Surg Endosc. 2007;21(12):2280–4. https://doi.org/10.1007/s00464-007-9384-8.
44. Hanyong S, Wanyee L, Siyuan F, et al. A prospective randomized controlled trial: comparison of two different methods of hepatectomy. Eur J Surg Oncol. 2015;41(2):243–8. https://doi.org/10.1016/j.ejso.2014.10.057.

45. Ichida A, Hasegawa K, Takayama T, et al. Randomized clinical trial comparing two vessel-sealing devices with crush clamping during liver transection. Br J Surg. 2016;103(13):1795–803. https://doi.org/10.1002/bjs.10297.
46. Sultan AM, Shehta A, Salah T, et al. Clamp-crush technique versus harmonic scalpel for hepatic parenchymal transection in living donor hepatectomy: a randomized controlled trial. J Gastrointest Surg. 2019;23(8):1568–77. https://doi.org/10.1007/s11605-019-04103-5.
47. El Shobary M, Salah T, El Nakeeb A, et al. Spray diathermy versus harmonic scalpel technique for hepatic parenchymal transection of living donor. J Gastrointest Surg. 2017;21(2):321–9. https://doi.org/10.1007/s11605-016-3312-y.
48. Badawy A, Seo S, Toda R, et al. Evaluation of a new energy device for parenchymal transection in laparoscopic liver resection. Asian J Endosc Surg. 2018;11(2):123–8. https://doi.org/10.1111/ases.12432.
49. Takayama T, Makuuchi M, Kubota K, et al. Randomized comparison of ultrasonic vs clamp transection of the liver. Arch Surg. 2001;136(8):922–8. https://doi.org/10.1001/archsurg.136.8.922.
50. Doklestic K, Karamarkovic A, Stefanovic B, et al. The efficacy of three transection techniques of the liver resection: a randomized clinical trial. Hepato-Gastroenterology. 2012;59(117):1501–6. https://doi.org/10.5754/hge11552.
51. Savlid M, Strand AH, Jansson A, et al. Transection of the liver parenchyma with an ultrasound dissector or a stapler device: results of a randomized clinical study. World J Surg. 2013;37(4):799–805. https://doi.org/10.1007/s00268-012-1884-6.
52. Hutchins R, Bertucci M. Experience with TissueLink™—radiofrequency-assisted parenchymal division. Dig Surg. 2007;24(4):318–21. https://doi.org/10.1159/000103665.
53. Arita J, Hasegawa K, Kokudo N, Sano K, Sugawara Y, Makuuchi M. Randomized clinical trial of the effect of a saline-linked radiofrequency coagulator on blood loss during hepatic resection. Br J Surg. 2005;92(8):954–9. https://doi.org/10.1002/bjs.5108.
54. Saiura A, Yamamoto J, Koga R, et al. Usefulness of LigaSure for liver resection: analysis by randomized clinical trial. Am J Surg. 2006;192(1):41–5. https://doi.org/10.1016/j.amjsurg.2006.01.025.
55. Ikeda M, Hasegawa K, Sano K, et al. The vessel sealing system (LigaSure) in hepatic resection: a randomized controlled trial. Ann Surg. 2009;250(2):199–203. https://doi.org/10.1097/SLA.0b013e3181a334f9.
56. Muratore A, Mellano A, Tarantino G, Marsanic P, De Simone M, Di Benedetto F. Radiofrequency vessel-sealing system versus the clamp-crushing technique in liver transection: results of a prospective randomized study on 100 consecutive patients. HPB (Oxford). 2014;16(8):707–12. https://doi.org/10.1111/hpb.12207.

57. Vollmer CM, Dixon E, Sahajpal A, et al. Water-jet dissection for parenchymal division during hepatectomy. HPB (Oxford). 2006;8(5):377–85. https://doi.org/10.1080/13651820600839449.
58. Schemmer P, Friess H, Hinz U, et al. Stapler hepatectomy is a safe dissection technique: analysis of 300 patients. World J Surg. 2006;30(3):419–30. https://doi.org/10.1007/s00268-005-0192-9.
59. Rahbari NN, Elbers H, Koch M, et al. Randomized clinical trial of stapler versus clamp-crushing transection in elective liver resection. Br J Surg. 2014;101(3):200–7. https://doi.org/10.1002/bjs.9387.
60. Schwarz C, Klaus DA, Tudor B, et al. Transection speed and impact on perioperative inflammatory response—a randomized controlled trial comparing stapler hepatectomy and CUSA resection. PLoS One. 2015;10(10):e0140314. Published 2015 Oct 9. https://doi.org/10.1371/journal.pone.0140314.
61. Fritzmann J, Kirchberg J, Sturm D, et al. Randomized clinical trial of stapler hepatectomy versus LigaSure™ transection in elective hepatic resection. Br J Surg. 2018;105(9):1119–27. https://doi.org/10.1002/bjs.10902.
62. Kaibori M, Matsui K, Ishizaki M, et al. A prospective randomized controlled trial of hemostasis with a bipolar sealer during hepatic transection for liver resection. Surgery. 2013;154(5):1046–52. https://doi.org/10.1016/j.surg.2013.04.053.
63. Iida H, Maehira H, Mori H, Tani M. Efficiency of a radiofrequency sealer (Aquamantys) for parenchymal transection during laparoscopic hepatectomy. Asian J Endosc Surg. 2020;13(4):505–13. https://doi.org/10.1111/ases.12785.
64. Gugenheim J, Bredt LC, Iannelli A. A randomized controlled trial comparing fibrin glue and PlasmaJet on the raw surface of the liver after hepatic resection. Hepato-Gastroenterology. 2011;58(107–108):922–5.
65. Nagano Y, Matsuo K, Kunisaki C, et al. Practical usefulness of ultrasonic surgical aspirator with argon beam coagulation for hepatic parenchymal transection. World J Surg. 2005;29(7):899–902. https://doi.org/10.1007/s00268-005-7784-2.
66. Frilling A, Stavrou GA, Mischinger HJ, et al. Effectiveness of a new carrier-bound fibrin sealant versus argon beamer as haemostatic agent during liver resection: a randomised prospective trial. Langenbeck's Arch Surg. 2005;390(2):114–20. https://doi.org/10.1007/s00423-005-0543-x.
67. Mueller GR, Wolf RF, Hansen PD, Gregory KW, Prahl SA. Hemostasis after liver resection improves after single application of albumin and argon beam coagulation. J Gastrointest Surg. 2010;14(11):1764–9. https://doi.org/10.1007/s11605-010-1262-3.
68. Ikegami T, Shimada M, Imura S, et al. Argon gas embolism in the application of laparoscopic microwave coagulation therapy. J Hepato-Biliary-Pancreat Surg. 2009;16(3):394–8. https://doi.org/10.1007/s00534-008-0039-5.

69. Brustia R, Granger B, Scatton O. An update on topical haemostatic agents in liver surgery: systematic review and meta analysis. J Hepatobiliary Pancreat Sci. 2016;23(10):609–21. https://doi.org/10.1002/jhbp.389.
70. Boonstra EA, Molenaar IQ, Porte RJ, de Boer MT. Topical haemostatic agents in liver surgery: do we need them? HPB (Oxford). 2009;11(4):306–10. https://doi.org/10.1111/j.1477-2574.2009.00065.x.
71. Huntington JT, Royall NA, Schmidt CR. Minimizing blood loss during hepatectomy: a literature review. J Surg Oncol. 2014;109(2):81–8. https://doi.org/10.1002/jso.23455.
72. Peralta E. Overview of topical hemostatic agents and tissue adhesives. In UpToDate, Post TW (Ed). Wolters Kluwer. https://www.uptodate.com. Accessed on 9 Oct 2023.
73. Peralta E. Fibrin sealants. In UpToDate, Post TW (Ed). Wolters Kluwer. https://www.uptodate.com. Accessed on 9 Oct 2023.

Robotic Approaches to Hepatic Transection

14

Miho Akabane, Brendan Visser, and Kazunari Sasaki

Introduction

Minimally invasive surgery has increasingly become popular in liver surgery, with laparoscopic liver resection becoming quite common worldwide. Minimally invasive approaches tend to involve less blood loss, quicker recovery periods, and reduced postoperative pain compared to the traditional open approach while maintaining comparable oncological results [1–8]. However, performing major liver resections laparoscopically con-

---

Copyright
The authors retain the copyright of this article, and the publisher is granted the license to publish this article. This means that the authors hold the final copyright and retain the rights for future works, such as the rights to create derivative works, and the rights to commercialize the work.

M. Akabane · K. Sasaki (✉)
Division of Abdominal Transplant, Department of Surgery, Stanford University Medical Center, Stanford, CA, USA
e-mail: sasakik@stanford.edu

B. Visser
Section of Hepatobiliary and Pancreatic Surgery, Division of General Surgery, Department of Surgery, Stanford University Medical Center, Stanford, CA, USA

© The Author(s), under exclusive license to Springer Nature Switzerland AG 2025
A. Alseidi et al. (eds.), *The SAGES Manual of Contemporary Indications and Management of Hepatic and Biliary Diseases*, https://doi.org/10.1007/978-3-032-04823-3_14

tinues to be challenging, in part due to inherent limitations including the restricted range of laparoscopic instruments, and the reduction in dexterity due to the fulcrum effect and instrument length [1, 9–12]. In this context, robotic liver resection has generated growing interest, presenting a promising alternative with a broad range of applications [2, 3, 11].

Robotic systems, designed to augment the surgeon's abilities, offer articulating instruments, motion stabilization, and a three-dimensional view controlled by the surgeon which offer improved dexterity of dissection [13]. Adoption of robotic liver resections has been hampered by limitations of existing robotic instrumentation for transection of the liver parenchymal. A variety of transection techniques have been described, pointing to a need for further research and perhaps instrument development [1, 8, 14].

In this section, we aim to outline the essentials of preoperative preparation and each step in robotic liver resection. Additionally, we shed light on common precautions to be noted during this procedure.

Preoperative Planning for Robotic Hepatic Resection

Anatomic Evaluation

Robotic hepatic resection follows the same initial directives as open or laparoscopic procedures. However, it is critical to highlight that converting to open surgery from robotic generally takes more time than from the laparoscopic approach, because additional time is required to undock the robot, rearrange the room for open surgery, and for the surgeon to scrub in. Therefore, all team members need to engage in meticulous preoperative planning. The key to this process is to understand a patient's anatomy through detailed analysis utilizing triphasic liver computed tomography (CT) or magnetic resonance (MR) imaging. In many individuals (55–75%), liver anatomy demonstrates the classic pattern, but there exists a substantial prevalence of vascular and biliary anatomic variations that require alterations to the operative plan and attention during the resection to avoid injury [15–19]. The most frequent anatomical artery variants are the replaced and accessory right or left hepatic arteries. While not all variations are significant in the surgery, a replaced or accessory left hepatic artery demands particular caution, especially when determining the ligation position during the left hepatectomy [15, 16, 18]. A replaced or accessory artery originating from the superior mesenteric artery also needs careful attention to avoid potential injury during the resection of the bile duct [18].

Understanding portal vein anatomy is equally essential. The classic anatomy is observed in approximately 65% of cases [19]. Anomalies, such as portal vein trifurcation or the presence of a Z-type pattern, where a right posterior branch arises as the first branch of the portal vein trunk, necessitate specific surgical strategies to prevent unintended devascularization of vital liver segments [15, 19, 20]. Furthermore, the presence of intrahepatic bifurcations requires parenchymal dissection to access the portal pedicles [21].

Awareness of the anatomy of the hepatic veins is crucial in ensuring adequate venous outflow from the remnant liver segments to avoid congestion and bleeding [15, 20, 22]. A noteworthy variant of right liver venous drainage is the presence of an accessory inferior right hepatic vein draining segments 5 and 6 into the inferior vena cava. For example, the presence of this vein allows the preservation of segments 5 and 6 with complete resection of segments 7 and 8 and the right hepatic vein [15, 20, 22]. Regarding the middle hepatic vein, it is advised to retain it whenever feasible to prevent potential venous congestion in the peripheral regions. Intriguingly, the right anterior section drains not solely through the right but also through the middle hepatic vein via the branches termed V5 and V8; Substantial V5 and V8 branches necessitate additional careful ligation during right hepatectomy with the transection plane to the right side of the middle hepatic vein.

The classic bile duct anatomy is apparent in 58% of individuals [23, 24]. MR cholangiography is a non-invasive tool that offers intricate details of anatomical structures [23]. A prevalent variation, occurring in 13% of the population, involves the right posterior duct draining into the left hepatic duct, a crucial consideration during a left hepatectomy [24]. Another common anomaly, observed in 11% of individuals, is the triple confluence of the hepatic ducts, where a distinct right hepatic duct is not present, complicating the process of a right hepatectomy [24]. Additionally, there exist rare variations including aberrant ducts demanding complex surgical procedures [24].

Fluorescence imaging with indocyanine green (ICG) is a useful adjunct during hepatectomy to accurately image the demarcation line after inflow occlusion and division [25, 26]. After inflow occlusion, 2.5 mg of ICG is injected followed by a 10 cc flush of saline while the liver is viewed under fluorescent light. The line of demarcation is easily visible (superior to visual assessment of the ischemic demarcation). This enhanced clarity facilitates a more accurate and safer liver resection by highlighting the anatomic plane with fewer intrahepatic vascular structures. Furthermore, ICG binds with plasma proteins in the blood and is selectively absorbed by the liver and then excreted through the bile [27]. This process allows for the distinct imaging of the bile duct's course sometime after the ICG injection, aiding in precisely locating the appropriate position for the bile duct incision.

Other Important Steps to Prepare for a Safe Robotic Liver Resection

Determining the suitability of robotic liver resection hinges partly on various factors, including tumor location and size, as well as its proximity to vital structures. Beyond this assessment, it is critical to employ CT volumetric software to estimate the future liver remnant volume, a practice that is also common in open liver surgery [28]. This process is essential in mitigating the significant risk of postoperative liver failure that is associated with major liver surgeries [29]. Da Vinci system (Intuitive Surgical, Inc., Sunnyvale, CA) can display three-dimensional images on its console during surgery, provided the appropriate settings are used [30].

Proper patient positioning and the efficient arrangement of surgical instruments are vital to prevent complications, especially collision/compression between the patient's body and the robotic arm. An integrated bed system enables surgeons to use gravity, making liver mobilization and adjusting liver transection to a robotic arm easier. During the liver transection phase, the anesthesiologist has a crucial role in maintaining the central venous pressure below 5 mmHg to foster a safe surgical environment [31]. Moreover, the team should be prepared for the immediate conversion to open surgery if necessary, especially in instances of severe bleeding that is hard to control or if the surgery encounters prolonged delays.

Each Step in Robotic Liver Resection

Set Up

Meticulous preparation is essential to ensure the smooth progression of the procedure. Here is a simple guide to the setup and the initial steps:

1. Patient positioning and anesthesia:
   - Induction and maintenance of general anesthesia are carried out.
   - An arterial line is placed. Central venous catheter (commonly in the internal jugular or subclavian vein) is placed very selectively only in high-risk patients.
   - For most resections (segments 1,2,3,4,5,8), the patient is placed in lithotomy with the thighs flat with the torso. Lithotomy facilitates access for the bedside assistant.
   - The patient is positioned with some degree of rotation (up to and including full lateral decubitus) depending on the planned resection for right posterior sector resections.
2. Preoperative preparations:
   - Orogastric tube insertion for gastric decompression.
   - Foley catheter insertion for urinary bladder decompression.
   - Sterile draping of the abdomen.

3. Robotic system setup:
    - The robot "patient cart" (robotic arms) is generally positioned on the patient's left side. If conversion to open surgery is required, it is easier to permit undocking and quick access for a surgeon to open operating on the patient's right.
    - The robotic surgical system is synced with the operating table to facilitate easy repositioning during the surgery without undocking the robot.
4. Initial incisions and diagnostic laparoscopy:
    - Pneumoperitoneum is established to achieve an intra-abdominal pressure of 15 mmHg for trocar placement (which can be selectively reduced after all trocars are positioned).
    - The first trocar is placed using an optical entry system, while subsequent trocars are placed under direct vision with the camera.
5. Trocar placement:
    - Four 8 mm robotic trocars are placed in a straight line 7 cm apart for most resections. If the surgeon chooses to use the robotic stapler, one of the trocars is substituted for a 12 mm trocar. Generally, we choose to operate with two right-hand instruments and one left-hand instrument. The camera trocar is typically positioned slightly to the patient's left of the planned transection line to allow both right-hand instruments to have good access as the liver transection plane is opened. The horizontal line formed by the trocars is perpendicular to the vertical line of the planned transection. For example, for a planned left or right lobectomy, the trocars are in a straight horizontal line across the abdomen. For a segment 6 resection, the line of the trocars would be turned diagonally to align the perpendicular to the planned transection more closely. The position of the line on the vertical axis of the patient's torso is adjusted according to the length of the torso, body habitus, and the degree of insufflation. However, generally, the line of trocars is positioned above the level of the umbilicus (and sometimes substantially so in men with a deeper "barrel" shape) to allow

the surgeon to look down (with the 30-degree camera) on the hepatoduodenal ligament for inflow dissection. Typically, the line of trocars is approximately 10 cm inferior to the planned inferior edge of the surgical field (which extends the cephalad as the hepatectomy progresses). Of note, if it is planned to use a robotic stapler, the trocars should be slightly more inferior (approximately 15 cm) because the stapler arm requires significantly more space to articulate and maneuver. Trocar placement is critical to success with the robotic platform (even more so than in laparoscopy) and should be carefully planned preoperatively.

6. Assistant Setup and Instrumentation:
   – A bedside assistant is positioned between the patient's legs.
   – An assistant trocar is placed in the lower abdomen, ensuring it is at least 10 cm below the line of robotic trocars. This placement is crucial to avoid collisions with the robotic arms. At the beginning of the procedure, we make the extraction incision—its size tailored to the extent of the planned resection—choosing between a low midline or Pfannenstiel incision. We then insert a GelPoint Mini® (Applied Medical, Rancho Santa Margarita, CA) and introduce a 12 mm trocar through the GelPoint. For patients with a particularly long torso, a short lower midline incision is preferred over a Pfannenstiel incision, as the latter may be positioned too low to provide safe and efficient assistance.
7. Robotic system docking:
   – The robot is docked, with the arms equipped with basic instruments. Our standard setup for the instruments, arranged from the patient's right to left, includes a fenestrated bipolar, the camera, monopolar scissors, and the Cadiere grasper.
8. Ultrasonographic examination:
   – A systematic ultrasonographic examination of the liver is conducted using a drop-in robotic ultrasound probe to confirm the tumor location and to scrutinize for any additional tumors that might alter the surgical plan.

Liver Mobilization

The surgical often (though not necessarily) begins with mobilization. This is a delicate procedure, requiring gentle handling of the liver to prevent any accidental tears, especially concerning the short hepatic veins that are prone to injury. The utilization of rolled gauze as a cushion is helpful when mobilizing liver parenchyma using robotic arms. Also, similar to other minimally invasive operations, the utilization of gravity is helpful in mobilizing the liver. However, the range of table rotation is limited in robotic liver surgery compared to the laparoscopic approach. One of the key tips for liver mobilization is that surgeons should swiftly modify approach angles and directions if they encounter difficulty. For instance, if there is resistance when mobilizing from the top, it is advisable to shift to the bottom or side immediately.

Pringle Maneuver and Hilar Dissection

The implementation of the Pringle maneuver and hilar dissection is determined case-by-case, influenced by the preferences of the surgeon. The Pringle maneuver involves dissecting the hepatoduodenal ligament and using tools such as a Foley catheter or vessel loop to intermittently control the flow in the hepatic hilum. This involves introducing a taping tool into the abdominal cavity. Initially, the hepatic round ligament is raised ventrally using forceps held by an assistant. Following this, the tool is inserted through the opened lesser omentum and maneuvered behind the hepatoduodenal ligament. The tool is then carefully advanced, guided by the probing action of robotic forceps. The tip of the taping tool is captured on the opposite side, enabling the taping of the hepatoduodenal ligament. This tape, once attached to the hepatoduodenal ligament, is threaded through a tourniquet catheter (measuring 21–23 cm in length) and brought out through the abdominal wall. Depending on the location of the lesion, the tourniquet catheter is positioned on the patient's left side for right lobe lesions, and on the right side for left lobe lesions. To obstruct hepatic inflow, the tape is pulled from outside the body, tightening the tourniquet. One of the disadvantages of robotic surgery is the lack of sensation, especially in the encircled liver hilum. Special attention is needed when encircling the liver hilum. When navigating behind the liver hilum, lifting the liver adequately using the falciform ligament is a key tip.

Parenchymal Transection

Following the delineation of the designated resection area—a process achieved through ischemic discoloration or negative fluorescence imaging after ICG injection—the transection of the liver commences [32]. Once this demarcation is established, ultrasonography is employed to re-examine the lesion, aligning it with the marks made during the cautery process, and these marks are visible in the ultrasonography images. Different tools can be used for the parenchymal dissection in robotic liver resection, including Cavitron Ultrasonic Surgical Aspirator (CUSA®) through assistant port, clamp-crushing method using bipolar forceps or Synchroseal® (Intuitive Surgical Inc., Sunnyvale, CA, USA), or Harmonic scalpel® (Ethicon Endo-Surgery) [14]. There is no standard liver parenchymal transection in robotic liver surgery similar to open and laparoscopic liver resection. Each technique has its advantages and disadvantages. CUSA® requires an expert at the bedside and careful tracer positioning to avoid collisions with the robotic arm. The Harmonic Scalpel® lacks articulation and is less effective at achieving hemostasis on larger vessels. The clamp-crushing method with Maryland bipolar forceps can result in burnt liver tissue accumulation. SynchroSeal® is a bipolar electrosurgical instrument designed for use with a compatible da Vinci surgical system and electro-surgical generator, capable of sealing and cutting vessels up to 5 mm in diameter and tissue bundles with a single pedal press. It features a refined, curved jaw for improved dissection and secure grasping, with an articulating wrist that allows for approaching anatomy from preferred angles. Currently, our dominant strategy is SynchroSeal®, acknowledging its deficiencies and the ongoing need for better instruments.

One of the biggest advantages of robotic surgery to the laparoscopic approach is the feasibility of suture repair in the robotic approach. Suture repair can control large vessel injuries or a bleeding spot hiding inside the parenchyma, which is usually difficult to control by energy devices. Furthermore, robotic hepatectomies present particular advantages, especially for resections in posterosuperior segments, such as segments 7 and 8, where laparoscopic resections are technically demanding [33]. Although robotic hepatectomies lack some of the flexibility inherent in open liver resections, they compensate with instruments capable of flexible bending. This adaptability simplifies access to segments that pose considerable technical challenges and require significant effort in laparoscopic resections [34, 35]. In addition, robotic surgeries retain the benefits of minimally invasive techniques seen in laparoscopic procedures, including an enhanced, magnified three-dimensional field of view and a caudal view [36, 37]. Ogiso et al. clarified this advantage with an analogy: in open surgery, the transection plane progresses from the ventral surface to the dorsal side, akin to "opening a book". In contrast, minimally invasive methods employ a caudo-cranial approach, as if "opening a door" [38]. Robotic methods may be considered for patients for whom laparoscopic approaches might be deemed too risky.

Conclusion

Robotic surgery has been growing rapidly as a tool to address some of the shortcomings of laparoscopy. In recent years, it has broadened its utility in this area significantly. This strategy is particularly beneficial in facilitating various stages of the operation, including hilum dissection, liver mobilization, and parenchymal transection. Moreover, the robotic setup potentially integrates with emerging technologies, promoting a safer operational environment. However, it is critical to note that there is no standardized method for robotic liver resection at present. Therefore, comprehensive preoperative assessments are vital, alongside ensuring the surgical team is uniformly prepared and aligned in their approach, which is central to achieving successful outcomes.

Declarations: Authors' Contributions Participated in research design; Akabane M, Sasaki K.
Participated in the writing of the paper; Akabane M, Sasaki K.
Participated in the critical review: Akabane M, Visser B, Sasaki K.

Availability of Data and Materials Not applicable

Financial Support and Sponsorship None.

Conflicts of Interest All authors declared that there are no conflicts of interest.

Ethical Approval and Consent to Participate Not applicable.

References

1. Choi GH, Chong JU, Han DH, Choi JS, Lee WJ. Robotic hepatectomy: the Korean experience and perspective. Hepatobiliary Surg Nutr. 2017;6(4):230–8. https://doi.org/10.21037/hbsn.2017.01.14.
2. Chen PD, Wu CY, Hu RH, et al. Robotic major hepatectomy: is there a learning curve? Surgery. 2017;161(3):642–9. https://doi.org/10.1016/j.surg.2016.09.025.
3. Liu R, Wakabayashi G, Kim HJ, et al. International consensus statement on robotic hepatectomy surgery in 2018. World J Gastroenterol. 2019;25(12):1432–44. https://doi.org/10.3748/wjg.v25.i12.1432.
4. Wong DJ, Wong MJ, Choi GH, Wu YM, Lai PB, Goh BKP. Systematic review and meta-analysis of robotic versus open hepatectomy. ANZ J Surg. 2019;89(3):165–70. https://doi.org/10.1111/ans.14690.
5. Chen PD, Wu CY, Hu RH, et al. Robotic versus open hepatectomy for hepatocellular carcinoma: a matched comparison. Ann Surg Oncol. 2017;24(4):1021–8. https://doi.org/10.1245/s10434-016-5638-9.
6. Kingham TP, Leung U, Kuk D, et al. Robotic liver resection: a case-matched comparison. World J Surg. 2016;40(6):1422–8. https://doi.org/10.1007/s00268-016-3446-9.
7. Jackson NR, Hauch A, Hu T, Buell JF, Slakey DP, Kandil E. The safety and efficacy of approaches to liver resection: a meta-analysis. JSLS. 2015;19(1):e2014.00186. https://doi.org/10.4293/jsls.2014.00186.
8. Giulianotti PC, Sbrana F, Coratti A, et al. Totally robotic right hepatectomy: surgical technique and outcomes. Arch Surg. 2011;146(7):844–50. https://doi.org/10.1001/archsurg.2011.145.
9. Buell JF, Cherqui D, Geller DA, et al. The international position on laparoscopic liver surgery: the Louisville statement, 2008. Ann Surg. 2009;250(5):825–30. https://doi.org/10.1097/sla.0b013e3181b3b2d8.
10. Wakabayashi G, Cherqui D, Geller DA, et al. Recommendations for laparoscopic liver resection: a report from the second international consensus conference held in Morioka. Ann Surg. 2015;261(4):619–29. https://doi.org/10.1097/sla.0000000000001184.

11. Croner RS, Perrakis A, Brunner M, Matzel KE, Hohenberger W. Pioneering robotic liver surgery in Germany: first experiences with liver malignancies. Front Surg. 2015;2:18. https://doi.org/10.3389/fsurg.2015.00018.
12. Croner RS, Perrakis A, Hohenberger W, Brunner M. Robotic liver surgery for minor hepatic resections: a comparison with laparoscopic and open standard procedures. Langenbeck's Arch Surg. 2016;401(5):707–14. https://doi.org/10.1007/s00423-016-1440-1.
13. Leung U, Fong Y. Robotic liver surgery. Hepatobiliary Surg Nutr. 2014;3(5):288–94. https://doi.org/10.3978/j.issn.2304-3881.2014.09.02.
14. Perrakis A, Rahimli M, Gumbs AA, et al. Three-Device (3D) technique for liver parenchyma dissection in robotic liver surgery. J Clin Med. 2021;10(22). https://doi.org/10.3390/jcm10225265.
15. Catalano OA, Singh AH, Uppot RN, Hahn PF, Ferrone CR, Sahani DV. Vascular and biliary variants in the liver: implications for liver surgery. Radiographics. 2008;28(2):359–78.
16. Covey AM, Brody LA, Maluccio MA, Getrajdman GI, Brown KT. Variant hepatic arterial anatomy revisited: digital subtraction angiography performed in 600 patients. Radiology. 2002;224(2):542–7.
17. Hiatt JR, Gabbay J, Busuttil RW. Surgical anatomy of the hepatic arteries in 1000 cases. Ann Surg. 1994;220(1):50.
18. Lowe MC, D'Angelica MI. Anatomy of hepatic resectional surgery. Surg Clin. 2016;96(2):183–95.
19. Covey AM, Brody LA, Getrajdman GI, Sofocleous CT, Brown KT. Incidence, patterns, and clinical relevance of variant portal vein anatomy. Am J Roentgenol. 2004;183(4):1055–64.
20. Sahani D, Mehta A, Blake M, Prasad S, Harris G, Saini S. Preoperative hepatic vascular evaluation with CT and MR angiography: implications for surgery. Radiographics. 2004;24(5):1367–80.
21. Schultz SR, LaBerge JM, Gordon RL, Warren RS. Anatomy of the portal vein bifurcation: intra-versus extrahepatic location—implications for transjugular intrahepatic portosystemic shunts. J Vasc Interv Radiol. 1994;5(3):457–9.
22. Barbaro B, Soglia G, Alvaro G, et al. Hepatic veins in presurgical planning of hepatic resection: what a radiologist should know. Abdom Imaging. 2013;38:442–60.
23. Mortelé KJ, Ros PR. Anatomic variants of the biliary tree: MR cholangiographic findings and clinical applications. Am J Roentgenol. 2001;177(2):389–94.
24. Puente SG, Bannura GC. Radiological anatomy of the biliary tract: variations and congenital abnormalities. World J Surg. 1983;7:271–6.
25. Landsman ML, Kwant G, Mook GA, Zijlstra WG. Light-absorbing properties, stability, and spectral stabilization of indocyanine green. J Appl Physiol. 1976;40(4):575–83. https://doi.org/10.1152/jappl.1976.40.4.575.

26. Chiow AKH, Rho SY, Wee IJY, Lee LS, Choi GH. Robotic ICG guided anatomical liver resection in a multi-Centre cohort: an evolution from "positive staining" into "negative staining" method. HPB (Oxford). 2021;23(3):475–82. https://doi.org/10.1016/j.hpb.2020.08.005.
27. Gao Y, Li M, Song Z-f, et al. Mechanism of dynamic near-infrared fluorescence cholangiography of extrahepatic bile ducts and applications in detecting bile duct injuries using indocyanine green in animal models. J Huazhong Univ Sci Technolog Med Sci. 2017;37:44–50.
28. Wang Y, Cao D, Chen SL, Li YM, Zheng YW, Ohkohchi N. Current trends in three-dimensional visualization and real-time navigation as well as robot-assisted technologies in hepatobiliary surgery. World J Gastrointest Surg. 2021;13(9):904–22. https://doi.org/10.4240/wjgs.v13.i9.904.
29. Akabane M, Shindoh J, Kobayashi Y, Okubo S, Matsumura M, Hashimoto M. Risk stratification of patients with marginal hepatic functional reserve using the remnant hepatocyte uptake index in gadoxetic acid-enhanced magnetic resonance imaging for safe liver surgery. World J Surg. 2023;47(4):1042–8. https://doi.org/10.1007/s00268-023-06888-8.
30. Takahara K, Kusaka M, Shiroki R. Novel three-dimensional workstation system for intraoperative navigation in robot-assisted partial nephrectomy: a single-arm study. JU Open Plus. 2023;1(9):e00048. https://doi.org/10.1097/ju9.0000000000000053.
31. Li Z, Sun YM, Wu FX, Yang LQ, Lu ZJ, Yu WF. Controlled low central venous pressure reduces blood loss and transfusion requirements in hepatectomy. World J Gastroenterol. 2014;20(1):303–9. https://doi.org/10.3748/wjg.v20.i1.303.
32. Berardi G, Wakabayashi G, Igarashi K, et al. Full laparoscopic anatomical segment 8 resection for hepatocellular carcinoma using the Glissonian approach with indocyanine green dye fluorescence. Ann Surg Oncol. 2019;26:2577–8.
33. Abu Hilal M, Tschuor C, Kuemmerli C, López-Ben S, Lesurtel M, Rotellar F. Laparoscopic posterior segmental resections: how I do it: tips and pitfalls. Int J Surg. 2020;82s, 178–186. https://doi.org/10.1016/j.ijsu.2020.06.052.
34. Ban D, Tanabe M, Ito H, et al. A novel difficulty scoring system for laparoscopic liver resection. J Hepatobiliary Pancreat Sci. 2014;21(10):745–53. https://doi.org/10.1002/jhbp.166.
35. Wakabayashi G. What has changed after the Morioka consensus conference 2014 on laparoscopic liver resection? Hepatobiliary Surg Nutr. 2016;5(4):281–9. https://doi.org/10.21037/hbsn.2016.03.03.
36. Tomishige H, Morise Z, Kawabe N, et al. Caudal approach to pure laparoscopic posterior sectionectomy under the laparoscopy-specific view.

World J Gastrointest Surg. 2013;5(6):173–7. https://doi.org/10.4240/wjgs.v5.i6.173.
37. Wakabayashi G, Cherqui D, Geller DA, Han HS, Kaneko H, Buell JF. Laparoscopic hepatectomy is theoretically better than open hepatectomy: preparing for the 2nd international consensus conference on laparoscopic liver resection. J Hepatobiliary Pancreat Sci. 2014;21(10):723–31. https://doi.org/10.1002/jhbp.139.
38. Ogiso S, Nomi T, Araki K, et al. Laparoscopy-specific surgical concepts for hepatectomy based on the laparoscopic caudal view: a key to reboot surgeons' minds. Ann Surg Oncol. 2015;22(Suppl 3):S327–33. https://doi.org/10.1245/s10434-015-4661-6.

Hemostasis and Basics of Hemorrhage Control

15

Alice Zhu, Brittany Greene, and Shiva Jayaraman

Introduction

Despite advances in surgical techniques and perioperative care for patients undergoing liver resection, intraoperative blood loss and need for blood transfusions remain a significant concern in hepatectomies and is a challenge to liver surgeons. Blood loss is independently associated with worse perioperative and long-term outcomes, thus it is paramount to minimize blood loss and blood transfusion in hepatic surgery [1–3]. This chapter will review the basics of hemostasis and hemorrhage control.

A. Zhu
Division of General Surgery, Department of Surgery,
University of Toronto, Toronto, ON, Canada

B. Greene · S. Jayaraman (✉)
Division of General Surgery, Department of Surgery,
University of Toronto, Toronto, ON, Canada

HPB Surgery Service, Division of General Surgery, St. Joseph's Health Centre, Unity Health Toronto, Toronto, ON, Canada
e-mail: Shiva.Jayaraman@unityhealth.to

© The Author(s), under exclusive license to Springer Nature Switzerland AG 2025
A. Alseidi et al. (eds.), *The SAGES Manual of Contemporary Indications and Management of Hepatic and Biliary Diseases*, https://doi.org/10.1007/978-3-032-04823-3_15

Preoperative Care and Planning

Minimizing blood loss starts outside of the operating room with patient preoperative optimization and careful planning.

Risk Assessment, Anemia Assessment, and Anemia Management

Individual patient transfusion risk should be assessed preoperatively using a validated hepatectomy transfusion risk score [4–6]. Identification of high-risk patients will direct the use of blood management interventions, such as iron supplementation and intraoperative pharmacologic agents such as topical hemostatic agents [4]. Preoperative anemia should be routinely assessed at the initial consultation to allow for adequate time to identify anemia and its cause [4, 7, 8]. Work-up for anemia should include complete blood count, and in patients with anemia, include ferritin, transferrin saturation, vitamin B12, and creatinine [4]. Preoperative anemia, defined by hemoglobin of </= 130 g/L should be treated to reduce the risk for intraoperative red blood cell transfusion. Patients with iron-deficient anemia (serum ferritin <30ug/L or serum ferritin <100ug/L if transferrin saturation < 20%) should be initiated on oral iron supplementation prior to surgery. If time to surgery is less than 4 weeks, or if patients cannot tolerate oral iron, intravenous iron is recommended [4, 8–10]. The routine use of erythropoiesis-stimulating agents and autologous blood donation prior to liver resection are currently not recommended [4].

Vascular Anatomy

Understanding of the patient's vascular anatomy and identification of variants plays an important role in operative planning. Routine computed tomographic angiography should be performed in all patients undergoing liver resection. Accurate preoperative delineation of hepatic vascular anatomy and evaluation of the parenchyma provide critical information to the surgeon [11]. In cases of hepatic tumor resection, multiplanar reformation and 3D reconstruction provide a vascular road map for understanding the relationship of the tumor and adjacent vasculature [11].

In the preoperative state, it is crucial to carefully review the inflow pedicles and outflow veins and identify any variant anatomy. Aberrant hepatic veins can be a source of excessive hemorrhage if not recognized prior to surgery. The most common venous variant is an accessory right hepatic vein (RHV), occurring in 52.5% of patients [11, 12]. Another venous variant is the early branching of the vein that drains segment VIII into the middle hepatic vein [11]. Common hepatic arterial variants include a replaced or accessory left hepatic artery (LHA), branching from the left gastric artery and replaced or accessory right hepatic artery, branching from the superior mesenteric artery [11]. Portal venous anatomy is also crucial for preoperative planning. Portal venous variants, including the trifurcation of the portal vein and separate origin of the right posterior portal vein may also affect surgical technique [11, 13]. We recommend a thorough review of vascular anatomy and discussion of cases at multi-disciplinary boards prior to all cases. Knowledge of vascular anatomy and variants, particularly sectoral and segmental pedicles, is key in preventing inadvertent injury to aberrant hepatic vessels, and avoiding undue hemorrhage and postoperative hepatic infarction.

Non-operative Techniques

In addition to refinement in surgical techniques, improvements in outcomes of liver resections are largely due to advancements in anesthetic and perioperative care.

Low Central Venous Pressure Anesthesia

Maintaining low central venous pressure (CVP) anesthesia has been demonstrated to result in decreased blood loss, transfusion requirements, and perioperative morbidity in liver resections

[14–16]. This is based on the premise that blood loss during hepatectomy is largely derived from the backflow from hepatic veins and the vena cava, and blood loss is therefore exacerbated from hypervolemic or normovolemic fluid resuscitation.

In the pretransection phase, low CVP is primarily established through restrictive volume administration. Here, intravenous fluids of <1 ml/kg/h and urine output of 25 ml/h is accepted [17]. Close communication with the anesthesiologist and preoperative nursing teams is important to prevent liberal crystalloid infusions prior to the patient's entry into the Operating Room. Trendelenburg positioning can also be used to increase venous return to the heart, while decreasing CVP in the vena cava [17]. Pharmacologic adjuncts, including loop diuretics, morphine, and intravenous nitroglycerin, have also been shown to assist in achieving a low CVP [17]. However, with judicious fluid administration, these agents are seldomly used. Hypoventilation to decrease intrathoracic pressures and subsequently CVP has also been demonstrated [18]. The results of a randomized control trial, however, do not support differences in bleeding despite reduction in CVP obtained via hypoventilation [18]. Clamping of infrahepatic inferior vena cava has also been shown to effectively decrease CVP and significantly reduce blood loss [19, 20]. This technique, however, has been associated with a significant increase in postoperative pulmonary embolism [19]. Hypovolemic phlebotomy has also been discussed to decrease CVP and blood loss [21]. Evidence however is limited to small sample size retrospective reviews and there is currently no consensus on recommendation for or against its routine use [4].

In the post-transection phase, once the specimen has been removed and hemostasis achieved. Restoration of euvolemia with fluids and normalization of blood pressure and urine output has been associated with decreased operative blood loss [17].

Autotransfusion and Cell-Salvage

Several strategies for autotransfusion have been described. First, preoperative autologous blood (PABD) donation, whereby patients donate blood in advance of surgery which can then be transfused in the perioperative period. In patients undergoing liver resections, however, PABD does not reduce the need for allogenic red blood cell transfusion or improve perioperative outcomes [22, 23]. Furthermore, this technique is limited by high processing costs, and a high rate of wasted blood prodcts [24].

Second, acute normovolemic hemodilution (ANH) whereby whole blood from patients is removed immediately before surgery and patients are autotransfused during the posttransection phase. Meta-analysis including 4 randomized trials demonstrates a significant reduction for allogenic transfusion with ANH [25]. Limitations of the technique include that it is labor intensive and can lead to transient hypotension [17]. In patients with intraoperative blood loss >/= 800 ml, ANH has been shown to reduce allogenic red cell transfusion as well as the need for fresh frozen plasma [26]. Its use should be considered in patients who are at high risk of major blood loss.

Thirdly, intraoperative cell salvage (ICS) is routinely used in high blood loss procedures and has been shown to reduce the allogenic red blood cell transfusion [27]. Concerns for this technique include oncologic safety of cell-salvage and availability of the equipment. Although there is a theoretical concern of dissemination of malignant cells, meta-analysis has failed to identify evidence that ICS increases the risk of tumor recurrence [28]. This data, however, is limited by retrospective study designs and oncological safety remains uncertain [28].

Pharmacologic Agents

The use of pharmacologic agents may reduce bleeding and transfusion requirements in surgery. There is strong evidence to support antifibrinolytic agents such as aprotinin and tranexamic acid to reduce blood loss and transfusion requirements in high blood loss procedures such as trauma and cardiac surgery [29, 30]. Although fewer trials have evaluated the effects of antifibrinolytics on hemostasis in elective liver resections, smaller randomized studies have shown both tranexamic acid and aprotinin can decrease intraoperative blood loss and transfusion requirements [31, 32]. However, the recent HeLIX trial, found that among patients undergoing liver resection for cancer-related indications, tranexamic acid did not reduce bleeding or blood transfusion, and was associated with an increased rate of perioperative complications, without a significant differences in thromboembolism events [33]. Concerns for thromboembolic complications have not been demonstrated in large prospective trials [34].

Procoagulant agents, including recombinant factor VIIa, antithrombin III, and desmopressin, have been studied with disappointing results in randomized controlled trials [29]. These drugs have not been shown to control perioperative bleeding, and is currently not recommended in patients undergoing hepatic resection [17].

Surgical Strategies

Vascular Occlusion

Intermittent inflow occlusion during hepatic resection is recommended to reduce blood loss during hepatic resection [4]. This involves placing a non-crushing vascular clamp on the porta hepatis to occlude the hepatic artery and portal vein (Pringle maneuver). Depending on the extent of the planned resection, selective clamping of the right, left, or sectoral pedicles can provide adequate inflow occlusion while limiting ischemia to the remnant liver. Intermittent pedicular clamping with 15–20 min clamping and alternating with 5-min reperfusion periods is safe and well tolerated in patients with both normal and abnormal liver parenchyma [35]. There is conflicting evidence to support hepatic vascular exclusion in minimizing blood loss or transfusion requirements [36]. As such, hepatic vascular exclusions are currently not recommended for routine liver resection [4].

Intraoperative Ultrasound

Intraoperative ultrasound is an invaluable tool in hepatic surgery that allows for the identification and characterization of vascular and biliary structures during liver resections. It is a safe and inexpensive technique that can be used dynamically in the operating room by the surgeon to map out vascular anatomy and avoid inadvertent bleeding. When used to guide resection, intraoperative ultrasound enables a three-dimensional hepatic vessel reconstruction, thereby accurately describing the hepatic segmental boundaries and anatomic variations.

Parenchymal Transection

The risk of blood loss is significant during parenchymal transection of the liver due to lack of mechanisms such as vasoconstriction within hepatic sinusoids. Considerable research have been done into transection method and transection device. It is generally recommended that surgeons choose the technique based on level of comfort, experience, and specific procedure [4]. Specific approaches are discussed in detail in the Chap. 13.

Remnant Surface Management and Topical Hemostatic Agents

Following transection, significant blood loss can occur from the raw liver surface leading to clinically significant hemorrhage. Surgeons must inspect the cut surface of liver remnant meticulously to identify small vessel bleeding, which can be easily controlled with suture ligation, clips, or other topical sealing techniques.

Topical hemostatic agents should be used as an adjunct after parenchymal transection [4]. Available agents can be classified as (1) hemostatic matrix agents, (2) coagulation factor-based agents, and (3) combination agents (Table 15.1).

Matrix agents provide a scaffold for endogenous coagulation to occur. They do not contain active coagulation factors. Typical composition includes collagen, cellulose, gelatin, and microporous polysaccharide spheres. Examples include Avitene, Instat, Surgicel, Gelfoam, Surgifoam, and Arista. Coagulation factor-

Table 15.1 Topical hemostatic agents

Agent	Mechanism	Active component	Examples
Matrix agents	Provides scaffold for endogenous coagulation	Collagen, cellulose, Gelatin, microporous polysaccharide spheres	Avitene, Instat, Surgicel, Gelfoam, Surgifoam, arista
Coagulation factor-based agents	Reenact endogenous coagulation cascade	Fibrin sealant, topical thrombin	Tisseel, Evithrom
Combination agents	Combination of the above	Gelatin/thrombin, collagen/fibrinogen/thrombin	Floseal, Surgiflo, Tachosil

Adopted from Eason and Karanicolas (2016), Surg Clin N Am, 96 (2) 219–229

based agents typically contain fibrin sealant (fibrinogen and thrombin) with other various coagulation co-factors. They serve to reenact the endogenous coagulation cascade. Common agents include Tisseel and Evithrom. Combination agents such as Floseal, Surgiflo, and TachoSil contain both active hemostatic components as well as a coagulation matrix. It is important to note that although these agents have been shown to reduce time to hemostasis and increase rates of obtaining complete intraoperative hemostasis, there is no evidence that topical agents reduce amount of blood loss, transfusion requirements, or peri-operative morbidity in liver resections [37, 38]. Thus, it is recommended that these agents be used as adjuncts [4]. Furthermore, no one particular agent demonstrates superiority over the others [4, 17].

Operative Toolbox

Preoperative planning as outlined above plays an important role in minimizing intraoperative blood loss. Bleeding, however, can occur unexpectedly and it is important to be prepared for it.

When bleeding is encountered unexpectedly, it is crucial to remain calm. Temporizing measures can be taken to minimize blood loss when unexpected bleeding is encountered, allowing time for resuscitation, assessment of the situation, and call for help if necessary. In this section, we describe operative techniques/useful tools for the surgeon when bleeding is encountered in open surgery and in laparoscopic surgery.

Open Surgery

Manual Compression and Peripheratic Packing

Manual compression with the surgeon's hand may help tamponade bleeding from raw liver surfaces. This allows rapid temporary control of the bleeding sufficient time for resuscitation. Perihepatic packing is a common technique used for hemostasis in liver trauma and hepatic injury. In elective liver resection, like manual compression, this technique is used to provide temporary control. Perihepatic packing can be accomplished via introducing a sponge at the site of bleeding.

Pringle Maneuver

If manual compression fails, a Pringle maneuver can be easily applied to control hemorrhage. The maneuver clamps across the porta hepatis, interrupting hepatic arterial and portal venous inflow into the liver. If clamping of the porta successfully reduces bleeding, hemorrhage is more likely related to hepatic inflow, whereas ongoing bleeding suggests a hepatic outflow source. As noted above, the Pringle maneuver should be temporary and not exceed 30 minutes at a time and temporary release to allow reperfusion is recommended.

Direct Liver Suturing

When there is ongoing bleeding from the liver, directly suturing the liver can be helpful. Depending on the situation, a single stitch or a continuous suture may be needed to obtain hemostasis. Regardless, all open surgical sets should have a hemostatic suture, such as a 5–0 prolene, loaded and ready to go in the event of unexpected bleeding.

Laparoscopic Surgery

Compression and Perihepatic Packing

Similar to open surgery, direct compression and perihepatic packing can be done as a first step when bleeding is encountered. Laparoscopically, one can introduce a sponge or a piece of Surgicel with hemostatic properties and apply direct pressure. If the bleeding stopped with pressure, it is important to release the pressure as well as the pneumoperitoneum for several minutes to reassess if bleeding reoccurs without pressure. If bleeding restarts, reapply pressure.

Lowering Central Venous Pressure and Increasing Pneumoperitoneum

Low central venous pressure (CVP) anesthesia is safe and has been demonstrated to decrease blood loss as described earlier in this chapter. In laparoscopy, positive pressure insufflation of the peritoneal cavity using carbon dioxide (CO_2) is required to allow visualization. Increasing pneumoperitoneum has also been shown to decrease hepatic perfusion [39], and can therefore be used to the surgeon's benefit when bleeding is encountered. The counterpressure exerted by pneumoperitoneum also contributes to hemostasis during laparoscopic hepatectomy by tamponade [40]. The combination of low CVP and positive pressure pneumoperitoneum during laparoscopic liver parenchymal resection, however, runs the theoretical risk of air emboli when insufflation pressures exceed CVP [41]. In animal models studying the association between CVP and pneumoperitoneum, gas embolisms occurred typically during dissection near the left hepatic vein, and tended to be transient and subclinical [42]. Regardless, care must be taken when dissecting around large veins and both the anesthesiology and surgical teams must be aware of the potential for CO_2 embolism.

Increasing Exposure and Improving Visualization

It is crucial to have adequate exposure and visualization when bleeding is encountered during parenchymal transection. This may necessitate the insertion of additional ports. In laparoscopic cases where the liver bed is bleeding, one can consider placing a Nathanson retractor through the epigastric port and/or placing a fan retractor on the porta hepatis to increase visualization. Mobilization of the falciform with an energy device can also be considered to allow maximum cephalad retraction and exposure.

Pringle Maneuver

In any laparoscopic liver resection where bleeding may be encountered, we recommend having tools for a Pringle maneuver set up and ready for inflow occlusion, prior to starting parenchymal transection. Even in cases that are seemingly straightforward such as a small wedge resection or left lateral sectionectomy, having a Pringle maneuver prepared can be helpful.

To establish the Pringle maneuver laparoscopically, a disposable 5 mm plastic trochar is first introduced into the left upper quadrant. An umbilical tape marked at its midpoint should be passed through the pars flaccida and foramen of Winslow, with the center of the tape aligned at the porta, and the ends brought through the disposable trochar. Should inflow occlusion be necessary, the trochar can quickly be advanced over the umbilical tape and secured with a clamp on the tape externally (Video 1, Laparoscopic Pringle Maneuver) [43].

Direct Liver Suturing—The "Quick Stitch"

Direct liver suturing can be used to control ongoing oozing from the liver parenchyma. In the laparoscopic liver set up, we recommend having at least two laparoscopic "quick stitches" readily available (Video 2, Laparoscopic Liver Quick-Stitch) [44]. We use a 2-0 or 3-0 silk suture cut to 20 cm with two metal clips applied perpendicular to the suture, near the end, loaded on a laparoscopic needle driver for expeditious placement of stitches when needed. The perpendicular clips at the end of the suture help compress bleeding once the stitch is deployed and prevent the stitch from pulling through, allowing for quick control of bleeding. A figure of eight or a running suture line may be necessary to achieve hemostasis with the stitch. In lieu of knot-tying, a clip is placed at the junction of the suture and the parenchyma to secure the stitch. This maneuver typically provides definitive control of bleeding. Additional sutures can be placed as needed.

Conversion to Open and Calling for Help
Bleeding in laparoscopy can be challenging to control. With patient safety as the top priority, it is crucial to remain calm and call for help early. If the above strategies do not obtain hemostasis or the surgeon does not feel comfortable to continue laparoscopically, conversion to open may be required. Conversion should not be seen as a failure, but rather another tool in the hemostatic toolbox.

Note on Energy Adjuncts

Conventional electrocautery or argon beam coagulation can be used to control mild bleeding from raw liver surface and can be used with topical hemostatic agents as adjuncts. Electrocautery works via desiccation and is only effective for small vessels (</= 5 mm). Argon plasma coagulation (APC) delivers electrical energy through an arc of ionized gas, providing monopolar electrothermal hemostasis. APC has the advantage of preventing the electrode to stick to the tissue [45], and has therefore become a standard tool used to achieve secondary hemostasis by sealing the cut edge of the liver. When used in confined spaces such as laparoscopic procedures, however, there is a risk of argon gas embolism and subsequent cardiac arrest caused by intra-abdominal over-pressurization [46]. Larger vessels should be clipped or suture ligated. See Chap. 13 for further details.

Summary

The potential for major blood loss remains a significant concern for patients undergoing liver surgery. Strategies to minimize intraoperative blood loss starts with preoperative care and planning, identification of high-risk patients, optimizing modifiable factors, and reviewing patient's anatomy. Intraoperatively, non-operative techniques such as lowering central venous pressure and increasing pneumoperitoneum in laparoscopy can help with minimizing blood loss and require cooperation between the surgeon and anesthesiologist. Surgeons should also be aware of operative techniques and tools available such that they are prepared when unexpected bleeding is encountered.

Laparoscopic Pearls

- Optimizing visualization and exposure is key.
- Have two laparoscopic "quick-stitches" readily available (Video 2—Laparoscopic Liver Quick-Stitch).
- Have a Pringle maneuver set up and ready around the porta prior to parenchymal transection (Video 1—Video-Pringle maneuver).
- Patient's safety should be the priority. Remain calm, recognize bleeding, and calling for help early is not a sign of weakness.
- Conversion to open in a laparoscopic case should not be seen as a failure.

Open Surgery Pearls

- Hemostatic sutures (i.e., 5–0 prolene) and topical agents should be easily accessible.
- Be prepared to apply a Pringle maneuver.
- Temporary measures such as manual compression and perihepatic packing are fast and effective ways to control bleeding until further assessments can be made.

References

1. Hallet J, Tsang M, Cheng ESW, et al. The impact of perioperative red blood cell transfusions on long-term outcomes after hepatectomy for colorectal liver metastases. Ann Surg Oncol. 2015;22:4038–45.
2. Bui LL, Smith AJ, Mark B, et al. Minimising blood loss and transfusion requirements in hepatic resection. HPB. 2002;4:5–10.
3. Jarnagin WR, Gonen M, Fong Y, et al. Improvement in perioperative outcome after hepatic resection. Ann Surg. 2002;236:397–407.
4. Hallet J, Jayaraman S, Martel G, et al. Patient blood management for liver resection: consensus statements using Delphi methodology. HPB. 2019;21:393–404.
5. Lemke M, Mahar A, Karanicolas PJ, et al. Three point transfusion risk score in hepatectomy: an external validation using the American College of Surgeons—National Surgical Quality Improvement Program (ACS-NSQIP). HPB. 2018;20:669–75.
6. HPB CONCEPT Team. Three-point transfusion risk score in hepatectomy. Br J Surg. 2017;104:434–42.
7. Kotzé A, Harris A, Baker C, et al. British Committee for Standards in haematology guidelines on the identification and management of preoperative anaemia. Br J Haematol. 2015;171:322–31.
8. Muñoz M, Acheson AG, Auerbach M, et al. International consensus statement on the peri-operative management of anaemia and iron deficiency. Anaesthesia. 2017;72:233–47.
9. Hallet J, Hanif A, Callum J, et al. The impact of perioperative iron on the use of red blood cell transfusions in gastrointestinal surgery: a systematic review and meta-analysis. Transfus Med Rev. 2014;28:205–11.
10. Froessler B, Palm P, Weber I, et al. The important role for intravenous iron in perioperative patient blood management in major abdominal surgery. Ann Surg. 2016;264:41–6.
11. Sahani D, Mehta A, Blake M, et al. Preoperative hepatic vascular evaluation with CT and MR angiography: implications for surgery. Radiographics. 2004;24:1367–80.
12. Soyer P, Heath D, Bluemke DA, et al. Three-dimensional helical CT of intrahepatic venous structures: comparison of three rendering techniques. J Comput Assist Tomogr. 1996;20:122.
13. Cheng YF, Huang TL, Lee TY, et al. Variation of the intrahepatic portal vein; angiographic demonstration and application in living-related hepatic transplantation. Transplant Proc. 1996;28:1667–8.
14. Melendez JA, Arslan V, Fischer ME, et al. Perioperative outcomes of major hepatic resections under low central venous pressure anesthesia: blood loss, blood transfusion, and the risk of postoperative renal dysfunction. J Am Coll Surg. 1998;187:620–5.

15. Wang W-D, Liang L-J, Huang X-Q, et al. Low central venous pressure reduces blood loss in hepatectomy. World J Gastroenterol. 2006;12:935–9.
16. Smyrniotis V, Kostopanagiotou G, Theodoraki K, et al. The role of central venous pressure and type of vascular control in blood loss during major liver resections. Am J Surg. 2004;187:398–402.
17. Eeson G, Karanicolas PJ. Hemostasis and hepatic surgery. Surg Clin N Am. 2016;96:219–28.
18. Hasegawa K, Takayama T, Orii R, et al. Effect of hypoventilation on bleeding during hepatic resection: a randomized controlled trial. Arch Surg. 2002;137:311–5.
19. Rahbari NN, Koch M, Zimmermann JB, et al. Infrahepatic inferior vena cava clamping for reduction of central venous pressure and blood loss during hepatic resection: a randomized controlled trial. Ann Surg. 2011;253:1102.
20. Zhu P, Lau W-Y, Chen Y-F, et al. Randomized clinical trial comparing infrahepatic inferior vena cava clamping with low central venous pressure in complex liver resections involving the Pringle manoeuvre. Br J Surg. 2012;99:781–8.
21. Ryckx A, Christiaens C, Clarysse M, et al. Central venous pressure drop after hypovolemic phlebotomy is a strong independent predictor of intraoperative blood loss during liver resection. Ann Surg Oncol. 2017;24:1367–75.
22. Hashimoto T, Kokudo N, Orii R, et al. Intraoperative blood salvage during liver resection: a randomized controlled trial. Ann Surg. 2007;245:686.
23. Park JO, Gonen M, D'Angelica MI, et al. Autologous versus allogeneic transfusions: no difference in perioperative outcome after partial hepatectomy. J Gastrointest Surg. 2007;11:1286–93.
24. Sima CS, Jarnagin WR, Fong Y, et al. Predicting the risk of perioperative transfusion for patients undergoing elective hepatectomy. Ann Surg. 2009;250:914–21.
25. Gurusamy KS, Li J, Vaughan J, et al. Cardiopulmonary interventions to decrease blood loss and blood transfusion requirements for liver resection. Cochrane Database Syst Rev. 2012; https://doi.org/10.1002/14651858.CD007338.pub3.
26. Jarnagin WR, Gonen M, Maithel SK, et al. A prospective randomized trial of acute Normovolemic Hemodilution compared to standard intraoperative management in patients undergoing major hepatic resection. Ann Surg. 2008;248:360.
27. Carless PA, Henry DA, Moxey AJ, et al. Cell salvage for minimising perioperative allogeneic blood transfusion. Cochrane Database Syst Rev. 3

28. Waters JH, Yazer M, Chen Y-F, et al. Blood salvage and cancer surgery: a meta-analysis of available studies. Transfusion. 2012;52:2167–73.
29. Gurusamy KS, Li J, Sharma D, et al. Pharmacological interventions to decrease blood loss and blood transfusion requirements for liver resection. Cochrane Database Syst Rev. 2009:CD008085.
30. CRASH-2 Trial Collaborators, Shakur H, Roberts I, et al. Effects of tranexamic acid on death, vascular occlusive events, and blood transfusion in trauma patients with significant haemorrhage (CRASH-2): a randomised, placebo-controlled trial. Lancet. 2010;376:23–32.
31. Wu C-C, Ho W-M, Cheng S-B, et al. Perioperative parenteral tranexamic acid in liver tumor resection: a prospective randomized trial toward a "blood transfusion"-free hepatectomy. Ann Surg. 2006;243:173.
32. Lentschener C, Benhamou D, Mercier FJ, et al. Aprotinin reduces blood loss in patients undergoing elective liver resection. Anesth Analg. 1997;84:875–81.
33. Karanicolas PJ, Lin Y, McCluskey SA, et al. Tranexamic Acid in Patients Undergoing Liver Resection: The HeLiX Randomized Clinical Trial. JAMA. 2024;332(13):1080–9.
34. Henry DA, Carless PA, Moxey AJ, et al. Anti-fibrinolytic use for minimising perioperative allogeneic blood transfusion. Cochrane Database Syst Rev. 2011; https://doi.org/10.1002/14651858.CD001886.pub4.
35. Belghiti J, Noun R, Malafosse R, et al. Continuous versus intermittent portal triad clamping for liver resection: a controlled study. Ann Surg. 1999;229:369–75.
36. Gurusamy KS, Kumar Y, Sharma D, et al. Methods of vascular occlusion for elective liver resections. Cochrane Database Syst Rev. 2007; https://doi.org/10.1002/14651858.CD006409.pub2.
37. Boonstra EA, Molenaar IQ, Porte RJ, et al. Topical haemostatic agents in liver surgery: do we need them? HPB. 2009;11:306–10.
38. Sanjay P, Watt DG, Wigmore SJ. Systematic review and meta-analysis of haemostatic and Biliostatic efficacy of fibrin sealants in elective liver surgery. J Gastrointest Surg. 2013;17:829–36.
39. Hashikura Y, Kawasaki S, Munakata Y, et al. Effects of peritoneal insufflation on hepatic and renal blood flow. Surg Endosc. 1994;8:759–61.
40. Are C, Fong Y, Geller DA. Laparoscopic liver resections. Adv Surg. 2005;39:57–75.
41. Lantz PE, Smith JD. Fatal carbon dioxide embolism complicating attempted laparoscopic cholecystectomy—case report and literature review. J Forensic Sci. 1994;39:1468–80.
42. Jayaraman S, Khakhar A, Yang H, et al. The association between central venous pressure, pneumoperitoneum, and venous carbon dioxide embolism in laparoscopic hepatectomy. Surg Endosc. 2009;23:2369–73.
43. Jayaraman S. Laparoscopic Pringle Maneuver: 3 ways. Youtube. Available from: https://www.youtube.com/watch?v=PEbUTLJm1qQ&t=4s

44. Jayaraman S. I love the liver quick stitch. Youtube. Available from: https://www.youtube.com/watch?v=BNiJAyUUvds
45. Raiser J, Zenker M. Argon plasma coagulation for open surgical and endoscopic applications: state of the art. J Phys D Appl Phys. 2006;39:3520.
46. Kono M, Yahagi N, Kitahara M, et al. Cardiac arrest associated with use of an argon beam coagulator during laparoscopic cholecystectomy. Br J Anaesth. 2001;87:644–6.

Assessment of the Hepatic Remnant and Preoperative Imaging

16

Matthew Dixon, Jordan Tasse, and Sam Pappas

Introduction

Hepatectomy can be considered for patients with both primary hepatic malignancies (such as hepatocellular carcinoma (HCC) and intrahepatic and perihilar cholangiocarcinoma) as well as secondary hepatic malignancies (such as metastases secondary to colorectal cancer and neuroendocrine tumors). Preparation for hepatectomy heavily relies on adequate preoperative imaging to identify number, size, and location of tumors, but also to adequately assess intrahepatic anatomy of the portal pedicles as well as the hepatic veins and their branches. Due to inflow or outflow involvement, or size and multiplicity of tumor burden, a major hepatectomy (resection of 3 or more segments) is often required. In such cases, the hepatobiliary surgeon must carefully consider the size of the future liver remnant (FLR) as well in order to miti-

M. Dixon (✉) · S. Pappas
Division of Surgical Oncology, Rush University Medical Center, Chicago, IL, USA
e-mail: Matthew_Dixon@rush.edu

J. Tasse
Department of Interventional Radiology, Rush University Medical Center, Chicago, IL, USA

© The Author(s), under exclusive license to Springer Nature Switzerland AG 2025
A. Alseidi et al. (eds.), *The SAGES Manual of Contemporary Indications and Management of Hepatic and Biliary Diseases*, https://doi.org/10.1007/978-3-032-04823-3_16

gate the incidence of post-hepatectomy liver failure (PHLF) [1–3]. This chapter will discuss preoperative imaging prior to hepatectomy, calculation and assessment of the FLR, and techniques to manipulate the volume of the FLR.

Preoperative Imaging

Diagnostic imaging for patients who are potential candidates for a hepatectomy is relied upon heavily for preoperative planning. First, it is important in the detection of any extrahepatic disease that may otherwise alter treatment planning for a major hepatectomy. It also allows for assessment of the size, location, and relationship to critical vascular inflow and outflow structures. In the case of colorectal liver metastases (CRLM), it also allows for assessment of multiplicity and distribution of disease [4]. Depending on the malignancy type, preoperative imaging practices can vary between centers and for several diseases, there is no consensus on optimal imaging strategy.

Ultrasound

Ultrasound is a versatile and inexpensive imaging modality that is not uncommonly the initial imaging modality ordered in the evaluation of patients with liver lesions. It is a useful screening tool for patients at an elevated risk of developing HCC. As a surveillance test, it has a sensitivity ranging from 58% to 89% for detecting HCC in high-risk patients [5, 6]. For HCC <5 cm, the lesions often appear hypoechoic, but may appear hyperechoic from fatty infiltration [7, 8]. Larger tumors can appear heterogenous because of tumor necrosis [9]. Intrahepatic cholangiocarcinoma can be hyperechoic or hypoechoic [10, 11]. Perihilar cholangiocarcinoma is often identified by the presence of upstream biliary dilation that converges at the biliary confluence and the tumors are usually isoechoic [12]. An initial diagnosis of CRLM on ultrasound is not typical, as these lesions are more often discovered on staging cross-sectional imaging [13, 14]. For the purposes of preoperative evaluation, however, ultrasound has a limited role as it suffers from low sensitivity, and inability to assess for extrahepatic disease [15, 16]. In contrast, intraoperative ultrasound is a very effective tool for performance of a safe hepatectomy and familiarity with this technique is a critical component of the hepatobiliary surgeon's armamentarium.

Multidetector Computed Tomography

Multidetector computed tomography (MDCT) is one of the most widely available, and therefore one of the most commonly used imaging modalities in the preoperative planning for hepatic tumors. Advantages include superior spatial resolution and with the use of intravenous (IV) contrast, portal pedicles and hepatic veins can be used as landmarks to localize tumors to specific segments, and are very useful for surgical planning [17]. Limitations of MDCT include difficulty with investigation of lesions <1 cm, as well as difficulty with evaluating hepatic lesions in the presence of steatosis, which can be common in patients with primary liver tumors arising in the setting of steatohepatitis, or patients who have had prior chemotherapy (as is the case with many CRLM patients). Other disadvantages include use of ionizing radiation as well as not infrequent allergies to the IV contrast. IV contrast use is contraindicated in renal insufficiency.

Use of IV contrast and the timing of image acquisition are important for lesion characterization and relationship to intrahepatic structures. Routine CT imaging will typically only use the portal venous phase, and because most hepatic tumors are hypovascular relative to the adjacent liver parenchyma, lesions are often most conspicuous on this phase [17]. Acquisition of a triple-phase (non-contrast, arterial phase, portal venous phase) or quadruple phase (triple-phase, plus a delayed venous phase) MDCT often leads to better lesion characterization and relationship to critical intrahepatic structures.

Useful information can be gathered from all phases. On non-contrast imaging, attenuation values of 54–80 Hounsfield units (HU) are normal. This value can be increased in the setting of hemochromatosis for example, and decreased in the setting of steatohepatitis [17]. Arterial phase images are typically acquired 30 seconds after administration of IV contrast. These images are useful for characterizing arterial anatomy, including aberrant hepatic arterial anatomy, as well as for lesion characterization, which is important as the majority of primary and secondary neoplasms receive most of their blood supply from the hepatic arterial system [17, 18]. Hypervascular neoplasms such as HCC or metastatic neuroendocrine tumors often enhance prominently on this phase with minimal enhancement of the normal parenchyma and have rapid washout and become isoattenuating to the rest of the liver on the portal venous phase. The portal phase is typically obtained 60–70 s after contrast administration. This phase provides the optimal contrast differential between hypovascular lesions such as CRLM, and the surrounding liver parenchyma (which unlike the arterial phase, enhances maximally on the portal phase). This phase also provides clear delineation of the portal veins and the hepatic veins. The delayed venous phase is typically obtained 3–5 min after administration of contrast. Hypervascular tumors, like HCC, will typically be hypoattenuating to the surrounding liver parenchyma on this phase, and more fibrotic tumors such as cholangiocarcinoma and some metastatic lesions will hold onto contrast longer and appear hyperattenuating to the normal parenchyma on this phase [17].

Magnetic Resonance Imaging

Magnetic resonance imaging (MRI), unlike MDCT, does not utilize ionizing radiation. With superior tissue contrast resolution, MRI is better suited to characterizing hepatic lesions, and is superior to MDCT for detecting lesions <1 cm in size. It can also offer similar ability as CT to delineate the relationship of hepatic lesions to critical hepatic inflow and outflow structures on the IV contrast phases.

MRI sequences are often grouped according to longitudinal (T1) relaxation along the magnetic axis, and transverse (T2) relaxation along the magnetic axis. There are differences in these relaxation times for various soft tissues, and this can be used to improve imaging contrast and diagnostic accuracy. Diffusion weighted imaging (DWI) measures the motion of water molecules in tissues, which can be affected by pathologic conditions, and is a part of standard liver MRI protocols. DWI images can be very useful for detecting and characterizing liver lesions as well as assessing treatment response. Use of IV contrast has also improved lesion detection and hepatic lesion characterization as well. Two commonly used IV contrast agents for characterizing hepatobiliary tumors include gadobenic acid (MultiHance; Bracco Imaging) and gadoxetic acid (Eovist; Bayer Healthcare). Both IV contrasts are preferentially taken up by hepatocytes and excreted by the biliary system. Thus, these contrasts are useful for detecting lesions as well as characterizing intrahepatic anatomy on the delayed phase (10–20 min after IV administration). On the 20-min delayed phases, hepatocytes have retained some of the contrast and appear bright, in contrast to lesions and intrahepatic vasculature which appear dark. Furthermore, some of the contrast has been excreted into the biliary system at this point, and the biliary anatomy can be assessed on this phase of the scan as well (Fig. 16.1). Utilization of hepatocyte-specific contrast has improved detection of more metastatic lesions compared to conventional MRI, and contrast-enhanced MDCT [19, 20]. By combining hepatobiliary phase

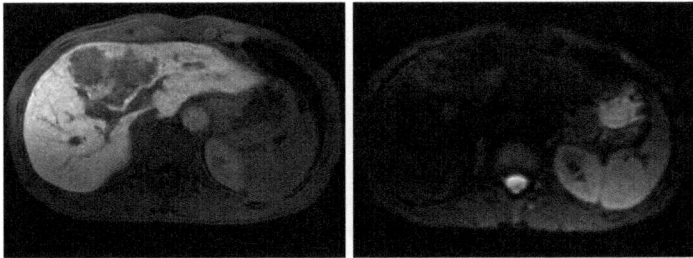

Fig. 16.1 MRI study of a patient with a single large colorectal liver metastasis. The left-hand panel depicts the 20 min delayed phase images after injection of Eovist IV contrast. The right-hand panel depicts the diffusion-weighted images

contrast sequences with DWI sequences, this achieves a high detection rate, in particular for small liver lesions, with a sensitivity of 95.5% [19].

Disadvantages of MRI include higher cost and longer acquisition time. This longer acquisition time can often be significant for patients who suffer from claustrophobia, as these patients will not be able to tolerate undergoing an MRI. An absolute contraindication to MRI is for patients with metallic implants that are not MRI compatible.

Determination of the Future Liver Remnant

Calculation of the FLR relies heavily on good preoperative imaging and volumetry. Several software programs exist that allow clinicians to outline individual segments of the liver, as well as the entire FLR, which allows an estimation of the actual volume in cm [3] of the FLR. This is a critical first step, however this absolute volume is of little value, and must be considered in the context of the overall liver volume.

In general, there are two methods for estimating volume of the FLR. The first method directly determines the FLR as a proportion of the non-tumor-bearing liver:

$$TLV_{Measured} = V_{Total\,Liver} - V_{Total\,Tumor}$$

$$FLR_{Measured} = LRV\,/\,TLV_{Measured} \times 100\%$$

Using this methodology, the measured total liver volume ($TLV_{Measured}$, expressed in cm [3]) is determined by first measuring the volume of the entire liver ($V_{Total\,Liver}$, expressed in cm [3]), and subtracting the total volume of all tumors ($V_{Total\,Tumor}$, expressed in cm [3]). Once $TLV_{Measured}$ is determined, the liver remnant volume (LRV, expressed in cm [3]) is divided by $TLV_{Measured}$ to determine $FLR_{Measured}$ (expressed as %). This methodology of determining the FLR likely intuitively makes the most sense, however there are several disadvantages of this method. These include errors in measurement due to partial volume effect as well as respiratory changes. Furthermore, calculation of all tumor volumes in patients with multiple liver metastases can be quite tedious with high inter-observer variability [21].

The second method employs a standardized approach across patients. In this approach, the LRV is derived in the same manner, estimating its volume based on CT or MRI images. However, the difference lies in how the TLV is estimated. In an effort to estimate the hepatic metabolic demands for individual patients, Vauthey et al. [21] examined the relationship between body surface area (BSA) and liver size, and demonstrated the presence of a linear relationship between BSA and TLV:

$$TLV_{Standard} = (1267.28 \times BSA) - 794.41$$

$$FLR_{Standard} = LRV / TLV_{Standard} \times 100\%$$

The standardized TLV (TLV$_{Standard}$, expressed in cm [3]) is estimated as a function of BSA,

which is often determined using the Mosteller formula:

$$BSA = \sqrt{\frac{[height(cm) \times weight(kg)]}{3600}}$$

The standardized liver volume (TLV$_{Standard}$) is estimated as a function of BSA rather than the measured nontumor-containing liver parenchyma volume on cross-sectional imaging. This standardized approach excludes confounding variables such as tumor volume, and keeps the denominator stable when growth is assessed over multiple scans (discussed later in this chapter) [21]. The FLR$_{Standard}$ is then the quotient of LRV and TLV$_{Standard}$, determined in the same manner as described above for FLR$_{Measured}$. This is the methodology most commonly utilized, and for the remainder of the chapter, FLR should be assumed to refer to FLR$_{Standard}$.

Optimal FLR Volumes

Minimum acceptable FLR volumes have been established in order to mitigate the risk of PHLF. These can include patients who have been exposed to cytotoxic chemotherapy, as well as patients with a history of cirrhosis. A careful assessment of the patient's history is critical in order to determine the minimum acceptable FLR volume for each individual patient.

For patients who have no history of cytotoxic chemotherapy exposure or cirrhosis and have an otherwise normal liver, the minimum acceptable FLR volume was established by a retrospective study by Kishi et al. [1] This study involved patients undergoing an extended right hepatectomy, with volumetric analysis by CT scan. The patients were organized into different categories based on their FLR: <20%, 20–30%, and >30%. For patients with an FLR ≤20%, 34% of them experienced PHLF, and 11% of them died from liver failure. For patients with an FLR of 20–30%, the incidence of PHLF and death from liver failure was 10% ($p < 0.001$) and 3% ($p = 0.038$) respectively. For patients with an FLR >30%, the incidence of PHLF and death from liver failure was 15% and 3%, which was also significantly better compared to patients with an FLR <20% ($p = 0.010$, $p = 0.021$), but not for patients with an FLR of 20–30%. When patients had an FLR <20%, the odds ratio of PHLF on multivariate analysis was 3.18 (95% CI 1.34–7.54). This study established an FLR of 20% as the absolute minimum necessary after extended right hepatectomy, although most hepatobiliary surgeons will still aim for a minimum FLR higher than 20%.

The minimum FLR volume also depends on exposure to cytotoxic chemotherapy, which is especially important to know for patients with colorectal liver metastases. For example, patients who have received oxaliplatin-containing regimens can acquire sinusoidal obstruction syndrome, and patients who have received irinotecan-containing regimens can develop chemotherapy-associated steatohepatitis (CASH) [22]. The negative effects of these chemotherapeutic agents must be taken into account when considering an adequate FLR volume in patients exposed to prior chemotherapy. Shindoh et al. performed a retrospective analysis of 194 patients who underwent an extended right hepatectomy after receiving preoperative chemotherapy [2]. Subgroups in the analysis included patients who had an FLR <30%, or ≥ 30%.

Each group was defined as having received no preoperative chemotherapy, short-course chemotherapy (≤12 weeks), or long-course chemotherapy (>12 weeks). For patients who received long-course chemotherapy and had an FLR <30%, 16.3% experienced PHLF, and 2.3% experienced death from liver failure. In comparison, patients who had an FLR <30% and underwent short-course chemotherapy, 5.1% experienced PHLF, and 1.3% experienced death from liver failure ($p = 0.006$ compared to long-course chemotherapy). For the patients had an FLR ≥30%, the patients who underwent long course chemotherapy experienced PHLF at a rate of 10%, with no cases of death from liver failure. For the patients who had an FLR ≥30% and underwent short-course chemotherapy, none of the patients experienced PHLF. In practice, for patients who had chemotherapy, especially long-course chemotherapy, and need to undergo a right or extended right hepatectomy, ensuring the FLR is >30% helps to reduce the rate of PHLF.

Patients with cirrhosis also require special consideration. When considering a patient's fitness for major liver resection, special consideration of the patient's history, etiology of fibrosis, and thorough work up are all important. Laboratory values can be used to compute one of many clinical scoring systems, such as the widely used Childs-Pugh score, and model for end-stage liver disease (MELD) score, as well as the Albumin-Bilirubin (ALBI) score [23], and most recently, the combined APRI/ALBI score [24]. In general, patients with Childs-Pugh score of A, and ALBI score of grade 1 are considered to have adequate hepatic functional reserve to tolerate a major hepatectomy while mitigating post-hepatectomy complications [23]. However, this must still be used in conjunction with determining the FLR volume, which remains the most important predictor of post-hepatectomy complications (Fig. 16.2). For these patients, an FLR cutoff of 40% has generally been accepted as the minimum FLR value [25, 26], though many hepatobiliary surgeons would still advocate for an even higher FLR prior to embarking on a major hepatectomy [27].

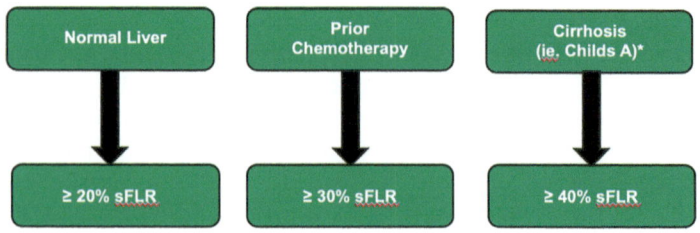

Fig. 16.2 Summary of minimum acceptable standardized future liver remnant volume required to minimize post-hepatectomy liver failure and death from liver failure

Embolization Techniques

Portal Vein Embolization

Portal vein embolization (PVE) was first described by Kinoshita et al. [28] At the time, this was used as a countermeasure to protect the liver from tumor thrombus growth due to hepatocellular carcinoma, thus blocking the tumor thrombus from continuing to grow into the main portal vein and contralateral portal vein. An unintended and beneficial consequence that they noted was hypertrophy of the contralateral lobe of the liver [28]. Makuuchi et al. later reported their experience with introducing PVE in the care of patients with cholangiocarcinoma who had a small liver remnant. They also noted atrophy of the tumor-bearing lobe with hypertrophy of the FLR [29]. The indications for PVE have since expanded to any disease where the FLR is found to be too small in size to safely perform a major hepatectomy.

All patients who are undergoing a right hepatectomy or extended right hepatectomy should have their volumetry calculated. PVE is indicated in any patient in whom their FLR is not large enough and does not meet the minimum size requirements summarized in Fig. 16.1. Contraindications to PVE include (1) patients who already have an adequate FLR that could otherwise proceed directly to surgery, (2) tumor invasion or tumor thrombus involving the ipsilateral portal vein. Portal hypertension is not considered a contraindication for performing PVE. For patients who have mild portal hypertension (approx. 10–15 mm Hg) that are asymptomatic, PVE is not considered a contraindication; however, it can elevate PV pressures and worsen symptoms associated with portal hypertension [30].

There are several approaches described for performing PVE. The original description involved performing a mini-laparotomy and accessing the portal vein through a branch of the ileocolic vein [31]. Disadvantages of this approach include its invasiveness, and with the advancement of interventional radiological techniques, this approach has been largely abandoned (Figs. 16.3 and 16.4). The percutaneous approaches for PVE include a transhe-

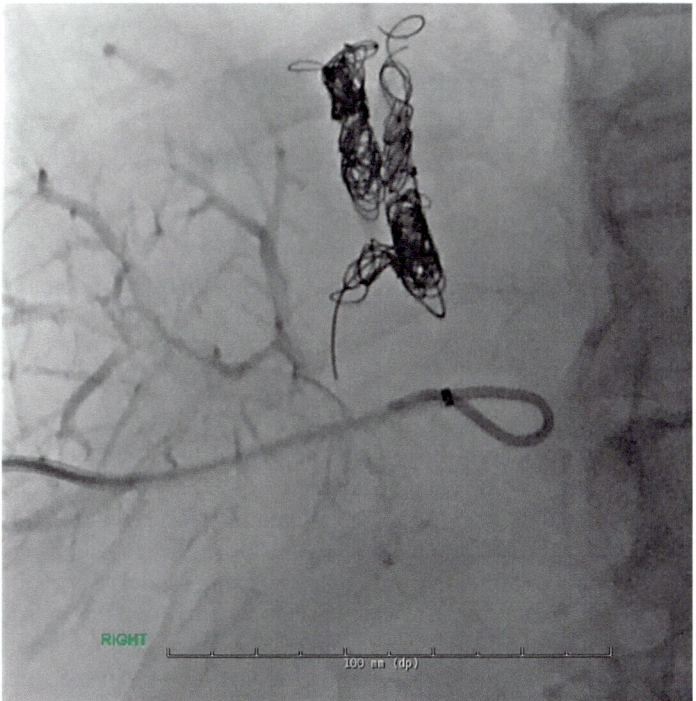

Fig. 16.3 Fluoroscopic images from a right portal vein embolization utilizing metallic coils. Note the coil deployment in the right anterior sector and right posterior sector portal venous branches

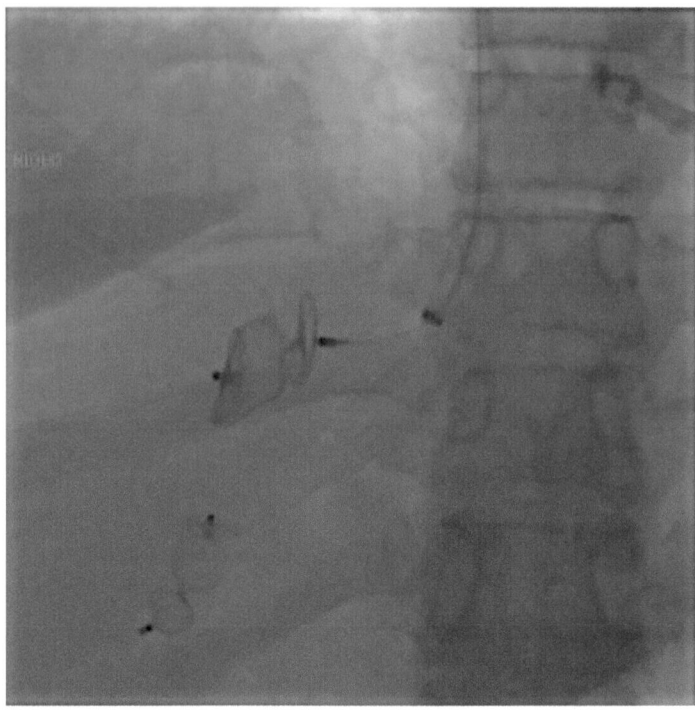

Fig. 16.4 Fluoroscopic images from a right hepatic vein embolization. Image demonstrates deployment of Amplatzer Vascular Plugs into the intrahepatic portion of the right hepatic vein

patic approach and a transsplenic approach. In the transhepatic approach, the portal vein is percutaneously accessed directly and the embolization is performed under venographic guidance. This approach can be performed by accessing either the ipsilateral side or the contralateral side. Accessing the ipsilateral side has benefits in that only the side to be resected is instrumented, and this avoids instrumenting the FLR. This technique, however, can be technically challenging due to the sharp angulation between the right anterior and posterior pedicles, requiring the use of specialized techniques and catheters for access. It also theoretically carries the risk of tumor seeding as well as non-target embolization on withdrawal of catheters [3]. Accessing the contralateral side is a technically easier embolization as it avoids any of the sharp angulation with the ipsilateral approach, and the right anterior and posterior pedicle branches of the portal vein can be accessed directly from the main portal vein. One of the disadvantages is that it involves instrumentation of the portal vein in the FLR which could theoretically expose the FLR to vascular injury. However, a meta-analysis by Abdulkhir et al. found no difference in the complication rates between the two approaches, with an overall morbidity of 2.2% [31].

Transsplenic access is a newer approach performed with vascular access into the portal venous system via direct puncture of the splenic vein through splenic parenchyma [32, 33]. Transsplenic access easily accesses the right anterior and posterior pedicle portal venous branches, and avoids the risk of tumor seeding and nontarget embolization with ipsilateral access, and avoids instrumentation and risk of injury to the FLR with contralateral access. Major complications are reported in only 3.8% of cases, and minor complications are reported in 7.4% of cases.

Various embolic agents have been described (Table 16.1). In their original manuscript, Kinoshita et al. used several different embolic agents, including gelatin sponges cut into 2 mm pieces and a mixture of thrombin, glucose, fibrin, and lipiodol [28]. Several embolic materials are available for PVE (see Table 16.1). The two most frequently used agents are gelfoam and cyanoacry-

Table 16.1 Embolic agents and combinations of agents used

Agents	Combinations reported
Cyanoacrylate	Cyanoacrylate + lipiodol
Lipiodol	Gelfoam + thrombin + urograffin
Gelfoam	Polyvinyl alcohol + coil + lipiodol + fibrin Glue
Thrombin	Fibrin glue + lipiodol + polyvinyl alcohol
Urograffin	Gelfoam + urograffin + gentamicin
Polyvinyl alcohol	Gelfoam + coils
Coils and microcoils	Polyvinyl alcohol + microcoils
Fibrin glue	
Gentamicin	
Embol-78	

late. Gelfoam is frequently combined with thrombin and urograffin to form an embolus that can occlude small outflow vessels as well. A notable disadvantage of gelfoam, however, is that there is a frequent recanalization of the portal vein that may lead to ineffective hypertrophy of the FLR [31, 34]. Cyanoacrylate can be combined with lipiodol, leading to reliable and effective hypertrophy of the FLR that rarely results in recanalization of the portal vein [31]. A disadvantage, however is that cyanoacrylate can produce a significant inflammatory reaction with peribiliary fibrosis that can make subsequent portal dissection and hepatic mobilization more difficult [31, 35, 36]. Polyvinyl alcohol leads to a minimal amount of inflammation and when combined with metallic coils can produce reliable embolization of the portal vein with minimal recanalization; however, it can cause peripheral fibrosis and necrosis as well as post-procedural pain that can be severe [31, 37]. No single agent has proven to be superior.

PVE is well tolerated overall. Minor complications can include abdominal discomfort or pain in up to 19% of cases, fever in 23% of cases, and nausea or vomiting in 2.4% of cases. Major complications are rare, and can include liver abscess (0.3%), cholangitis (0.2%), main or FLR portal vein thrombus (0.2%), subcapsular hematoma (0.2%), portal hypertension (0.1%), and septic necrosis from hepatic artery injury (0.1%) [31].

Hepatic Vein Embolization

Hepatic vein embolization (HVE) has been introduced both as a salvage technique to induce further growth in the FLR if PVE fails to produce adequate hypertrophy, as well as a technique combined with PVE, such that HVE is performed at the same setting as PVE, in a strategy known as liver venous deprivation (LVD). Hwang et al. observed that occlusion of one graft hepatic vein during portal flow deprivation accelerated atrophy of the ipsilateral liver and resulted in further hypertrophy of the contralateral liver and hypothesized that a right HVE would lead to further growth in the FLR in patients who had already undergone a right PVE prior to a planned right hepatectomy [38]. They reported their experience with 12 patients who underwent PVE followed by HVE. The mean FLR prior to PVE was 34.8% ± 1.6%. Two weeks after the PVE, the FLR increased to 39.7% ± 0.6%. These patients then underwent HVE 13.5 ± 4.2 days after PVE. They had no significant complications after HVE. FLR volumetry was determined 2 weeks after HVE and demonstrated a mean FLR of 44.2% ± 1.1%. This represents an overall degree of hypertrophy of 9.4% [38]. They then examined results of PVE with subsequent HVE in a larger cohort [39]. In this series of 42 patients, the pre-PVE FLR volume was 33.9% ± 2.2%, which increased to 38.4% ± 1.5% after PVE. After a median of 11.5 ± 6.7 days, HVE was then performed and FLR increased to 43.7 ± 2.1% [40].

In 2016, Guiu et al. examined the safety and efficacy of performance of right PVE and right HVE during the same procedure, and introduced the term LVD, where both the hepatic venous inflow and outflow were simultaneously occluded [41]. In their series of 7 patients, there were no complications observed from this combined procedure. After a mean interval of 23 days (range: 13–30 days) from the LVD procedure, repeat imaging was obtained and demonstrated that the FLR volume increased from 28.2% (22.4–33.3%) to 40.9% (33.6–59.3%), resulting in a mean degree of hypertrophy of 12.7%. The patients who are candidates for LVD is a matter of ongoing investigation. Some centers continue to utilize HVE as a salvage technique after inadequate FLR growth only, and reserve LVD for patients who have a particularly limited FLR from the outset [39]. The international DRAGON-1 trial is a phase II multicenter trial with the primary endpoint being a composite of the safety of LVD, 90-day mortality and 1 year accrual monitoring of each participating center [42]. This trial has finished accrual, and we are awaiting results. The DRAGON-2 trial is a phase III trial which will compare PVE to LVD for patients with CRLM, and is now open and accruing patients [43].

In the series by Guiu et al., the technique they utilized for LVD was through a single stick by accessing the right hepatic vein percutaneously under ultrasound guidance. After accessing the distal right hepatic vein under ultrasound guidance, and after placement of an Aprima introducer set, a trans-hepatic 7F Destination sheath was placed over a guidewire, and an Amplatzer Vascular Plug II (St Jude Medical) of between 18 and 22 mm in size was deployed, with the distal part 1 cm or greater away from the junction of the right hepatic vein with the inferior vena cava. A venogram was performed to check for right hepatic vein occlusion by the plugs, and patent distal branches and potential veno-venous collaterals were embolized using a 1:1 mixture of lipiodol and N-butylcyanoacrylate [41]. The right hepatic venous access tract is then embolized using the same embolic material. Two alternatives to this approach, as described in the DRAGON 1 protocol, include a transjugular or transfemoral approach where, after access to the right hepatic vein is obtained, appropriately sized Amplatzer Vascular Plugs (type I, II, or IV) are then introduced into the right hepatic vein, and sometimes the segment 5 and segment 8 branches of the middle hepatic vein [42]. Our center favors the transjugular approach for LVD procedures with the advantage being direct access into the right hepatic vein without having to take any high-angle approaches to gain access to the right hepatic vein.

Assessing Response After Embolization

After patients have undergone volume augmenting procedures, it must be determined whether adequate hypertrophy to the FLR has occurred prior to embarking on the intended liver resection. It is important to note, however that the rate of growth of the FLR over time is not linear, as there appears to be an initial rapid hypertrophy phase in the first 2–2.5 weeks following PVE/LVD, which is followed by a plateau phase characterized by a much slower rate of increase in size of the FLR volume (Fig. 16.5). For this reason, repeat volumetry is ideally calculated between 3 and 4 weeks after PVE/LVD.

Two important parameters to determine adequacy of hypertrophy should be determined and documented for each patient. The first parameter measures the amount of growth of the FLR, known as the degree of hypertrophy (DoH). In a study by Ribero et al., they examined the FLR before PVE, and after PVE, and the incre-

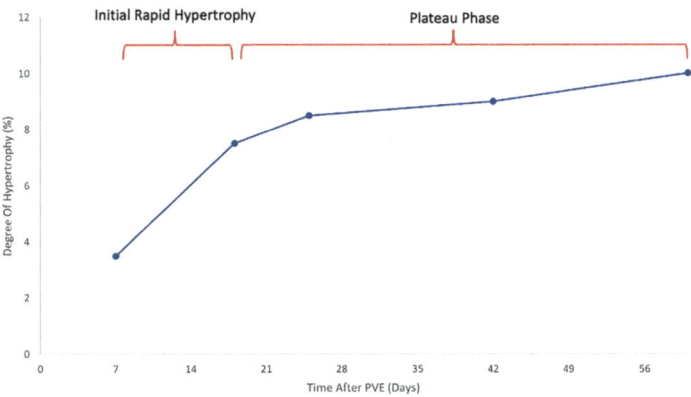

Fig. 16.5 Figure adapted from Ribero et al. [44] highlighting the kinetics of growth of the FLR, including an initial rapid hypertrophy phase in the first 2 to 2.5 weeks, followed by a longer plateau phase

mental increase in volume of the FLR is the DoH [44]. Through a sensitivity analysis of the receiver operating characteristic (ROC) curve, an optimal DoH cutoff value of 5% was determined. Patients were dichotomized into having an FLR of ≤20% or >20%. Among patients who had an FLR <20% with a DoH of <5%, all patients experienced PHLF. Among patients with an FLR >20%, if their DoH was <5%, 60% of patients experienced PHLF, however if their DoH was >5%, only 6% experienced PHLF ($P < 0.001$). When patients had an FLR ≤20% and a DoH <5%, this combination of factors had a sensitivity of 80% and a specificity of 94% in predicting PHLF [44].

The second parameter to consider in patients who have undergone volume augmentation procedures looks at the rate of growth of the FLR over time. This important parameter is known as the kinetic growth rate (KGR) which was described by Shindoh et al. [45] The KGR is essentially the DoH averaged out over the number of weeks after PVE (which, as mentioned above, is most often determined between 3 and 4 weeks after). Through a sensitivity analysis, a KGR of 2% per week provided the optimal balance between sensitivity and specificity. When KGR <2%, the sensitivity and specificity for predicting PHLF were 100% and 71%, respectively. When this was applied to their cohort of patients, the authors found that in patients who had a KGR >2%, no patients experienced post hepatectomy liver failure or death from liver failure. However, in patients who had a KGR <2% per week, 21.6% of patients experienced PHLF ($P = 0.0001$), and 8.1% of patients experienced death from liver failure ($P = 0.04$). The KGR has therefore emerged as a powerful predictor of adequate response of the FLR to PVE, and performance of major hepatectomy in patients with a KGR <2% is not advisable [45].

Managing Inadequate Growth of the FLR

Inadequate growth of the FLR, as determined by DoH and KGR can be a challenge. Several potential reasons may exist, such as re-canalization of the right portal vein that has interrupted the hypertrophy response of the FLR, and this should be one of the first issues to be ruled out. If the right portal vein has re-canalized, then repeat PVE should be attempted if possible. Assuming there has not been recanalization of the right portal vein, several rescue maneuvers are available. In cases where an extended right hepatectomy is required, embolization of the segment 4 branches can be pursued if not already done [46]. Performing right hepatic vein (+/− middle hepatic vein) embolization, if it has not already been done, should be pursued next. While controversial, radioembolization with Y90 may be an option. This technique is considered minimally embolic to the arterial system, so the risk of hepatocyte and biliary ischemia may be low, but should still be a consideration when selecting this technique. Theoretical advantages include generation of further hypertrophy of the FLR (though this is over a longer time course compared to PVE/LVD) [47, 48], and has the potential added benefit of a targeted treatment to the tumor in the embolized liver while awaiting further hypertrophy of the FLR [49, 50]. Finally, though an in-depth discussion is beyond the scope of this chapter, associating liver partition and portal vein occlusion for staged hepatectomy (ALPPS) as a rescue procedure may be an option for highly selected patients [51].

Summary

Optimal preoperative imaging is critical prior to major hepatectomy, not only for determining resectability, but also for adequate assessment of the FLR. These data can then be used to determine whether any additional measurements need to be taken in order to augment the volume of the FLR via the embolization techniques discussed in this chapter for purposes of minimizing the incidence of post-hepatectomy liver failure.

References

1. Kishi Y, Abdalla EK, Chun YS, et al. Three hundred and one consecutive extended right hepatectomies: evaluation of outcome based on systematic liver volumetry. Ann Surg. 2009;250(4):540–8.
2. Shindoh J, Tzeng C-WD, Aloia TA, et al. Optimal future liver remnant in patients treated with extensive preoperative chemotherapy for colorectal liver metastases. Ann Surg Oncol. 2013;20(8):2493–500.
3. Dixon M, Cruz J, Sarwani N, et al. The future liver remnant: definition, evaluation and management. Am Surg. 2021;87(2):275–86.
4. Adams RB, Aloia TA, Loyer E, et al. Selection for hepatic resection of colorectal liver metastases: expert consensus statement. HPB. 2013;15(2):91–103.
5. Bolondi L. Screening for hepatocellular carcinoma in cirrhosis. J Hepatol. 2003;39(6):1076–84.
6. Singal A, Volk ML, Waljee A, et al. Meta-analysis: surveillance with ultrasound for early-stage hepatocellular carcinoma in patients with cirrhosis. Aliment Pharmacol Ther. 2009;30(1):37–47.
7. Caturelli E, Pompili M, Bartolucci F, et al. Hemangioma-like lesions in chronic liver disease: diagnostic evaluation in patients. Radiology. 2001;220(2):337–42.
8. Choi BI, Takayasu K, Han MC. Small hepatocellular carcinomas and associated nodular lesions of the liver: pathology, pathogenesis, and imaging findings. AJR Am J Roentgenol. 1993;160(6):1177–87.
9. Tanaka S, Kitamura T, Imaoka S, et al. Hepatocellular carcinoma: sonographic and histologic correlation. AJR Am J Roentgenol. 1983;140(4):701–7.
10. Chung YE, Park MS, Park YN, et al. Hepatocellular carcinoma variants: radiologic-pathologic correlation. AJR Am J Roentgenol. 2009;193(1):W7–W13.

11. Soyer P, Bluemke DA, Reichle R, et al. Imaging of intrahepatic cholangiocarcinoma: 1. Peripheral cholangiocarcinoma. AJR Am J Roentgenol. 1995;165(6):1427–31.
12. Bloom CM, Langer B, Wilson SR. Rule of US in the detection, characterization and staging of cholangiocarcinoma. Radiographics. 1999;19(5):1199–218.
13. Kruskal JB, Thomas P, Nasser I, et al. Hepatic colon cancer metastases in mice: dynamic in vivo correlation with hypoechoic rims visible at US. Radiology. 2000;215(3):852–7.
14. Wernecke K, Henke L, Vassallo P, et al. Pathologic explanation for hypoechoic halo seen on sonograms of malignant liver tumors: an invitro correlative study. AJR Am J Roentgenol. 1992;159(5):1011–6.
15. Floriani I, Torri V, Rulli E, et al. Performance of imaging modalities in diagnosis of liver metastases from colorectal cancer: a systematic review and meta-analysis. J Magn Reson Imaging. 2010;31(1):19–31.
16. Castisani V, Ricci P, Erturk M, et al. Detection of hepatic metastases from colorectal cancer: prospective evaluatioin of grayscale US versus SonoVue® low mechanical index real time-enhanced US as compared with multidetector-CT or Gd-BOPTA-MRI. Ultraschall Med. 2010;31(5):500–5.
17. Katz SS. Computed tomography of the liver, biliary tract, and pancreas. In: Jarnagin WR, editor. Blumgart's surgery of the liver, biliary tract and pancreas, 2-Volume Set. 6th ed. Elsevier; 2017. p. 316–357.e6. ISBN 9780323340625.
18. Fournier LS, Cuenod CA, de Bazelaire C, et al. Early modifications of hepatic perfusion measured by functional CT in a rat model of hepatocellular carcinoma using a blood pool contrast agent. Eur Radiol. 2004;14(11):2125–33.
19. Vilgrain V, Esvan M, Ronot M, et al. A meta-analysis of diffusion-weighted and gadoxetic acid-enhanced MR imaging for the detection of liver metastases. Eur J Radiol. 2016;26(12):4595–615.
20. Zech CJ, Korpraphong P, Huppertz A, et al. Randomized multicentre trial of gadoxetic acid-enhanced MRI versus conventional MRI or CT in the staging of colorectal cancer liver metasteases. Br J Surg. 2014;101(6):613–21.
21. Vauthey J-N, Abdalla EK, Doherty DA, et al. Body surface area and body weight predict total liver volume in Western adults. Liver Transpl. 2002;8(3):233–40.
22. Morris-Stiff G, Tan Y-M, Vauthey JN. Hepatic complications following preoperative chemotherapy with oxaliplatin or irinotecan for hepatic colorectal metastases. Eur J Surg Oncol. 2008;34(6):609–14.
23. Fagenson AM, Gleeson EM, Pitt HA, et al. Albumin-bilirubin score vs model for end-stage liver disease in predicting post-hepatectomy outcomes. J Am Coll Surg. 2020;230(4):637–45.

24. Starlinger P, Ubl DS, Hackl H, et al. Combined APRI/ALBI score to predict mortality after hepatic resection. BJS Open. 2021;5(1):zraa043.
25. Azoulay D, Castaing D, Smail A, et al. Resection of nonresectable liver metastases from colorectal cancer after per- cutaneous portal vein embolization. Ann Surg. 2000;231(4):480–6.
26. Kubota K, Makuuchi M, Kusaka K, et al. Measurement of liver volume and hepatic functional reserve as a guide to decision-making in resectional surgery for hepatic tumors. Hepatology. 1997;26(5):1176–81.
27. Clavien P-A, Petrowsky H, DeOliveira ML, et al. Strategies for safer liver surgery and partial liver transplantation. N Engl J Med. 2007;356(15):1545–59.
28. Kinoshita H, Sakai K, Hirohashi K, et al. Preoperative portal vein embolization for hepatocellular carcinoma. World J Surg. 1986;10(5):803–8.
29. Makuuchi M, Thai BL, Takayasu K, et al. Preoperative portal embolization to increase safety of major hepatectomy for hilar bile duct carcinoma: a preliminary report. Surgery. 1990;107(5):521–7.
30. Vauthey JN, Dixon E, Abdalla EK, et al. Pretreatment assessment of hepatocellular carcinoma: expert consensus statement. HPB. 2010;12(5):289–99.
31. Abulkhir A, Limongelli P, Healey AJ, et al. Preoperative portal vein embolization for major liver resection: a meta-analysis. Ann Surg. 2008;247(1):49–57.
32. Ko HK, Ko GY, Sung KB, et al. Portal vein embolization via percutaneous transsplenic access prior to major hepatectomy for patients with insufficient future liver remnant. J Vasc Interv Radiol. 2016;27(7):981–6.
33. Sarwar A, Brook OR, Weinstein JL, et al. Trans-splenic portal vein embolization: a technique to avoid damage to the future liver remnant. Cardiovasc Intervent Radiol. 2016;39(10):1514–8.
34. De Baere T, Roche A, Vavasseur D, et al. Portal vein embolization: utility for inducing left hepatic lobe hypertrophy before surgery. Radiology. 1993;188(1):73–7.
35. De Baere T, Roche A, Elias D, et al. Preoperative portal vein embolization for extension of hepatectomy indications. Hepatology. 1996;24(6):1386–91.
36. Imamura H, Shimada R, Kubota M, et al. Preoperative portal vein embolization: an audit of 84 patients. Hepatology. 1999;29(4):1099–105.
37. Shimamura T, Nakajima Y UY, et al. Efficacy and safety of preoperative percutaneous transhepatic portal embolization with absolute ethanol: a clinical study. Surgery. 1997;121(2):135–41.
38. Hwang S, Lee SG, Ko GY, et al. Sequential preoperative ipsilateral hepatic vein embolization after portal vein embolization to induce further liver regeneration in patients with hepatobiliary malignancy. Ann Surg. 2009;249(4):608–16.

39. Ayabe RI, Vauthey JN, Newhook TE. Optimizing the future liver remnant: portal vein embolization, hepatic venous deprivation, and associating liver partition and portal vein ligation for staged hepatectomy. Surgery. 2023;174(1):116–8.
40. Hwang S, Ha TY, Ko GY, et al. Preoperative sequential portal and hepatic vein embolization in patients with hepatobiliary malignancy. World J Surg. 2015;39(12):2990–8.
41. Guiu B, Chevallier P, Denys A, et al. Simultaneous trans-hepatic portal and hepatic vein embolization before major hepatectomy: the liver venous deprivation technique. Eur Radiol. 2016;26(12):4259–67.
42. Korenblik R, Olij B, Aldrighetti LA, et al. Dragon 1 protocol manuscript: training, accreditation, Implementation and safety evaluation of portal and hepatic vein embolization (PVE/HVE) to accelerate future liver remnant (FLR) hypertrophy. Cardiovasc Intervent Radiol. 2022;45(9):1391–8.
43. The DRAGON 2 Trial (DRAGON 2); 2022. https://clinicaltrials.gov/ct2/show/NCT05428735?term1/4DRAGON-2&draw1/42&rank1/41. Accessed 12 June 2023.
44. Ribero D, Abdalla EK, Madoff DC, et al. Portal vein embolization before major hepatectomy and its effects on regeneration, resectability and outcome. Br J Surg. 2007;94(11):1386–94.
45. Shindoh J, Truty MJ, Aloia TA, et al. Kinetic growth rate after portal vein embolization predicts posthepatectomy outcomes: toward zero liver-related mortality in patients with colorectal liver metastases and small future liver remnant. J Am Coll Surg. 2013;216(2):201–9.
46. Kishi Y, Madoff DC, Abdalla EK, et al. Is embolization of segment 4 portal veins before extended right hepatectomy justified? Surgery. 2008;144(5):744–51.
47. Teo JY, Allen JC, Ng DC, et al. A systematic review of contralateral liver lobe hypertrophy after unilobar selective internal radiation therapy with Y90. HPB. 2016;18(1):7–12.
48. Garlipp B, de Baere T, Damm R, et al. Left-liver hypertrophy after therapeutic right-liver radioembolization is substantial but less than after portal vein embolization. Hepatology. 2014;59(5):1864–73.
49. Kulik LM, Carr BI, Mulcahy MF, et al. Safety and efficacy of 90Y radiotherapy for hepatocellular carcinoma with and without portal vein thrombosis. Hepatology. 2008;47(1):71–81.
50. Salem R, Lewandowski RJ, Mulcahy M, et al. Radioembolization for hepatocellular carcinoma using Yttrium-90 microspheres: a comprehensive report of long-term outcomes. Gastroenterology. 2010;138(1):52–64.
51. Enne M, Schadde E, Bjornsson B, et al. ALPPS as a salvage procedure after insufficient future liver remnant hypertrophy following portal vein occlusion. HPB. 2017;19(12):1126–9.

Hilar Dissection

Federico Gaudenzi, Taiga Wakabayashi, and Go Wakabayashi

Introduction

Modern liver surgery, at its core, aims to maximize patient survival while minimizing the risks of intraoperative and postoperative complications. Since the first successful liver resection performed in 1888 by Langenbach, the first right hepatectomy reported by Ichio Honjo from Japan in 1949 and the first case series described by Lortat-Jacob from France in 1952 [1], intraoperative bleeding has remained a significant concern, closely linked to surgical outcomes. Consequently, acquiring vascular control before, during, and/or after parenchymal transection has always been a crucial step in performing liver resections [2, 3]. Accurate identification of the hepatic vascular anatomy in each case is essential for gaining vascular control, particularly when undertaking anatomical, parenchymal-sparing resections. These procedures are pivotal in modern, safe liver surgery as they preserve adequate remnant liver volume and enable re-resection in case of recurrence [4].

Supplementary Information The online version contains supplementary material available at https://doi.org/10.1007/978-3-032-04823-3_17.

F. Gaudenzi · T. Wakabayashi (✉) · G. Wakabayashi
Center for Advanced Treatment of Hepatobiliary and Pancreatic Diseases, Ageo Central General Hospital, Saitama, Japan
e-mail: gowaka@ach.or.jp

Since the first experiences, control of both the inflow and outflow vessels before parenchymal transection was deemed necessary. As far as hepatic outflow is concerned, for their first right hepatectomies Honjo and Lortat-Jacob reported a complete mobilization of the right liver before liver transection to secure the right hepatic vein (RHV). In 1984, Makuuchi et al. underlined the importance of dividing the inferior vena cava (IVC) ligament for extrahepatic dissection and division, which could reduce massive bleeding around IVC. Their approach has therefore been named the "conventional approach". In the same years, Takasaki et al. described an alternative approach to RHV without mobilization of the right liver and with parenchymal transection before accessing the RHV. During the following decades, Takasaki's "anterior approach" or "non-touch isolation method" has been demonstrated to reduce massive bleeding from IVC and to provide better survival rates and disease-free survival rates compared to the conventional approach, especially when dealing with huge lesions of the right liver [5].

On the other hand, approaches to hepatic inflow during surgery can significantly vary based on factors such as the procedure's purpose (e.g., transplant vs. oncologic surgery), location and extent of resection, operative setting (e.g., open vs. minimally invasive surgery), and the surgeon's expertise. Generally, these approaches can be categorized into three main categories as described by Coinaud C [6].: intrafascial, extrafascial, and extrafascial transfissural approaches.

The intrafascial approach was introduced by Honjo and Lortat-Jacob in the 1950s. These two early pioneers, at about the same time even though thousands of miles apart, independently described their first successful right hepatectomies and the related necessity of obtaining vascular control before parenchymal transection, by addressing the hepatic hilum and individually preparing each element (hepatic artery, portal vein, and common bile duct) within the vasculobiliary sheath of the hepatoduodenal ligament [1]. Since this technique was the first one suggested for anatomical major liver resections and it allowed for vascular control prior to parenchymal transection, it is also referred to as "control method" or "standard hilar dissection".

Conversely, the extrafascial and extrafascial transfissural approaches are referred to as the "Glissonean (or Glisson's or Glissonian) pedicle approach" according to Takasaki's 1986 definition [7]. The extrafascial approach includes two sub-categories: the extrafascial extrahepatic approach (namely, the proper Takasaki's approach) and the extrafascial intrahepatic approach, each suitable for different types of resections. Lastly, the extrafascial and transfissural approach, or Ton That Tung approach, involves major parenchymal transection followed by intrahepatic isolation and division of Glissonean pedicles [6, 8–12]. These surgical approaches have evolved over decades, based on innovative insights into liver anatomy that have been gained through histopathological and surgical research. Modern liver surgeons must familiarize themselves with this knowledge to optimize resection precision, procedural safety, and ultimately, surgical outcomes.

According to Sugioka's comprehensive theory of surgical liver anatomy [10], known as the "Gate theory," the Glissonean sheath, also known as the Walaeus sheath, encapsulates the hepatic artery, portal vein, and bile duct, forming the Glissonean pedicle. This capsule forms a thick plate at the inferior part of the liver, referred to as the hilar plate, and extends itself into the liver parenchyma, continuing to follow and cover each pedicle; this bundle, originated from the hepato-duodenal ligament, ramifies inside the liver parenchyma and is named Glissonean tree, with branches that are classified into three main orders according to Brisbane 2000 terminology [13].

It is crucial to distinguish the Glissonean/Walaeus sheath from the peritoneal serosa that wraps the Glissonean pedicle at the hepatoduodenal ligament and covers nearly the entire liver's surface except for the bare area. These two entities are separated from the Laennec's capsule, first described in 1802 [14] and then demonstrated by Hyashi's [15] and Sugioka's studies. This capsule consists in a dense fibrous layer beneath the serosa, extended on the entire liver's surface, including the bare area and the intrahepatic parenchyma surrounding the Glissonean pedicles. Bearing that in mind, it is easy to understand that a space between Laennec's capsule and the Glissonean pedicle can be individuated and accessed, allowing for the extrahepatic, selective pedicle isolation without parenchymal destruction. This space can be accessed through specific gates, accounting for 6 and defined from 4 essential anatomical landmarks, namely the cystic plate, the Arantius plate, the umbilical plate, and the pedicle for the caudate process (G1c). The Gates are located as follows: Gate 1, caudal end of the Arantius plate; gate II, junction between the round ligament and umbilical plate; Gate III, the right edge of the root of umbilical portion; Gate IV, left edge of the right anterior Glissonean pedicle and cystic plate; Gate V, bifurcation of the right Glissonean pedicle; Gate VI, between the posterior right Glissonean pedicle and G1c [10, 12].

Understanding this anatomy is crucial for performing selective pedicle isolation without parenchymal destruction. These studies backboned the Tokyo 2020 terminology of liver anatomy and resections that established important updates of the Brisbane 2000 system [4]: Sugioka's gate theory and his reevaluation of liver anatomy therefore provide an ideal background for the systematic extrahepatic Glissonean approach in modern liver surgery.

Pre-op and Preparation Pearls

Given all the aforementioned considerations and the pivotal role of hilar dissection in ensuring a safe liver resection, it becomes evident how crucial it is to carefully evaluate the anatomy of the portal triad and its possible variations in each specific case. In this context, two-dimensional (2D) computed tomography (CT) and magnetic resonance imaging (MRI) are fundamental tools for diagnosing and planning operations for space-occupying liver lesions. They allow surgeons to mentally reconstruct three-dimensional (3D) images, facilitating the assessment of specific conditions and the generation of ideal surgical plans. However, since these stereoscopic images are temporary and unstable in the human brain, representing them to the treatment team is extremely challenging, and their match with the actual anatomical structure presents specific limitations for complex surgeries.

In this context, the recent rapid evolution of digital medical technology has led to the development of increasingly refined 3D reconstruction visualization models. This technology transforms 2D sectional image sequences from ultrasound, CT, and MRI into 3D images, analyzing massive image data files through computer image processing systems. The result is an intuitive, clear, multi-angled, and objective model that accurately indicates lesion locations, surgical margins, and anatomical relationships with the vasculobiliary system. These models enable preoperative evaluations, surgical planning, and provide useful guidance for precise liver resection strategies. Furthermore, a recent meta-analysis by Liu et al. demonstrated that 3D reconstruction visualization models can significantly reduce operative time, blood transfusion volume, hospital stay, and postoperative complications in liver surgery [16].

Moreover, surgeons must accurately acknowledge their patients' medical history to complete their understanding of relevant anatomy in each specific case. Past episodes of acute cholangitis, biliary strictures, fibrosis, cholecystitis, cholelithiasis, liver cirrhosis, adjuvant chemotherapy, as well as the size and location of tumors, can all alter hilar anatomy and affect surgical approaches. Knowing as many details as possible about the expected scenario will ensure that instrumentation, operating room staff, and expertise are adequate for the procedure.

All the aforementioned information is essential for safely planning correct resection plans and determining the best routes to reach them. Liver surgeons can choose from several approaches to obtain safe and effective control of the vascular pedicles nourishing the parenchyma to be resected. The debate over which approach is the best in terms of safety and perioperative outcomes has persisted for several years. Since the first description of the Glissonean approach by Takasaki et al. [7, 11], several studies have investigated the potential advantages and drawbacks of this technique compared to standard hilar dissection. Concerns were initially raised about the risk of bile duct injury related to accidental stapling of the liver remnant's pedicle [17]. However, the first prospective randomized trial comparing hilar dissection and the Glissonean approach did not observe any bile duct injuries.

Particularly, while observing a shorter hilar dissection time for Glissonean approach, the study reported shorter pedicular clamping time, less cytolysis, and cheaper equipment for traditional hilar dissection compared to *en bloc* stapling transection of Glissonean pedicles [18]. On the other hand, retrospective studies in patients with hepatocellular carcinoma demonstrated that the Glissonean approach in open hepatectomies was an important oncological prognostic indicator, leading to significantly higher 5-year survival rates [19].

In the subsequent years, with the advent of minimally invasive surgery, retrospective and prospective studies investigated the implications of these techniques in laparoscopic liver resections. Surprisingly, the first retrospective studies not only demonstrated "not inferiority" but also several advantages of laparoscopic Glissonean approach compared with laparoscopic standard hilar dissection: shorter operative time, lower need for blood transfusions, fewer postoperative complications, fewer cases of positive surgical margins, and more cases of major liver resections were observed in the Glissonean group compared to the standard group in the laparoscopic setting [20]. Additionally, the first randomized controlled trial comparing the two approaches proved laparoscopic Glissonean approach hemihepatectomies to offer notable advantages in terms of hilar dissection time and overall operative time, without enhancing postoperative overall complication rates or intraoperative blood loss, and without significant differences regarding the 1-year, 3-year, and 5-year disease-free survival and overall survival rates.

In conclusion, various techniques can be used to gain vascular control before and during hepatic resection. The extrafascial approach has demonstrated substantial advantages compared to intrafascial or standard hilar dissection, especially in a minimally invasive setting. Indications may vary depending on the specific disease being treated, the procedure to be performed (e.g., liver transplant vs. hepatic resection), and the operative setting (e.g., open liver surgery vs. laparoscopic and robot-assisted liver resections). The key steps and fundamental setups are described below.

Key Steps

Open Surgery—Setup and Pitfalls

After thorough abdominal exploration and liver exposure but before commencing hepatectomy, regardless of its purpose, achieving hepatic inflow control is crucial to ensure procedural safety by minimizing blood loss and ensuring adequate vascularization and biliary drainage of the remnant liver.

Understanding the relational anatomy of structures in the hepatic hilum, including potential variations specific to each case, is imperative. Considerable variability exists in the arterial and biliary systems, which should be anticipated during preoperative assessment and defined during hilar dissection, particularly when planning an intrafascial approach. This vascular control technique remains indispensable not only in transplant surgery, where each main vascular structure must be fully isolated to enable safe anastomoses, but also in cases of perihilar cholangiocarcinoma. However, dissection of the hepatoduodenal ligament may be challenging in patients with adhesions from previous surgeries. Careful division of adhesions, mobilization of the duodenum, and intermittent palpation of the region of the porta hepatis to identify hepatic artery pulses can facilitate approaching the hepatoduodenal ligament from the right, using the common bile duct as an initial landmark [21]. Reverse Trendelenburg positioning, ranging from 0 to 30 degrees, may aid in adequate lowering of inframesocolic viscera and correct straightening and tension of the porta hepatis' vascular structures. Essential instrumentation includes straight or angled DeBakey forceps to minimize vascular manipulation injuries, bipolar scissors for coagulation and section of surrounding tissues, while monopolar cautery should be carefully used due to its risk of thermal damage of the vessels themselves and the surrounding tissues and organs. Fibrous scarring and adhesions can be divided using bipolar or ultrasonic energy devices. Damage control instruments such as thin monofilament sutures and vascular DeBakey clamps are crucial, along with silicone, rubber, or cotton loops to encircle isolated structures.

However, potential pitfalls exist with the traditional hilar approach. Although dissection of first-order portal pedicles can be safely performed, safe access to second or more peripheral pedicles is not well established [22]. This may pose challenges, especially in liver resections involving second or third-order Glissonean pedicles. Alternatively, these pedicles can be isolated from the hilar plate and detached from the liver parenchyma using the existing space between the pedicles and the Laennec capsule, thereby performing an extrafascial approach [12]. Various techniques can ease parenchymal transection once the pedicle nourishing the tumor-bearing area is encircled. For example, temporary clamping with a Bulldog clamp can help identify a demarcation line on the liver's surface, and contrast-enhanced ultrasound (CEUS) can confirm the correctness of the clamped pedicle.

Furthermore, navigating the correct plane during deeper parenchymal transection has always been challenging. Staining techniques, initially using methylene blue [23] but later replaced with indocyanine green (ICG) [24, 25], can assist in clarifying the shape and borders of segments to be resected. ICG emits fluorescence when intravenously administered, aiding in identifying respective portal territories and performing anatomic liver resections through image-guided navigation systems [12, 26]. The main methods of intraoperative ICG administration include negative staining, where ICG is administered after clamping the portal pedicle of target segments, and positive staining, where the dye is injected directly into portal venous branches of the target segments. Glissonean approach can be particularly useful for ICG-guided negative staining. After clamping the Glissonean pedicle nourishing the tumor-bearing area and administering ICG intravenously, fluorescent images can be displayed on a television monitor, allowing real-time verification of the adequacy of the transection plane. However, this method achieves its maximum immediacy with overlay image systems available in laparoscopy.

Minimally Invasive Surgery

The advancement of minimally invasive surgery (MIS) over the past two decades has inevitably ignited debate regarding the optimal approach to hilar dissection in terms of safety and intraoperative and postoperative outcomes. Given the demonstrated advantages of anatomical resections (AR) over non-anatomical parenchymal-sparing resections in oncological outcomes, including lower rates of recurrence and remnant liver ischemia (RLI)— recently identified as a prognostic factor linked to worse long-term outcomes [27], precise MIS techniques can facilitate parenchymal sparing anatomical resections such as sectionectomy, segmentectomy, and subsegmentectomy [4]. It is evident how the Glissonean approach, especially extrahepatically, can be advantageous in MIS, facilitated by the caudal and magnified view of key anatomical structures [22].

Comparing the Glissonean approach to traditional hilar dissection in the context of minimally invasive anatomical liver resection (MIALR), several studies have reported shorter operative times, lower transfusion rates, reduced R1 resection rates, decreased morbidity, and shorter hospital stays [20, 22, 28]. Various pathophysiological mechanisms may underlie these advantages, including selective clamping of the addressed Glissonean pedicle, which may decrease the risk of ischemia-reperfusion damage following intermittent Pringle maneuver, leading to improved liver function tests, decreased postoperative ascites, and shorter hospital stays. Consequently, the Glissonean approach has the potential to further enhance the established benefits of MIALR compared to open liver resections, particularly in terms of postoperative morbidity rates and length of hospital stay.

Laparoscopy—Setup and Pitfalls

Compared to open surgery, the laparoscopic setting posed new challenges to the surgeon's work, since it is characterized by lack of tactile sensation, particular movement restrictions and requires specific anatomical knowledge, offering new and different views of the surgical field. However, the extraordinary advances in laparoscopic techniques, surgical instruments, and experience all have allowed laparoscopic Glissonean approach anatomical hepatectomies (LGAH) to be increasingly performed recently, thus creating the possibility to assess their outcomes and compare them to those of laparoscopic hilar approach hepatectomies (LHAH). Interestingly, a recent prospective, randomized controlled trial, comparing 96 LGAH to 94 LHAH that were performed during a 7-year span time, demonstrated significantly shorter hilar dissection time and overall operative time in favor of LGAH group, while no significant differences were observed between the two groups as regarding as 1-, 3-, and 5-year disease-free and overall survival rates [29].

Furthermore, according to Takasaki's concept of the "cone unit," which comprises the smallest resectable anatomical part of the liver supplied by a tertiary Glissonean pedicle, with the base on the hepatic surface and the apex toward the hilum, identifying the pedicle feeding the narrowest anatomical area allows for anatomical and parenchymal sparing resection, which is an important prognostic factor for hepatocellular carcinoma (HCC) and colorectal liver metastases (CLRM) resections [30, 31].

With these concepts in mind, surgeons can plan laparoscopic parenchymal sparing anatomical liver resections using the laparoscopic Glissonean approach. Preoperative fundamentals include a 3D reconstruction visualization model of the case, evaluating liver anatomy, portal territories, tumor location, and the relationship with surrounding anatomy and Glissonean pedicles. This enables planning of resection targeting the narrowest and oncologically safe anatomical tumor-bearing area and its feeding pedicle, respecting the "cone unit" principle [32].

Inside the operating room, under general anesthesia, the patient is positioned with legs closed, supine with arms open, or in a 45° left-lateral semi-decubitus position with the right arm on an elevated armrest for segment 7 segmentectomies and right posterior sectionectomy. The operating surgeon stands on the patient's right side. An 8 to 12 mmHg pressure carbon dioxide pneumoperitoneum may suffice, while an endoscope optimized for both high-definition white light and near-infrared fluorescence (NIRF) is essential. Preoperative administration of ICG (intravenous,

0.5 mg/kg) two weeks before surgery can aid in tumor detection on the liver surface, in addition to intraoperative ultrasound (IOUS).

A "cystic plate cholecystectomy", detaching the cystic plate from Laennec's capsule as described by Sugioka et al. [10] is crucial in most cases except for tumors located in the left lateral section, to better visualize essential landmarks guiding access to the gates. The hilar plate detachment from Laennec's capsule can be performed using bipolar scissors and bipolar electrocautery, preserving Laennec's capsule as much as possible. If pedicle isolation is challenging to find extrahepatically (e.g., for deep tertiary branches such as G4a, G7, and G8 dorsal and ventral), a small parenchymal dissection can be performed using cavitron ultrasonic energy. Throughout the dissection, the Pringle maneuver is useful to minimize bleeding and keep the surgical field clean, enhancing the precision of dissection itself. Once the pedicle is isolated, it should be encircled with a silicon loop and temporarily clamped with an endoscopic bulldog to draw a demarcation line on the liver surface.

IOUS is then carried out to confirm whether the ischemic area corresponds to the tumor-bearing one: if not, the dissection/isolation/encircling/clamping can be repeated until the correct pedicle is achieved. Further confirmation of the correct ischemic area can be given by contrast-enhanced IOUS. At this point, ICG negative staining can be obtained with a 0.5 mg intravenous bolus of ICG: using the innovative "overlay mode," a superimposed image will be generated by projecting the ICG-NIRF data onto the white light image, avoiding the need to look at two different images alternately. The ischemic area will appear cyanotic dark while the future liver remnant will shine green. This image system allows direct transection of the superficial parenchyma following the demarcation line using ultrasonic shears, while the deepest layers can be separated with cavitron ultrasonic energy following the plane between the "shining green" and the "cyanotic dark" parenchyma. Additionally, a preoperative 3D model repeatedly checked on a dedicated screen, as well as the repetition of IOUS especially during Pringle-free time, can help to maintain the correct transection plane. When the Glissonean pedicle is finally found again during transection, it can be divided between clips or through a vascular stapler [27]. With the described technique, an image-guided anatomical parenchymal sparing resection for each cone unit, regardless of its location, can be pursued.

Concerns have been raised about the risk of portal triad injuries of segments adjacent to the resected area, caused by inadvertently stapling their Glissonean pedicles, thereby increasing the incidence of arteriovenous fistula and biliary complication rates. However, recent studies have not shown any significant difference between Glissonean approach laparoscopic liver resections (LLRs) and traditional hilar approach LLRs. Several methods can be applied to avoid injury to adjacent pedicles, including clear identification of the anatomic space between the Laennec capsule and Glissonean pedicles bifurcation through a clean surgical field using the Pringle maneuver, as well as grasping an appropriate angle to insert the curved forceps and avoiding any forceful maneuvers.

Finally, as defined for open liver resections, the Glissonean approach still presents some limitations: lesions infiltrating the liver hilum, Klatskin tumors, the second stage of ALPPS (associating liver partition and portal vein ligation for staged hepatectomy), liver resections required for complex bile duct injuries with vascular involvement, and living donor hemihepatectomies can all represent contraindications to this inflow control technique, thus necessitating traditional hilar dissection [29]. Essential instrumentation includes bipolar scissors and forceps, laparoscopic bulldog clamps, vascular clips, and tapes.

Robot-Assisted Liver Surgery—Setup and Pitfalls

Robotic liver resections (RLRs) have recently gained widespread acceptance and a wider range of applications. Compared to laparoscopy, the robotic approach offers several advantages such as tools with seven degrees of freedom, steady three-dimensional vision, and tremor filtration [33]. However, RLRs still face difficulties toward global and uniform adoption due to several reasons, including the high costs of instrumentation, the high level of required experience in open and minimally invasive surgery, as well as the absence of instruments that some surgeons consider essential for safe resection, such as the cavitron ultrasonic surgical aspirator (CUSA) and waterjet[34]. Robotic liver transection currently relies on bipolar forceps, clamp-crush technique, and harmonic scalpel, as laparoscopic CUSA and waterjet can only be used by the first assistant at the patient's side. Consequently, the first experiences of robotic liver resections using the Glissonean approach have been described only recently, while comparative studies, both retrospective and prospective, among the possible inflow control techniques in RLRs, are still lacking.

Nevertheless, the feasibility and safety of the Glissonean approach have already been demonstrated [33–38]. All published experiences reported the use of minor liver transection to gain access to the Glissonean pedicle, thus pursuing an extrafascial intrahepatic approach. The same basic steps mentioned for laparoscopy, including cystic plate cholecystectomy, detachment of the hilar plate from Laennec's capsule through bipolar energy, selective pedicle encircling and clamping, and the use of IOUS and ICG guidance, can allow for safe anatomical parenchymal sparing liver resections even in the robot-assisted setting. Regarding ICG guidance, a main limitation compared to laparoscopy is that the overlay mode cannot be applied to the robotic system: ICG staining can only be visualized without normal white light and just superimposed on grayscale background images [26]. However, a significant advantage compared to LLRs is that with the robotic approach, the Glissonean pedicle can be encircled with ease comparable to the open technique [37], thus overcoming the movement and view limitations of laparoscopy while preserving a minimally invasive approach.

Certainly, a key point in the RLR setup is the port positioning. Adequate distance among the ports themselves and in relation to the surgical target must be ensured by proper preoperative evaluation of CT scans. A useful tip could be to draw the future port sites, accurately measured from one another, on the patient's skin before the procedure begins. If robotic arms are too close, several instrumentation conflicts will occur; moreover, insufficient distance of the port sites from the surgical target can significantly increase the procedure's technical difficulty.

In conclusion, robotic liver surgery, with its greater ergonomics and range of motion, can facilitate complex and delicate maneuvers, including hilar dissection, with the identification and control of individual structures from the hepatoduodenal ligament. However, traditional hilar dissection presents limitations inherited from open surgery, particularly for anatomical segmentectomies and subsegmentectomies, especially for tumor-bearing areas located in posterosuperior segments, which is also a typical feature of minimally invasive surgery. On the other hand, the Glissonean approach can be easier for cirrhotic cases due to capsular retraction that facilitates visualization and extrahepatic isolation of the Glissonean pedicle [37]; it can also be extremely useful in repeat surgeries with previous manipulation of the hepatic hilum, and generally speaking, it can find its exquisite indications in cases that require excellent accuracy and dexterity [34, 35]. However, there is still a lack of high-level evidence, and further studies are needed to assess the intraoperative and postoperative short- and long-term outcomes related to the aforementioned inflow control techniques in robotic liver resections.

The presented case is a symptomatic 10-cm nodule consistent with focal nodular hyperplasia and involving the whole left hemi liver. A minimally invasive left hepatectomy with left and middle hepatic vein resection and using Da Vinci Xi system (Intuitive Surgical, Inc., Sunnyvale, California, USA) is planned.

The first step consists of resecting the round ligament and encircling it with an endoloop, in order to direct traction as needed. Secondly, intraoperative ultrasound (IOUS) is carried out to confirm the number and extent of the nodule and to verify its relationship with the nearby vessels, according to preoperative imaging.

The hepatoduodenal ligament is encircled and taped to setup the Pringle maneuver from the left hypochondrium, in an extracorporeal fashion. At this point the dissection of Gate I and Gate III can be pursued: Gate I is identified as the caudal end of the Arantius plate, while Gate III as the right edge of the Glissonean pedicle root of the umbilical portion. In this way, the left main Glissonean pedicle (G2 + 3 + 4) can be isolated from the Laennec capsule and encircled with a yellow tape.

The left hemi liver is fully mobilized and the common trunk of middle and left hepatic veins (MHV and LHV) is isolated and encircled with a blue tape.

The left main Glissonean pedicle is then clamped with a laparoscopic bulldog clamp: IOUS, together with the demarcation line appearing on parenchymal surface, confirms the absence of blood inflow toward the tumor-bearing area.

A 0.5 mg intravenous bolus of ICG is then administered and through Da Vinci Xi's Firefly® mode the dark cyanotic tumor-bearing area can be distinguished from the shining green liver remnant on a grayscale background, according to the negative staining technique. Under ICG guidance, the transection line can be easily identified and tracked with bipolar forceps.

Parenchymal transection is then performed by using harmonic scalpel and bipolar forceps, according to the crush-clamp technique. The adequacy of transection plane is constantly re-assessed by checking on the preoperative 3D model and by repeating IOUS. When the left Glissonean pedicle is finally found again during transection, it is divided through a vascular stapler.

After division of MHV-LHV common trunk with a vascular stapler, the resection can be completed. A Doppler-IOUS is finally performed, in order to assess the adequate perfusion and venous drainage of the liver remnant.

The presented case is a nonalcoholic steatohepatitis-related hepatocellular carcinoma located at segment 3. The preoperative preparation includes a 3D reconstruction visualization model based on the preoperative CT scan: the anatomical relationship between the nodule and the two subsegmental Glissonean pedicles nourishing segment 3 can be identified as G3a and G3b. In sight of a possible future HCC recurrence, a minimally invasive anatomical parenchymal-sparing resection using Da Vinci Xi system (Intuitive Surgical, Inc., Sunnyvale, California, USA) is planned.

The first step consists of taping the hepatoduodenal ligament in order to setup the Pringle maneuver from the right hypochondrium, in an extracorporeal fashion. Secondly, G3a and G3b pedicles are distinctly identified near the junction between the umbilical plate and the root of round ligament, which is pulled ventrally and caudally to ensure adequate tension and to ease clear exposure of the addressed pedicles. After encircling G3b and G3a with a yellow tape, they are selectively clamped with two laparoscopic bulldog clamps: intraoperative ultrasound (IOUS), together with the demarcation line appearing on parenchymal surface, confirms the absence of blood inflow toward the tumor-bearing area.

A 0.5 mg intravenous bolus of ICG is then administered and through Da Vinci Xi's Firefly® mode the dark cyanotic tumor-bearing area can be distinguished from the shining green liver remnant on a grayscale background, according to the negative staining technique. Under ICG guidance, the transection line can be easily identified and tracked with bipolar forceps.

Superficial transection is then performed by using harmonic scalpel, while the deeper transection plane is followed with bipolar forceps, according to the crush-clamp technique. When the G3b and G3a Glissonean pedicles are finally found again during transection, they are divided through monopolar scissors or harmonic scalpel between vascular clips. The adequacy of transection plane is constantly re-assessed by checking on the ICG staining and repeated IOUS. Finally, after segment 3 hepatic vein (V3) isolation with a blue tape and its division with a vascular stapler, the resection can be completed.

References

1. Nanashima A, Ariizumi SI, Yamamoto M. East meets west: east and west pioneers of "anatomical right hepatectomy" – period of dawn to establishment. J Hepatobiliary Pancreat Sci. 2018;25:214–6. https://doi.org/10.1002/jhbp.531.
2. Arish A, Eshkenazy R, Bismuth H. Milestones in the evolution of hepatic surgery. Rambam Maimonides Med J. 2011;2 https://doi.org/10.5041/rmmj.10021.
3. Cho SC, Kim JH. Laparoscopic left Hemihepatectomy using the hilar plate-first approach (with video). World J Surg. 2022;46:2454–8. https://doi.org/10.1007/s00268-022-06654-2.

4. Wakabayashi G, et al. The Tokyo 2020 terminology of liver anatomy and resections: updates of the Brisbane 2000 system. J Hepatobiliary Pancreat Sci. 2022;29:6–15. https://doi.org/10.1002/jhbp.1091.
5. Ariizumi SI, Nanashima A, Yamamoto M. Anterior approach in right hepatectomy. J Hepatobiliary Pancreat Sci. 2018;25:351–2. https://doi.org/10.1002/jhbp.567.
6. Coinaud C. Surgical anatomy of the liver revisited. Self-printed; 1989.
7. Takasaki K, K S, Tanaka S. Newly developed systematized hepatectomy by Glissonean pedicle transection method (in Japanese). Shujutu (Operation). 1986:7–14.
8. Jegadeesan MJ, a. R. Anatomical basis of approaches to liver resection. Acta Sci Gastroin Disorder. 2020;3:12.
9. Van Ha Q, Nguyen TH, Van Nguyen H, Le XA, Tran KH. Hepatectomy using a combination of extrafascial extrahepatic (Takasaki approach) and extrafascial intrahepatic pedicle approaches (ton that Tung approach). J Surg Case Rep. 2021;2021 https://doi.org/10.1093/jscr/rjab419.
10. Sugioka A, Kato Y, Tanahashi Y. Systematic extrahepatic Glissonean pedicle isolation for anatomical liver resection based on Laennec's capsule: proposal of a novel comprehensive surgical anatomy of the liver. J Hepatobiliary Pancreat Sci. 2017;24:17–23. https://doi.org/10.1002/jhbp.410.
11. Takasaki K. Glissonean pedicle transection method for hepatic resection: a new concept of liver segmentation. J Hepato-Biliary-Pancreat Surg. 1998;5:286–91. https://doi.org/10.1007/s005340050047.
12. Wakabayashi T, Colella M, Berardi G, Wakabayashi G. In: Ielpo B, Rosso E, Anselmo A, editors. Glissonean pedicles approach in minimally invasive liver surgery. Springer; 2023. p. 155–60.
13. Strasberg SM, et al. The Brisbane 2000 terminology of liver anatomy and resections. HPB. 2000;2:333–9. https://doi.org/10.1016/s1365-182x(17)30755-4.
14. Laennec RTHL. Lettre sur des Tuniques qui enveloppent certains visceres, et fournissent des gaines membraneuses a leurs vaisseaux. Journ De Med Chir et Pharm Vendemiaire. 1802:539–75.
15. Hayashi S, et al. Connective tissue configuration in the human liver hilar region with special reference to the liver capsule and vascular sheath. J Hepato-Biliary-Pancreat Surg. 2008;15:640–7. https://doi.org/10.1007/s00534-008-1336-8.
16. Liu Y, et al. A meta-analysis of the three-dimensional reconstruction visualization technology for hepatectomy. Asian J Surg. 2023;46:669–76. https://doi.org/10.1016/j.asjsur.2022.07.006.
17. Fong Y, Blumgart LH. Useful stapling techniques in liver surgery. J Am Coll Surg. 1997:93–100. https://doi.org/10.1016/s1072-7515(01)00889-4.

18. Figueras J, et al. Hilar dissection versus the "glissonean" approach and stapling of the pedicle for major hepatectomies: a prospective, randomized trial. Ann Surg. 2003;238:111–9. https://doi.org/10.1097/01.SLA.0000074981.02000.69.
19. Tsuruta K, Okamoto A, Fau-Toi M, Toi M, Fau-Saji H, Saji H, Fau-Takahashi T, Takahashi T. Impact of selective Glisson transection on survival of hepatocellular carcinoma. Hepato-Gastroenterology. 2002;49:1607.
20. Machado MA, et al. The laparoscopic Glissonean approach is safe and efficient when compared with standard laparoscopic liver resection: results of an observational study over 7 years. Surgery. 2016;160:643–51. https://doi.org/10.1016/j.surg.2016.01.017.
21. Chapman WC, Kelly Wright J, Wise PE, Wright Pinson C. Techniques of exposure, hilar dissection, and parenchymal division in hepatic surgery. Oper Tech Gen Surg. 2002;4:13–32. https://doi.org/10.1053/otgn.2002.30437.
22. Morimoto M, et al. Glissonean approach for hepatic inflow control in minimally invasive anatomic liver resection: a systematic review. J Hepatobiliary Pancreat Sci. 2022;29:51–65. https://doi.org/10.1002/jhbp.908.
23. Makuuchi M, Fau-Hasegawa H, Hasegawa H, Fau-Yamazaki S, Yamazaki S. Ultrasonically guided subsegmentectomy. Surg Gynecol Obstet. 1985;161:346–50.
24. Tanaka T, et al. Is a fluorescence navigation system with indocyanine green effective enough to detect liver malignancies? J Hepatobiliary Pancreat Sci. 2014;21:199–204. https://doi.org/10.1002/jhbp.17.
25. Aoki T, et al. Image-guided liver mapping using fluorescence navigation system with indocyanine green for anatomical hepatic resection. World J Surg. 2008;32:1763–7. https://doi.org/10.1007/s00268-008-9620-y.
26. Wakabayashi T, et al. Indocyanine green fluorescence navigation in liver surgery: a systematic review on dose and timing of administration. Ann Surg. 2022;275:1025–34. https://doi.org/10.1097/SLA.0000000000005406.
27. Berardi G, et al. Parenchymal sparing anatomical liver resections with full laparoscopic approach: description of technique and short-term results. Ann Surg. 2021;273:785–91. https://doi.org/10.1097/SLA.0000000000003575.
28. Liu F, et al. The extrahepatic Glissonean versus hilar dissection approach for laparoscopic formal right and left Hepatectomies in patients with hepatocellular carcinoma. J Gastrointest Surg. 2019;23:2401–10. https://doi.org/10.1007/s11605-019-04135-x.
29. Liao KX, et al. Laparoscopic Glissonean pedicle versus hilar dissection approach hemihepatectomy: a prospective, randomized controlled trial. J Hepatobiliary Pancreat Sci. 2022;29:629–40. https://doi.org/10.1002/jhbp.1129.

30. Kobayashi K, et al. Parenchyma-sparing liver resection for hepatocellular carcinoma in left lateral section is associated with better liver volume recovery. HPB (Oxford). 2018;20:949–55. https://doi.org/10.1016/j.hpb.2018.03.020.
31. Evrard S, Torzilli G, Caballero C, Bonhomme B. Parenchymal sparing surgery brings treatment of colorectal liver metastases into the precision medicine era. Eur J Cancer. 2018;104:195–200. https://doi.org/10.1016/j.ejca.2018.09.030.
32. Wakabayashi T, et al. Laparoscopically limited anatomic liver resections: a single-center analysis for oncologic outcomes of the conceptual procedure. Ann Surg Oncol. 2024;31:1243–51. https://doi.org/10.1245/s10434-023-14462-8.
33. Fujikawa T, Uemoto Y, Matsuoka T. Intrahepatic Glissonean approach for robotic anatomical liver resection of segment 7 using the saline-linked Monopolar cautery scissors (SLiC-scissors) method: a technical case report with videos. Cureus. 2023;15:e38470. https://doi.org/10.7759/cureus.38470.
34. Machado MA, Makdissi F. ASO author reflections: Glissonean approach is useful in robotic liver resections. Ann Surg Oncol. 2022;29:8452–3. https://doi.org/10.1245/s10434-022-12404-4.
35. Machado MAC, Ardengh AO, Lobo Filho MM, Mattos BH, Makdissi FF. Robotic anatomical resection of liver segment 4 with Glissonean approach and selective hepatic artery clamping. Arq Gastroenterol. 2021;58:127–8. https://doi.org/10.1590/S0004-2803.202100000-21.
36. Machado MA, Mattos BH, Lobo Filho M, Makdissi F. Intrahepatic Glissonean approach for robotic left hepatectomy. Surg Oncol. 2021;38:101601. https://doi.org/10.1016/j.suronc.2021.101601.
37. Machado MA, Mattos BH, Filho ML, Makdissi F. Intrahepatic Glissonean approach for robotic right hepatectomy. Surg Oncol. 2021;38:101579. https://doi.org/10.1016/j.suronc.2021.101579.
38. Machado MAC, Mattos BV, Lobo Filho MM, Makdissi F. Glissonean approach during robotic Mesohepatectomy for recurrent colorectal liver metastasis. Ann Surg Oncol. 2022;29:8449–51. https://doi.org/10.1245/s10434-022-12331-4.

Part V

Basic Maneuvers Procedure

Liver Mobilization and Ultrasound

18

James M. McDermott, Jonathan C. Delong, and Monica M. Dua

Relevant Surgical Anatomy

The liver is anchored within the abdominal cavity by several key attachments to the diaphragm, retroperitoneum, inferior vena cava (IVC), and stomach. During hepatic resection, these ligamentous and anatomic attachments must be systematically divided to achieve adequate mobilization. The falciform ligament connects the anterior surface of the liver to the ventral abdominal wall and anterior diaphragm. Its free inferior edge contains the round ligament (ligamentum teres), which extends to the umbilicus. The coronary ligament secures the superior surface of the liver to the diaphragm, while the right and left triangular ligaments are lateral condensations of the coronary ligament that anchor the respective lobes of the liver to the right and left hemidiaphragm. The hepatogastric ligament, a component of the lesser omentum, connects the left lobe of the liver to the lesser curvature of the stomach.

J. M. McDermott · M. M. Dua (✉)
Department of Surgery, Stanford University, Stanford, CA, USA
e-mail: jmcderm@stanford.edu; mdua@stanford.edu

J. C. Delong
Department of Surgery, University of Tennessee Medical Center Knoxville, Knoxville, TN, USA
e-mail: JCDeLong@utmck.edu

© The Author(s), under exclusive license to Springer Nature Switzerland AG 2025
A. Alseidi et al. (eds.), *The SAGES Manual of Contemporary Indications and Management of Hepatic and Biliary Diseases*, https://doi.org/10.1007/978-3-032-04823-3_18

Posteriorly, the hepatorenal ligament attaches the liver to the anterior surface of the right kidney. The right adrenal gland resides beneath the right posterior liver and must be meticulously identified and dissected free during mobilization. Once the hepatorenal ligament is divided, the retroperitoneum drops posteriorly, enhancing exposure of the retrohepatic IVC, a critical structure during liver mobilization and resection.

Intraoperative Ultrasound

Intraoperative ultrasound is a crucial component of any major liver resection. It is widely utilized to locate lesions in the liver, determine if additional tumors are present that were not seen on preoperative imaging, stage disease, and locate vascular and biliary structures. With current transducer resolutions, the sensitivity of intraoperative ultrasound has been reported as 90–95% for lesions larger than 2 mm. Intraoperative ultrasound is considered the gold standard of imaging with superior sensitivity to liver-specific magnetic resonance imaging (MRI), computed tomography (CT), and fluorodeoxyglucose-positron emission tomography (FDG-PET) [1–4]. The immediate imaging and high spatial resolution of intraoperative ultrasound provides information to guide resection, improve safety through identification of critical structures, and evaluate tumor relationships to planned surgical margins [2, 4, 5]. In some cases, this real-time information may even change or alter the surgical plan. Due to its immediate availability and ease of use, intraoperative ultrasound can be used frequently throughout the case to check progress and verify the dissection is on its intended course.

Open Liver Mobilization

Right Liver Mobilization

Depending on body habitus and tumor location, the incision for a right hepatectomy can be a generous midline laparotomy incision which would need to go past the umbilicus for adequate exposure and mobilization of the right liver or more standardly a modified Makuuchi incision (reverse L). The reverse L Makuuchi incision consists of a vertical midline component and a right subcostal (horizontal) component, forming an inverted "L" shape:

1. Midline Vertical Limb:
   - Begins at the xiphoid process and extends inferiorly along the midline.
   - Typically ends just above the umbilicus, though it may be extended below if additional exposure is needed based on patient body habitus or tumor size.
   - Horizontal Limb (Right Subcostal Component):
   - Originates from the inferior end of the midline incision.
   - Extends laterally to the right, as a straight line to two fingerbreadths below the costal margin or following a curved or slightly oblique path that parallels the right costal margin.

Mobilization begins with identification and division of the ligamentum teres and falciform ligament using electrocautery (Fig. 18.1). A tie is placed on the ligamentum teres to serve as a handle for cephalad retraction of the liver. For major liver resections, the Thompson Retractor is our preferred self-retaining retractor due to its strength, stability, and broad selection of blades. The retractor is positioned to achieve both anterior and cephalad retraction of the ribs, which provides optimal exposure of the suprahepatic inferior vena cava (IVC) and facilitates mobilization of the right lobe [5].

Three-point retraction is critical:

- Upward retraction of the left costal margin at the 1 o'clock position.
- Superior retraction of the right costal margin at 11 o'clock.
- Inferior retraction of the lower abdomen at 7 o'clock.

Failure to provide anterior retraction in addition to cephalad tension will limit working space at the hepatic dome. Dissection

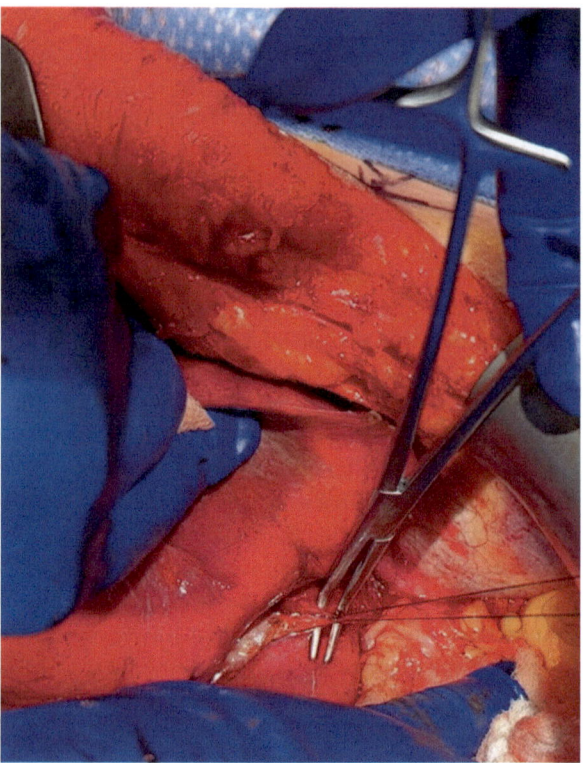

Fig. 18.1 Open mobilization of the liver using a midline incision begins with identification and division of the ligamentum teres and falciform ligament using electrocautery. A tie can be placed on the ligamentum teres to serve as a handle for cephalad retraction of the liver

of the falciform ligament is extended onto the right coronary ligament, exposing the suprahepatic IVC, which is cleared of fibrous attachments up to the level of the right hepatic vein. The right hepatic vein and the common trunk of the middle and left hepatic veins are exposed anteriorly using sharp dissection. Dissection between the middle and right hepatic veins can be continued to reveal the longitudinal groove at the origin of the right hepatic vein.

In larger patients or those with a deep or heavy right lobe, complete mobilization may require division of the left lobe ligamentous attachments to facilitate rotation of the right lobe out of the abdomen. The right lobe is retracted medially, while the right costal margin is retracted cephalad and laterally to expose the right triangular ligament, which is divided in a lateral-to-medial direction from the liver's inferior surface. Instead of simple lateral retraction, the assistant must progressively roll the liver out of the abdominal cavity to optimize tension and visualization. A laparotomy sponge positioned over the dome of the liver provides improved grip and protects the parenchyma during this maneuver. Dissection continues inferiorly to separate the right adrenal gland and expose the right lateral wall of the IVC. The retrohepatic IVC is then dissected in an inferior-to-superior direction (Fig. 18.2). Careful identification and division of short hepatic veins and retrohepatic branches from the caudate lobe and right liver is performed using clips, ties, or a vascular stapler for larger vessels. In some patients, a sizable accessory right hepatic vein may be encountered and can often be preserved to maintain venous drainage from the posterior sector—particularly important in cases requiring resection of the right and middle hepatic veins.

As dissection proceeds superiorly, the hepatocaval ligament (Makuuchi's ligament) is identified lateral to the right hepatic vein and divided, typically using a vascular stapler due to the frequent presence of an associated small vein. Division of this ligament exposes the lateral border of the right hepatic vein. Dissection of the inferior border of the vein establishes a tunnel between the right and middle hepatic veins, which connects to the groove created superiorly by division of the coronary ligament. A right-angle clamp can then be used to pass a vessel loop or suture around the right hepatic vein within this tunnel. Division of the hepatocaval ligament increases the mobility of the right lobe, facilitating leftward and caudal retraction for completion of mobilization. For bulky right-sided tumors not amenable to conventional mobilization, the anterior approach or "hanging maneuver" can be employed [6]. This involves blunt dissection of a narrow, avascular tunnel anterior to the IVC,

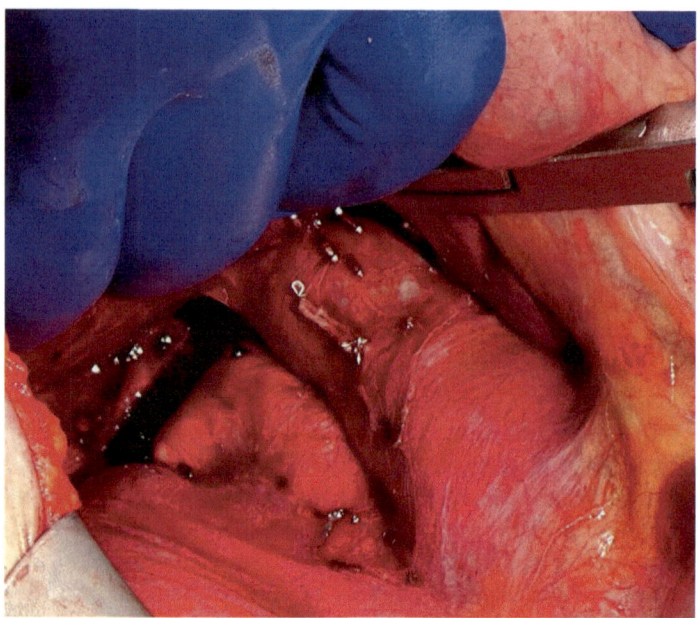

Fig. 18.2 The retrohepatic IVC is dissected in an inferior-to-superior direction. Careful division of short hepatic veins and retrohepatic branches from the caudate lobe and right liver is performed using clips, ties, or a vascular stapler for larger vessels

allowing passage of an umbilical tape or Penrose drain between the liver and IVC. This tape suspends the liver during parenchymal transection, enabling a controlled anterior-to-posterior (A–P) dissection from the liver surface down to the hilum and IVC. This technique minimizes the risk of tumor rupture or bleeding during mobilization of large masses. However, one must be cautious—deep parenchymal bleeding from the middle hepatic vein can be difficult to control if the liver has not been fully mobilized, as the ability to lift the liver for compression or rapid hemostasis is limited [6, 7].

Left Liver Mobilization

For left-sided liver resections, a midline laparotomy incision is typically sufficient, extending at least to the umbilicus. In some cases, the incision may need to be extended several centimeters below the umbilicus to ensure adequate retraction and exposure. With appropriate superior retraction, the ligamentum teres and falciform ligament are identified and divided using electrocautery, continuing the dissection up to the suprahepatic inferior vena cava (IVC) and the hepatic veins. Mobilization proceeds with division of the left coronary ligament, which is divided close to the liver surface. Right-angle forceps are then used to develop the groove between the middle and left hepatic veins, a key step for establishing control of venous outflow. The left lobe of the liver is then reflected medially, exposing the hepatogastric ligament, which is divided to open the lesser sac. It is important to note that a replaced or accessory left hepatic artery may traverse this ligament and should be identified and preserved when appropriate. The ligamentum venosum, visible over the caudate lobe, is then divided to open the space anterior to the IVC and posterior to the left hepatic vein. Blunt dissection is performed within this plane to connect with the previously developed dissection between the middle and left hepatic veins, thereby facilitating control of the left hepatic vein. In cases where a common trunk of the middle and left hepatic veins precludes safe extrahepatic dissection of the left hepatic vein, the remaining portion of the vein can be isolated intrahepatically following parenchymal transection.

Laparoscopic Mobilization of the Liver

Positioning and Port Placement

For both right and left liver mobilizations done laparoscopically, the patient is positioned supine on a split-leg table or lithotomy position with both arms padded and tucked by their sides. Hips are abducted to allow the surgeon to stand between the patient's legs. Reverse Trendelenburg and leftward tilt should be used and modified as needed throughout the procedure to allow the bowel to fall into the lower abdomen and improve exposure of the liver. Port placement for laparoscopic right and left hepatectomy is shown in Fig. 18.3.

Laparoscopic Right Liver Mobilization

Once port placement is complete, laparoscopic intraoperative ultrasound is utilized to evaluate the target lesion, assess the remainder of the liver parenchyma, and identify key anatomical landmarks, including the right and middle hepatic veins and the inflow pedicle. Right liver mobilization begins with the identification and division of the ligamentum teres and falciform ligament, using monopolar electrocautery or a laparoscopic vessel sealer. These structures should be divided high along the anterior abdominal wall to prevent residual tissue from obstructing the operative field.

Dissection proceeds toward the right hepatic vein. Tilting the operating table to the left allows the liver to fall away from the

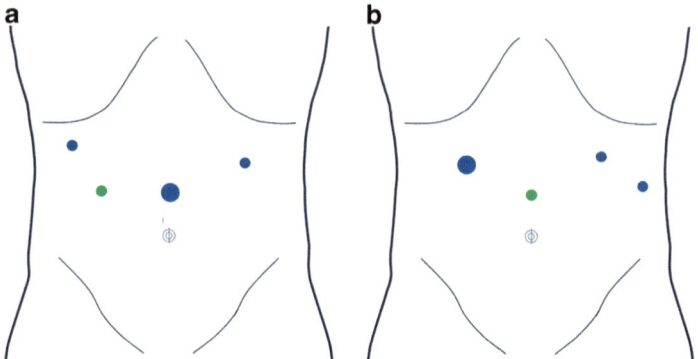

Fig. 18.3 One option for laparoscopic port placement for (**a**) Right hepatectomy and (**b**) Left hepatectomy. The small circles represent 5 mm ports and the larger circle is for the 10 mm ports. The green circle indicates where the laparoscope would be for the majority of the case

diaphragm, improving exposure of the right triangular ligament and right hepatic vein. With downward traction applied to the liver using a grasper or triangular liver retractor, the coronary and right triangular ligaments are divided in a medial-to-lateral direction through the epigastric port. This direction of dissection reduces the risk of injuring phrenic vessels and diaphragmatic collaterals, particularly in patients with cirrhosis [8]. Once superior ligamentous attachments are released, the right liver lobe is rotated medially using the retractor or Endo-paddle. Retraction may also be assisted by grasping the gallbladder fundus or round ligament. Dissection of the inferior right triangular ligament is completed in a medial-to-lateral fashion. The right adrenal gland, often adherent to the posterior aspect of the liver, is carefully dissected using electrocautery. Through the right lateral ports, dissection of the retroperitoneum is initiated to mobilize the liver from the inferior vena cava (IVC), proceeding from inferior to superior, as in the open approach. Short hepatic veins encountered along the retrohepatic IVC are controlled with a laparoscopic vessel sealer, clip applier, or when necessary, a laparoscopic stapler.

Laparoscopic Left Liver Mobilization

Laparoscopic mobilization of the left liver is initiated in a similar fashion to right liver mobilization. After dividing the ligamentum teres and falciform ligament, a medial-to-lateral dissection of the left coronary and left triangular ligaments is carried out to allow medial rotation of the left lobe of the liver [9]. In laparoscopic left lateral segmentectomy, this approach permits the left triangular ligament to be preserved initially to provide effective traction until the parenchymal transection is complete and the left hepatic vein is divided with a stapler. Additional retraction of the liver toward the right can be achieved using the gallbladder or the ligated falciform ligament. The gastrohepatic ligament is then divided using a laparoscopic vessel sealer, extending the dissection superiorly toward the diaphragm to complete exposure.

Robotic Mobilization of the Liver

Positioning and Port Placement

The patient is positioned supine in the lithotomy or split-leg position with a slight reverse Trendelenburg tilt to allow gravitational retraction of the bowel. One commonly used robotic configuration involves placement of an 8 mm robotic trocar—designated as the camera port—approximately two fingerbreadths superior and two fingerbreadths to the right of the umbilicus. Three additional 8 mm robotic working ports are inserted in a horizontal alignment, spaced approximately 7 cm apart to optimize instrument triangulation and range of motion. The bedside assistant is positioned between the patient's legs, with an assistant port placed inferior to the umbilicus. This port facilitates the introduction of instruments, suctioning, and stapling, and allows for active assistance throughout the procedure [9].

Robotic Right Liver Mobilization

Mobilization is started by dividing the ligamentum teres near the connection to the anterior abdominal wall. The ligament is clipped and used as a retraction lever to be pulled by one of the robotic arms. Using a grasper or vessel sealer to apply downward pressure to the anterior liver and tension on the ligamentum teres, the other working arm is equipped with an electrocautery hook or monopolar scissors to divide the falciform ligament up to the level of the hepatic veins (Fig. 18.4). While maintaining downward pressure, the left working arm divides the superior right coronary ligament. If required, the gallbladder can be mobilized from adhesions at this time to allow for additional traction from the retractor holding the ligamentum teres. Following dissection of the coronary ligament, the left retraction arm is used to elevate the right side of the liver to enable access to the inferior right triangular ligament. The inferior right triangular ligament is divided from medial to lateral until it meets the prior dissection of the right

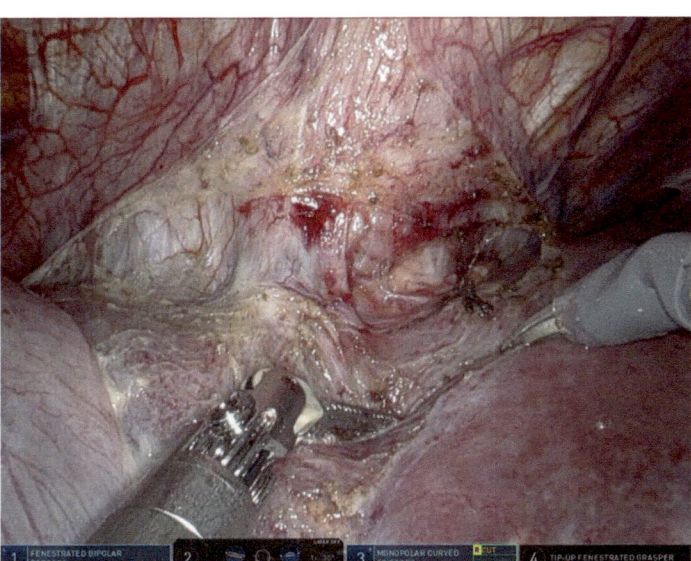

Fig. 18.4 In robotic mobilization of the liver, a robotic caudle grasper or vessel sealer can be used to apply downward pressure to the anterior liver while the other working arm is equipped with an electrocautery hook or monopolar scissors to divide the falciform ligament up to the level of the hepatic veins

coronary ligament. During division of the triangular ligament, exposure and traction can be improved with leftward rotation of the bed, increased traction from the ligamentum teres and gallbladder, or use of a triangular retractor. The use of a Ray-Tec surgical sponge in the interface between the retracting arm and the liver can help maintain traction while protecting the liver parenchyma from unintended damage. The retrohepatic inferior vena cava will be exposed by short hepatic veins which can be ligated with a vessel sealer if small or with clips if larger. As the inferior vena cava is further dissected in an inferior to superior direction, the inferior vena cava ligament (Makuuchi's ligament) is identified and divided with an endoscopic stapler. As the surgeon continues to move superiorly, the right border of the right hepatic vein is identified.

Robotic Left Liver Mobilization

Like the right-sided mobilization, the ligamentum teres is divided near its attachment to the anterior abdominal wall using the robotic electrocautery hook or the monopolar scissors. Using a grasper or vessel sealer to apply downward pressure to the anterior liver and tension on the ligamentum teres, the other working arm is used to divide the falciform ligament up to the hepatic veins with the electrocautery hook or the monopolar scissors. Dissection continues with division of the left coronary and triangular ligaments, with care taken to avoid injury to phrenic nerve branches or phrenic vein. An accessory or replaced left hepatic artery may be identified in the gastrohepatic ligament which is the superior access to the lesser sac.

Summary

Liver mobilization is a foundational component of safe and effective hepatic surgery. Whether performed through an open, laparoscopic, or robotic approach, meticulous attention to anatomic detail and stepwise dissection of the liver's ligamentous and vascular attachments are critical for optimal exposure and operative success. Mastery of mobilization techniques—including identification of major hepatic veins, preservation or division of short hepatic vessels, and safe manipulation around the inferior vena cava—provides the surgeon with a stable and controlled operative field. Intraoperative ultrasound complements mobilization by guiding resection planes, identifying key vascular structures, and confirming parenchymal and biliary anatomy, particularly in complex resections. While the principles remain constant across surgical platforms, technological advancements in minimally invasive and robotic-assisted surgery have expanded the surgeon's ability to safely mobilize the liver with enhanced visualization and precision. Ultimately, thoughtful mobilization tailored to the patient's anatomy and pathology is integral to minimizing complications and achieving oncologic and technical success in liver surgery.

Intraoperative Ultrasound—Open Surgery

Setup and Settings

Surgeons must familiarize themselves with the ultrasound device so common settings are well-understood and can be adjusted accordingly.

Frequency Frequency is directly related to the resolution of the image, with increased frequency resulting in improved image resolution. While it may seem that higher frequency probes (15 MHz) should be used for improved resolution, these probes have limited depth of penetration when compared to that seen with the lower frequency probes (3–5 MHz). The greater image depth seen with lower frequency probes makes them the more useful tool for intraoperative liver ultrasound.

Gain Gain in intraoperative ultrasound can be thought of as brightness. Increased gain will amplify the echoes returning to the ultrasound to increase image brightness but will also introduce or increase noise.

Time Gain Compensation (TGC) TGC allows the surgeon to adjust the gain at various levels of the ultrasound imaging to compensate for the relative dampening of echoes returned from deeper levels. The controls to adjust TGC are usually located at the top right of the ultrasound keyboard. With the controls centered, there will be uniform gain throughout the image. Having them instead positioned in a slight backslash (\) will increase the gain in a stepwise fashion for each increase in depth.

Depth: Depth is the distance to which the ultrasound will display an image. Depth is inversely related to image resolution, where increased depth will decrease image resolution. Whereas decreasing the depth will increase the image resolution, but at the cost of a more limited field of view.

Focus Focus is used to improve the image at a certain depth to allow for improved visualization of a particular point of interest.

Freeze This will hold the current image on the ultrasound screen.

Measure This will measure the distance between two selected points.

Evaluating the Liver Parenchyma

Intraoperative ultrasound should be performed early during abdominal exploration to corroborate preoperative imaging findings and guide operative planning. Particular attention should be paid to the future liver remnant (FLR) to identify any occult lesions that may alter the surgical approach or render the disease unresectable. Ultrasound evaluation is ideally conducted prior to extensive liver mobilization, as dissection can introduce artifact at the probe–liver interface, compromising image quality. A systematic survey of the hepatic parenchyma should be performed using overlapping vertical strokes—commonly referred to as the "lawn mower" technique—progressing across the liver from either side. For evaluation of the superior hepatic dome, which may be difficult to visualize directly, the probe can also be applied to the inferior surface of the liver to achieve optimal imaging [10].

Identifying Anatomical Landmarks

To delineate the hepatic venous anatomy, the ultrasound probe can be placed centrally in the liver, just to the patient's right of the falciform ligament. From this position, tilting the probe superiorly will typically reveal the junction of the hepatic veins as they enter the suprahepatic inferior vena cava (Fig. 18.5). Tilting the probe inferiorly from the same position exposes the bifurcation of the right and left portal veins. From this vantage point, the probe can be maneuvered: inferiorly to visualize the main portal vein, to the right to follow the right portal vein and its division into ante-

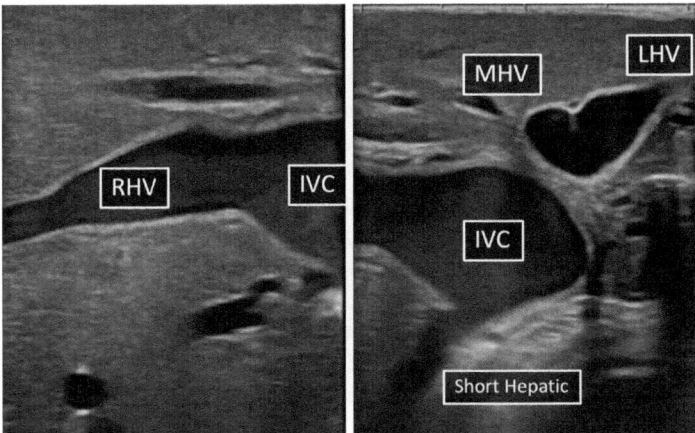

Fig. 18.5 The ultrasound probe can be placed centrally in the liver, just to the patient's right of the falciform ligament. From this position, tilting the probe superiorly will typically reveal the junction of the hepatic veins as they enter the suprahepatic inferior vena cava

rior and posterior branches, or to the left to trace the left portal vein and its segmental branches [11]. Once the falciform ligament is divided, the probe can also be placed over the dome of the liver, and a gentle rocking motion can be used to better visualize venous structures, including short hepatic veins.

In a right trisegmentectomy, intraoperative ultrasound is essential to ensure adequate outflow through the left hepatic vein before resecting the middle hepatic vein, as these typically converge prior to draining into the IVC. Doppler ultrasound can be used to assess left hepatic vein flow; diminished flow or venous congestion may indicate compromised outflow. Upon completion of the resection, Doppler imaging is again used to confirm adequate inflow and outflow in the remnant liver. During a central hepatectomy, intraoperative ultrasound is first used to survey the hepatic parenchyma for additional lesions, confirm tumor location in segments IV, V, and VIII, and evaluate for vascular and biliary anatomical variants. This operation involves two major planes of parenchymal transection: between segments VI/VII and V/VIII, and between segments II/III and IV. Although technically demanding, central resections preserve maximal liver parenchyma by sparing uninvolved segments. To plan the anterior-posterior plane between the anterior and posterior sectors, the right hepatic vein can be mapped using ultrasound. This same anatomical landmark is crucial when planning right anterior or posterior sectorectomies. Complete liver mobilization is critical, as the right hepatic vein naturally courses in a horizontal plane within the liver. By rotating the right lobe 90 degrees out of the abdomen, the hepatic vein is reoriented into a more accessible anterior-posterior plane for safer and more controlled dissection.

Distinguishing hepatic veins from portal triad structures can be challenging, particularly in the presence of dilated bile ducts. Portal structures are encased in Glisson's capsule and therefore appear with a characteristic thick, echogenic border or "halo" on ultrasound [12], in contrast to hepatic veins, which lack these features. Additional identification tools include Doppler imaging: the portal vein demonstrates steady, monophasic flow, arterial waveforms are typically triphasic, and dilated bile ducts will show no flow (Fig. 18.6). Accurate interpretation is essential prior to transecting any inflow structures. Preoperative biliary drainage of the future liver remnant—via percutaneous transhepatic catheters or internal-external stents—not only optimizes liver function but also aids intraoperative identification of biliary structures. On ultrasound, biliary stents produce posterior acoustic shadowing, making them readily identifiable. In cases requiring biliary reconstruction, these stents can be preserved intraoperatively to serve as a guide or temporary internal stent across the hepaticojejunostomy.

Intraoperative ultrasound is also indispensable for precise targeting during needle-based procedures, such as liver biopsy or tumor ablation. With one hand stabilizing the probe on the liver surface, the needle or ablation probe should be introduced in the same plane as the ultrasound beam. Maintaining the probe and needle in plane ensures continuous visualization of the needle tip throughout its course, improving targeting accuracy and minimizing the risk of injury [11].

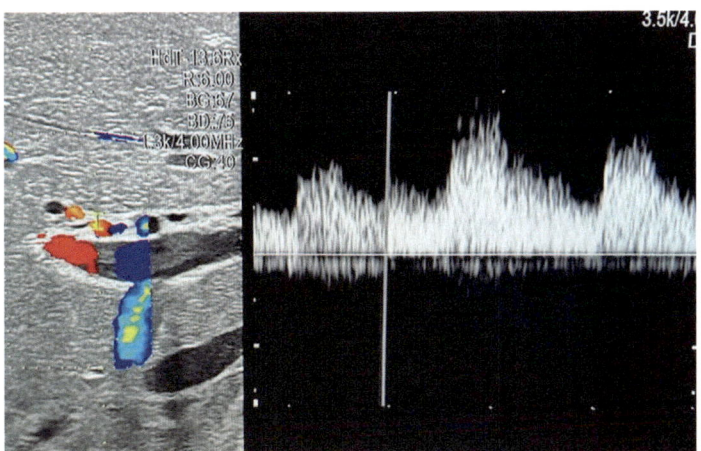

Fig. 18.6 Doppler ultrasound can be used to assess vascular structures in the liver. The portal vein demonstrates steady, monophasic flow, arterial waveforms are typically triphasic, and dilated bile ducts will show no flow

Ultrasound in Minimally Invasive Approaches

Laparoscopic Ultrasound

Unlike in open procedures, the use of intraoperative ultrasound in laparoscopic liver surgery is inherently limited by trocar placement, which often results in probe angles that are vertical or oblique rather than horizontal or transverse. These unique angles can make image interpretation and spatial conceptualization more challenging, particularly for surgeons with limited experience in laparoscopic ultrasound. To mitigate these limitations and improve probe maneuverability, a linear flexible side-viewing laparoscopic probe is preferred over a rigid side-viewing probe. The flexible design allows for better navigation through a laparoscopic port and adapts more easily to the required imaging angles. A right subcostal port is commonly used and provides the most accurate approximation of a transverse image. Additional commonly utilized trocar sites include the periumbilical and subxiphoid/epigastric regions. As described previously, the patient is positioned on a split-leg table in lithotomy, with the hips abducted to allow the surgeon to stand between the patient's legs. The laparoscopic ultrasound probe can articulate up to 180 degrees in both horizontal and vertical directions via two lever controls. A clear sterile drape placed over the ultrasound console allows the surgeon to adjust settings—such as Doppler mode, measurement tools, depth, and gain—while simultaneously handling the laparoscope and ultrasound probe.

Two visualization strategies can be employed to display both the laparoscopic and ultrasound images. One option is to position the laparoscopic and ultrasound monitors side-by-side, providing the surgeon with two full-sized, separate displays. Alternatively, a "picture-in-picture" mode can be activated on the laparoscopic monitor, allowing for concurrent visualization of both video feeds on a single screen. While the latter option offers improved ergonomics, it may compromise image size and resolution. The overall ultrasound approach parallels that of open procedures, beginning with a comprehensive assessment of the liver parenchyma to identify the target lesion, exclude disease in the future liver remnant, and localize critical vascular structures, including portal inflow and hepatic outflow. The "lawn mower" technique, using overlapping vertical strokes, remains an effective method for systematic parenchymal evaluation in the laparoscopic setting. Stand-off scanning may be employed to assess the superior dome and capsular edges of the liver. In this technique, saline is instilled between the dome and the diaphragm to create an acoustic medium that enhances visualization of difficult-to-reach areas. Doppler ultrasound can further assist in identifying hepatic arteries, portal veins, and hepatic veins.

For right and left hepatectomies, the middle hepatic vein can be visualized and used as a landmark to define the transection plane. In central hepatectomy or left hepatic trisegmentectomy, the right hepatic vein may serve this role. After initial ultrasound mapping, the planned transection plane can be marked on the liver surface with electrocautery. It is advisable to repeat ultrasound evaluation along this line prior to parenchymal transection to confirm anatomical landmarks and lesion margins. Intraoperative ultrasound should also be utilized throughout the resection to guide dissection and maintain orientation. A surgical sponge placed in the transection plane midway through the procedure may further enhance visualization of margins and transection direction on ultrasound. During left hepatectomy, intraoperative ultrasound is particularly helpful when mobilizing the left triangular ligament. It allows for visualization of the suprahepatic inferior vena cava and left hepatic vein trunk to determine whether an extrahepatic portion of the left hepatic vein is at risk of injury during mobilization. The left phrenic vein can also serve as a helpful anatomical landmark, as it drains directly into the left hepatic vein and marks the path toward the cava.

Robotic Ultrasound

Intraoperative ultrasound during robotic-assisted liver surgery utilizes a drop-in linear probe of varying lengths, which is inserted through an assistant port and manipulated by one of the robotic instruments. Unlike laparoscopic ultrasound, where probe mobility is limited by the rigid shaft and port alignment, robotic ultrasound offers enhanced dexterity due to the articulation of the robotic arms and the ability to maneuver the probe freely within the abdomen. This setup more closely replicates the full range of motion available during open surgery. The probe is controlled directly by the surgeon at the console, allowing real-time manipulation and interpretation of the ultrasound while simultaneously viewing both the operative field and ultrasound images on a single integrated screen. Although the general principles of laparoscopic ultrasound apply, the robotic interface provides improved ergonomics and precision. A potential limitation, however, is that the ultrasound system settings (e.g., gain, depth, Doppler mode) still need to be adjusted manually on the machine itself, requiring the surgeon to step away from the console or rely on the bedside assistant for these adjustments.

Summary

Intraoperative ultrasound is an indispensable tool in hepatic surgery, offering real-time, high-resolution imaging that enhances surgical precision, improves oncologic outcomes, and reduces the risk of complications. From confirming preoperative imaging findings and identifying occult lesions to delineating critical vascular and biliary anatomy, intraoperative ultrasound plays a central role in operative planning and intraoperative decision-making. Its utility spans open, laparoscopic, and robotic platforms, each with distinct advantages and technical nuances. Mastery of ultrasound fundamentals—such as probe selection, image optimization settings, and Doppler interpretation—is essential for effective use. Whether guiding parenchymal transection, confirming vascular inflow and outflow, or enabling precise ablation and needle targeting, intraoperative ultrasound provides unparalleled anatomic clarity. As technology continues to evolve, its integration into all forms of minimally invasive liver surgery will only deepen, underscoring the need for all hepatobiliary surgeons to develop and maintain proficiency in its use.

Disclosures All authors have nothing to disclose.

References

1. Langella S, Ardito F, Russolillo N, et al. Intraoperative ultrasound staging for colorectal liver metastases in the era of liver-specific magnetic resonance imaging: is it still worthwhile? J Oncol. 2019;1369274:1–8.
2. Joo I. The role of intraoperative ultrasound staging for colorectal liver metastases in the era of liver-specific magnetic resonance imaging: is it still worthwhile? Ultrasonography. 2015;34(4):246–57.
3. Coco D, Leanza S. Routine intraoperative ultrasound for the detection of liver metastases during resection of primary colorectal cancer—a systematic review. Maedica (Bucur). 2020;15(2):250–2.
4. Lubner MG, Gettle LM, Kim DH, et al. Diagnostic and procedural intraoperative ultrasound: technique, tips and tricks for optimizing results. 2021;94:20201406, 1–10.
5. Aragon and Solomon. Techniques of hepatic resection. J Gastrointest Oncol. 2012;3(1):28–40.

6. Liu CL, Fan ST, Lo CM, et al. Anterior approach for major right hepatic resection for large hepatocellular carcinoma. Ann Surg. 2000;232(1):25–31.
7. Nanashima A, Sumida Y, Abo T, et al. Usefulness and application of the liver hanging maneuver for anatomical liver resections. World J Surg. 2008;32(9):2070–6.
8. Ikoma N, Itano O, Oshima G, et al. Laparoscopic liver mobilization: tricks of the trade to avoid complications. Surg Laparosc Endosc Percutan Tech. 2015;25(1):e21–3.
9. Giulianotti PC, Bianco FM, Daskalaki D. Robotic liver surgery: technical aspects and review of the literature. Hepatobiliary Surg Nutr. 2016;5(4):311–21.
10. Kruskal JB, Kane RA. Intraoperative US of the liver: techniques and clinical applicatitons. Radiographics. 2006;26(4):1067–84.
11. Hagopian EJ. Liver ultrasound: a key procedure in the surgeon's toolbox. J Surg Oncol. 2020;122(1):61–9.
12. Kesimal U, Ceken K, Kabaalioglu A. The role of intraoperative ultrasonography in detection of hepatic vein variations. J Ultrasound. 2021;25(1):19–25.

Minimally Invasive Pringle Maneuvers

19

Hemasat Alkhatib, Ali M. Kara, Ahmad Abou Abbass, and Kevin El-Hayek

Introduction

In recent years, minimally invasive liver resection (using laparoscopic, robotic, or hybrid techniques) has become popular for treating both benign and malignant liver diseases. It offers lower complication rates and better oncological outcomes compared to traditional open surgery [1–3]. The success of minimally invasive

Supplementary Information The online version contains supplementary material available at https://doi.org/10.1007/978-3-032-04823-3_19.

H. Alkhatib · A. M. Kara
Department of General Surgery, The MetroHealth System,
Cleveland, OH, USA

A. A. Abbass
South Orange County Surgical Medical Group, Mission Viejo, CA, USA

K. El-Hayek (✉)
Department of General Surgery, The MetroHealth System, Cleveland, OH, USA

Case Western Reserve University School of Medicine, Cleveland, OH, USA
e-mail: kelhayek@metrohealth.org

© The Author(s), under exclusive license to Springer Nature Switzerland AG 2025
A. Alseidi et al. (eds.), *The SAGES Manual of Contemporary Indications and Management of Hepatic and Biliary Diseases*,
https://doi.org/10.1007/978-3-032-04823-3_19

liver resection has encouraged skilled surgeons to undertake more intricate procedures that involve dealing with various challenges during surgery. One critical aspect is the preservation of hemostasis at the liver transection site. The Pringle maneuver, originally described by James Hogarth Pringle in 1908, involves occluding the portal triad to control bleeding in liver surgery [4]. This maneuver improves visibility, reduces blood loss, and minimizes the risk of damage to biliary structures [5, 6]. Routine use of the Pringle maneuver during minimally invasive liver resection lowers conversion rates without harming the liver [7].

Various techniques for performing the minimally invasive Pringle maneuver exist, categorized as intracorporeal and extracorporeal approaches, but there's no consensus on the best method due to individual advantages and disadvantages [8]. Various techniques will be demonstrated in the supplemental videos included in this chapter.

Extracorporeal Techniques

- The hepatoduodenal ligament is identified, and the pars flaccida of the gastrohepatic ligament is opened.
- A tape is passed through the foramen of Winslow behind and around the hepatoduodenal ligament. The tape is then brought out extracorporeally through the minimally invasive port. A laparoscopic articulating instrument can be used to facilitate the passage of the tape behind the foramen of Winslow.
- The port is then removed, and the tape is threaded through a Rummel tourniquet. The tourniquet is then advanced to the level of the hepatic pedicle, with the end of the tourniquet remaining extracorporeally.
- To perform the Pringle maneuver, an assistant at bedside tightens the tourniquet.

Alternatives

- An umbilical/cotton tape, penrose drain, cotton gauze, or infusion tubing can be used as alternative material to create the sling around the hepatoduodenal ligament [7, 9, 10].
- A 24-French chest tube, or any double-ended catheter can be used as an alternative to the traditional Rummel Tourniquet [7, 10, 11].

Intracorporeal Techniques

- The hepatoduodenal ligament is identified, and the pars flaccida of the gastrohepatic ligament is opened.
- A 14-French foley catheter is shortened to 15 cm and placed intraperitoneally.
- The tip of the catheter is passed behind the foramen of Winslow and pulled around from the lesser sac.
- A grasper is placed through the foley side hole, and the other end of the catheter is pulled through, creating a circular loop.
- The loop is tightened to perform the Pringle maneuver. A surgical clip can be used to hold the tension [12].

Alternatives

- A liver circle device described by Gao et al. [13] a device made of medical silica gel with a tapered stem and a circular hole that put together form a loop around the hepatoduodenal ligament.
- A six-loop Pringle maneuver using a T-tube and 10-French foley catheter described by Chao et al. [14]. Briefly, all arms of the T-tube are trimmed to 1–2 cm. The foley is trimmed to 12 cm, and the cut end is inserted and sutured into the main stem of the T-tube. The other end of the foley catheter is then placed within the T-tube arms, forming the six-loop.

- A penrose drain, elastic rim of surgical glove or a vessel loop can be used to pass around the hepatoduodenal ligament and a hemo-o-lock clip is used to clamp down and perform the Pringle maneuver [15, 16].

Vascular Clamp Techniques

- Extracorporeal Satinsky clamp [17]: This method is particularly useful in reoperative surgery when dissection of the hepatoduodenal ligament can be challenging. The clamp can either be introduced through the left lateral abdominal wall if a space behind the hepatoduodenal ligament was able to be dissected. If adhesions are severe, the clamp can alternatively be introduced vertically, clamping the structures anteriorly.
- Intracorporeal bulldog clamp [18]: The matched forceps are used to insert the bulldog clamp intraperitoneally through a 12 mm port. This method is useful when the hepatoduodenal ligament is dissected and lymphadenectomy performed, skeletonizing the porta hepatis structures. Alternative methods pose a higher risk of injury due to the loss of the protective soft tissue.

Discussion

Minimally invasive Pringle maneuver techniques exhibit variability, each offering unique advantages and drawbacks [8]. Intracorporeal methods offer the advantage of eliminating the need for an additional port site. In contrast, extracorporeal techniques may facilitate maneuvering and exposure but may compromise the surgical view and lead to instrument clustering. Some methods necessitate the creation of a posterior plane to the hepatoduodenal ligament, which can pose challenges. In such cases, an extracorporeal Satinsky clamp may prove useful, as it obviates the need for this dissection. Consequently, it is imperative for surgeons to be well-versed in the repertoire of minimally invasive

Pringle maneuver techniques, enabling them to adapt to various surgical scenarios. Currently, no high-level data definitively establishes the superiority of one method over another. Hence, a surgeon's proficiency in a chosen maneuver remains paramount for achieving optimal outcomes in these procedures.

References

1. Kamarajah SK, Gujjuri RR, Hilal MA, Manas DM, White SA. Does minimally invasive liver resection improve long-term survival compared to open resection for hepatocellular carcinoma? A systematic review and meta-analysis. Scand J Surg. 2022;111:14574969211042455.
2. Chen J, Li H, Liu F, Li B, Wei Y. Surgical outcomes of laparoscopic versus open liver resection for hepatocellular carcinoma for various resection extent. Medicine. 2017;96:e6460.
3. Uemoto Y, Taura K, Nishio T, Kimura Y, Nam NH, Yoshino K, Yoh T, Koyama Y, Ogiso S, Fukumitsu K, Ishii T, Seo S, Uemoto S. Laparoscopic versus open liver resection for hepatocellular carcinoma: a case controlled study with propensity score matching. World J Surg. 2021;45:2572–80.
4. Pringle JH. V. Notes on the arrest of hepatic hemorrhage due to trauma. Ann Surg. 1908;48:541–9.
5. Belghiti J, Noun R, Zante E, Ballet T, Sauvanet A. Portal triad clamping or hepatic vascular exclusion for major liver resection. A controlled study. Ann Surg. 1996;224:155–61.
6. Al-Saeedi M, Ghamarnejad O, Khajeh E, Shafiei S, Salehpour R, Golriz M, Mieth M, Weiss KH, Longerich T, Hoffmann K, Büchler MW, Mehrabi A. Pringle maneuver in extended liver resection: a propensity score analysis. Sci Rep. 2020;10:8847.
7. Dua MM, Worhunsky DJ, Hwa K, Poultsides GA, Norton JA, Visser BC. Extracorporeal Pringle for laparoscopic liver resection. Surg Endosc. 2015;29:1348–55.
8. Mownah OA, Aroori S. The Pringle maneuver in the modern era: a review of techniques for hepatic inflow occlusion in minimally invasive liver resection. Annals Hepato-Biliary-Pancreatic Surg. 2023;27:131–40.
9. Okuda Y, Honda G, Kurata M, Kobayashi S. Useful and convenient procedure for intermittent vascular occlusion in laparoscopic hepatectomy. Asian J Endoscop Surg. 2013;6:100–3.
10. Rotellar F, Pardo F, Bueno A, Martí-Cruchaga P, Zozaya G. Extracorporeal tourniquet method for intermittent hepatic pedicle clamping during laparoscopic liver surgery: an easy, cheap, and effective technique. Langenbeck's Arch Surg. 2012;397:481–5.

11. Peng Y, Wang Z, Wang X, Chen F, Zhou J, Fan J, Shi Y. A novel very simple laparoscopic hepatic inflow occlusion apparatus for laparoscopic liver surgery. Surg Endosc. 2019;33:145–52.
12. Huang JW, Su WL, Wang SN. Alternative laparoscopic Intracorporeal Pringle maneuver by Huang's loop. World J Surg. 2018;42:3312–5.
13. Gao Z, Li Z, Zhou B, Chen L, Shen Z, Jiang Y, Zheng X, Xiang J, Zhang Q, Wang W, Yan S. A self-designed liver circle for on-demand Pringle's manoeuver in laparoscopic liver resection. J Minim Access Surg. 2021;17:120–6.
14. Chao Y-J, Wang C-J, Shan Y-S. Technical notes: a self-designed, simple, secure, and safe six-loop intracorporeal Pringle's maneuver for laparoscopic liver resection. Surg Endosc. 2012;26:2681–6.
15. Cai J, Zheng J, Xie Y, Kirih MA, Jiang G, Liang Y, Liang X. A novel simple intra-corporeal Pringle maneuver for laparoscopic hemihepatectomy: how we do it. Surg Endosc. 2020;34:2807–13.
16. Choi YI. The usefulness of the totally intra-corporeal Pringle maneuver with Penrose drain tube during laparoscopic left side liver resection. Annals Hepato-Biliary-Pancreatic Surg. 2020;24:252–8.
17. Onda S, Haruki K, Furukawa K, Yasuda J, Shirai Y, Sakamoto T, Gocho T, Ikegami T. Newly-revised Pringle maneuver using laparoscopic Satinsky vascular clamp for repeat laparoscopic hepatectomy. Surg Endosc. 2021;35:5375–80.
18. He L, Li W, Zhou D, Wang L, Hou H, Geng X. Comparative analysis of vascular bulldog clamps used in laparoscopic liver resection. Medicine. 2021;100:e26074.

20. Intraoperative Cholangiography, Choledochoscopy, and Fluorescent Cholangiography

Domenech Asbun, Levan Tsamalaidze, and Horacio Asbun

Introduction

It is fundamental for hepatobiliary surgeons to master the skills necessary to assess and access the biliary tree. Intraoperative cholangiography, choledochoscopy, and fluorescent cholangiography are three mainstay techniques. Ongoing technological advancements have not only increased the instruments and techniques available but have also expanded the indications for their use.

In this chapter we will review the technical details of these procedures, as well as an overview of the state-of-the-art and current decision-making considerations.

Supplementary Information The online version contains supplementary material available at https://doi.org/10.1007/978-3-032-04823-3_20.

D. Asbun (✉) · L. Tsamalaidze · H. Asbun
Division of Hepatobiliary and Pancreas Surgery, Miami Cancer Institute, Miami, FL, USA
e-mail: domenech.asbun@baptisthealth.net

© The Author(s), under exclusive license to Springer Nature Switzerland AG 2025
A. Alseidi et al. (eds.), *The SAGES Manual of Contemporary Indications and Management of Hepatic and Biliary Diseases*, https://doi.org/10.1007/978-3-032-04823-3_20

Intraoperative Cholangiogram

Background

Since the introduction of intraoperative cholangiograms (IOC) in 1937 by Mirizzi [1], this technique of imaging the biliary tree has been widely accepted as a reliable diagnostic modality in hepato-pancreatobiliary (HPB) surgery. IOC involves accessing the biliary tree and obtaining contrast-enhanced images by injecting contrast through the access point. Usually, the cystic duct or common bile duct (CBD) are cannulated. IOC is used to delineate anatomy, evaluate for choledocholithiasis or other intraductal abnormalities, and to assess for injury to the biliary tree.

Up to 22% of patients with cholelithiasis are estimated to have concomitant choledocholithiasis [2]. If left untreated, retained CBD stones may cause unfavorable sequelae, such as biliary obstruction, cholangitis, and pancreatitis. Diagnostic accuracy of IOC for choledocholithiasis is 99%, which allows surgeons the possibility to prevent these sequelae [3, 4].

Safe cholecystectomy multi-society practice guidelines strongly recommend surgeons have a low threshold to perform IOC during cholecystectomy when faced with unclear anatomy, possible choledocholithiasis, or possible bile duct injury (BDI) [5]. Although it is not entirely clear that routine use of IOC decreases the risk of BDI, its use can benefit patients through prompt identification and treatment of BDI [6, 7]. Thus, it is crucial for surgeons to be facile and comfortable with the use of IOC. Additionally, IOC has been widely used in liver surgery for evaluation of normal and variant anatomy of the intra- and extra-hepatic biliary tree, localization of the optimal bile duct transection site, and identification of post-hepatectomy biliary leakage [8–10].

Equipment

- Cholangiogram catheter, usually 3 or 4 French
- Laparoscopic cholangiogram forceps (optional)
- Injectable radiopaque contrast agent with tubing and 3-way stopcock
- Intraoperative X-ray machine or fluoroscopic C-arm, as well as radiation protection for the surgical team and the operating room staff

Technique

Overview of Steps
1. Access and cannulate biliary tree intraoperatively
2. Inject contrast
3. Obtain fluoroscopic X-ray images, or flat-plate X-ray images if fluoroscopy not available
4. Interpret cholangiogram: contrast goes from cystic duct distally into duodenum and proximally into right and left liver segments
5. Closure of access to biliary tree

1. Access/Cannulation of Biliary Tree
   - IOC is most commonly performed during laparoscopic cholecystectomy. After obtaining the Critical View of Safety [11], the cystic duct is clipped proximally (gallbladder side) and a partial ductotomy is made on the cystic duct.
     - Assure the ductotomy is wide enough for passage of the cholangiogram catheter, but ideally not so wide as to risk completely transecting the cystic duct.
     - The ductotomy should be close to the proximal clip. Cutting too distally risks injury to CBD or difficulty in closure after IOC.

- Pass the catheter gently through the ductotomy and advance distally until it is well positioned. Secure it with a partially closed clip or cholangiogram forceps (Fig. 20.1).
    - The catheter should be near, but not through, the cystic duct-CBD junction. Avoid placing the end of the catheter against the side-wall of the CBD.
    - Some catheters are specifically manufactured for use in cholangiograms. However, less costly options may be use of a 3 or 4 French ureteral catheter or vascular catheter.
    - Some manufacturers provide a laparoscopic grasper with a channel for the catheter (cholangiogram forceps). These can be used to gently grasp the duct at the ductotomy site and allow easier feeding of the catheter. Other manufacturers make cholangiogram kits that

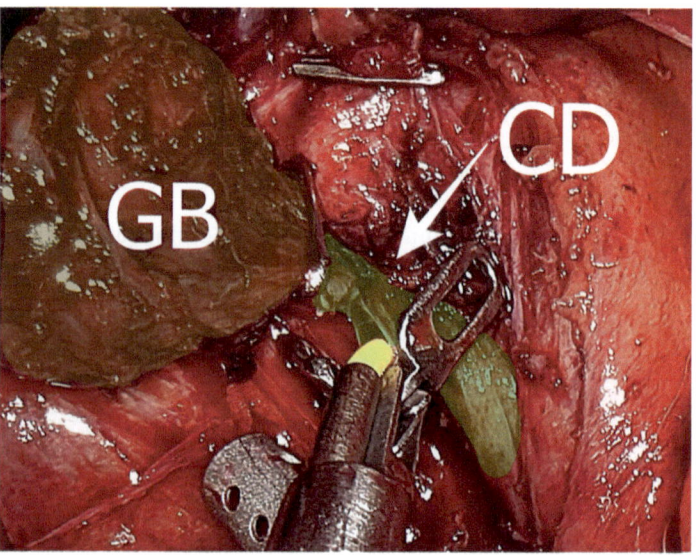

Fig. 20.1 Cholangiogram catheter through cystic ductotomy, secured with cholangiogram forceps. Cystic duct in light green, gallbladder in dark green. *CD* cystic duct. *GB* gallbladder. (Courtesy of D Asbun)

include a sheath for directing the catheter through the port and up to the ductotomy.
- After securing the catheter, the patient is usually positioned flat, and any retracted anatomic structures are released.

2. Inject Contrast
   - Inject sterile water/saline to confirm a seal at the ductotomy, followed by contrast agent.
     - Usually, a scout image is obtained with fluoroscopy/X-ray prior to injecting any contrast to confirm catheter location and fluoroscopy machine positioning.
     - Contrast diluted in 1:1 ratio with injectable saline or sterile water ("50–50 contrast") can be used initially, as full-concentration contrast may obscure anatomic structures.
   - Tubing most commonly used is repurposed intravenous (IV) tubing, connected to a three-way stopcock.
     - One end of stopcock is connected to a syringe with contrast, one to the IV tubing that is connected to the cholangiogram catheter, and the third end to a syringe with injectable saline/water.
   - Checking for leakage with saline/water is important, as inadvertent leakage of contrast early on can make subsequent interpretation more difficult.
   - Assure all tubing is free of air bubbles prior to injection into the biliary tree. Air bubbles can appear as filling defects and confound cholangiogram results.

3. Intraoperative Image Capture
   - Obtain intraoperative image with fluoroscopic C-arm or X-ray imaging.
   - Can obtain single still images, and/or ongoing "live" fluoroscopy.
     - If 50–50 contrast does not provide a clear picture, repeat imaging with full-strength contrast.
   - Avoid a delay between contrast injection and fluoroscopy, as the contrast will not remain in the biliary tree.
   - Consider the surgeon's position at bedside and the position of the screens showing the cholangiogram, especially dur-

ing continuous fluoroscopy. Assure the screens are in clear view of the surgeon, maintaining ergonomic principles.
4. Interpret Cholangiogram
    - A proper cholangiogram allows for visualization of contrast from cystic duct into CBD, distally into the duodenum, and proximally into the common, left, and right hepatic ducts, as well as segmental branches (Fig. 20.2).
    - Detailed understanding of biliary anatomy is crucial. Common aberrancies in anatomy involve the right hepatic ductal system, which is a frequent cause of BDI. Assure that the right anterior and posterior hepatic ducts are seen, as well as the left ductal system.
        – Careful assessment for areas of contrast leakage is important, as it may signal a site of BDI.
    - It is equally important to assure all above-mentioned anatomic structures are visualized. Inability to do so may indicate BDI through inadvertent biliary occlusion.
    - Persistent filling defects in the cholangiogram can be a sign of choledocholithiasis and must be further evaluated and managed. This is most commonly done via a laparoscopic common bile duct exploration or post-operative endoscopic retrograde cholangiopancreatogram.
5. Closure of Biliary Access
    - After successful cholangiogram, any clips/graspers holding the catheter are removed, the catheter gently withdrawn, and the distal cystic stump is doubly clipped or ligated.

Tips and Troubleshooting

- Patient positioning: If a cholangiogram does not show all structures clearly, attempt to reposition the patient to help with contrast flow. Usually this means placing the patient in Trendelenburg position to help with retrograde contrast flow into the liver.
- Catheter position: Another issue can arise if the distal end of the catheter is against the cystic duct or bile duct wall, if it is

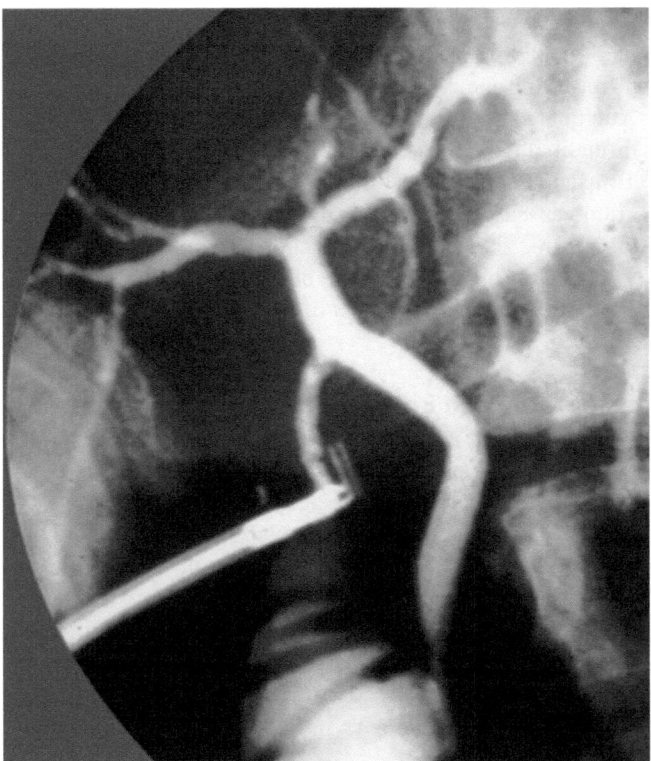

Fig. 20.2 Normal intraoperative cholangiogram shows contrast passing through the cystic duct, distally into the common bile duct and duodenum, and proximally into the common hepatic duct and intrahepatic bile ducts. There are no intraluminal filling defects and no leakage of contrast

compressed by a clip/grasper, or kinked. Assure all equipment is working well and the catheter is well-positioned. Slight adjustments in the catheter position, such as withdrawing or advancing a few millimeters, may solve problems with catheter function.
- Glucagon: Glucagon can be given intravenously (1 mg) to aid in Sphincter of Oddi relaxation, which can help pass contrast into the duodenum.

- Cholecystocholangiography: If the cystic duct is not easily identifiable, it is safer to perform a cholecystocholangiogram, by inserting the cholangiogram catheter into the gallbladder. Attempts should be made to advance the catheter toward the infundibulum and occlude the gallbladder body/fundus.
- Transcholedochal/transbiliary cholangiogram: A cholangiogram can be performed through any established access in the biliary tree. For example, the catheter can be placed through the CBD during common bile duct exploration, or to delineate anatomy of a transected duct of unknown origin.

Considerations in Robotic-Assisted Operations

The above steps are similar when IOC is performed during robotic-assisted operations. Passage of the cholangiogram catheter may be easier due to the robotic platform's articulating instruments. Care must be taken not to tear the cystic duct, cystic artery, or other anatomic structures, given the loss of haptic feedback and strength of robotic instruments. The surgeon or a qualified assistant must be present at bedside to inject contrast. Usually, one or a few robotic arms must be repositioned or removed to allow for positioning of the C-arm.

Choledochoscopy

Background

The first published description of using an optical instrument to visualize the lumen of the biliary tree dates back to 1899, although its more widespread use by surgeons was not established until the latter half of the following century [12, 13]. Choledochoscopy is used not only to inspect the bile ducts but also to allow access for further instrumentation and therapeutic procedures, such as clearing of choledocholithiasis. The term "choledochoscopy" is sometimes used specifically for endoluminal visualization of the extrahepatic biliary tree, with the term "cholangioscopy" used for the intrahepatic biliary tree. Here we will use "choledochoscopy" to describe both. The discussion will be limited to intra-operative, trans-abdominal techniques, excluding others such as per-oral endoscopic or percutaneous transhepatic approaches.

The bile ducts are accessed through a transected cystic duct ("transcystic" approach) or through a choledochotomy ("transcholedochal"). Transcystic choledochoscopy is most commonly used in patients with a dilated cystic duct, small choledochal stones, and a non-dilated CBD. Transcholedochal choledochoscopy is more common with a smaller cystic duct, a parallel-running cystic duct, larger stones, a dilated CBD, and often when the transcystic approach fails [14].

Choledochoscopes (or cholangioscopes) are long, thin, flexible endoscopes that allow for illumination, visualization, and instrumentation of the biliary tree. Current choledochoscopes rely on either digital or fiberoptic technology for endoluminal visualization. Outer diameters generally range from 2.8 to 3.6 mm [13]. There is an accessory working channel that allows for passage of accessory instruments, such as retrieval baskets, biopsy forceps, and guidewires.

The surgeon usually holds the choledochoscope handle in their left hand, using the knobs to control the direction of the tip. The right hand advances the choledochoscope and is also used to control its axial rotation.

There has been increasing interest in choledochoscopy as a possible tool during laparoscopic common bile duct exploration (LCBDE) in patients undergoing cholecystectomy with choledocholithiasis. Historically, many patients with choledocholithiasis undergo endoscopic retrograde cholangiopancreatogram (ERCP) as a separate procedure, typically before cholecystectomy. However, there is a growing body of evidence to suggest that LCBDE during cholecystectomy may provide benefits over separate ERCP and cholecystectomy. These benefits include shorter hospital stay, lower rates of retained stones or lithiasis recurrence, and decreased perioperative complications [15, 16]. Choledochoscopy is not necessary for all LCBDE, but it is an important technique to know well.

Equipment

- Choledochoscope and basic equipment per manufacturer (e.g., light source, digital controller, etc.)
- Saline for irrigation, usually with pressure bag
- Accessories if needed (e.g., retrieval basket, balloon catheter, guidewire, forceps, etc.)
- Additional screens for viewing the choledochoscope image

Technique

> **Overview of Steps**
> 1. Plan for trajectory of choledochoscope
> 2. Access and cannulate biliary tree intraoperatively
> 3. Advance choledochoscope to target area
> 4. Further intervention as indicated using choledochoscope accessory channel
> 5. Closure of access to biliary tree

1. Trajectory of Choledochoscope
   - Choledochoscope may be introduced through an existing port, or with placement of an additional 5 mm port. Plan for a trajectory of the choledochoscope that minimizes turns and acute angles.
     - Right-sided and subxiphoid approaches are usually preferred.
     - Introducer sheaths are available from some manufacturers, although they will not compensate for an overly acute angle of passage into the biliary tree.
   - Consider the surgeon's position at bedside and the position of the screens showing the choledochoscope view. Assure the screens are in clear view of the surgeon, maintaining ergonomic principles.

2. Access/Cannulation of Biliary Tree
    - Transcystic access is obtained after achieving the Critical View of Safety and isolating the cystic duct. A clip is placed on the gallbladder side, and a partial ductotomy is made with laparoscopic shears on the cystic duct side. The choledochoscope is advanced into the cystic duct.
        – Introducer sheath may be used if available from manufacturer.
        – Avoid cystic ductotomy too close to CBD, as it may injure the CBD or make eventual closure of cystic duct difficult.
    - Cystic duct may need to be gently dilated, although not always. The cystic duct should usually be at least 5 mm in diameter.
        – Dilation is especially helpful for spiraling cystic ducts or those with pronounced spiral valves of Heister.
        – Dilation preferentially done with a balloon catheter, or gently with a Maryland or right-angle grasper.
        – May do under fluoroscopic guidance, especially during balloon dilation.
        – No need to dilate larger than largest choledochal stone, if choledochoscopy being done to aid in stone extraction.
        – Avoid dilating larger than common bile duct diameter.
    - Transcholedochal access is obtained through a longitudinal incision on the anterior aspect of the CBD (Fig. 20.3).
        – A longitudinal incision avoids injury to the choledochal vascular plexus.
        – Incision should be approximately 5 mm in length. If stone extraction is anticipated, incision is extended to accommodate the stone diameter.
        – Choledochotomy ideally made with a scalpel tip or harmonic scalpel. Avoid excessive energy use during choledochotomy, which may otherwise lead to strictures.
3. Advance Choledochoscope
    - Right hand gently advances the choledochoscope and twists as needed, as the left hand maneuvers the direction of the tip (Fig. 20.4).

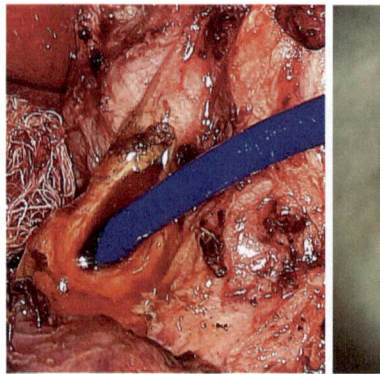 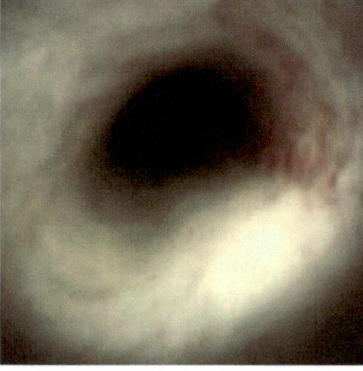

Fig. 20.3 Left: Transcholedochal choledochoscopy in a patient with a benign biliary stricture and choledocholithiasis prior to choledochoduodenostomy. Choledochoscope is passing distally through a vertical incision in common bile duct. Right: Intraluminal view of CBD confirming clearance of stones. (Courtesy of D Asbun)

- Assistant may be necessary to hold tissue or the choledochoscope loosely in place, without restricting its advancement.
- Different knobs on the left hand generally control either "up-down" motion or "left-right" motion.
  - Familiarize yourself with controls on the choledochoscope beforehand.
- Keep the ductal lumen in the center of the choledochoscope view to avoid significant pressure on the sidewall of the biliary duct (Fig. 20.3).
- Continuous irrigation through choledochoscope is usually employed for better visualization and dilation of the ductal lumen.
- Inspection begins immediately and continues both while advancing choledochoscope and while drawing it back.
- Choledochoscope is generally advanced both proximally into the right and left hepatic ducts and distally past the ampulla into the duodenum. However, full course of choledochoscope depends on the indication for its use.

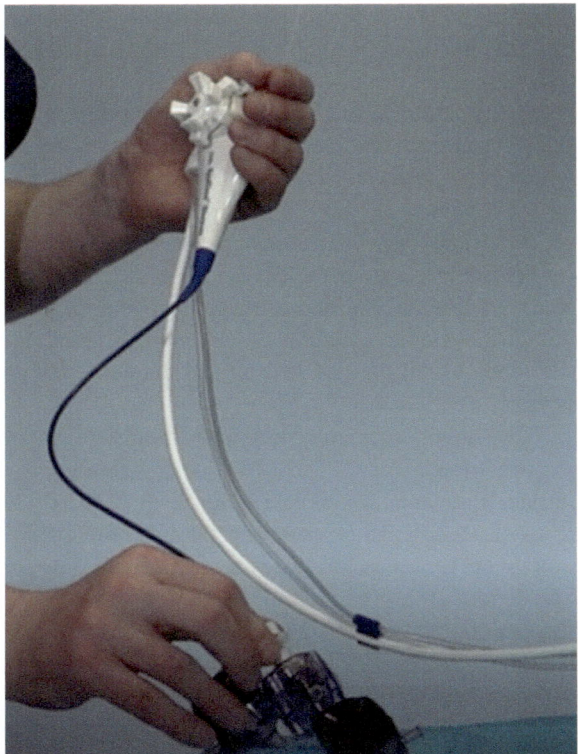

Fig. 20.4 Surgeon holding the choledochoscope in a training model

4. Further Interventions Through Accessory Channel
   - Depending on pathology and on available accessories, multiple further interventions are possible, as illustrated below.
   - Guidewire: A 0.035″ flexible-tip hydrophilic guidewire can be used to pass the choledochoscope into the biliary tree, or to aid in advancing the choledochoscope beyond difficult angles, strictures, or stones. Maintain control of the wire at all times.
   - Cholangiogram: Contrast may be injected through the accessory port, or through a catheter passed through the accessory port. Can assess anatomy and check for stones, strictures, leaks, etc.

- Flushing of stones: Stones can sometime be flushed through the ampulla using injectable saline or sterile water. May use glucagon to relax the sphincter of Oddi (see "Troubleshooting" in Cholangiogram section above).
- Basket retrieval: Choledochal stones and other intraluminal objects can be retrieved using a retrieval basket through the accessory port.
    - If through transcystic access, assure the extracted objects are not larger in diameter than the cystic duct.
- Balloon dilation: Balloon catheters can be passed to gently dilate the ampulla, strictures, or to push stones distally. Balloons usually are of 4–6 mm in diameter and 4 cm in length.
    - Take much care to avoid overdilation of any biliary structures.
- Stone fragmentation: Forceps, retrieval baskets, or lithotripsy catheters can be used to break up choledochal stones into smaller pieces for easier retrieval or passage into the duodenum.
- Biopsy: Forceps can be used for biopsy of abnormal intraductal tissue.

5. Closure of Access to Biliary Tree
    - If a transcystic approach was used, double clip or ligate the cystic duct after completion of choledochoscopy.
    - If a transcholedochal approach was used, suture close the ductotomy using interrupted or running sutures.
        - Size 4–0 or 5–0 absorbable sutures (polyglactin, polydioxanone, etc.) are usually used.
        - Smaller ducts are usually closed with interrupted sutures.

Tips and Troubleshooting

- Patient positioning: A reverse-Trendelenburg position with left-side down is helpful to expose the right-upper quadrant.
- Trocar positioning: If a LCBDE is expected, placing the mid clavicular port more lateral may facilitate the manipulation and canulation of the duct with the choledochoscope.

- Driving the choledochoscope: Use of the choledochoscope is similar to using larger endoscopes, and experience with these is helpful when learning to use the choledochoscope. Important principles include avoiding loops and turns in the scope (including the section near the handle), maintaining the lumen toward the center of view, and avoiding over-torquing the scope.
- Passage over a wire: Often choledochoscopy follows intraoperative cholangiogram. In these cases, a guidewire can sometimes be placed through the cholangiogram catheter, and the choledochoscope later advanced over the guidewire. This may assist in passage of the choledochoscope. Typically, a 0.035″ flexible-tip hydrophilic guidewire is used.
- Retention sutures on CBD: For transcholedochal access, retention sutures can be placed on either side of the choledochotomy to aid in opening it during introduction of the choledochoscope. Care must be taken to avoid excessive traction or ripping of the CBD.
- Stone clearance: The authors prefer to pass stones distally into the CBD if possible, as this decreases the risk of intra-abdominal spillage, choledochotomy enlargement, etc. As above, stones can be passed distally via flushing, pushing past the ampulla with a balloon, grasping with a basket or forceps and advancing past the ampulla, or fragmentation. However, undo force should be avoided whenever manipulating stones inside a bile duct and care must be taken to avoiding injury or perforation of the ducts.

Considerations in Robotic-Assisted Operations

Choledochoscopy is feasible during robotic-assisted operations. The articulating instruments of the robotic platform may assist in advancing the choledochoscope. However, the loss of haptic feedback and strength of the robotic instruments may increase the risk of inadvertent biliary injury, and extra care must be taken while manipulating cystic and bile ducts, and to avoid damaging the choledochoscope. With the aid of a bedside assistant, the surgeon can use the robot to position the choledochoscope inside the bile ductotomy, but they must be at bedside for the actual choledochoscopy. Some surgeons will suture the gallbladder to the anterior abdominal wall to aid in retraction, although the authors prefer to use a robotic arm to do so.

Fluorescent Cholangiography

Background

Fluorescent cholangiography (FC) refers to the fluorescent visualization of the biliary tree. This is achieved by intravenous administration of indocyanine green (ICG), which is excreted hepatically and subsequently excited by near-infrared light. Using specific imaging systems, the fluorescent ICG can be delineated in the biliary tree, aiding in detection and delineation of anatomic structures. FC is most commonly used during laparoscopic or robotic cholecystectomy, but can be employed in any operations where identifying bile ducts may be helpful, including other biliary operations and liver resections [17–19]. Video 20.1 demonstrates a difficult hepatic hilar dissection in a patient with hepatomegaly undergoing laparoscopic right hepatectomy (Video 20.1). Here, FC is helpful in delineating the course of the common hepatic duct.

FC was first described as an adjunct to cholecystectomy in 2009 by Ishizawa et al. [20]. Since then, multiple studies have emerged to show its utility in identifying biliary structures during cholecystectomy, including a multinational randomized controlled trial [21–23]. Advocates of FC cite the ease with which fluorescence imaging can be turned on/off, the low risk profile of ICG, and the real-time guidance that can be obtained throughout an operation [24, 25]. In comparison to IOC (another established method of visualizing the biliary tree), FC appears to be more cost-effective, does not expose the patient or medical staff to radiation, and does not require additional trained personnel, such as an X-ray technician [25, 26]. However, FC does not allow access to the biliary tree, and thus intraluminal interventions—for example, flushing the biliary tree to clear stones—are not possible.

Fluorescence imaging in hepatobiliary surgery can be used for purposes other than biliary ductal identification. For example, ICG is often used to delineate hepatic segmental anatomy, either through direct injection into a portal venous branch ("positive staining"), or by peripheral venous injection after ligating the target portal pedicle ("negative staining") [17, 27]. Furthermore, certain liver tumors can be identified through fluorescence by administering ICG days or weeks before an operation [28, 29]. Other uses include preoperative evaluation of hepatic function [30, 31] and to aid in lymphadenectomy [32, 33]. Details about these and other uses of fluorescence beyond anatomic identification of the biliary tree are outside the scope of this chapter.

Equipment

- ICG.
- FC laparoscopic imaging platform: allows for visualization in both normal white light as well as near-infrared imaging to capture fluorescence.

Technique

> **Overview of Steps**
> 1. Inject ICG preoperatively.
> 2. Activate fluorescence-imaging as needed during operation.

1. Inject ICG.
   - ICG is reconstituted into a solution per the manufacturer's instructions.
     - Usually, a 25 mg vial of powder ICG is reconstituted in 10 mL of sterile water.
     - Dosing is historically up to 2.5 mg per operation, although the authors prefer a much lower dose.

Furthermore, a recent randomized controlled trial showed benefits to using a lower dose of 0.05 mg [34].
- ICG is given as an IV injection between 30 minutes and two hours before the operation.
2. Activate fluorescence imaging as needed.
   - During the operation, the fluorescence imaging mode is activated, usually through buttons on the laparoscopic camera. It can be turned on/off as needed for real-time visualization of biliary anatomy.
   - Different imaging modes are possible, with types and names that depend on the manufacturer (Fig. 20.5). Examples of these include:
     – Overlay—A white-light image is mixed with fluorescence imaging to provide an "overlay" of fluorescent tissues on the usual non-fluorescent (white-light) view. Fluorescence appears as bright green.
     – Monochromatic—A black-and-white image is created, with fluorescence appearing as bright white.
     – Monochromatic + overlay—A gray-scale image with an overlay of the green-colored fluorescent tissue.
     – Fluorescence intensity color map—The intensity of fluorescence is demonstrated through different colors, providing a "heat map" that correlates with the degree of fluorescence demonstrated by the tissues. Usually presented as overlay on a grayscale or a white-light image.
   - Many manufacturers allow for adjustment of other fluorescence settings, including the sensitivity (or gain) with which fluorescence is captured.

Tips and Troubleshooting

- Dose: As mentioned above, it appears that lower doses achieve equally good delineation of the biliary tree, without unwanted fluorescence from other tissues (such as the liver). The authors prefer to use a 0.05 mg dose primarily for this reason.

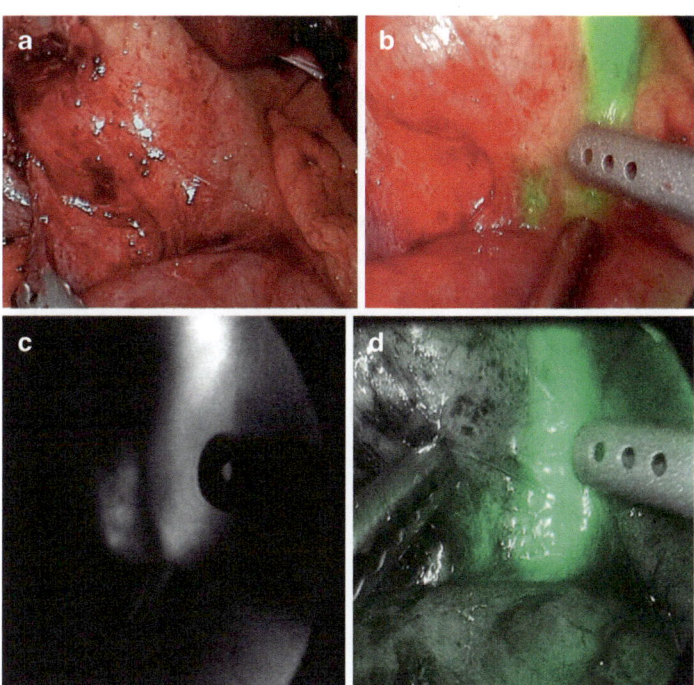

Fig. 20.5 Various modes of fluorescence imaging. Pictured views are: (**a**) standard white light; (**b**) fluorescence overlay; (**c**) monochromatic; (**d**) monochromatic + fluorescence overlay. (Courtesy of D Asbun)

- The distance between the laparoscope and the target issue can influence the visualization of the ICG and must be taken into account when adjusting the fluorescence intensity.
- Liver hyper-fluorescence: Exaggerated fluorescence of liver parenchyma can make delineation of bile ducts problematic, especially during liver resections. This can happen when ICG is administered too soon before an operation, when the sensitivity/gain setting on the camera is set too high, or when the administered dose is too high. Adjusting these factors can decrease the interference of hepatic parenchymal fluorescence when evaluating the bile ducts.

- Tissue penetration: Tissue with significant edema, fatty infiltration, or fibrotic changes may decrease the visualization of underlying fluorescence in bile ducts or other structures.
- Critical View of Safety: Although FC can aid significantly in identifying biliary structures during laparoscopic cholecystectomy, it is not a substitute for obtaining the Critical View of Safety before clipping the cystic duct or artery [5, 11].
- Bile leaks: FC can be used to identify areas of subtle bile leakage, which may be a sign of biliary injury, incomplete occlusion of a biliary or cystic duct, or a leaking duct of Luschka (subvesical duct).
- Safety and contraindications: A maximum recommended dose of ICG is 2 mg/kg, which is much higher than what a patient is expected to receive during the above-mentioned indications. Patients in whom ICG administration is generally contraindicated include those with iodine allergies, severe renal dysfunction, and hyperthyroidism.

Considerations in Robotic-Assisted Operations

The adoption of the robotic surgical platform has contributed to further adoption of FC by surgeons, as newer platforms use robotic laparoscopes equipped with near-infrared imaging technology. The fluorescent imaging view is toggled on and off with ease at the surgeon's console. The above-mentioned concepts apply.

Conclusion

Technological developments in general and HPB surgery have allowed for important adjunct techniques. Mastering the principles of intraoperative cholangiogram, choledochoscopy, and fluorescent cholangiography is vital for surgeons operating on the liver and bile ducts. These techniques can aid in intraoperative identification of anatomy, diagnosis of pathology, management of complications, and can improve outcomes.

References

1. Mirizzi P. Operative cholangiography. Surg Gynecol Obstet. 1932;65:702–10.
2. Molvar C, Glaenzer B. Choledocholithiasis: evaluation, treatment, and outcomes. Semin Intervent Radiol. 2016;33(4):268–76.
3. Videhult P, Sandblom G, Rasmussen IC. How reliable is intraoperative cholangiography as a method for detecting common bile duct stones? A prospective population-based study on 1171 patients. Surg Endosc. 2009;23(2):304–12.
4. Hope WW, Fanelli R, Walsh DS, Narula VK, Price R, Stefanidis D, et al. SAGES clinical spotlight review: intraoperative cholangiography. Surg Endosc. 2017;31(5):2007–16.
5. Brunt LM, Deziel DJ, Telem DA, Strasberg SM, Aggarwal R, Asbun H, et al. Safe cholecystectomy multi-society practice guideline and state-of-the-art consensus conference on prevention of bile duct injury during cholecystectomy. Surg Endosc. 2020;34(7):2827–55.
6. Buddingh KT, Nieuwenhuijs VB, van Buuren L, Hulscher JBF, de Jong JS, van Dam GM. Intraoperative assessment of biliary anatomy for prevention of bile duct injury: a review of current and future patient safety interventions. Surg Endosc. 2011;25(8):2449–61.
7. Ford JA, Soop M, Du J, Loveday BPT, Rodgers M. Systematic review of intraoperative cholangiography in cholecystectomy. Br J Surg. 2012;99(2):160–7.
8. Tuysuz U, Aktas H, Batı IB, Emıroglu R. The role of intraoperative cholangiography (IOC) and methylene blue tests in reducing bile leakage after living donor hepatectomy. Asian J Surg. 2021;44(1):147–52.
9. Hwang S, Choi BH, Song GW, Park GC, Park YH, Moon DB, et al. Technique of antegrade intraoperative cholangiography not requiring hepatic hilar dissection during repeated hepatectomy for hepatocellular carcinoma. Hepato-Gastroenterology. 2012;59(115):878–80.
10. Gao F, Xu X, Zhu YB, Wei Q, Zhou B, Shen XY, et al. Impact of intraoperative cholangiography and parenchymal resection to donor liver function in living donor liver transplantation. Hepatobiliary Pancreat Dis Int. 2014;13(3):259–63.
11. Strasberg SM, Brunt LM. Rationale and use of the critical view of safety in laparoscopic cholecystectomy. J Am Coll Surg. 2010;211(1):132–8.
12. Madden JL, Vanderheyden L, Kandalaft S. The nature and surgical significance of common duct stones. Surg Gynecol Obstet. 1968;126(1):3–8.
13. Lee T, Teng TZJ, Shelat VG. Choledochoscopy: an update. World J Gastrointest Endosc. 2021;13(12):571–92.
14. Yamakawa T, Sakai S, Mu ZB, Pineres G. Laparoscopic management of common bile duct stones. J Hep Bil Pancr Surg. 2000;7(1):9–14.

15. Singh AN, Kilambi R. Single-stage laparoscopic common bile duct exploration and cholecystectomy versus two-stage endoscopic stone extraction followed by laparoscopic cholecystectomy for patients with gallbladder stones with common bile duct stones: systematic review and meta-analysis of randomized trials with trial sequential analysis. Surg Endosc. 2018;32(9):3763–76.
16. Pan L, Chen M, Ji L, Zheng L, Yan P, Fang J, et al. The safety and efficacy of laparoscopic common bile duct exploration combined with cholecystectomy for the Management of Cholecysto-choledocholithiasis: an up-to-date meta-analysis. Ann Surg. 2018;268(2):247–53.
17. Aoki T, Yasuda D, Shimizu Y, Odaira M, Niiya T, Kusano T, et al. Image-guided liver mapping using fluorescence navigation system with Indocyanine green for anatomical hepatic resection. World J Surg. 2008;32:1763–7.
18. Abu Hilal M, Aldrighetti L, Dagher I, Edwin B, Troisi RI, Alikhanov R, et al. The Southampton consensus guidelines for laparoscopic liver surgery: from indication to implementation. Ann Surg. 2018;268(1):11.
19. Wang X, Teh CSC, Ishizawa T, Aoki T, Cavallucci D, Lee SY, et al. Consensus guidelines for the use of fluorescence imaging in hepatobiliary surgery. Ann Surg. 2021;274(1):97.
20. Ishizawa T, Tamura S, Masuda K, Aoki T, Hasegawa K, Imamura H, et al. Intraoperative fluorescent cholangiography using Indocyanine green: a biliary road map for safe surgery. J Am Coll Surg. 2009;208(1):e1.
21. Dip F, LoMenzo E, Sarotto L, Phillips E, Todeschini H, Nahmod M, et al. Randomized trial of near-infrared incisionless fluorescent cholangiography. Ann Surg. 2019;270(6):992.
22. Ishizawa T, Bandai Y, Ijichi M, Kaneko J, Hasegawa K, Kokudo N. Fluorescent cholangiography illuminating the biliary tree during laparoscopic cholecystectomy. Br J Surg. 2010;97(9):1369–77.
23. Osayi SN, Wendling MR, Drosdeck JM, Chaudhry UI, Perry KA, Noria SF, et al. Near-infrared fluorescent cholangiography facilitates identification of biliary anatomy during laparoscopic cholecystectomy. Surg Endosc. 2015;29(2):368–75.
24. Dip F, Roy M, Menzo EL, Simpfendorfer C, Szomstein S, Rosenthal RJ. Routine use of fluorescent incisionless cholangiography as a new imaging modality during laparoscopic cholecystectomy. Surg Endosc. 2015;29(6):1621–6.
25. Ishizawa T, Bandai Y, Kokudo N. Fluorescent cholangiography using Indocyanine green for laparoscopic cholecystectomy: an initial experience. Arch Surg. 2009;144(4):381–2.
26. Dip F, Asbun D, Rosales-Velderrain A, Lomenzo E, Simpfendorfer C, Szomstein S, et al. Cost analysis and effectiveness comparing the routine use of intraoperative fluorescent cholangiography with fluoroscopic cholangiogram in patients undergoing laparoscopic cholecystectomy. Surg Endosc. 2014;11:28.

27. Ishizawa T, Zuker NB, Kokudo N, Gayet B. Positive and negative staining of hepatic segments by use of fluorescent imaging techniques during laparoscopic hepatectomy. Arch Surg. 2012;147(4):393–4.
28. Terasawa M, Ishizawa T, Mise Y, Inoue Y, Ito H, Takahashi Y, et al. Applications of fusion-fluorescence imaging using indocyanine green in laparoscopic hepatectomy. Surg Endosc. 2017;31(12):5111–8.
29. Nakaseko Y, Ishizawa T, Saiura A. Fluorescence-guided surgery for liver tumors. J Surg Oncol. 2018;118(2):324–31.
30. Winkler K, Tygstrup N. Determination of hepatic blood flow in man by cardio green. Scand J Clin Lab Invest. 1960;12:353–6.
31. Levesque E, Martin E, Dudau D, Lim C, Dhonneur G, Azoulay D. Current use and perspective of indocyanine green clearance in liver diseases. Anaes Crit Care Pain Med. 2016;35(1):49–57.
32. Ruzzenente A, Conci S, Isa G, Campagnaro T, Pedrazzani C, De Bellis M, et al. The LIver SEntinel LYmph-node (LISELY) study: a prospective intraoperative real time evaluation of liver lymphatic drainage and sentinel lymph-node using near-infrared (NIR) imaging with Indocyanine green (ICG). Eur J Surg Oncol. 2022;48(12):2455–9.
33. Zhang Y, Zhang Y, Zhu J, Tao H, Liang H, Chen Y, et al. Clinical application of indocyanine green fluorescence imaging in laparoscopic lymph node dissection for intrahepatic cholangiocarcinoma: a pilot study (with video). Surgery. 2022;171(6):1589–95.
34. Ladd AD, Zarate Rodriguez J, Lewis D, Warren C, Duarte S, Loftus TJ, et al. Low vs standard-dose Indocyanine green in the identification of biliary anatomy using near-infrared fluorescence imaging: a multicenter randomized controlled trial. J Am Coll Surg. 2023;236(4):711–7.

Part VI

Partial Hepatectomy (Non-anatomical) – Procdure

Liver Core Needle Biopsies and Wedge Resection

21

Tyler D. Robinson and Erin W. Gilbert

Overview

Liver biopsy is central to the diagnosis, evaluation and management of a spectrum of liver diseases, including those of infectious, inflammatory, hereditary, toxic, metabolic, posttransplant or malignant etiologies. The first liver biopsy was performed in 1883 by the Nobel Prize-winning German physician Paul Ehrlich, but it was not until Italian internist Georgio Menghini reported the first percutaneous technique in 1958 that the procedure was more widely adopted [1].

While biopsy remains the diagnostic gold standard, the indications for performing liver biopsy have changed in recent decades. The evolution of highly effective treatment for two common causes of cirrhosis, viral hepatitis B and C infection, and advances in noninvasive radiological, immunological, biochemical, and genetic markers of hepatic disease have led to the decrease in the number of liver biopsies performed globally [2].

T. D. Robinson
Mercy Medical Group, Sacramento, CA, USA

E. W. Gilbert (✉)
Department of Surgery, Louisiana State University Health & Science University, New Orleans, LA, USA
e-mail: egilb3@lsuhsc.edu

© The Author(s), under exclusive license to Springer Nature Switzerland AG 2025
A. Alseidi et al. (eds.), *The SAGES Manual of Contemporary Indications and Management of Hepatic and Biliary Diseases*,
https://doi.org/10.1007/978-3-032-04823-3_21

Nonetheless, biopsy remains essential in the diagnosis of uncertain or cryptogenic liver diseases and is useful in the staging and prognosis of parenchymal diseases including cirrhosis. The surgeon should be familiar with the current indications, contraindications, limitations, alternatives, techniques, and complications of liver biopsy.

Indications

Over 100 diseases of the liver may benefit from liver biopsy and histopathologic tissue examination. In the 2009 consensus guidelines for liver biopsy, the American Association for the Study of Liver Diseases (AASLD) published the following indications:

- Diagnosis:
  - Multiple parenchymal liver diseases.
  - Abnormal liver tests of unknown etiology.
  - Fever of unknown origin.
  - Focal or diffuse abnormalities on imaging studies.
- Prognosis: staging of known parenchymal liver disease.
- Management: developing treatment plans based on histologic analysis.

The most common liver diseases likely to be encountered by the surgeon include viral hepatitis, alcoholic cirrhosis, fatty liver disease, posttransplant dysfunction, and malignancy [3].

The most recent multi-society consensus guidelines for the use of liver biopsy in clinic practice were published in 2020 as a joint statement from the British Society of Gastroenterology, Royal College of Radiologists, and Royal College of Pathology [4]. This guideline supports liver biopsy for histopathological interpretation when unable to identify diagnosis, management or prognosis using noninvasive methods, and for research purposes with appropriate ethics approval.

Most indications for liver biopsy can be accomplished by radiology using percutaneous techniques. In some instances it is advantageous to perform percutaneous biopsy as with larger, resectable nonmetastatic but malignant appearing masses to decrease the risk of peritoneal seeding from laparoscopic biopsy. However, several indications might be better served by surgical biopsy. Certainly, if already operating for another reason, an indicated biopsy of liver parenchyma can be performed during surgery if the surgeon is comfortable doing so. Caution is advised in patients with cirrhosis or a fibrotic appearing liver. Second, when evaluating the potential for metastatic gastrointestinal malignancy, the peritoneum and hepatic surface may be biopsied during surgery. Prior to definitive surgical resection or palliative procedure, as in diversion for an obstructing cancer, any concerning peritoneal or hepatic lesions should be biopsied (if no evidence of metastatic disease on imaging) and sent for pathologic analysis.

A circumstance particular to the surgeon might be described as a "incidental indication" for liver biopsy, or whether to perform a liver biopsy when an unexpected abnormal hepatic finding is encountered during surgery for another reason. With the prevalence of high-quality cross-sectional imaging, this situation is encountered less frequently. Common benign hepatic irregularities such as hepatic cysts and hemangiomas can usually be visually identified, and do not require biopsy. More concerning lesions, including focal areas of fibrosis, retraction of Glisson's capsule, adherence to neighboring structures, or discoloration, should raise suspicion. If an unexpected hepatic lesion is encountered that is not readily identifiable, it is best to have a hepatobiliary surgeon view the lesion intraoperatively. If the hepatobiliary surgeon is not available, the primary surgeon should take multiple intraoperative pictures of the lesion, obtain high-quality, liver protocol (multiphase) cross-sectional imaging following surgery, and provide the patient with a referral to a hepatobiliary surgeon for evaluation and consideration of biopsy if deemed appropriate.

Contraindications

Absolute contraindications to percutaneous liver biopsy include uncontrolled ascites and uncorrectable coagulopathy. Relative contraindications include morbid obesity and failure of previous percutaneous biopsy.

Limitations

Limitations of liver biopsy include small tissue samples, heterogenous variation in liver parenchyma, location of the liver lesion, and variation in histopathologic diagnosis.

As the diagnostic yield increases with the quality and size of the pathologic specimen, small fragmented specimens, more commonly from transjugular or endoscopic biopsy techniques, may not be diagnostic due to inadequacy of the specimen. One study demonstrated that when specimen length from percutaneous biopsy increased from 15 to 25 mm, the percentage of specimens yielding the correct diagnoses increased from 55 to 75% [5]. Interoperator variability exists among all biopsy techniques. When performing liver biopsy, the technician should endeavor to provide the largest, most complete sample possible while minimizing potential complications.

A second limitation is that tissue heterogeneity can exist within the liver, and therefore a single sample might not entirely rule in or rule out the disease within other hepatic segments or the entire organ. One study demonstrated that variations between right and left lobe liver biopsies in Hepatitis C underdiagnosed cirrhosis in 14.5% of patients [6].

Finally, interoperator variability exists during the histopathologic diagnosis of liver disease. In one study of second opinion pathology in liver biopsy, 28% of biopsies had major discrepancies between pathologic interpretation [7].

Alternatives

Several noninvasive techniques for evaluation of the liver have developed in recent years and have increased the diagnostic accuracy and prevalence of use. The extent of parenchymal liver disease can be assessed by serologic or radiologic approaches. The former has the advantage of being a quantitative test denoting hepatic function, while the latter merely identifies the extent of fibrosis or fatty changes.

Examples of serologic testing for liver function include HepaScore and FibroSure (FibroTest), which are used to assess liver fibrosis in chronic viral hepatitis B or C, alcoholic liver disease, and fatty liver disease. Five or more biochemical assays, including bilirubin, gamma glutamyl transpeptidase, apolipoprotein A1, among others, are used to calculate a score that is proportional to the severity of fibrosis [8].

Liver elastography can be performed by either ultrasound or magnetic resonance imaging to evaluate the extent of liver fibrosis. The most common liver ultrasonographic elastography test uses a shear wave emitted from an ultrasound probe to estimate the degree of liver fibrosis. This device transduces a 50 MHz ultrasonographic wave into the liver, which is measured to calculate the shear wave as a proxy for liver stiffness, expressed in kilopascals [9].

Techniques

Liver biopsy can be accomplished by percutaneous, transjugular, endoscopic, or surgical approaches.

Percutaneous liver biopsy should be approached using external landmarks as and when biopsy is indicated for evaluation of parenchymal architecture in the absence of a discrete lesion (i.e., cirrhosis). This is most commonly performed from a right posterolateral approach through the eighth, ninth, or tenth intercostal spaces, taking care to avoid the neurovascular bundle running inferior to the rib. Image-guided percutaneous biopsy, most commonly utilizing ultrasonography, can be utilized to target hepatic masses when needed. Percutaneous core needle biopsies are frequently obtained using a spring-loaded needle requiring a single pass, but suction or cutting needles may also be utilized. A comparative study found that 16-gauge needles significantly increased diagnostic yield without increasing complications, when compared to 18-gauge needles [10].

Transjugular liver biopsies are performed by interventional radiologists using fluoroscopic venography. An introducer sheath typically placed through the right jugular vein allows a catheter to be wedged into one of the hepatic veins, and a cutting needle is advanced through the vein wall into parenchyma. As the specimens rendered by transjugular biopsy can often be fragmented and smaller, the diagnostic yield of transjugular biopsy is more limited than other approaches and may be nondiagnostic or inconclusive [2].

Endoscopic liver biopsy performed during upper endoscopy has been demonstrated in recent years to be a safe procedure with high diagnostic yield [10, 11]. Endoscopic biopsies are usually performed using ultrasonographic guidance, and are typically performed with 19-gauge core cutting needles. The lateral part of the left lobe of the liver can be accessed from the stomach and a portion of the right lobe from the duodenal bulb.

Surgical liver biopsy can be performed during laparoscopy or laparotomy. The most common reason for surgical biopsy is evaluation of surface lesions concerning for metastasis during staging laparoscopy for a gastrointestinal malignancy. Any grossly abnormal appearing discrete hepatic lesion may prompt the surgeon to obtain a biopsy. Wedge resections can be performed sharply using cold scissors or a scalpel, and can also be performed using electrosurgical instruments such as a laparoscopic L-hook, an oscillating ultrasonic scalpel, or a bipolar energy device. The diagnostic yield from these surgical specimens can be limited by a preponderance of Glissen's capsule, damage to the tissue during biopsy (coagulative artifact), and wider portal tracts in the hepatic subcapsule. When assessing liver parenchyma, one should consider performing a core needle biopsy prior to surgical biopsy, as recommended by some pathologists [2]. A variety of techniques for achieving hemostasis following biopsy have been described and studied, and in practice are largely dependent on surgeon preference. A 2019 systematic review and meta-analysis of 22 randomized controlled trials evaluating hepatic parenchymal transection techniques concluded that bipolar cautery was best at reducing blood loss and was associated with shortest operating time, but that the ultrasonic oscillating scalpel was best overall in transecting the parenchyma and had the fewest major complications [12]. Argon beam electrocoagulation is also considered an efficient and effective means to achieve a durable surface coagulum with minimal deep tissue injury. Our recommendation for surgical liver biopsy of small incidental lesions is the use of cold scissors to perform an excisional wedge resection inclusive of normal subcortical parenchyma to ensure adequate biopsy, followed by hemostasis with an electrosurgical device. Liver hemostasis can be reliably achieved with monopolar electrocautery set to coagulation mode and a power setting of between 60 and 100 W. This rapidly coagulates extruded blood into a thick eschar on the hepatic cortex, which inhibits further bleeding. Since bleeding is often from low pressure hepatic venules, topical hemostatic agents, including a hydrocellulose matrix, especially in combination with direct pressure, is frequently helpful.

An endoscopic retrieval bag may be used to extract larger specimens during laparoscopy. Surgical liver biopsies, especially when frozen section is required for metastatic evaluation, are sent as fresh specimens to the pathologist. Direct communication with the surgical pathology team is strongly recommended.

Complications

The overall complication rate varies by approach, but with each is acceptably low. Overall mortality rate of percutaneous liver biopsy was estimated at 0.2% in a study of over 60,000 patients. The majority of complications occur within 6 h following procedure, and up to 90% within 24 h [13], with approximately 2–3% of patients requiring hospitalization [14]. The two most common complications following percutaneous liver biopsy are pain and bleeding. Severe pain is uncommon following an uncomplicated procedure, and should be further evaluated by serologic testing and imaging using either ultrasonography or computed tomography to evaluate for hemoperitoneum. The incidence of bleeding requiring transfusion or angiographic intervention is 0.5% [15, 16]. Hypotension or tachycardia following liver biopsy should prompt workup for bleeding as the diagnostic imperative. Symptomatic bleeding is typically managed supportively, but angioembolization may be required in severe cases. In addition to subcapsular hematoma and hemoperitoneum, other complications from liver biopsy can include hemobilia, biloma, bile peritonitis, and transient bacteremia. Other organ injury is infrequent but can occur, such as pneumothorax, lung injury, or injury to other abdominal organs (Table 21.1, Figs. 21.1, 21.2, and 21.3).

Table 21.1 Summary of the American Association for the Study of Liver Diseases (AASLD) liver biopsy recommendations

Focal disease and mass lesions
Liver biopsy should be considered in patients in whom diagnosis is in question, and when knowledge of a specific diagnosis is likely to alter the management plan
Liver histology is an important adjunct in the management of patients with known liver disease, particularly in situations where (prognostic) information about fibrosis stage may guide subsequent treatment; the decision to perform liver biopsy in these situations should be closely tied to consideration of the risks and benefits of the procedure
Technical issues, contraindications, and complications
Prior to the performance of liver biopsy, patients should be educated about their liver disease and about investigations other than liver biopsy (if any) that may also provide diagnostic and prognostic information
Prior to performance of liver biopsy, patients must be carefully informed about the procedure itself including alternatives (as above), risks, benefits, and limitations; written informed consent should be obtained

(continued)

Table 21.1 (continued)

Management of medications
Antiplatelet medications should be discontinued several to 10 days before liver biopsy, although there is uncertainty surrounding the need for their discontinuation. Management of specific compounds should be handled on a case-by-case basis, taking into account their clinical indications, as well as the potential bleeding risk associated with their use in the setting of liver biopsy
Anticoagulant medications should be discontinued prior to liver biopsy. Warfarin should generally be discontinued at least 5 days prior to liver biopsy. Heparin and related products should be discontinued 12–24 h prior to biopsy. In all patients, the risk of discontinuing anticoagulant medications must be weighed against the (potential) risk of bleeding during/after liver biopsy
Antiplatelet therapy may be restarted 48–72 h after liver biopsy
Warfarin may be restarted the day following liver biopsy
Liver biopsy procedure
Performance of liver biopsy requires an adequate sized and dedicated physical space suitable for focused physician effort as well as safe patient recovery
The use of sedation, preferably light sedation, is safe and does not lead to increased procedural risk
Vital signs must be frequently monitored (at least every 15 min for the first hour) after liver biopsy
The recommended observation time after biopsy is between 2 and 4 h and will vary depending on local expertise and practice
Ultrasound guidance with marking of the optimal biopsy site performed immediately preceding biopsy, by the individual performing the biopsy, is preferred, though not mandatory, because it likely reduces the risk of complications from liver biopsy
Contraindications
Percutaneous liver biopsy with or without image guidance is appropriate only in cooperative patients, and this technique should not be utilized in uncooperative patients
Uncooperative patients who require liver biopsy should undergo the procedure under general anesthesia or via the transvenous route
In patients with clinically evident ascites requiring a liver biopsy, a transvenous approach is generally recommended, although percutaneous biopsy (after removal of ascites) or laparoscopic biopsy are acceptable alternatives

(continued)

Table 21.1 (continued)

Patients who require liver biopsy and who have a large vascular lesion identified on imaging should undergo the procedure using real-time image guidance
The decision to perform liver biopsy in the setting of abnormal laboratory parameters of hemostasis should continue to be reached as the result of local practice(s) and consideration of the risks and benefits of liver biopsy because there is no specific PT-INR and/or platelet count cutoff at or above which potentially adverse bleeding can be reliably predicted
Complications
Those performing liver biopsy must be cognizant of multiple potential complications (including death) that may occur after liver biopsy and discuss these appropriately with their patients beforehand
Platelet transfusion should be considered when levels are less than 50,000 to 60,000/mL (this applies whether one is attempting biopsy transcutaneously or transvenously)
The use of prophylactic or rescue strategies such as plasma, fibrinolysis inhibitors, or recombinant factors should be considered in specific situations, although their effectiveness remains to be established
In patients with renal failure or on hemodialysis, desmopressin (DDAVP) may be considered, although its use appears to be unnecessary in patients on stable dialysis regimens
Patients on chronic hemodialysis should be well dialyzed prior to liver biopsy, and heparin should be avoided if at all possible
Radiological considerations
Image-guided liver biopsy is recommended in certain clinical situations including in patients with known intrahepatic lesions (real-time imaging is strongly preferred) and in those with previous intra-abdominal surgery who may have adhesions. Image-guided liver biopsy should also be considered in the following situations: Patients with small livers that are difficult to percuss, obese patients, and patients with clinically evident ascites
Pathological considerations
Because diagnosis, grading, and staging of nonneoplastic, diffuse parenchymal liver disease is dependent on an adequate sized biopsy, a biopsy of at least 2–3 cm in length and 16-gauge in caliber is recommended

(continued)

Table 21.1 (continued)

It is recommended that if applicable, the presence of fewer than 11 complete portal tracts be noted in the pathology report, with recognition that diagnosis, grading, and staging may be incorrect due to an insufficient sample size
If cirrhosis is suspected, a cutting rather than a suction needle is recommended
In clinical practice, the use of a simple (e.g., Metavir or batts-Ludwig) rather than complex (e.g., Ishak) scoring system is recommended
Noninvasive alternatives to liver biopsy
Liver biopsy is currently a fundamentally important tool in the management of patients with liver disease, important for diagnosis as well as staging of liver disease and its use is recommended until clearly superior methodologies are developed and validated
Training for liver biopsy
Specific training for liver biopsy is essential and is recommended for those who perform it
Liver biopsy should be taught to trainees by experts, highly experienced in the practice of liver biopsy and management of its potential complications
Although the number of biopsies required to become adequately trained is unknown, it is recommended that operators perform at least 40 biopsies
Training in percutaneous liver biopsy should include specific training in ultrasound interpretation of fundamental liver anatomy and other landmarks
Image-guided liver biopsy should be taught to trainees by experts who themselves have adequate training and experience with the technique

Data summarized from: Rockey DC, Caldwell SH, Goodman ZD, et al. Liver biopsy. Hepatology 2009; 49:1017

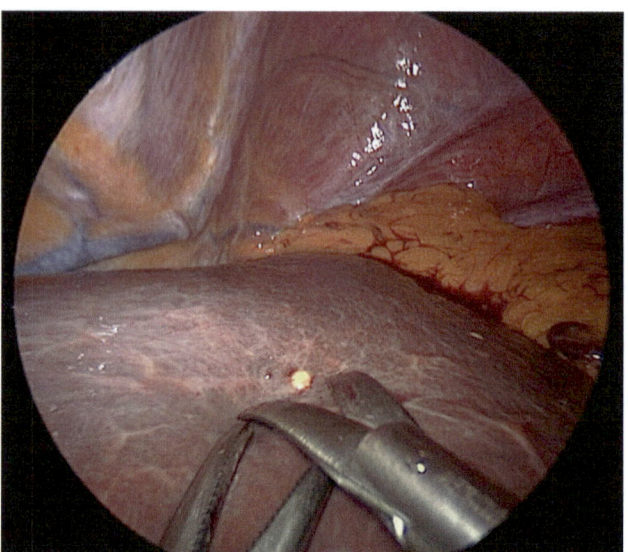

Fig. 21.1 Small peripheral liver lesion

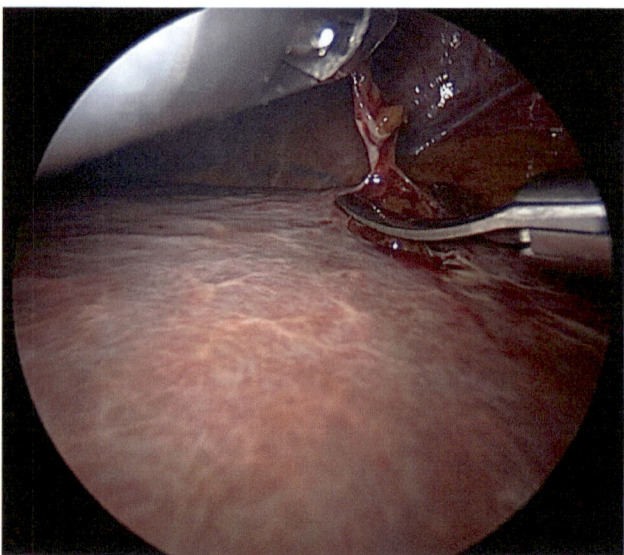

Fig. 21.2 Sharp excision of small peripheral liver lesion

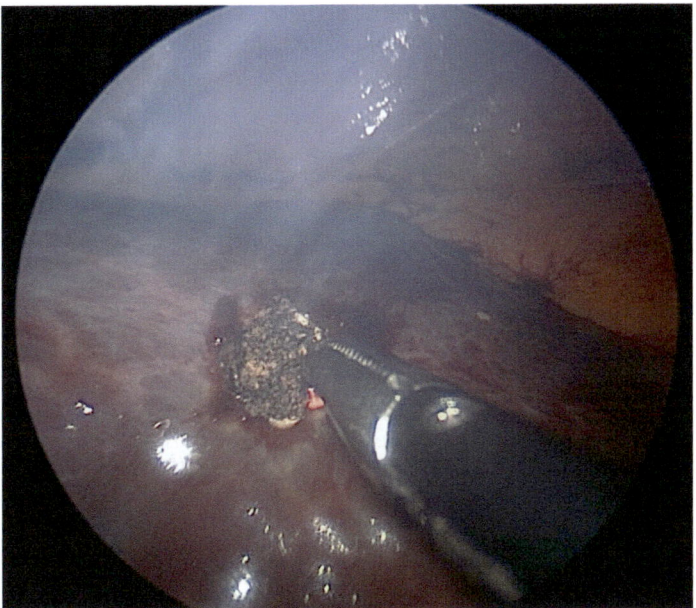

Fig. 21.3 Electrosurgical hemostasis of resection bed

Conclusion

Liver biopsy has historically been essential to the diagnosis, staging, and management of a wide range of liver pathologies. Since the procedure became widespread in the mid-twentieth century, the percutaneous core needle biopsy has reached global utilization and is now the gold standard for tissue diagnosis. Several other approaches, including transjugular, endoscopic, and surgical, have been developed and are frequently used when percutaneous biopsy is not favored. In the past several decades, noninvasive serologic and radiologic examination of the liver as well as effective medical treatments for viral hepatitis have lessened the importance of liver biopsy and have led to an overall decrease in the number of biopsies performed worldwide. The procedure is nonetheless well tolerated. The surgeon should be aware of several infrequent but pathognomonic complications including pain and bleeding, as well as the techniques, limitations, timing, and rationale for liver biopsy.

Conflicts of Interest The authors declare no conflicts of interest regarding this publication.

References

1. Bravo A, Sheth SG, Chopra S. Liver Biopsy. N Engl J Med. 2001;344(7):495–500.
2. Jain D, Torres R, Celli R, Koelmel J, Charkoftaki G, Vasiliou V. Evolution of the liver biopsy and its future. Transl Gastroenterol Hepatol. 2021:1–21.
3. Rockey DC, Caldwell SH, Goodman ZD, Nelson RC, Smith AD. Liver biopsy. Hepatology. 2009;49((3):1017–44. https://doi.org/10.1002/hep.22742.
4. Neuberger J, Patel J, Caldwell H, et al. Guidelines on the use of liver biopsy in clinical practice from the British society of gastroenterology, the royal college of radiologists and the royal college of pathology. Gut. 2020;69(8):1382–403.
5. Bedossa P, Dargère D, Paradis V. Sampling variability of liver fibrosis in chronic hepatitis C. Hepatology. 2003;38(6):1449–57.
6. Regev A, Berho M, Jeffers LJ, et al. Sampling error and intraobserver variation in liver biopsy in patients with chronic HCV infection. Am J Gastroenterol. 2002;97(10):2614–8.
7. Bejarano PA, Koehler A, Sherman KE. Second opinion pathology in liver biopsy interpretation. Am J Gastroenterol. 2001;96(11):3158–64.
8. Zeremski M, Dimova RB, Benjamin S, et al. FibroSURE as a noninvasive marker of liver fibrosis and inflammation in chronic hepatitis B. BMC Gastroenterol. 2014;14:118.
9. Afdhal NH. Fibroscan (transient elastography) for the measurement of liver fibrosis. Gastroenterol Hepatol (N Y). 2012;8(9):605–7.
10. Kumar M, Andi A, Lucas S, et al. PWE-120 liver biopsy using 16 G needle: a comparative study. Gut [Internet]. 2013;62(Suppl 1):A179 LP–A180. Available from: http://gut.bmj.com/content/62/Suppl_1/A179.2.abstract
11. Kd J, Laoveeravat P, Eu Y, et al. REVIEW 83 endoscopic ultrasound guided liver biopsy: recent evidence 98 impact of a simulation-based induction programme in gastroscopy on trainee outcomes and learning curves CASE REPORT 111 gallbladder perforation due to endoscopic sleeve gastroplasty. World J Gastro Endosc World J Gastrointest Endosc

[Internet]. 2020;12(3):83–118. Available from: https://www.wjgnet.com/bpg/gerinfo/240
12. Kamarajah SK, Wilson CH, Bundred JR, et al. A systematic review and network meta-analysis of parenchymal transection techniques during hepatectomy: an appraisal of current randomised controlled trials. Hpb [Internet]. 2020;22(2):204–14. Available from: https://doi.org/10.1016/j.hpb.2019.09.014.
13. West J, Card TR. Reduced mortality rates following elective percutaneous liver biopsies. Gastroenterology. 2010;139(4):1230–7.
14. Piccinino F, Sagnelli E, Pasquale G, Giusti G. Complications following percutaneous liver biopsy. A multicentre retrospective study on 68,276 biopsies. J Hepatol. 1986;2(2):165–73.
15. Janes CH, Lindor KD. Outcome of patients hospitalized for complications after outpatient liver biopsy. Ann Intern Med. 1993;118(2):96–8.
16. Boyum JH, Atwell TD, Schmit GD, et al. Incidence and risk factors for adverse events related to image-guided liver biopsy. Mayo Clin Proc. 2016;91(3):329–35.

Inferior Partial Hepatectomy and Superior Partial Hepatectomy

22

Aleksandr Kalabin, John Martinie, and Erin Baker

Introduction

"A backbone" of successful liver surgery is careful preoperative planning and detailed understanding of Couinaud's segmental anatomy and their critical structures, namely portal vein, biliary tree, hepatic arteries, and veins. The liver is classically divided into the right and left lobes by the Cantlie's line (extending from the gallbladder fossa cephalad to the inferior vena cava) and further subdivided into eight liver segments where each segment is fed by an independent portal branch. The true anatomic left lobe has medial segment IV and lateral segments II and III and could be subdivided into a superior (segments II and IVa) and inferior (segments III and IVb) sectors. The segments of the right liver lobe (segments V–VIII) are also split into superior (segments VII and VIII) and inferior (segment V and VI) sectors. The term "anatomical" liver resection is usually used if one or more Couinaud's segments along with its corresponding portal pedicles are removed, whereas if only a portion of liver parenchyma is resected

A. Kalabin (✉) · J. Martinie · E. Baker
Charlotte, NC, USA
e-mail: Aleksandr.Kalabin@atriumhealth.org;
John.Martinie@atriumhealth.org; Erin.Baker@atriumhealth.org

© The Author(s), under exclusive license to Springer Nature Switzerland AG 2025
A. Alseidi et al. (eds.), *The SAGES Manual of Contemporary Indications and Management of Hepatic and Biliary Diseases*, https://doi.org/10.1007/978-3-032-04823-3_22

independently of vascular segmental anatomy, it is called "nonanatomical" or wedge resection.

Posterior–superior segments of the liver, traditionally referred to segments I (Couinaud), IVa, VII, and VIII are located in the difficult-to-expose regions near the diaphragm and in close proximity to important vascular structures including the hepatic veins and inferior vena cava. For years, segmentectomy and wedge resections of the posterior–superior liver segments were considered more technically challenging as compared to anterior–inferior segments (II, III, IVb, V, and VI) due to their less accessible anatomic location, challenges with exposure, and ability to control possible intraoperative bleeding. Anterior–inferior segments have been classically described as less technically challenging from a surgical standpoint [1, 2]. With growing emphasis on liver parenchyma preservation, major hepatectomy procedures can be avoided in favor of nonanatomic partial (wedge) resections and anatomic minor resections. For many disease processes, these can be performed safely and feasibly with minimally invasive techniques [3]. In our opinion, if no major contraindications exist, laparoscopic or robotic approaches both should be primarily regarded as a preferable alternative to open technique for major or minor liver resection [4].

Preoperative Imaging

Optimal surgical strategy of any liver resection procedure starts long before the operating room and accurate understanding of the number, size, and exact location of liver lesions is paramount. High quality modern preoperative imaging (CT or MRI) is an invaluable tool in careful surgical planning with a goal of preserving as much unaffected liver tissue as possible. Present-day imaging modalities provide detailed assessment of feasibility of liver resection with identification of very small lesions and clear understanding of anatomical relationship of the portal vein, hepatic artery, and hepatic veins. Although several variants of hepatic arterial anatomy do exist and should be acknowledged, the anatomy of the portal and hepatic veins are more relevant as it relates to nonanatomic liver resections. Standard portal vein bifurcation at the hilum to the left and right liver lobes is seen in 65% of cases. However, portal "trifurcation" and "Z-type" portal vein (absent right portal vein with right sectorial branches originating from the main trunk) as well as left portal vein feeding the segment VIII can be encountered [5]. The preservation of outflowing hepatic veins of a future liver remnant is particularly important to avoid postoperative venous congestion and related complications. The right hepatic vein (RHV) classically drains segments VI and VII and occasionally segments V and VII. The left hepatic vein (LHV) drains segments II and III, and occasionally the segment IV. And the middle hepatic vein drains the central part of the liver and receives tributaries from segments IV, V, and VII. De Chicchis proposed four morphological variants of RHV [6] that have to be delineated and reviewed on preoperative scans for proper operative planning as transecting the middle hepatic vein (MHV) could be associated with potentially severe postoperative congestion of the so-called "marginal zones" in both liver lobes. While type 1 and type 2 RHV conventionally drain segments V, VI, and VII, type 3 RVH drains the total right hemiliver as segmental venous drainage from segment VIII empties in the RHV. This particular variant of RHV drainage as well as distal RHV confluence in type 3 RHV is important to recognize when planning resections of posterior–superior liver segments. Another important variant is the accessory right hepatic vein (ARHV) or type IV based on De Chicchis classification. Cheng et al. found that in 400 normal livers studied with ultrasound, an inferior right hepatic vein (IRHV) was found to drain segment VI of the liver and flow into the inferior vena cava (IVC) in 18% of the cases [7]. Koc et al. described the presence, type, and number of variants or anomalies of the hepatic veins based on localization and segmental venous drainage [8]. Proper delineation of the complex outflow liver anatomy allowed Makuuchi to perform first resection of segments VII and VIII, sparing segments V and VI (with the presence of ARHV) reported in 1987 [9]. Anatomical variations do exist for the left hepatic vein (LHV) with variable venous outflow for segment IV either draining into the MHV or the LHV. Again, the venous anatomy and drainage should be recognized to avoid unnecessary hepatic tissue congestion after the surgery.

Surgical Approach/Preoperative Preparation

Historically, an open abdominal approach was used for posterior–superior liver lesions when laparoscopic liver resections were most commonly performed for small, solitary, anterior–inferior segment lesions [10, 11]. However, more recent studies have reported that lesions located in restricted and difficult-to-expose hepatic areas (posterior–superior—Couinaud segments VII–VIII) are technically amenable for minimally invasive approach most likely due to the recent technological improvements, increasing experience and development of more innovative techniques. Over the last decade, minimally invasive approaches have been increasingly utilized for many minor and major hepatectomies regardless of the tumor location. Given that multiple studies have demonstrated safety, feasibility, and efficacy of performing major and minor hepatectomy laparoscopically and/or robotically, both approaches should be considered standard technique unless contraindications exist otherwise [11–13].

Considering that many patients may have underlying chronic liver disease, perioperative management cannot be overestimated. Preoperative optimization of liver function, improving the nutritional and functional status of the patient, and correcting the coagulopathy are of uppermost importance. Close intraoperative communication with anesthesia colleagues and maintenance of low central venous pressure including limiting fluids and decreasing intrathoracic pressure has a crucial role in patients' outcomes. Establishment of large-bore venous access and arterial line for continuous systemic blood pressure monitoring is advised.

Open Surgery—Setup and Pitfalls

Open Approach

Standard upper midline laparotomy incision is usually done for left-sided hepatic lesions. Midline laparotomy incision with extension over the xyphoid process or right subcostal incision with midline extension allows exposure of the right-sided and posterior–superior liver lesions as well as extrahepatic inferior vena cava. Right thoracoabdominal incision have more of historical interest and rarely utilized in this day and age. Bilateral subcostal incision (Chevron) is rarely used at present and could be considered for larger tumors where spatial challenges and exposure are problematic.

Once the abdominal cavity is entered, thorough inspection for signs of metastatic disease is performed. One or two small newly discovered colorectal liver metastatic lesion(s) in a favorable location could be excised or ablated during the same procedure. This may not be true for hepatocellular carcinoma or intrahepatic cholangiocarcinoma. Diffuse metastatic disease should be considered as a contraindication for liver resection. Next the falciform, ipsilateral (depends on the location of the lesion) coronal and triangular ligaments are divided to facilitate extensive liver mobilization. Intraoperative ultrasound is an invaluable tool and is utilized routinely. Three major components of the ultrasound evaluation should be ascertained: evaluation of liver segments with delineation of correspondent portal and hepatic venous anatomy, visualization and characterization of all visible liver lesions, and outlining of the resection plane with marking of the liver capsule along the line of transection (electrocautery). Next, dissection of porta hepatis is executed and the portal triad is encircled with a tape in preparation for Pringle maneuver (inflow occlusion). The next step is parenchymal transection, and it can be performed by multiple techniques (finger fracture, clamp-fracture, sharp dissection, Harmonic Scalpel (Ethicon Endo-Surgery, Cincinnati, OH, USA), TissueLink (Salient Surgical Technologies, Portsmouth, NH, USA), Cavitron Ultrasonic Surgical Aspirator

[CUSA, Valleylab, Boulder, CO, USA], Radiofrequency dissector sealer, Water-jet dissection, etc.). After parenchymal transection is done, meticulous hemostasis should be obtained. Visible bleeding vessel could be controlled with nonabsorbable fine sutures or clips. Electrocautery and argon beam coagulation are effective adjuncts for small vessels and raw surfaces. Hemostatic fibrin and thrombin-based agents (Surgifoam Absorbable Gelatin Sponge and Surgiflo Hemostatic Matrix Kit—both Ethicon Inc., Somerville, NJ, USA; Floseal Hemostatic Matrix—Baxter International Inc., Fremont, CA, USA) are effective and can assist with management of oozing from the cut parenchymal liver surface.

Occult biliary leaks should be identified and controlled. Completion ultrasound to document adequate inflow and outflow to the liver remnant is performed at the completion of the case. In general, we infrequently leave drains after liver resection. In rare cases, drains may be placed for more extensive resection, significant hepatic abscess, problematic perihilar dissection, or biliary reconstruction. Attention is also paid to the expected pathology and potential need for reoperation in the future.

Laparoscopic Surgery—Setup and Pitfalls

Although some authors recently proposed a semi-prone patient position [14] or even an intercostal trocar approach [15, 16], our group approaches most of the anterior–inferior lesions with a standard supine position, posterior–superior liver lesions either with a patient in a split leg supine position (segment VIII), or in a left lateral decubitus position (segment VII). For most posterior–superior hepatectomies, we use 45 cm long laparoscopic instruments, whereas regular length instruments are utilized for anterior–inferior liver lesions (nonobese patients). A footboard could be installed depending on the exact location of the lesion and patient's habitus. Patient is then placed in reverse Trendelenburg position and slight right-sided tilted up position. Occasionally, for more posterior liver lesions (segments VII and VIII), patient could be placed in a semi-lateral position with an intent to place the trocars more laterally on the abdominal wall [17]. In this instance, the right arm is carefully supported up and over the chest to expose and open the distance between the inferior border of the rib cage and the anterior superior iliac crest. Alternative positioning techniques include a split leg table (with or without supportive footboards) or lithotomy position with stirrups. The surgeon stands on the left side of the patient or between the legs.

Abdominal access is usually achieved with an open technique, with a 12 mm blunt tip Hasson trocar is placed above the umbilicus and pneumoperitoneum established and maintained throughout the surgery at 12–15 mmHg. For patients with a history of cirrhosis and periumbilical varices, a cut down approach (open Hasson technique) may be performed over the rectus sheath to avoid excessive bleeding from periumbilical varices. A second 12 mm trocar may be placed in the subxiphoid area (or midclavicular line depending on lesion location) and two additional 5 mm trocars are usually inserted in the right midclavicular and midaxillary lines along the subcostal margins. 12 mm subxiphoid and 5 mm midclavicular trocars are the main working ports, with the camera inserted through the initial 12 mm paraumbilical port and operated by the assistant along with another 5 mm port in the midaxillary line. For tumors in segments VII and VIII, sometimes a hand-access port (Gelport Applied Medical, Rancho Santa Margarita, CA, USA) is placed in the right upper quadrant to facilitate retraction and mobilization of the liver from the retroperitoneum.

Next, laparoscopic ultrasonography is performed and all liver lesions as well as inflow and outflow segmental anatomy are identified. The same principles of laparoscopic ultrasonography are applied as with an open approach. Anterior–inferior liver segments are readily assessable for laparoscopic surgery and usually no additional maneuvers are required. For right-sided posterior–superior lesions, the right liver lobe should be fully mobilized, with exposure of the inferior vena cava. The liver should be separated from the diaphragm superiorly and posterior ligaments should be taken down. After the right lobe is mobilized, it could be retracted medially, sometimes a liver retractor (additional

5 mm trocar can be placed) is utilized for that purpose or one of the right upper quadrant ports could be extended and hand-access port placed for manual liver retraction. A sling technique for laparoscopic resection of segment VII lesion was also described [18]. Briefly, the right liver lobe is mobilized until the right lateral wall of the inferior vena cava could be identified. A 1-inch packing tape sling is laparoscopically wrapped around segment 6 and externalized through a separate stab incision at the left-upper quadrant. The right hemi-liver is then gently pulled anterior and cephalad, and triangular ligament is fully divided in order to further advance the sling over the segment VIII. The liver should be amenable for retraction away from the diaphragm. Then the dorsal hepatic ligament is divided, and the right liver lobe should be completely mobile at that stage of the surgery. The sling is used to rotate the liver and the segment VII could be fully released.

Once the resection line is determined with the help of the laparoscopic ultrasound, it is marked and the resection groove is executed with electrocautery. To facilitate the exposure, especially with lesions in posterior aspects of segments VI and VII, suture retraction could be employed. For that, sutures are placed to the lateral or superior/inferior edges of the resection line and tails are brough out through the previously placed trocars or separate stab incisions for forceful retraction and fixed to the operative drape. The hepatoduodenal ligament is encircled with an umbilical tape with a tourniquet for an intermittent inflow occlusion (Pringle maneuver), and parenchymal transection is done with one or combination of the techniques/equipment (Harmonic Scalpel—Ethicon, Cincinnati, OH, USA), Aquamantys (Medtronic, Minneapolis, MN, USA), TissueLink (Salient Surgical Technologies, Portsmouth, NH, USA), or CUSA (Tyco Healthcare, Mansfield, MA), laparoscopic electrocautery device, laparoscopic staplers, or other methods mentioned previously. Hemostasis, assessment for bile leak, and completion ultrasound should be performed similar to the open technique. The specimen is placed into a laparoscopic bag and retrieved trough one of the 12 mm or hand-assisted ports. Large specimen could be retrieved through additional suprapubic incision.

Robotic Surgery—Setup and Pitfalls

The Da Vinci Xi robotic platform is most commonly used for minimally invasive liver surgery. Patient is placed in supine position with both arms extended. The pneumoperitoneum is obtained with Veress needle inserted below the umbilicus and maintained at 12–15 mmHg throughout the procedure. The abdominal access is obtained with the 12 mm trocar below the umbilicus (blunt vs. Optiview), once the Veress needle is removed and is subsequently utilized as an assistant port. For left-sided liver lesions, we place four 8 mm trocars for four robotic arms—3–4 cm above the umbilicus at the midclavicular lines and anterior axillary lines bilaterally. Occasionally, for left lateral liver lesions (segments II and III), right-sided trocars may be positioned more medially. For right-sided liver lesions, two left-sided 8 mm ports are usually placed more cranially, 6–8 cm above the umbilicus. Then the robot is docked. The liver is completely mobilized by taking down falciform, coronary, and triangular ligaments. For segments VII–VIII liver lesions, retro-hepatic inferior vena cava should be exposed. Robot-integrated intraoperative ultrasound is done to localize the lesions and delineate the anatomy. The line of transection is marked with electrocautery with ultrasound guidance to ensure appropriate oncological margins. Porta hepatis is dissected, and inflow portal vein and hepatic artery are identified. Pringle maneuver could be performed with intermittent occlusion of the inflow vessels with bulldog clamps introduced into the abdomen through the assistant port. Liver parenchyma is divided with bipolar forceps with intermittent saline irrigation. Large portal branches and hepatic veins are controlled with hem-o-lock clips and/or an endoscopic stapler. The specimen is removed through a separate Pfannenstiel incision, and a closed suction drain may be placed. Recent reports confirmed that robotic approach for resection of posterior–superior liver segment is safe and feasible [19, 20].

Transthoracic Approach

Transthoracic approach for posterior–superior liver lesions was recently described [17, 21]. This approach could be particularly convenient in patient with morbid obesity or patients with multiple previous abdominal surgeries. The patient is placed in a modified French or left lateral decubitus position, and single lung ventilation is obtained. Access to the right thoracic cavity is obtained after the lung is deflated with a standard thoracoscopic technique and thoracic cavity explored. At that stage, transthoracic transdiaphragmatic intraoperative sonography could be performed to localize the liver lesion. Transthoracic hepatic resection with partial resection of the diaphragm is done and the diaphragm later is repaired primarily with a chest tube placed at the end of the case.

Although the technique was originally described in 2003 [22], it is still considered innovative and evolving, and recent studies reported a lot of variability in technical details. Minimally invasive transthoracic liver resection (MITTLR) approach has not been standardized and the data on long-term outcomes is still underreported [23]. MITTLR is not uniformly adopted, and more studies are needed to validate its safety and reproducibility.

Conclusion

Nonanatomical inferior and superior partial hepatectomies have emanated as a safe and advantageous alternative over major hepatectomies, especially in patients with limited hepatic function/reserve. Moreover, partial hepatectomies performed with minimally invasive techniques are considered a standard approach in a majority of high-volume tertiary facilities in the United States.

References

1. Kaneko H, Takagi S, Otsuka Y, Tsuchiya M, Tamura A, Katagiri T, Maeda T, Shiba T. Laparoscopic liver resection of hepatocellular carcinoma. Am J Surg. 2005;189(2):190–4. https://doi.org/10.1016/j.amjsurg.2004.09.010. PMID: 15720988.
2. Cho JY, Han HS, Yoon YS, Shin SH. Outcomes of laparoscopic liver resection for lesions located in the right side of the liver. Arch Surg. 2009;144(1):25–9. https://doi.org/10.1001/archsurg.2008.510. PMID: 19153321.
3. Kabir T, Syn N, Goh BKP. Current status of laparoscopic liver resection for the management of colorectal liver metastases. J Gastrointest Oncol. 2020;11(3):526–39. https://doi.org/10.21037/jgo.2020.02.05. PMID: 32655931; PMCID: PMC7340801
4. Fruscione M, Pickens R, Baker EH, Cochran A, Khan A, Ocuin L, Iannitti DA, Vrochides D, Martinie JB. Robotic-assisted versus laparoscopic major liver resection: analysis of outcomes from a single center. HPB (Oxford). 2019;21(7):906–11. https://doi.org/10.1016/j.hpb.2018.11.011. Epub 2019 Jan 5. PMID: 30617001.
5. Agostini A, Borgheresi A, Floridi C, Carotti M, Grazzini G, Pagnini F, Guerrini S, Palumbo P, Pradella S, Carrafiello G, Vivarelli M, Giovagnoni A. The role of imaging in surgical planning for liver resection: what the radiologist need to know. Acta Biomed. 2020;91(8-S):18–26. https://doi.org/10.23750/abm.v91i8-S.9938. PMID: 32945275; PMCID: PMC7944681
6. De Cecchis L, Hribernik M, Ravnik D, Gadzijev EM. Anatomical variations in the pattern of the right hepatic veins: possibilities for type classification. J Anat. 2000;197(Pt 3):487–93. https://doi.org/10.1046/j.1469-7580.2000.19730487.x. PMID: 11117632; PMCID: PMC1468147
7. Cheng YF, Huang TL, Chen CL, Chen TY, Huang CC, Ko SF, Yang BY, Lee TY. Variations of the middle and inferior right hepatic vein: application in hepatectomy. J Clin Ultrasound. 1997;25(4):175–82. https://doi.org/10.1002/(sici)1097-0096(199705)25:4<175::aid-jcu4>3.0.co;2-b. PMID: 9142616.
8. Koc Z, Ulusan S, Oguzkurt L, Tokmak N. Venous variants and anomalies on routine abdominal multi-detector row CT. Eur J Radiol. 2007;61(2):267–78. https://doi.org/10.1016/j.ejrad.2006.09.008. Epub 2006 Oct 17. PMID: 17049792.
9. Makuuchi M, Hasegawa H, Yamazaki S, Takayasu K. Four new hepatectomy procedures for resection of the right hepatic vein and preservation of the inferior right hepatic vein. Surg Gynecol Obstet. 1987;164(1):68–72. PMID: 3026059.

10. Buell JF, Cherqui D, Geller DA, O'Rourke N, Iannitti D, Dagher I, Koffron AJ, Thomas M, Gayet B, Han HS, Wakabayashi G, Belli G, Kaneko H, Ker CG, Scatton O, Laurent A, Abdalla EK, Chaudhury P, Dutson E, Gamblin C, D'Angelica M, Nagorney D, Testa G, Labow D, Manas D, Poon RT, Nelson H, Martin R, Clary B, Pinson WC, Martinie J, Vauthey JN, Goldstein R, Roayaie S, Barlet D, Espat J, Abecassis M, Rees M, Fong Y, McMasters KM, Broelsch C, Busuttil R, Belghiti J, Strasberg S, Chari RS, World Consensus Conference on Laparoscopic Surgery. The international position on laparoscopic liver surgery: the Louisville statement, 2008. Ann Surg. 2009;250(5):825–30. https://doi.org/10.1097/sla.0b013e3181b3b2d8. PMID: 19916210
11. Giuliani A, Aldrighetti L, Di Benedetto F, Ettorre GM, Bianco P, Ratti F, Tarantino G, Santoro R, Felli E. Total abdominal approach for posterosuperior segments (7, 8) in laparoscopic liver surgery: a multicentric experience. Updat Surg. 2015;67(2):169–75. https://doi.org/10.1007/s13304-015-0305-4. Epub 2015 Jun 16. PMID: 26076916.
12. Kose E, Kahramangil B, Aydin H, Donmez M, Aucejo F, Quintini C, Fung J, Berber E. Minimally invasive resection of posterosuperior liver tumors in the supine position using intra-abdominal trocars. Surg Endosc. 2020;34(2):536–43. https://doi.org/10.1007/s00464-019-06789-9. Epub 2019 Apr 8. PMID: 30963261.
13. Guro H, Cho JY, Han HS, Yoon YS, Choi Y, Jang JS, Kwon SU, Kim S, Choi JK. Laparoscopic liver resection of hepatocellular carcinoma located in segments 7 or 8. Surg Endosc. 2018;32(2):872–8. https://doi.org/10.1007/s00464-017-5756-x. Epub 2017 Jul 20. PMID: 28730274.
14. Ikeda T, Toshima T, Harimoto N, Yamashita Y, Ikegami T, Yoshizumi T, Soejima Y, Shirabe K, Maehara Y. Laparoscopic liver resection in the semiprone position for tumors in the anterosuperior and posterior segments, using a novel dual-handling technique and bipolar irrigation system. Surg Endosc. 2014;28(8):2484–92. https://doi.org/10.1007/s00464-014-3469-y. Epub 2014 Mar 13. PMID: 24622763; PMCID: PMC4077249
15. Hirokawa F, Hayashi M, Asakuma M, Shimizu T, Inoue Y, Uchiyama K. Intercostal trocars enable easier laparoscopic resection of liver tumors in segments 7 and 8. World J Surg. 2017;41(5):1340–6. https://doi.org/10.1007/s00268-016-3867-5. PMID: 28097410.
16. Lee W, Han HS, Yoon YS, Cho JY, Choi Y, Shin HK. Role of intercostal trocars on laparoscopic liver resection for tumors in segments 7 and 8. J Hepatobiliary Pancreat Sci. 2014;21(8):E65–8. https://doi.org/10.1002/jhbp.123. Epub 2014 May 19. PMID: 24841194.

17. Moisan F, Gayet B, Ward MA, Tabchouri N, Fuks D. Segment 7 laparoscopic liver resection: is it possible to resect when metastatic lesions border Suprahepatic veins? J Gastrointest Surg. 2018;22(9):1643–4. https://doi.org/10.1007/s11605-018-3824-8. Epub 2018 May 31. PMID: 29855869.
18. Mashchenko I, Trtchounian A, Buchholz C, de la Torre AN. A sling technique for laparoscopic resection of segment seven of the liver. JSLS. 2018;22(2):e2018.00017. https://doi.org/10.4293/JSLS.2018.00017. PMID: 29977110; PMCID: PMC6020890.
19. Machado MAC, Mattos BH, Lobo Filho MM, Makdissi FF. Robotic Resection of Postero-Superior Liver Segments (7,8) (with Video). J Gastrointest Surg. 2021;25(2):574–5. https://doi.org/10.1007/s11605-020-04799-w. Epub 2020 Sep 18. PMID: 32948960.
20. Zhao Z, Yin Z, Pan L, Li C, Hu M, Lau WY, Liu R. Robotic hepatic resection in postero-superior region of liver. Updat Surg. 2021;73(3):1007–14. https://doi.org/10.1007/s13304-020-00895-3. Epub 2020 Oct 8. PMID: 33030697.
21. Yamashita S, Loyer E, Kang HC, Aloia TA, Chun YS, Mehran RJ, Eng C, Lee JE, Vauthey JN, Conrad C. Total transthoracic approach facilitates laparoscopic hepatic resection in patients with significant prior abdominal surgery. Ann Surg Oncol. 2017;24(5):1376–7. https://doi.org/10.1245/s10434-016-5685-2. Epub 2016 Nov 22. PMID: 27878479.
22. Teramoto K, Kawamura T, Takamatsu S, Noguchi N, Nakamura N, Arii S. Laparoscopic and thoracoscopic partial hepatectomy for hepatocellular carcinoma. World J Surg. 2003;27(10):1131–6. https://doi.org/10.1007/s00268-003-6936-5. Epub 2003 Aug 18. PMID: 12917768.
23. Pathak S, Main BG, Blencowe NS, Rees JRE, Robertson HF, Abbadi RAG, Blazeby JM. A systematic review of minimally invasive trans-thoracic liver resection to examine intervention description, governance, and outcome reporting of an innovative technique. Ann Surg. 2021;273(5):882–9. https://doi.org/10.1097/SLA.0000000000003748. PMID: 32511126.

23. Anatomic Metastasectomy/Segmentectomy and Left Lateral Sectionectomy

Gabriella Lionetto, Avril Kaye Coley, and Cristina R. Ferrone

Hepatic resection for the treatment of colorectal cancer metastases has been established as potentially curative [1] and improvement in long-term outcomes for metastatic neuroendocrine tumors, sarcomas, and other malignancies has been demonstrated [2, 3]. The key principles of liver resection are complete removal of the disease while preserving future liver function. While preservation of hepatic parenchyma is important for all patients, it is essential for those with underlying liver disease, as is often the case in patients with hepatocellular carcinoma or in patients with liver metastases who have received hepatotoxic chemotherapy.

G. Lionetto
Department of Surgery, Unit of General and Pancreatic Surgery,
University of Verona Hospital Trust, Verona, Italy
e-mail: gabriella.lionetto@univr.it

A. K. Coley
Department of Surgery, Massachusetts General Hospital, Harvard Medical School, Boston, MA, USA
e-mail: akcoley@mgh.harvard.edu

C. R. Ferrone (✉)
Department of Surgery, Cedars Sinai Medical Center,
Los Angeles, CA, USA
e-mail: cristina.ferrone@cshs.org; CFERRONE@mgh.harvard.edu

© The Author(s), under exclusive license to Springer Nature Switzerland AG 2025
A. Alseidi et al. (eds.), *The SAGES Manual of Contemporary Indications and Management of Hepatic and Biliary Diseases*,
https://doi.org/10.1007/978-3-032-04823-3_23

Anatomic metastasectomy/hepatic segmentectomy is a favorable option for achieving a satisfactory oncologic outcome while preserving liver parenchyma.

Preoperative Considerations

Chemotherapy-Induced Hepatotoxicity

In addition to the usual preoperative assessment of patient functional status and comorbidities, careful consideration must be given to patients with liver metastases who have received preoperative chemotherapy. The incidence of chemotherapy-induced steatosis and steatohepatitis increases with the number of cycles of chemotherapy administered, as well as the interval of time after cessation of systemic therapy [4]. Evaluation of these patients by multidisciplinary tumor boards is critical for determining an individualized approach that will avoid prolonged chemotherapy administration and delays in proceeding to hepatic resection once disease is resectable.

Synchronous Colon Cancer Primary and Liver Metastases

In patients with synchronous colorectal liver metastases, careful consideration must be given to the optimal sequence of their liver and colon resection and the timing of systemic therapy. Timing of therapy depends on location and symptoms of the colorectal cancer and the number and location of the hepatic metastases. If the colon cancer is asymptomatic, most patients will receive 3 months of systemic therapy followed by hepatic resection. Three months of systemic therapy have become the standard due the results of the EORTC 40983 trial—the only randomized evidence in this area—comparing surgery alone vs perioperative FOLFOX (6 cycles before and after liver resection), which showed improved disease-free survival in the chemotherapy group, although no overall survival advantage possibly due to a lack of power [5, 6].

However, it is noteworthy that chemotherapy for CRLM may induce changes to the liver parenchyma [7, 8] and, specifically, administration of 6 cycles or more of Oxaliplatin-based chemotherapy has been linked to an increased risk of sinusoidal obstruction syndrome, finally leading to poorer postsurgical morbidity and disease-specific outcomes [9, 10].

The management of synchronous colorectal cancer and liver metastases requires careful consideration of surgical complexity, patient comorbidities, and tumor biology [11]. While simultaneous resection offers logistical advantages, they can be associated with higher rates of complications, including postoperative ileus, anastomotic failure, and liver failure [12]. Current evidence and guidelines recommend careful patient selection, reserving combined surgery for cases where both resections are minor and low risk. When either procedure is complex, a staged approach is preferred, prioritizing the more challenging resection first—often the liver (the so-called "liver first" approach)—to confirm the feasibility of an R0 resection and guide further treatment. Preoperative systemic therapy plays a key role in assessing tumor biology, as progression during chemotherapy may preclude surgery, as disease progression on chemotherapy portends a poorer overall prognosis, while evidence of radiographic response may indicate a better prognosis [13, 14]. Minimally invasive techniques and optimization of patient comorbidities can mitigate risks, but individualized strategies remain essential to balance oncologic outcomes with surgical morbidity [15].

Hepatocellular Carcinoma and Cholangiocarcinoma

Most patients with hepatocellular carcinoma and cholangiocarcinoma have underlying chronic liver disease. Therefore, careful consideration must be given to the patient's performance status and baseline liver function when evaluating them for a potential liver resection. In general, patients with good performance status and Child-Pugh Class A liver function without portal hypertension are able to tolerate an anatomic liver resection. In patients with Child-Pugh Class B liver function, however, careful consideration must be given to whether patients should undergo locoregional therapies, such as ablation or arterial ablation, rather than a more limited nonanatomic hepatic resection. There have been randomized control trials that indicate fewer complications with radiofrequency ablation and similar survival outcomes compared to surgery for lesions <3 cm [16–18]. However, a Cochrane meta-analysis of these and other non-randomized trials indicates that liver resection may provide better overall survival and a lower local recurrence rate [19].

For the treatment of intrahepatic cholangiocarcinoma, surgical resection currently remains the only curative intervention. Though patients frequently present with advanced disease or large tumors requiring anatomic resections, parenchymal-sparing resections have shown similar outcomes when compared to anatomic resections as long as clear margins can be obtained and a portal lymphadenectomy is performed [20].

Imaging

All patients should have cross-sectional abdominal imaging within 1 month of their operation to assess the number and location of the hepatic lesions and their relationship to vascular structures. Quadruple-phase contrast helical computed tomography (CT) is more reliable for detecting extrahepatic disease, while MRI is more specific for small liver lesions. When assessing preoperative imaging for a patient undergoing an anatomical hepatic resection, these elements need to be evaluated relative to the hepatic lesion:

- Inflow and outflow vessels including the portal veins, hepatic arteries, and hepatic veins.
- Biliary anatomy.
- Variant vascular or biliary anatomy.
- Functional liver remnant.
- Tumor margin relative to essential structures.

- *Note*: A 1 cm margin is generally accepted for hepatic lesions [21]. A close margin does not necessarily preclude resection if an R0 resection can still be achieved.

General Operative Steps

The patient should be positioned supine on the operating room table with both arms out to allow the anesthesia team easy access to the patient's arms throughout the operation.

Hepatic resection can be performed open or minimally invasively [22, 23]. For an open operation, a right subcostal or a midline incision can be utilized. The first step in the operation is a thorough exploration of the abdomen to assess for extrahepatic disease. Next, an intraoperative ultrasound (IOUS) is performed to fully outline the lesion(s) including assessment of the portal veins and their branches, the course of the hepatic veins, and finally a full parenchymal assessment, looking for any occult lesions. The planned margin and transection line should be outlined after fully defining the lesion(s) and its relationship to surrounding structures.

To mobilize the liver, the falciform ligament is taken down, leaving enough to reattach it to the anterior abdominal wall if a right or extended right hepatectomy is performed. Depending on the location of the lesion, the left or right triangular ligaments may need to be taken down. Care should be taken to avoid injury to the diaphragm, phrenic nerves, and phrenic veins at this step. After mobilization of the liver, parenchymal transection is initiated. Several methods for parenchymal transection include bipolar forceps, vessel sealers, ultrasonic dissectors, and staplers. Our approach utilizes the Harmonic surgical scalpel activated just before the active tine contacts the liver tissue on the anterior surface; the inactive blade is then gradually closed to achieve simultaneous hemostasis and tissue transection. While approaching the dissection plane, care is taken to proceed slowly from superficial to deep keeping the transection line at the same depth. An ultrasonic dissector and bipolar can be utilized to compliment the Harmonic and allow for careful dissection and identification of vital structures. Control of the inflow and outflow to the segment of interest is obtained using a tristapler (2 mm/2.5 mm/3.5 mm) or clips when the vessels are encountered within the liver parenchyma.

Anatomical Segmentectomy (Fig. 23.1)

"Anatomical" resection of the liver refers to removal of a functional *segment* of hepatic parenchyma with defined boundaries dictated ("réglées" [24]) by the vascular and biliary anatomy supplying the Glissonian branches. This technique has the advantage of completely removing the tumor-bearing portal territory to achieve a radical resection, while simultaneously maximizing the amount of remnant liver which, as mentioned, is of utmost importance in patients with underlying liver disease or with altered liver function due to systemic treatment-related toxicity.

Anatomical segmentation of the liver, as initially described by Couinaud [25, 26], states that the first bifurcation of the Glissonian pedicle—the first-order branches of the portal vein (PV)—divides the organ into right and left hemi-livers. The secondary bifurca-

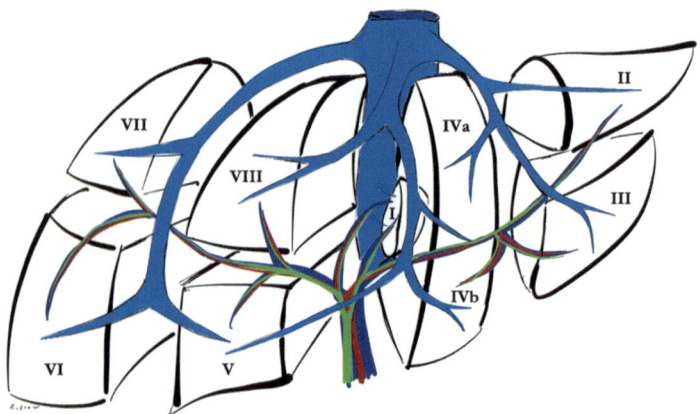

Fig. 23.1 Scheme of the anatomical segmental division of the liver according to Couinaud

tion originates the second-order branches for the right anterior/posterior and the left medial/lateral sections. The third-order branches refer to the segmental branches; however, in many cases, each segment is fed by two or more independent pedicles.

While nowadays the Couinaud scheme is accepted as a simplification [27], the improvement in preoperative radiological assessment and surgical technique has led us to extend the concept of anatomical resection to the "*cone unit*," the smallest anatomical part of the liver supplied by a third-order branch with the base on the hepatic surface and the apex pointing to the hilum [28]. However, given the knowledge of the highly variable PV branching patterns, it is imperative when planning an anatomical resection to confirm the actual anatomy of the segment of interest by detailed preoperative imaging and/or IOUS.

Before parenchymal dissection, an umbilical tape is passed around the hepatoduodenal ligament for inflow occlusion—Pringle maneuver—if needed. Dissection lines are generally determined by using IOUS, by injecting dye in the PV ("staining technique") [29] or by Indocyanine Green Dye (ICG) negative staining after pedicle clamping [30–32].

The key steps of each anatomical resection according to the involved segment are outlined in the following table.

Segment	Key steps	Pitfalls
S1	Division of the gastro-hepatic ligament; Posterior dissection of the hepatoduodenal ligament to identify, dissect, and divide the portal pedicles to S1 (**P1**s); Mobilization of the caudate lobe from the left side and along the anterior aspect of the IVC, dividing the **short hepatic veins**; Division of the **proper hepatic vein**; Exposure of the confluence of the LHV and MHV with the **IVC**; Dissection of the liver parenchyma toward the IVC exposing the posterior aspect of the **MHV**.	Preservation of the accessory LHA running through the gastro-hepatic ligament, if present. Depending on the tumor location, the duct of Arantius can be cut or preserved.

(continued)

Segment	Key steps	Pitfalls
S2	Identification of the root of the **LHV** behind the left lobe; Parenchymal dissection along the LHV, dividing the superficial hepatic veins draining S2 at their confluence; Intraparenchymal division of **P2**.	LHV can give left extrahepatic branch running through the left coronary ligament
S3	Division of the Glisson's capsule of S3 on the left side of the round ligament in the umbilical fossa; Identification and division of **P3**; Parenchymal dissection along the demarcation line, exposing the **LHV**.	A variably sized UFV draining S3 and S4 into the LHV is exposed during dissection of the medial side of S3.
S4a	Parenchymal dissection on the right side of the falciform ligament toward the confluence of the LHV and MHV; Identification and division of **P4a**; Further dissection along the area of demarcation on the surface, exposing the **MHV** toward its confluence with the IVC.	Care must be taken not to injure the UFV running between S3 and S4. Small veins draining S4a may directly open in the suprahepatic cava close to the main trunk of the MHV and LHV.
S4b	Identification and division of **P4b** in the umbilical fissure; Parenchymal dissection along the area of demarcation. S4 segmentectomy can be performed by the combination of the subsegmentectomy of its apical and basal component.	
S5	Dissection of the triangle of Calot and division of the cystic duct and artery; The transverse boundary is determined under US guidance; Medial aspect dissection along the **MHV** from the liver edge toward the hilum, dividing the MHV tributaries; Lateral aspect dissection along the **RHV** from the liver edge toward the hilum, exposing the right paramedian sector Glisson's capsule; Identification and division of **P5** from the right paramedian branch; Further parenchymal dissection along the area of demarcation.	

(continued)

Segment	Key steps	Pitfalls
S6	Mobilization of the right liver from the diaphragm and the right adrenal gland; Division of the **short hepatic veins** draining into the IVC; Parenchymal dissection exposing the **RHV**; Identification and division of **P6s** posteriorly to the RHV; The cranial boundary is determined by the area of demarcation on the liver surface.	Before dividing P6s, the blood supply to S7 should be confirmed.
S7	Exposure of the root of the RHV; The longitudinal dissection line along the RHV and the horizontal boundary above the bifurcation of the portal pedicles for S6 and S7 are determined under US guidance; Parenchymal dissection exposing the **RHV**; Identification and division of **P7s**; Identification and division of thick tributaries of the RHV.	Extrahepatic exposure of the RHV requires the division of the right retrocaval ligament [28].
S8	Exposure of the root of the RHV and the MHV; The longitudinal dissection lines along the RHV and MHV are determined under US guidance; Parenchymal dissection along the **RHV** and **MHV** toward the root of the ventral (**P8v**) and dorsal (**P8d**) branches of S8 portal pedicles; Identification and division of thick tributaries of the RHV and MHV.	Given the complete absence of anatomical landmarks on the liver surface and the high anatomical variation of his portal pedicles, anatomical resection of S8 is generally considered a demanding procedure. Craniocaudal hepatic vein dissection allows a major vascular control to avoid severe intraoperative bleeding [33, 34].

IVC inferior vena cava, *LHV* left hepatic vein, *MHV* middle hepatic vein, *P1–8* portal pedicles to segment 1–8, *RHV* right hepatic vein, *S1–8* segment 1–8, *UFV* umbilical fissural vein, *US* ultrasound

Left Lateral Sectionectomy

The lateral part of the left liver is an easily accessible anatomical portion with a very consistent anatomy, well individualized by the round ligament and the falciform ligament. Resection of this part of the liver was the first anatomical liver resection performed at the hands of the German surgeon Carl Johann August Langenbuch in 1888 (notably the pathological examination of the specimen revealed only normal parenchyma) [35]. Despite the terminological controversies, left lateral *section*ectomy or *segment*ectomy (LLS) refers to the en bloc resection of the liver segments II–III according to Couinaud [24, 36].

The intrahepatic vascular and biliary anatomy of the left lateral section tends to be very consistent. During preoperative planning, it is essential to assess whether the LHV and the MHV form a common trunk for drainage into the inferior vena cava (IVC) and how close the confluence is to the theoretical surgical margin, especially when dealing with S2 lesions. It is also important to identify any potential relevant anatomical variants, in particular the presence of a *type 3* left bile duct variant where the proper or an accessory duct from S4 drains into the S3 duct [37].

After the Louisville statement, laparoscopy has been acknowledged as the standard and preferred method for LLS [38]. In the setting of different difficulty scoring systems, LLS locates among the low/intermediate difficulty procedures and therefore represents a landmark operation in the learning curve of the laparoscopic liver surgeon [39–41].

Key Operative Steps

Left lateral sectionectomy can be divided into five phases [41–43]:

- Patient positioning and access.
- Continuous assessment.
- Mobilization.
- Parenchymal transection.
- Hemostasis.

Patient Positioning and Access

The most adopted patient positions are outlined in Fig. 23.2. The modified Lyod–Davis position can also be utilized especially in the setting of combined colorectal and liver resection.

In addition, a slight reverse Trendelenburg is utilized to improve the caudal exposure by gravitationally shifting the visceral structures away from the liver hilum, as well as decreasing hepatic venous return and pressure.

A schematic of most common port sites is described in Fig. 23.3.

According to the patient morphology, the lesion location, and the left lateral section dimensions, a general tip is to position the trocars high enough or to use instruments long enough to fully mobilize the left portion of the triangular ligament, which in some cases could extend to the upper lobe of the spleen.

Continuous Assessment

As previously mentioned, IOUS is performed to scan the rest of the liver parenchyma to assess the theoretical surgical margins and to explore the relationship between the target lesion and the

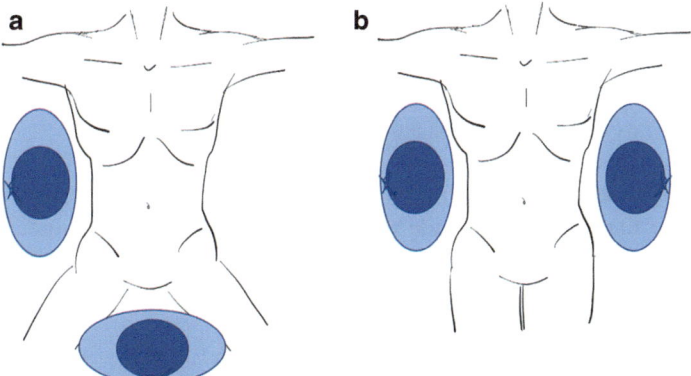

Fig. 23.2 (**a**) Supine straight split-leg position (the "French" position). The main surgeon stands between patient's legs. (**b**) Supine straight position. The main surgeon stands on patient's right side

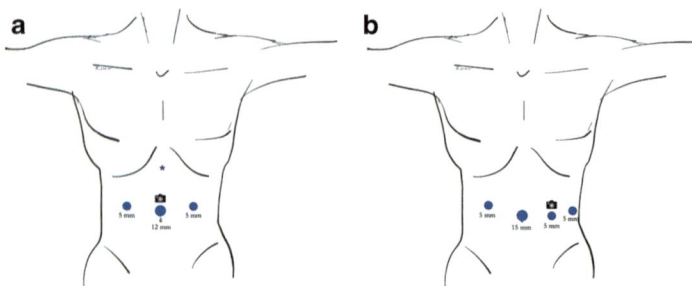

Fig. 23.3 (a) In the straight split-leg setting, the first port placement is usually the supraumbilical 12 mm port (for the camera) with an additional 5 mm right working port (for falciform retraction and to facilitate the use of the linear stapler) and a 5 mm left operating port. According to the patient's xiphoid–umbilical distance, the optical trocar can be shifted further away from the umbilicus. A further 5 mm epigastric trocar is optional. (b) In the second setting, a 15 mm port is positioned through the umbilicus, an additional 5 mm port in the RUQ (for falciform retraction); a 5 mm camera is positioned in the left midclavicular line to align the resection line along the falciform ligament; an additional 5 mm port is positioned in the left anterior axillary line (helpful to mobilize the left tip of the liver and provide retraction)

portal and hepatic veins. The limits of the planned resection are usually marked superficially on the liver parenchyma under US guidance to direct the resection. US should be performed multiple times during the operation to confirm location of the lesion and vicinity of significant vasculature.

Mobilization

The first step is to divide the falciform ligament in its highest insertion against the abdominal wall. Then the ligament is progressively transected closer to the liver surface when approaching the IVC.

The phrenic veins and the LHV must be identified to avoid inadvertent injury. *IOUS is a useful tool to identify and avoid injury of the vessels.* To complete the mobilization of the left lateral section, the left lateral portion of the triangular ligament is then divided.

Transection
Dividing the "bridge" between S3 and S4b allows for better identification of the hilar plate. This maneuver exposes the point of access of the left portal pedicle into the liver, which might be further dissected and isolated in order to perform a selective Pringle. A Glissonian approach allows for early control of the inflow.

The Lesion and the Margin Guide Everything Generally, the parenchymal transection is performed along the left side of the falciform ligament with an anterior approach. If the need to achieve a negative margin requires to extend the resection to the right side of the falciform, the transection line should always hit the biliary plate on the left side to preserve the portal inflow for S4.

The parenchyma is dissected, as described, as much as possible by means of energy devices, saving the stapler for the control of the main vasculature: the goal is to use two to three loads in total (one to two loads for the left lateral pedicle and the biliary plate and one load for the LHV). Care must be taken to approach the LHV with a 90° angle with the stapler to avoid caval injuries while minding the location of the esophagus. Depending on the location of the lesion relative to the left hepatic vein, the length of vein should be maximized so that a staple misfire can be salvaged.

Hemostasis
Hemostasis is usually performed by argon beam and/or cautery—either bipolar or monopolar according to the surgeon's preference and expertise, taking care to avoid touching the staple lines. Whenever using the Argon beam, caution must be taken to avoid a significant increase in the pneumoperitoneum, potentially leading to argon gas embolism. A stepwise decrease in pneumoperitoneum at the end of the intervention is recommended to carefully inspect for any focus of bleeding.

References

1. Fong Y, Cohen AM, Fortner JG, et al. Liver resection for colorectal metastases. J Clin Oncol Off J Am Soc Clin Oncol. 1997;15(3):938–46. https://doi.org/10.1200/JCO.1997.15.3.938.

2. Tran CG, Sherman SK, Chandrasekharan C, Howe JR. Surgical management of neuroendocrine tumor liver metastases. Surg Oncol Clin N Am. 2021;30(1):39–55. https://doi.org/10.1016/j.soc.2020.08.001.
3. Adam R, Chiche L, Aloia T, et al. Hepatic resection for noncolorectal nonendocrine liver metastases: analysis of 1,452 patients and development of a prognostic model. Ann Surg. 2006;244(4):524–35. https://doi.org/10.1097/01.sla.0000239036.46827.5f.
4. Vauthey J-N, Pawlik TM, Ribero D, et al. Chemotherapy regimen predicts steatohepatitis and an increase in 90-day mortality after surgery for hepatic colorectal metastases. J Clin Oncol Off J Am Soc Clin Oncol. 2006;24(13):2065–72. https://doi.org/10.1200/JCO.2005.05.3074.
5. Nordlinger B, Sorbye H, Glimelius B, et al. Perioperative chemotherapy with FOLFOX4 and surgery versus surgery alone for resectable liver metastases from colorectal cancer (EORTC intergroup trial 40983): a randomised controlled trial. Lancet (London, England). 2008;371(9617):1007–16. https://doi.org/10.1016/S0140-6736(08)60455-9.
6. Nordlinger B, Sorbye H, Glimelius B, et al. Perioperative FOLFOX4 chemotherapy and surgery versus surgery alone for resectable liver metastases from colorectal cancer (EORTC 40983): long-term results of a randomised, controlled, phase 3 trial. Lancet Oncol. 2013;14(12):1208–15. https://doi.org/10.1016/S1470-2045(13)70447-9.
7. Nakano H, Oussoultzoglou E, Rosso E, et al. Sinusoidal injury increases morbidity after major hepatectomy in patients with colorectal liver metastases receiving preoperative chemotherapy. Ann Surg. 2008;247(1):118–24. https://doi.org/10.1097/SLA.0b013e31815774de.
8. Brouquet A, Benoist S, Julie C, et al. Risk factors for chemotherapy-associated liver injuries: a multivariate analysis of a group of 146 patients with colorectal metastases. Surgery. 2009;145(4):362–71. https://doi.org/10.1016/j.surg.2008.12.002.
9. Soubrane O, Brouquet A, Zalinski S, et al. Predicting high grade lesions of sinusoidal obstruction syndrome related to oxaliplatin-based chemotherapy for colorectal liver metastases: correlation with post-hepatectomy outcome. Ann Surg. 2010;251(3):454–60. https://doi.org/10.1097/SLA.0b013e3181c79403.
10. Tamandl D, Klinger M, Eipeldauer S, et al. Sinusoidal obstruction syndrome impairs long-term outcome of colorectal liver metastases treated with resection after neoadjuvant chemotherapy. Ann Surg Oncol. 2011;18(2):421–30. https://doi.org/10.1245/s10434-010-1317-4.
11. Mayo SC, Pulitano C, Marques H, et al. Surgical management of patients with synchronous colorectal liver metastasis: a multicenter international analysis. J Am Coll Surg. 2013;216(4):707–8. https://doi.org/10.1016/j.jamcollsurg.2012.12.029.
12. Giuliante F, Viganò L, De Rose AM, et al. Liver-first approach for synchronous colorectal metastases: analysis of 7360 patients from the

LiverMetSurvey registry. Ann Surg Oncol. 2021;28(13):8198–208. https://doi.org/10.1245/s10434-021-10220-w. Epub 2021 July 1. PMID: 34212254; PMCID: PMC8590998.
13. Ali SM, Pawlik TM, Rodriguez-Bigas MA, Monson JRT, Chang GJ, Larson DW. Timing of surgical resection for curative colorectal cancer with liver metastasis. Ann Surg Oncol. 2018;25(1):32–7. https://doi.org/10.1245/s10434-016-5745-7.
14. Siriwardena AK, Mason JM, Mullamitha S, Hancock HC, Jegatheeswaran S. Management of colorectal cancer presenting with synchronous liver metastases. Nat Rev Clin Oncol. 2014;11(8):446–59. https://doi.org/10.1038/nrclinonc.2014.90. Epub 2014 June 3. PMID: 24889770.
15. Vreeland TJ, Collings AT, Ozair A, et al. SAGES/AHPBA guidelines for the use of minimally invasive surgery for the surgical treatment of colorectal liver metastases (CRLM). Surg Endosc. 2023;37(4):2508–16. https://doi.org/10.1007/s00464-023-09895-x. Epub 2023 Feb 21. PMID: 36810687.
16. Chen M-S, Li J-Q, Zheng Y, et al. A prospective randomized trial comparing percutaneous local ablative therapy and partial hepatectomy for small hepatocellular carcinoma. Ann Surg. 2006;243(3):321–8. https://doi.org/10.1097/01.sla.0000201480.65519.b8.
17. Huang J, Yan L, Cheng Z, et al. A randomized trial comparing radiofrequency ablation and surgical resection for HCC conforming to the Milan criteria. Ann Surg. 2010;252(6):903–12. https://doi.org/10.1097/SLA.0b013e3181efc656.
18. Feng K, Yan J, Li X, et al. A randomized controlled trial of radiofrequency ablation and surgical resection in the treatment of small hepatocellular carcinoma. J Hepatol. 2012;57(4):794–802. https://doi.org/10.1016/j.jhep.2012.05.007.
19. Wang Y, Luo Q, Li Y, Deng S, Wei S, Li X. Radiofrequency ablation versus hepatic resection for small hepatocellular carcinomas: a meta-analysis of randomized and nonrandomized controlled trials. PLoS One. 2014;9(1):e84484. https://doi.org/10.1371/journal.pone.0084484.
20. Zhang X-F, Bagante F, Chakedis J, et al. Perioperative and long-term outcome for intrahepatic Cholangiocarcinoma: impact of major versus minor hepatectomy. J Gastrointest Surg Off J Soc Surg Aliment Tract. 2017;21(11):1841–50. https://doi.org/10.1007/s11605-017-3499-6.
21. Pawlik TM, Scoggins CR, Zorzi D, et al. Effect of surgical margin status on survival and site of recurrence after hepatic resection for colorectal metastases. Ann Surg. 2005;241(5):715–722, discussion 722–4. https://doi.org/10.1097/01.sla.0000160703.75808.7d.
22. Ishizawa T, Gumbs AA, Kokudo N, Gayet B. Laparoscopic segmentectomy of the liver: from segment I to VIII. Ann Surg. 2012;256(6):959–64. https://doi.org/10.1097/SLA.0b013e31825ffed3.
23. Berardi G, Igarashi K, Li CJ, et al. Parenchymal sparing anatomical liver resections with full laparoscopic approach: description of technique and

short-term results. Ann Surg. 2021;273(4):785–91. https://doi.org/10.1097/SLA.0000000000003575.
24. Bismuth H, Houssin D, Castaing D. Major and minor segmentectomies "réglées" in liver surgery. World J Surg. 1982;6(1):10–24. https://doi.org/10.1007/BF01656369.
25. Couinaud C. [Liver lobes and segments: notes on the anatomical architecture and surgery of the liver]. Presse Med. 1954;62(33):709–712.
26. Couinaud C. [Surgical anatomy of the liver. Several new aspects]. Chirurgie. 1986;112(5):337–342.
27. Majno P, Mentha G, Toso C, Morel P, Peitgen HO, Fasel JHD. Anatomy of the liver: an outline with three levels of complexity – a further step towards tailored territorial liver resections. J Hepatol. 2014;60(3):654–62. https://doi.org/10.1016/j.jhep.2013.10.026.
28. Takasaki K. Glissonean pedicle transection method for hepatic resection: a new concept of liver segmentation. J Hepato-Biliary-Pancreat Surg. 1998;5(3):286–91. https://doi.org/10.1007/s005340050047.
29. Makuuchi M, Hasegawa H, Yamazaki S. Ultrasonically guided subsegmentectomy. Surg Gynecol Obstet. 1985;161(4):346–50.
30. Berardi G, Wakabayashi G, Igarashi K, et al. Full laparoscopic anatomical segment 8 resection for hepatocellular carcinoma using the Glissonian approach with Indocyanine green dye fluorescence. Ann Surg Oncol. 2019;26(8):2577–8. https://doi.org/10.1245/s10434-019-07422-8.
31. Makuuchi M, Yamamoto J, Takayama T, et al. Extrahepatic division of the right hepatic vein in hepatectomy. Hepato-Gastroenterology. 1991;38(2):176–9.
32. Gotohda N, Cherqui D, Geller DA, et al. Expert consensus guidelines: how to safely perform minimally invasive anatomic liver resection. J Hepatobiliary Pancreat Sci. 2022;29(1):16–32. https://doi.org/10.1002/jhbp.1079. Epub 2021 Nov 29. PMID: 34779150.
33. Ferrero A, Lo Tesoriere R, Giovanardi F, et al. Laparoscopic right posterior anatomic liver resections with Glissonean pedicle-first and venous craniocaudal approach. Surg Endosc. 2021;35(1):449–55. https://doi.org/10.1007/s00464-020-07916-7. Epub 2020 Aug 24. PMID: 32833101.
34. Anselmo A, Sensi B, Bacchiocchi G, Siragusa L, Tisone G. All the routes for laparoscopic liver segment VIII resection: a comprehensive review of surgical techniques. Front Oncol. 2022;12:864867. https://doi.org/10.3389/fonc.2022.864867.
35. Langenbuch C. Ein Fall von Resection Eines Linksseitigen Schnürlappens Der Leber. (Berl Klin Wochenschr, ed.).; 1888.
36. Bismuth H. Revisiting liver anatomy and terminology of hepatectomies. Ann Surg. 2013;257(3):383–6. https://doi.org/10.1097/SLA.0b013e31827f171f.
37. Reichert PR, Renz JF, D'Albuquerque LA, et al. Surgical anatomy of the left lateral segment as applied to living-donor and split-liver transplanta-

tion: a clinicopathologic study. Ann Surg. 2000;232(5):658–64. https://doi.org/10.1097/00000658-200011000-00007.
38. Buell JF, Cherqui D, Geller DA, et al. The international position on laparoscopic liver surgery: the Louisville statement, 2008. Ann Surg. 2009;250(5):825–30. https://doi.org/10.1097/sla.0b013e3181b3b2d8.
39. Ban D, Tanabe M, Ito H, et al. A novel difficulty scoring system for laparoscopic liver resection. J Hepatobiliary Pancreat Sci. 2014;21(10):745–53. https://doi.org/10.1002/jhbp.166.
40. Lin H, Bai Y, Yin M, Chen Z, Yu S. External validation of different difficulty scoring systems of laparoscopic liver resection for hepatocellular carcinoma. Surg Endosc. 2022;36(6):3732–49. https://doi.org/10.1007/s00464-021-08687-5.
41. Wakabayashi G, Cherqui D, Geller DA, et al. Recommendations for laparoscopic liver resection: a report from the second international consensus conference held in Morioka. Ann Surg. 2015;261(4):619–29. https://doi.org/10.1097/SLA.0000000000001184.
42. Goumard C, Farges O, Laurent A, et al. An update on laparoscopic liver resection: the French Hepato-Bilio-pancreatic surgery association statement. J Visc Surg. 2015;152(2):107–12. https://doi.org/10.1016/j.jviscsurg.2015.02.003.
43. Soubrane O, Cherqui D, Scatton O, et al. Laparoscopic left lateral sectionectomy in living donors: safety and reproducibility of the technique in a single center. Ann Surg. 2006;244(5):815–20. https://doi.org/10.1097/01.sla.0000218059.31231.b6.

Part VII

Major Hepatectomy

Open Right and Left Hepatectomy

24

Daniel W. Nelson
and Ching-Wei D. Tzeng

Introduction

Hemihepatectomy is a common operation for the treatment of primary and metastatic tumors of the liver and biliary tract. Due to their technical complexity and significant risk of postoperative morbidity and mortality, right and left hemihepatectomy (simplified nomenclature as "hepatectomy") are often described as major (≥3 segments) hepatic resections. Recent nomenclature and risk stratification schema have classified a left hepatectomy closer to minor rather than major hepatectomy due to the relatively small volume that is resected in most cases. In the modern era, parenchymal-sparing operations are generally preferred, as data have consistently demonstrated an improved safety profile without compromise of oncologic outcomes compared to more

D. W. Nelson · C.-W. D. Tzeng (✉)
Department of Surgical Oncology, The University of Texas M.D. Anderson Cancer Center, Houston, TX, USA
e-mail: CDTzeng@mdanderson.org

extensive "anatomic" operations [1]. However, when tumor anatomy involves inflow and/or outflow vasculature or Glissonian pedicles, removal of an entire hemiliver is mandated. With thorough preoperative planning to include high-quality multiphasic (arterial and portal venous phases) cross-sectional imaging for individualized characterization of vascular anatomy and accurate volumetric assessment, right and left hepatectomy may be performed in large-volume centers with 90-day mortality rates of less than 5% [2].

Anatomy

Liver anatomy is highly variable, and a complete description of the major vascular and biliary variations is beyond the scope of this chapter. However, a basic overview of relevant hepatic anatomy is warranted. As described by Couinaud in 1957, the liver may be divided into eight anatomic segments defined by portal segmentation. This anatomical definition provides the basis for safe hepatic resection while preserving vascular inflow, outflow, and biliary drainage to the remaining hepatic parenchyma, defined as the future liver remnant (FLR). The right liver may be divided into anterior (segments V and VIII) and posterior (segments VI and VII) sections, while the left liver is divided into medial (segment IV) and lateral (segments II and III) sections. While dual vascular inflow occurs via the hepatic arterial and portal venous systems, vascular outflow is achieved through drainage from the right, left, and middle hepatic veins and their tributaries. The middle hepatic vein (MHV) represents a critical anatomic landmark for the performance of hepatectomy as its course defines the main plane of division between the right and left liver. A true anatomic hepatectomy reveals the MHV on the final transection surface (Fig. 24.1). Careful review of preoperative cross-sectional imaging and liberal use of intraoperative ultrasound (IOUS) are essential for surgeons to familiarize themselves with each patient's vascular anatomy and facilitate safe hepatic resection.

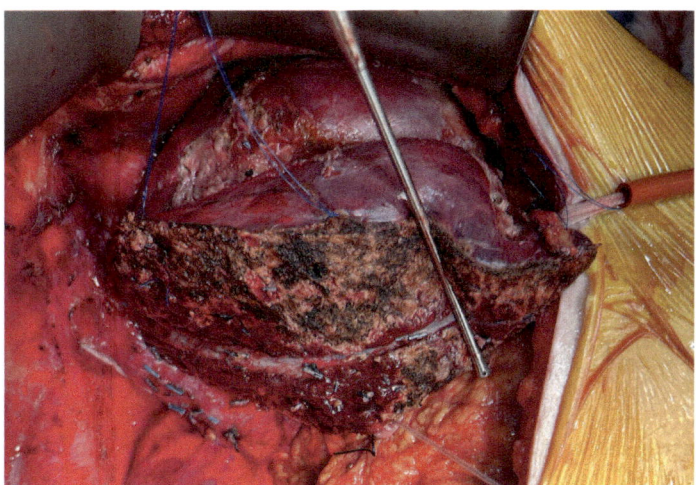

Fig. 24.1 A true anatomic hepatectomy reveals the middle hepatic vein on the final transection surface

Determinants of Postoperative Liver Function

Determination of resectability relies on one major principle that guides all liver resections. After removal of the tumor(s) with appropriate margins, there must be sufficient residual liver volume with adequate inflow, outflow, and biliary drainage to handle the burden of liver function proportionate to the patient's body size. Preoperatively, surgeon is estimating and counting on the regenerative capacity and anticipated volume of the FLR. The quality and functional reserve of the liver should be assessed using composite scoring systems such as the Child-Pugh classification system for liver disease. In addition, patients should be screened for clinical signs of portal hypertension, including the presence of ascites, evidence of venous collaterals, splenomegaly, or thrombocytopenia. However, the most reliable approach for predicting outcomes among candidates for major liver resection consists of formal assessment of FLR volume.

In the absence of underlying liver disease, the volume of the FLR can be measured directly with three-dimensional computed tomography (CT) volumetrics. However, in the setting of underlying liver disease such as cirrhosis, cholestasis from biliary obstruction, or extended chemotherapy exposure, CT volumetry is less reliable. In this case, the estimated total liver volume (TLV) can be calculated using a formula based on the linear correlation between TLV and body surface area (BSA) [3]:

$$TLV(cm^3) = -794.41 + 1267.28 \times BSA(m^2)$$

A standardized FLR (sFLR) volume can then be calculated using the measured FLR volume from CT volumetry divided by the calculated TLV:

$$sFLR = measured\ FLR\ volume\ /\ TLV$$

Among patients with normal livers undergoing right hepatectomy, hepatic insufficiency is rare, with an sFLR $\geq 20\%$ [4]. However, two caveats are relevant. It is important to note that in as many as 10% of patients, the left hemiliver will contribute $\leq 25\%$ of the TLV, and thus a straightforward right hepatectomy should not be assumed to be straightforward 100% of the time [5]. Second, with the ubiquity of steatosis, one must think twice before assuming that a patient has a normal liver and relying on that 20% rule. Larger sFLR volumes are necessary to reduce risk of postoperative hepatic insufficiency in patients with underlying liver disease or hepatic injury. For patients receiving extensive preoperative chemotherapy (>12 weeks) and/or steatosis at baseline, an sFLR $\geq 30\%$ has been associated with decreased rates of postoperative hepatic insufficiency and 90-day mortality [6]. Finally, an sFLR $\geq 40\%$ is recommended in patients undergoing resection with marked underlying liver disease such as fibrosis or cirrhosis [7].

Portal Vein Embolization and Hepatic Vein Embolization

For patients with insufficient preoperative FLR of the left liver, right portal vein embolization (PVE) has been demonstrated to be a safe and effective tool for promoting compensatory hypertrophy of the FLR, thereby permitting curative resection in patients previously considered unresectable [8]. During PVE the ipsilateral branch of the portal vein supplying the hemiliver planned for resection is cannulated under fluoroscopic guidance and occluded using embolic microparticles followed by coils. Hypertrophy of the contralateral liver segments is measured 4–6 weeks later. Although sFLR and a degree of hypertrophy of ≥5% have been shown to correlate with patient outcomes [9], the kinetic growth rate (KGR) (degree of hypertrophy at initial post-PVE assessment divided by the number of weeks after PVE) represents the most reliable and accurate predictor of postoperative outcomes, with a KGR of ≥2% per week associated with negligible rates of post-hepatectomy liver failure and liver-related 90-day mortality [10].

Although a majority of patients who undergo PVE will attain sufficient FLR hypertrophy to proceed to definitive surgery, up to 20% of patients with low baseline sFLR (<20%) will fail to achieve adequate hypertrophy from PVE alone. This risk is particularly high among heavily pretreated metastatic colorectal cancer patients. Hepatic vein embolization (HVE) has been a recent addition to PVE to augment inadequate hypertrophy and has been shown to be a safe and effective tool for inducing additional hypertrophy in patients with inadequate FLR following PVE [11]. Because of its success in augmentation, some have proposed doing both from the start, rather than as rescue. This has been described as "radiological simultaneous portohepatic vein embolization (RASPE)" [12] or liver venous deprivation (LVD). There is no consensus on what pre-procedure sFLR threshold is so low that it requires LVD instead of PVE alone, although we have used sFLR 20% as that pragmatic cutoff. In addition to this dilemma the additional option of Y-90 radioembolization and there is even less consensus. What is agreed upon is that sFLR must be adequate before right hepatectomy to avoid postoperative hepatic insufficiency.

Incision and Exposure

Mastery of incisions and exposure techniques are necessary to ensure safety and quality of exploration in a modern era that expects transfusion-free and mortality-free liver surgery. While traditional incisions used for hepatectomy have included the inverted-T (Mercedes), bilateral subcostal (Chevron), right and left subcostals (Kocher and Kehr), and the J (Makuuchi) incisions, incision selection should be dictated by the anatomic location of the tumor and planned operation with the goal of achieving optimal exposure to facilitate safe hepatic surgery.

The midline laparotomy is highly reproducible given the presence of easily identifiable landmarks based on the decussation of fascial components at the linea alba. This incision has the advantages of sparing muscular abdominal wall components and is optimal for left hepatectomy, provided it is extended to at least the level of the umbilicus. It can also be augmented by resection of the xyphoid process to provide exposure to the hepatic venous confluence and esophageal hiatus.

However, the midline laparotomy can be inadequate for right hepatectomy in cases with large diaphragmatic involvement, right liver atrophy, and inferior vena cava (IVC) or retroperitoneal involvement. In these scenarios, a reverse L (modified Makuuchi) incision provides optimal exposure of critical structures, including the IVC, hepatocaval junction, and esophageal hiatus. First described more than a century ago by George Clemens Perthes [13], the modern application of this incision differs from the original description in that the posterior sheath is entered at the same level as the anterior sheath and muscle, and does not include suture fixation of the rectus muscle. The upper midline portion of the incision curves laterally as a reverse L at the level of the umbilicus and proceeds ideally within a natural abdominal skin fold and ends at the midpoint between the anterior superior iliac spine (ASIS) and the lowest rib. This incision is similar to the traditional J incision, but has the advantages that it does not divide intercostal muscles and remains between dermatomal distributions of the nerves innervating the skin and musculature of the abdominal wall, thus reducing skin numbness, paresthesia, pain, and muscle atrophy [14].

Optimal exposure may be fully realized with strategic retractor placement. The oncology Thompson retractor is our preference (Thompson Surgical Instruments, Inc., Traverse City, Michigan). The Thompson retractor allows for ratcheted exposure of the left and right upper quadrants and the lower abdomen should that be required [14].

The right sidebar is positioned toward the floor and angled laterally to facilitate downward and right-sided retraction providing excellent view of right retroperitoneal structures and an *en face* view of the IVC. The placement of the right and left upper quadrant bladder blades facilitate retraction of the bilateral costal margins cephalad. Additionally, a malleable retractor may be placed over the right kidney for downward retraction, facilitating exposure of the right adrenal gland and IVC.

Open Right Hepatectomy

Principle steps of right hepatectomy in the way we perform are typically divided into five phases: mobilization, inflow ligation, outflow division, parenchymal transection, and hepatic duct transection last. While some surgeons advocate early transection of the entire right Glissonian pedicle, it is our bias to transect the right hepatic duct last once the parenchyma transection is completed.

Patients are positioned supine with the arms out laterally to permit peripheral vascular access. While low central venous pressure (CVP) surgery is key to reducing blood loss in liver surgery, we do not use CVP lines. Instead, we opt for two peripheral IV's and an arterial line for noninvasive hemodynamic monitoring. We use the reverse L incision beginning in the midline extending from the xyphoid down to 1 cm above the umbilicus and then carrying the incision laterally to the right between the most inferior rib and the ASIS. The round ligament (ligamentum teres) and falciform ligament are divided to the hepatic vein junction. A fixed retractor system is then installed as previously described. The right coronary and triangular ligaments are then divided to the confluence of the hepatic veins. For all right hepatectomies, we mobilize the left lateral liver to allow full rotation of the liver without squeezing the future liver remnant. Dissection proceeds to the origin of the right and middle hepatic vein, and the groove between these veins is developed using a right-angled instrument. The liver is then turned to the left and inferiorly and the remaining broad triangular ligament is divided exposing the bare area of the right liver. From here the right liver can further be mobilized off the retroperitoneum exposing the IVC and caval (Makuuchi) ligament. Commencing caudally to cephalad, dissection is continued along the anterior border of the IVC. Small retrohepatic caval branches draining the right hemiliver and paracaval process into the IVC may be ligated with clips or ties and divided. Larger vessels such as an inferior right hepatic vein should be suture ligated or divided using an endovascular stapler. Superiorly, the caval ligament will be encountered along the lateral border of the vena cava. The space between this ligament and the vena cava can be developed with a pediatric suction tip or curved blunt clamp and then divided with an endovascular stapler if robust with liver tissue or simply tied and sutured if thin. Development of the tunnel between the right and middle hepatic veins is completed and the right hepatic vein encircled with a vessel loop or loose tie for division later.

Attention is then turned to inflow control. We begin with IOUS to delineate right portal vein branching [15]. A cholecystectomy is performed, leaving the cystic duct stump long for later air cholangiogram. Dissection started on the posterolateral edge of the main portal vein by taking down the station 12p node. Sometimes, this space can be relaxed by performing a mini-Kocher to mobilize under the duodenum and right side of the hepatoduodenal ligament to show the IVC. Moving up the right side of the portal vein, the takeoff of the left portal vein should be exposed but not instrumented too much to avoid thrombosis. The caudate branch of the right portal vein is ligated and divided to allow room for a vascular stapler. Once the right portal vein is encircled, it can be clamped and inflow to the left liver confirmed via IOUS. With contralateral flow confirmed, the right portal vein may be stapled (most commonly) or suture ligated if there is not enough space for a stapler. The right hepatic artery is most commonly identified between the bile duct and portal vein before it splits into anterior and posterior branches. Depending on which one is easier to address, it can be ligated after the right PV transection or before. The ligation of either structure naturally opens the space for the second vascular structure. Once encircled, the right hepatic artery should be clamped, and flow palpated through the left hepatic artery at the base of the umbilical fissure and confirmed with IOUS. The right hepatic artery may then be ligated and divided.

With the inflow vessels divided, the right hepatic vein may be divided at the vena cava junction (which is our usual open technique to create laxity to lift the entire right hemiliver) or alternatively, it may be taken at the end of parenchymal transection (as is done in minimally invasive surgery or during an open anterior approach/hanging maneuver when the view over the top is not feasible). IOUS is repeated to mark the line of transection extending from the gallbladder fossa up to the IVC exactly along the right aspect of the middle hepatic vein. Care is taken to identify "V5" and "V8" tributaries to the middle hepatic vein to anticipate these vessels that are usually larger and require ties, sutures, and/ or even staplers [16]. Then three to four stay sutures are placed on each side of the planned transection line. An umbilical tape or vessel loop are then passed around the hepatoduodenal ligament and fastened with a Rummel tourniquet for planned Pringle maneuvers. Transection is performed with routine Pringle maneuver on at an interval of 15 min on and 5 min off. Multiple techniques and devices have been utilized to perform parenchymal transection. We use the previously described "two-surgeon technique" combining cavitron ultrasonic aspirator (CUSA, Integra) dissection and saline-linked cautery sealing, thereby dividing the tasks of parenchymal division and hemostasis between two surgeons, which has the advantages of minimizing the passing of

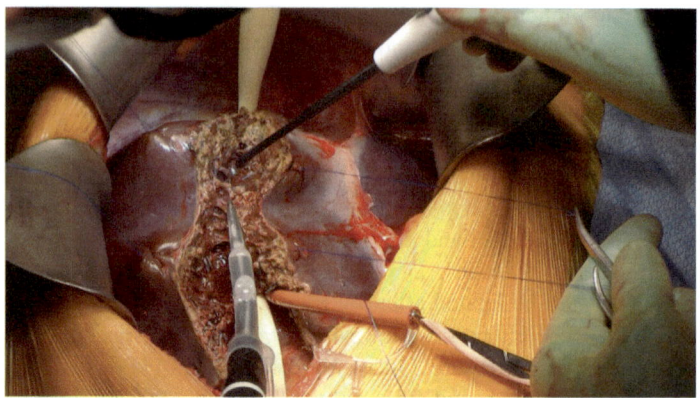

Fig. 24.2 Demonstration of simultaneous use of the cavitron ultrasonic aspirator (CUSA, Integra) dissection and saline-linked cautery sealing (Penrose hanging demonstrated along the line of transection)

instruments and allowing for the simultaneous performance of dissection and hemostasis (Fig. 24.2) [17]. One surgeon performs parenchymal dissection using the CUSA, while the partner operates the saline-linked cautery to coagulate and divide dissected vessels 3 mm or smaller. Larger vessels are controlled with clips or ties and divided. This two-surgeon technique has been shown to be associated with lower rates of intraoperative blood loss and blood transfusion [18]. Transection commences toward the right Glissonian pedicle. Once this is exposed, then the paracaval process is split and transected in the midline under the right Glissonian pedicle. One useful technique to stay in a straight line is to use a Penrose tape to "hang" the liver as if it were an anterior approach or hanging maneuver. Once we clear the right Glissonian sheath enough to show the bifurcation of right anterior and posterior, we can clamp down the stapler. One maneuver we have lately incorporated is to modify the air cholangiogram to use it at this point by injecting air into the left liver via the cystic duct with the stapler clamped but not fired (Fig. 24.3). Once air is shown in the left liver (Fig. 24.4), the stapler can be fired with assurance that there is no left hepatic duct injury.

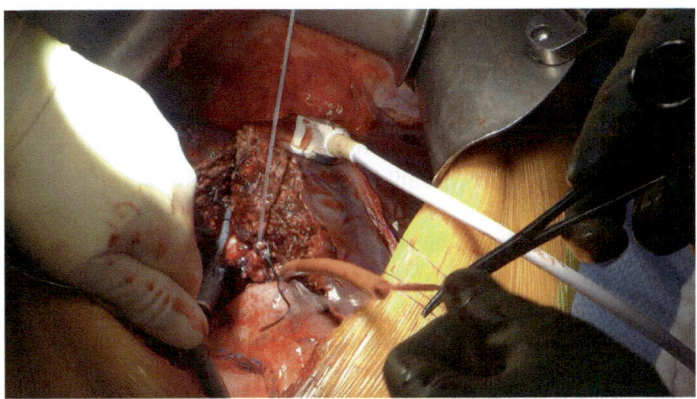

Fig. 24.3 Setup for the modified air cholangiogram. Air is injected into the left liver via the cystic duct with the stapler clamped but not fired

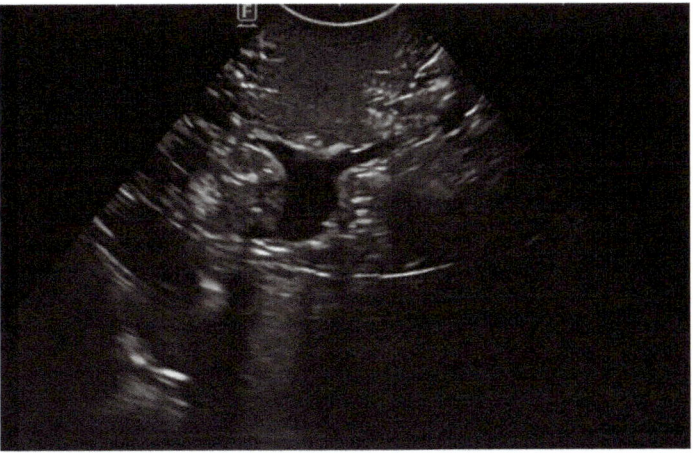

Fig. 24.4 Once air is shown in the left liver under ultrasound, the stapler can be fired with assurance that there is no left hepatic duct injury

Open Left Hepatectomy

Similar to the right hepatectomy, the round ligament and falciform ligament are divided back to the hepatic veins, but with a target of the junction between middle and left hepatic veins, which usually share a common trunk. A fixed retractor system is installed. The left liver is fully mobilized (as done with right hepatectomy). The right liver does not need to be mobilized unless there is a portion of the tumor that extends into the caudate or into the right liver. The left lateral section can now be reflected to the right and the gastrohepatic space opened. If there is an accessory or replaced left hepatic artery off the left gastric artery, it can be ligated once you confirm that the operation will be performed. IOUS should be used early on to confirm resectability and allow freedom to start taking vascular structures. The ligamentum venosum is identified and divided to open up the space to get under the left hepatic vein (LHV). Through a combination of dissection from above and below, tunnels are then developed to encircle the LHV.

The portal dissection is next. A cholecystectomy is performed with a long cystic duct stump for air cholangiogram at the end. The left hepatic artery comes off usually very early after the gastroduodenal artery (GDA) but can be ligated farther away if there is no pathology in the hepatoduodenal ligament. One can ensure right hepatic artery flow prior to ligating the left hepatic artery using palpation and IOUS. Once the artery is ligated and divided, a variable amount of soft tissue can be dissected to expose the left portal vein with the portal vein bifurcation delineated. The left portal vein should be encircled, and test clamped, and right portal inflow ensured by IOUS. Demarcation should become apparent as well at this point. The left portal vein is then stapled or ligated and divided.

The left hepatic vein may be stapled, or suture ligated and divided at this time, or taken at the end of parenchymal transection. Our preference is to staple it now to create more laxity to lift the left hemiliver. IOUS is repeated to cauterize and mark the line of transection extending from the gallbladder fossa up to the IVC along the left side of the middle hepatic vein. Stay sutures are

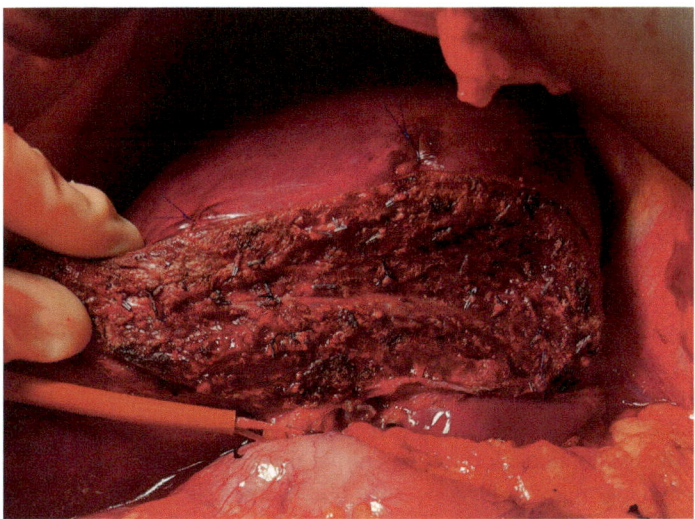

Fig. 24.5 Final transection surface following left hepatectomy demonstrating middle hepatic vein along the transection surface

placed on each side of the planned transection line. Pringle maneuver is again used with the two-surgeon technique. Transection continues toward the left Glissonian pedicle. Similar to the description of the stapler clamping for the right hepatectomy, the left hepatic duct can be clamped with the stapler and air injected into the cystic duct to prove right biliary patency before firing the stapler. Again, a true anatomic hepatectomy reveals the MHV on the final transection surface (Fig. 24.5).

Prevention of Bile Leak with Two-Step Air Leak Test

Postoperative bile leaks represent a primary source for potentially preventable morbidity following hepatectomy. Development of postoperative fluid collections and delays in treatment may result in sepsis and impact regenerative capacity of the FLR. Postoperative bile leaks may be anticipated in as many as 7.3% of patients undergoing hepatic resection based on prospective multicenter international data [19]. In efforts to mitigate this complication, prophylactic drains are placed in upward of half of all hepatectomies in the United States [20]. However, prospective and retrospective studies argue against this practice for routine cases. In a randomized controlled trial of 400 patients across seven centers in Japan, routine drain placement versus no drain was directly compared among patients undergoing uncomplicated hepatectomy and demonstrated zero bile leaks in the no-drain group versus 8% in the drain group with the authors concluding that drains should not be routinely placed after uncomplicated hepatectomy [21]. Systematic review and meta-analysis of the surgical literature have shown that various intraoperative leak tests (methylene blue, fat emulsion (with saline flushes), ICG, and air) are all safe and effective options for intraoperative detection and mitigation of clinically relevant postoperative bile leaks [22].

A novel "air leak test" or "air cholangiogram" was developed and is routinely utilized at the MD Anderson Cancer Center. Originally described to be used after specimen removal, the cystic duct stump is intubated with a 6.5 Fr (or smaller if needed) cholangiogram catheter. The tip of the catheter is secured with a 2–0 tie to prevent air leaking out of the cystic duct. The surgeon's left index finger and thumb are used to clamp the distal bile duct as air is injected. IOUS will demonstrate air in the ducts shining through and then once filled may look like "bright lights in a night sky." This view confirms biliary tree patency. Air is injected until the catheter has a "bounce" or recoil of 1 mL on the syringe. This allows an objective barometric test of the 1 mL "bounce" without producing excess barotrauma, since the goal is simply to expose occult leaks and not to disrupt ties and clips. Once the liver is filled with air, the remnant is dunked under sterile water to look for bubbles. Bubbles represent biliary tree leaks, which should be repaired with 6–0 polypropylene sutures, often times directly in the clear water. In our experience the most common areas of an occult leak are the edges of the hepatic duct staple line due to malformed or misaligned staples. Hemostatic agents (our preference is oxidized regenerated cellulose sheets) can be placed. This is a safe, fast, inexpensive, and repeatable test that has been associated with reductions in clinically relevant bile leaks and organ space infection rates in our experience [23, 24]. With an air leak test that is either negative or fixed until negative, one can be more confident in not leaving a surgical drain.

Conclusion

In summary, open right and left hepatectomy are common yet potentially challenging operations that require careful preoperative planning and intraoperative technique to be performed safely. Careful attention to preoperative planning, including accurate measurement of the FLR and selective use of PVE, HVE, or Y-90 is crucial for guide patient selection. However, a thorough knowledge of the vascular anatomy of the liver and meticulous surgical technique on the part of the surgeon remain essential to mitigating serious complications.

References

1. Nelson DW, Vreeland TJ. Parenchymal preservation in the operative management of colorectal liver metastases. In: Vauthey J-N, Kawaguchi Y, Adam R, editors. Colorectal liver metastasis. Cham: Springer; 2022. p. 29–34.
2. Vigano L, Torzilli G, Aldrighetti L, et al. Stratification of major hepatectomies according to their outcome: analysis of 2212 consecutive open resections in patients without cirrhosis. Ann Surg. 2020;272(5):827–33.
3. Vauthey JN, Abdalla EK, Doherty DA, et al. Body surface area and body weight predict total liver volume in Western adults. Liver Transpl. 2002;8(3):233–40.
4. Kishi Y, Abdalla EK, Chun YS, et al. Three hundred and one consecutive extended right hepatectomies: evaluation of outcome based on systematic liver volumetry. Ann Surg. 2009;250(4):540–8.
5. Abdalla EK, Denys A, Chevalier P, Nemr RA, Vauthey JN. Total and segmental liver volume variations: implications for liver surgery. Surgery. 2004;135(4):404–10.
6. Shindoh J, Tzeng CW, Aloia TA, et al. Optimal future liver remnant in patients treated with extensive preoperative chemotherapy for colorectal liver metastases. Ann Surg Oncol. 2013;20(8):2493–500.

7. Kubota K, Makuuchi M, Kusaka K, et al. Measurement of liver volume and hepatic functional reserve as a guide to decision-making in resectional surgery for hepatic tumors. Hepatology. 1997;26(5):1176–81.
8. Abdalla EK, Barnett CC, Doherty D, Curley SA, Vauthey JN. Extended hepatectomy in patients with hepatobiliary malignancies with and without preoperative portal vein embolization. Arch Surg. 2002;137(6):675–680; discussion 680–671.
9. Ribero D, Abdalla EK, Madoff DC, Donadon M, Loyer EM, Vauthey JN. Portal vein embolization before major hepatectomy and its effects on regeneration, resectability and outcome. Br J Surg. 2007;94(11):1386–94.
10. Shindoh J, Truty MJ, Aloia TA, et al. Kinetic growth rate after portal vein embolization predicts posthepatectomy outcomes: toward zero liver-related mortality in patients with colorectal liver metastases and small future liver remnant. J Am Coll Surg. 2013;216(2):201–9.
11. Niekamp AS, Huang SY, Mahvash A, et al. Hepatic vein embolization after portal vein embolization to induce additional liver hypertrophy in patients with metastatic colorectal carcinoma. Eur Radiol. 2020;30(7):3862–8.
12. Laurent C, Fernandez B, Marichez A, et al. Radiological simultaneous portohepatic vein embolization (RASPE) before major hepatectomy: a better way to optimize liver hypertrophy compared to portal vein embolization. Ann Surg. 2020;272(2):199–205.
13. Perthes G, Chir Z. Zur Schnittführung bei Operationen an den Gallenwegen. Zentralbl f Chir. 1912;39:1252–6.
14. Chang SB, Palavecino M, Wray CJ, Kishi Y, Pisters PW, Vauthey JN. Modified Makuuchi incision for foregut procedures. Arch Surg. 2010;145(3):281–4.
15. Vauthey JN, Yamashita S. Perfecting a challenging procedure: the Nagoya portal vein guide to left trisectionectomy. Surgery. 2017;161(2):355–6.
16. Ogiso S, Okuno M, Shindoh J, et al. Conceptual framework of middle hepatic vein anatomy as a roadmap for safe right hepatectomy. HPB (Oxford). 2019;21(1):43–50.
17. Aloia TA, Zorzi D, Abdalla EK, Vauthey JN. Two-surgeon technique for hepatic parenchymal transection of the noncirrhotic liver using saline-linked cautery and ultrasonic dissection. Ann Surg. 2005;242(2):172–7.
18. Palavecino M, Kishi Y, Chun YS, et al. Two-surgeon technique of parenchymal transection contributes to reduced transfusion rate in patients undergoing major hepatectomy: analysis of 1,557 consecutive liver resections. Surgery. 2010;147(1):40–8.
19. Brooke-Smith M, Figueras J, Ullah S, et al. Prospective evaluation of the international study group for liver surgery definition of bile leak after a liver resection and the role of routine operative drainage: an international multicentre study. HPB (Oxford). 2015;17(1):46–51.
20. Spolverato G, Ejaz A, Kim Y, et al. Patterns of care among patients undergoing hepatic resection: a query of the National Surgical Quality

Improvement Program-targeted hepatectomy database. J Surg Res. 2015;196(2):221–8.
21. Arita J, Sakamaki K, Saiura A, et al. Drain placement after uncomplicated hepatic resection increases severe postoperative complication rate: a Japanese multi-institutional randomized controlled trial (ND-trial). Ann Surg. 2021;273(2):224–31.
22. Vaska AI, Abbas S. The role of bile leak testing in liver resection: a systematic review and meta-analysis. HPB (Oxford). 2019;21(2):148–56.
23. Zimmitti G, Vauthey JN, Shindoh J, et al. Systematic use of an intraoperative air leak test at the time of major liver resection reduces the rate of postoperative biliary complications. J Am Coll Surg. 2013;217(6):1028–37.
24. Tran Cao HS, Phuoc V, Ismael H, et al. Rate of organ space infection is reduced with the use of an air leak test during major hepatectomies. J Gastrointest Surg. 2017;21(1):85–93.

Major Hepatectomy: MIS Left Hepatectomy and Right Hepatectomy

Christine Chung, Camilla Gomes, Paige-Ashley Campbell, and Adnan Alseidi

Introduction

There has been increased utilization of minimally invasive surgery (MIS) in hepatopancreaticobiliary (HPB) surgery as it has proven to be safer, more efficient, and without compromise to oncologic outcomes. MIS also allows for improved visualization and magnification, optimal retraction, ease of dissection, and enhanced ergonomics.

MIS hepatectomy has a favorable short-term outcome, including shorter length of hospitalization, less operative blood loss, less transfusion and analgesic requirements, faster return to oral intake, and fewer postoperative adhesions [1–3]. In fact, both MIS left and right hepatectomy have been associated with as much as 50% decreased length of stay compared to open techniques [4–6].

C. Chung (✉)
Virginia Mason Medical Center, Seattle, WA, USA

C. Gomes · P.-A. Campbell · A. Alseidi
Department of Surgery, University of California, San Francisco, San Francisco, CA, USA
e-mail: camilla.gomes@ucsf.edu; paigeashley.campbell@ucsf.edu; Adnan.Alseidi@ucsf.edu

Decreased intraoperative blood loss, which is likely due to improved visualization for hepatic inflow control, is of particular significance as it is one of the most dreaded complications of liver surgery and closely associated with increased morbidity and mortality [7]. Of note, the OSLO-COMET randomized controlled trial demonstrated that 30-day morbidity (Accordion grade 2 or higher) was noted to be significantly decreased in the laparoscopic versus the open liver resection group [8].

Long-term outcomes between MIS and open approaches are mostly equivalent, with no significant difference in overall survival or disease-free survival [9]. For example, for colorectal liver metastases, a multi-institutional analysis of patients undergoing laparoscopic versus open liver resection with approximately the same median number of metastases showed no difference in the R_0 rate, 5-year disease-free survival, or 5-year overall survival between the two groups [10]. Comparable findings were noted in a similar study analyzing patients with hepatocellular carcinoma [11]. In contrast, when comparing laparoscopic versus open approaches for intrahepatic cholangiocarcinoma, the former was associated with lower rates of margin positivity and recurrence [12].

Overall, MIS hepatectomy is associated with decreased surgical morbidity without compromising long-term and oncologic outcomes when compared to open hepatectomy [13, 14]. The MIS approach to hepatectomies is a safe and reasonable alternative when performed by an experienced surgeon.

Preoperative and Preparation Pearls

- Pertinent imaging clues
  - Identify the course of hepatic veins (i.e., right hepatic vein, segment 8 branch) as well as hepatic ducts in relation to the planned line of transection.
  - Mass size (5 cm or less is ideal).
  - Location (peripheral location in segments 2–6 is easiest).
- Contraindications

- Patient unable to tolerate procedure because of medical comorbidities.
- Insufficient oncologic margin.
- Hilar cholangiocarcinoma.
• Basics
  - 5 or 10 mm, 45° (or articulating) laparoscope and high-definition camera
  - Maintain low central venous pressure (CVP) while remaining cognizant of CO_2 tolerance.
  - Intermittent clamping of hepatic pedicle (Pringle) when necessary.
    Different ways to perform the Pringle maneuver.
      • Clamp technique with the Chitwood Debakey Clamp.
        - Dissect window around porta hepatis, place vessel loop, clamp on hepatoduodenal ligament.
      • Laparoscopic/robotic.
        - Make window in pars flaccida.
        - Trocar inserted with fiber tape, wrap tape around hepatoduodenal ligament through pars flaccida and foramen of Winslow.
        - Ends of fiber tape brought through the trocar to outside.
        - Advance trocar over fiber tape and clamp to perform Pringle versus ends of fiber tape brought through trocar to outside and Rummel tourniquet placed.
        - Video clip: getting the Pringle setup (courtesy of Dr. Adnan Alseidi, UCSF).
  - Pneumoperitoneum: higher versus lower.
    Higher
      • Higher pneumoperitoneum may prevent bleeding.
      • Steps:
        - Decrease PEEP.
        - Anesthesia monitors capnography. If it changes by 8 in either direction, notify the surgeon.
        - Increase pneumoperitoneum to 18.

- Pringle every 5 min.
- Parenchymal transection.
- If capnography decreases by 8—CO_2 is overwhelming the lungs. Decrease pneumoperitoneum to 12, increase peep, and evaluate for hole in hepatic vein.
- If capnography increases by 8—evaluate for a hole in the hepatic vein, but can keep all settings the same.

  Lower
  - Lower pneumoperitoneum may prevent holes in hepatic veins, but may have increased bleeding.
- Instruments needed.
  - Clip appliers.
  - Ultrasonic dissector.
  - Vascular stapler.
  - Hem-o-lock clips.
  - Large specimen bag.
  - Needle drivers/holders.
  - Laparoscopy specific:
  CUSA.
  Ratcheted, fenestrated, and atraumatic bowel forceps.
  Curved and right-angled dissectors.
  Scissors.
  Bipolar forceps.
  Harmonic scalpel (can cut through capsule) or Ligasure (seals small vessels).
  Liver retractor.
  - Robotic specific:
  Harmonic scalpel.
  Vessel sealer.
  Fenestrated bipolar.

Key Steps

- **MIS surgery**
  - Supine, legs apart, 15° reverse Trendelenburg.
  - Pitfalls.
    Inadvertent bowel or vascular injury with laparoscopic tools.
    Limited range of motion with instruments.
    Narrowed scope of vision that may distort anatomy.
- **Laparoscopy** (Fig. 25.1).
- **Caudal approach** [16]: Right hepatectomy
  Primary vascular control of right portal pedicle.
    - Encircle hepatic pedicle with tourniquet to allow for intermittent clamping.
    - *Pearls & Pitfalls: Ensure this is set up effectively and tested prior to further dissection*

  Intrafascial dissection of right portal vein and right hepatic artery.
    - Dissect backward up to the right portal pedicle with the right portal vein and hepatic artery, encircling each. Retract the cystic duct to the patient's left and gallbladder to the right, exposing the short course of the extrahepatic right pedicle. Make sure to visualize the bifurcation and left portal branch prior to transection. When transecting the right portal vein, displace the bifurcation to the left and lengthen the right branch, preventing narrowing of the left portal branch.

  Anterior approach without mobilization of right liver.
    - Open liver capsule with harmonic scalpel, then divide the parenchyma from bottom using ultrasonic dissector with bipolar or harmonic scalpel.
    - *Pearls & Pitfalls: While creating a "crater" with the harmonic scalpel, make sure to stay superficial to avoid deeper veins and ducts*
    - When parenchymal transection reaches the hilar plate, segment I is divided along the right aspect of the inferior vena cava. Once the right hepatic vein is reached, it is

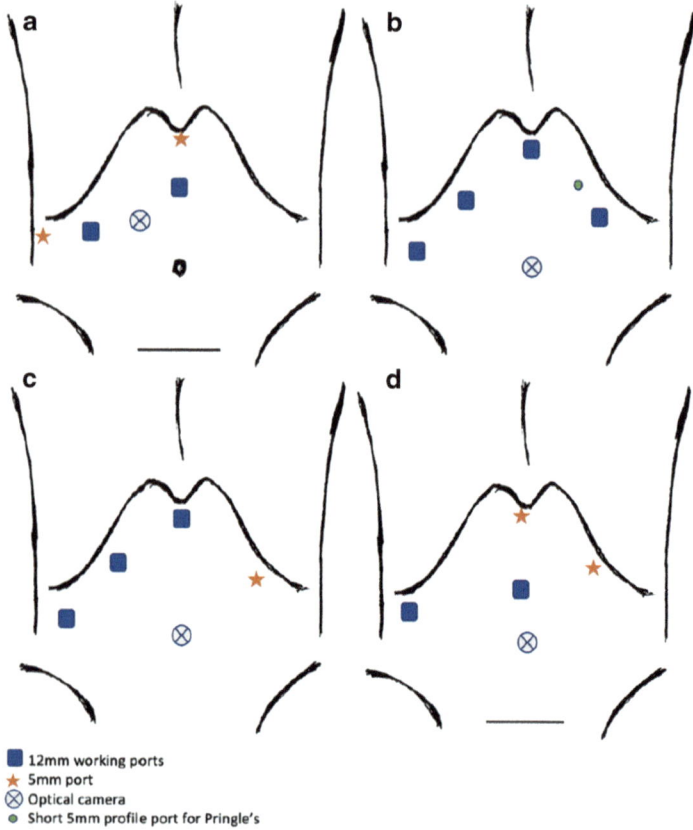

- ■ 12mm working ports
- ★ 5mm port
- ⊗ Optical camera
- ● Short 5mm profile port for Pringle's

Fig. 25.1 Laparoscopic port site examples [15]

dissected-free and stapled with a vascular stapler. Mobilize the devascularized right liver by freeing the right triangular ligament. Externalize the specimen in a plastic bag through the suprapubic incision.

Pearls & Pitfalls: Use an ultrasound to identify the middle hepatic vein to check for safety margin. Make sure to identify any branches coming off of the right hepatic vein

Challenges.
- The lack of wristed instruments in laparoscopy contributes to challenges with dissection. It is also difficult to reach the posterior and superior segments with laparoscopic instruments. Finally, the ability to quickly and effectively control bleeding laparoscopically is limited due to the current tools at our disposal.

Example of laparoscopic left hepatectomy: video clip courtesy of Dr. Adnan Alseidi.

- **Robotic** (Fig. 25.2).
  - **Robotic approach** [18].
    Positioning
    - 12° reverse Trendelenburg with a bump on the right side for right hepatectomy
    - Pfannenstiel incision with a hand port and 12-mm Airseal port.
    - Robotic ports placed across upper abdomen.
    - 12 mm assistant port placed between camera port and most lateral right-sided port for use of CUSA during parenchymal transection

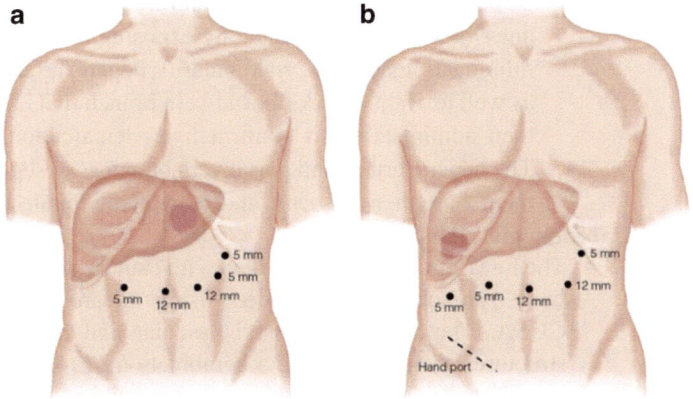

Fig. 25.2 Robotic port sites for (**a**) right hepatectomy and (**b**) left hepatectomy [17]

Inflow control
- *Right*
    The right hepatic artery is isolated as it enters the liver. The right portal vein is then isolated. Indocyanine green (ICG) is given to confirm liver demarcation following inflow control.
    Pearls & Pitfalls: Occlude the right hepatic artery before dividing it and use a doppler to confirm left hepatic artery flow. Identify the portal bifurcation and ensure the left portal vein is not compromised prior to right portal vein ligation
- *Left*
    Expose the left liver hilum below umbilical fissure. The left hepatic artery is isolated as it enters the umbilical fissure, then clipped and divided. The left portal vein is isolated. ICG is administered to confirm liver demarcation.
    Pearls & Pitfalls: Identify the portal bifurcation to ensure the right portal vein is not compromised.
- *Central*
    Inflow control of the right anterior sector and segment is performed. Extrahepatic control of the right anterior sector is performed by exposing the right hilum and ligating the right anterior hepatic artery as well as right anterior portal vein branch. ICG is then administered to confirm liver demarcation. The hepatic artery and portal vein branches to segment 4 are then dissected and individually ligated.

Parenchymal division
- The line of transection is marked with cautery and the liver parenchyma is divided using laparoscopic CUSA. The intraparenchymal vascular and biliary structures are divided with a combination of robotic vessel sealer, clips, and endovascular staplers. The specimen is then extracted through a Pfannenstiel incision.

- **Challenges**
 As the robotic trocars are longer, the CUSA instrument cannot be used for parenchymal transection. A new CUSA made specifically for the Robotic platform, however, is coming. Additionally, reliable instruments for dividing liver parenchyma and sealing blood vessels and bile ducts are still lacking.

References

1. Lillemoe K, Jarnagin W. Master techniques in surgery: hepatobiliary and pancreatic surgery. Philadelphia: Wolters Kluwer; 2020. ISBN 9781496385574
2. Schiffman S, Kim K, Tsung A, Marsh J, Geller D. Laparoscopic versus open liver resection for metastatic colorectal cancer: a meta-analysis of 610 patients. Surgery. 2015;157(2):211–22.
3. Cipriani F, Alzoubi M, Fuks D, Ratti F, Kawai T, Berardi G, Barkhatov L, Lainas P, Van der Poel M, Faoury M, Besselink M, D'Hondt M, Dagher I, Edwin B, Troisi R, Scatton O, Gayet B, Aldrighetti L, Hilal M. Pure laparoscopic versus open hemihepatectomy: A critical assessment and realistic expectations. A propensity score based analysis of right and left hemihepatectomies from 9 European tertiary referral centers. HPB. 2020;22:S404–5.
4. Park J, Kwon DCH, Choi GS, Kim SJ, Lee SK, Kim JM, et al. Safety and risk factors of pure laparoscopic living donor right hepatectomy: comparison to open technique in propensity score-matched analysis. Transplantation. 2019;103(10):e308–16.
5. Lee B, Choi Y, Han HS, Yoon YS, Cho JY, Kim S, et al. Comparison of pure laparoscopic and open living donor right hepatectomy after a learning curve. Clin Transpl. 2019;33(10):e13683.
6. Nguyen KT, Marsh JW, Tsung A, Steel JJL, Gamblin TC, Geller DA. Comparative benefits of laparoscopic vs open hepatic resection: a critical appraisal. Arch Surg. 2011;146(3):348–56.
7. Romano F, Garancini M, Uggeri F, Degrate L, Nespoli L, Gianotti L, Nespoli A, Uggeri F. Bleeding in hepatic surgery: sorting through methods to prevent it. HPB Surg. 2012;2012:1–12.
8. Chan A, Jamdar S, Sheen A, Siriwardena A. The OSLO-COMET randomized controlled trial of laparoscopic versus open resection for colorectal liver metastases. Ann Surg. 2018;268(6):e69.

9. Castaing D, Vibert E, Ricca L, Azoulay D, Adam R, Gayet B. Oncologic results of laparoscopic versus open hepatectomy for colorectal liver metastases in two specialized center. Ann Surg. 2009;250(5):849–55.
10. Beppu T, Wakabayashi G, Hasegawa K, Gotohda N, Mizuguchi T, Takahashi Y, Hirokawa F, Taniai N, Watanabe M, Katou M, Nagano H, Honda G, Baba H, Kokudo N, Konishi M, Hirata K, Yamamoto M, Uchiyama K, Uchida E, Kusachi S, Kubota K, Mori M, Takahashi K, Kikuchi K, Miyata H, Takahara T, Nakamura M, Kaneko H, Yamaue H, Miyazaki M, Takada T. Long-term and perioperative outcomes of laparoscopic versus open liver resection for colorectal liver metastases with propensity score matching: a multi-institutional Japanese study. J Hepatobiliary Pancreat Sci. 2015;22(10):711–20.
11. Takahara T, Wakabayashi G, Beppu T, Aihara A, Hasegawa K, Gotohda N, Hatano E, Tanahashi Y, Mizuguchi T, Kamiyama T, Ikeda T, Tanaka S, Taniai N, Baba H, Tanabe M, Kokudo N, Konishi M, Uemoto S, Sugioka A, Hirata K, Taketomi A, Maehara Y, Kubo S, Uchida E, Miyata H, Nakamura M, Kaneko H, Yamaue H, Miyazaki M, Takada T. Long-term and perioperative outcomes of laparoscopic versus open liver resection for hepatocellular carcinoma with propensity score matching: a multi-institutional Japanese study. J Hepatobiliary Pancreat Sci. 2015;22(10):721–7.
12. Ziogas I, Esagian S, Giannis D, Hayat M, Kosmidis D, Matsuoka L, Montenovo M, Tsoulfas G, Geller D, Alexopoulos S. Laparoscopic versus open hepatectomy for intrahepatic cholangiocarcinoma: An individual patient data survival meta-analysis. Am J Surg. 2021;222(4):731–8.
13. Ciria R, Cherqui D, Geller DA, Briceno J, Wakabayashi G. Comparative short-term benefits of laparoscopic liver resection: 9000 cases and climbing. Ann Surg. 2016;263(4):761–77.
14. Fretland A, Dagenborg V, Bjornelv G, Kazaryan A, Kristiansen R, Fagerland M, Hausken J, Tonnessen T, Abildgaard A, Barkhatov L, Yaqub S, Rosok B, Bjornbeth B, Andersen M, Flatmark K, Aas E, Edwin B. Ann Surg. 2018;267(2):199–207.
15. Thiruchelvam N, Lee SY, Chiow A. Patient and port positioning in laparoscopic liver resections. Hepatoma Res. 2021;7:22. https://doi.org/10.20517/2394-5079.2020.144.
16. Soubrane O, Schwarz L, Cauchy F, et al. A conceptual technique for laparoscopic right hepatectomy based on facts and oncologic principles: the caudal approach. Ann Surg. 2015;261(6):1226–30.
17. Labadie K, Sullivan KM, Park JO. Surgical resection in HCC. In: Liver cancer. IntechOpen; 2018. https://doi.org/10.5772/intechopen.81345.
18. Hawksworth J, Radkani P, Nguyen B, et al. Improving safety of robotic major hepatectomy with extrahepatic inflow control and laparoscopic CUSA parenchymal transection: technical description and initial experience. Surg Endosc. 2022;36(5):3270–6. https://doi.org/10.1007/s00464-021-08639-z.

Right Posterior Sectionectomy, Anterior Sectionectomy, and Central Hepatectomy

Chase J. Wehrle, Alejandro Pita, Jaekeun Kim, and Choon Hyuck David Kwon

Introduction

Advancements in surgical techniques and the availability of locoregional and systemic therapies have led to more precise hepatic resections for either benign or malignant conditions [1–3]. The overarching principles of hepatic resection include negative margins and maximizing preservation of hepatic parenchyma. The parenchymal preservation is increasingly important as operations are being offered to patients with compromised baseline

---

C. J. Wehrle · J. Kim · C. H. D. Kwon (✉)
Department of Liver Transplantation, Cleveland Clinic Foundation, Cleveland, OH, USA

Department of General Surgery, Section of HPB Surgery, Cleveland Clinic Foundation, Cleveland, OH, USA
e-mail: wehrlec@ccf.org; kimj30@ccf.org; kwonc2@ccf.org

A. Pita
Department of Liver Transplantation, Cleveland Clinic Foundation, Cleveland, OH, USA
e-mail: pitaa@ccf.org

liver function and repeat hepatectomy becomes more prevalent. Depending on the tumor etiology and location, anatomic resection may often be preferred to the nonanatomic approach whenever feasible, due to improved oncologic outcomes and reduced complication rates, particularly in hepatocellular carcinoma (HCC) [4, 5]. This goal may compete with preservation of sufficient functional liver remnant (FLR), where parenchyma should be spared where possible [6]. The right posterior sectionectomy (RPS), right anterior sectionectomy (RAS), and central hepatectomy (CH) represent technically challenging but highly effective approaches to the management of right posterior or centrally located lesions, respectively. These operations aim to achieve optimal negative margins through the anatomic resection, while simultaneously ensuring maximal preservation of the liver function.

Right Posterior Sectionectomy

Pitfalls and Pearls

In cases where the tumor is located in the right posterior region, the RPS is a viable alternative to the formal right hepatectomy designed to preserve hepatic parenchyma. Indications for the RPS include solitary or multiple tumors involving segments 6 and 7 or that involve the right posterior sectoral branches [7]. Historically, RPS has primarily been performed using open surgical techniques due to complex surgical technique, but recent advances and improved dissection techniques using the Glissonian-pedicle approach has allowed for the increased use of laparoscopic RPS (LRPS) [7–10]. Indeed, studies have demonstrated equivalent-to-improved outcomes of the laparoscopic or robotic approach when performed by experienced surgeons [10–12].

Surgeons may consider either robotic (RRPS) or laparoscopic RPS (LRPS). Primarily, the consideration with minimally invasive techniques should be surgeon experience and comfort level. As with laparoscopic approaches, the robotic technique has demonstrated nearly equivalent outcomes to the open approach [13, 14]. While robotic techniques are relatively newer and less studied, it offers the advantage of articulating instruments and improved ergonomics. The robotic technique may also offer more routine access to three-dimensional camera systems that can assist in a better assessment of hepatic architecture. In all cases of minimally invasive approaches, the surgeon and the surgical team should be prepared for rapid conversion to open in case it becomes necessary. These situations includes uncontrollable bleeding or concerns about compromising oncologic curability. When considering open conversion for bleeding control, maintain bleeding control either by focal compression with a sponge or clamping with an instrument while transitioning to an open procedure. This prevents increased bleeding during the conversion process, as the conversion will remove the pneumatic compression, exacerbating bleeding.

When a nonanatomic hepatectomy is planned, the transection plane is designed using intraoperative ultrasound. The necessary resection margin and important vascular structures found along the plane is identified and marked. However, when an anatomic posterior sectionectomy is planned, using intraoperative ultrasound alone for mapping can lead to incorrect transection planes and finding the ischemic plane after interruption of the inflow is essential to get the correct anatomic boundary. Individual dissection and identification of the right posterior arterial and portal branches can be done but it is technically complex and time consuming, so the Glissonian approach is a preferred method used by many surgeons [12]. Specifically, this approach involves up-front identification and ligation of the right posterior Glissonian pedicle, subsequently allowing for ischemic demarcation along the parenchyma supplied by the targeted pedicle [15]. Additionally, intravenous injection of indocyanine green after controlling the inflow can further enhance the visualization of the ischemic demarcation for proper anatomic resection.

Dissection of the Glissonian pedicle can be technically challenging, particularly when performed robotically or laparoscopically because of limitations of motions. Multiple techniques have been described to improve safety and reduce technical demand. Hilar dissection, which involves the identification of the hilum and concurrent cholecystectomy, serves as a starting point. In many cases, Rouviere's sulcus proves useful in locating the right posterior Glissonian pedicle, as it runs through this space in approximately 70–82% of cases [7]. By employing a blunt grasper or dissector, dissection can be initiated between the Laennec's capsule of the liver parenchyma and the Glissonian sheath wrapping the portal triad at the level of Rouviere's sulcus. This process is easier for cirrhotic livers since the liver capsule is sturdier due to fibrosis. Normal livers, or livers with steatosis or with previous chemotherapy, tend to be fragile and are prone to cause parenchymal tear and bleeding. Small branches may be encountered, necessitating their division to effectively isolate the main pedicle. In instances where the right posterior pedicle cannot be identified from the liver surface and runs deeper within the liver parenchyma, parenchymal dissection along the Rouviere's sulcus at the hilar area can facilitate the exposure of the Glissonian pedicle.

Traditionally, during extra-Glissonian approach, the right posterior branch is identified, ligated, and divided before parenchymal transection. The author prefers the temporary inflow control of the Glisson (TICGL) technique [16]. In brief, once the right posterior branch is exposed, a bulldog clamp is applied and the ischemic plane is identified. Parenchymal transection is initiated along the ischemic plane at this point and after approximately half of the parenchyma transection is done, the right posterior pedicle becomes relatively well exposed. The bulldog clamp is now removed and the pedicle is stapled and divided. The application of bulldog clamp before the parenchymal transection allows less blood loss and provides the correct anatomic transection, while the delayed application of stapler until the pedicle is exposed allows safer division of the right posterior pedicle. This technique provides surgeons to effectively address the challenges encountered during minimally invasive approach for an easier and safer procedure.

Other alternative options can be utilized. D'Hondt and Machado described anterior and posterior hepatotomies, followed by test-clamping of the pedicle and finally stapled pedicle transection [7, 17]. Homma advocated a caudate-first approach, wherein the caudate lobe is separated from the inferior vena cava (IVC) and divided posteriorly in parallel with the right lateral portion of the IVC and then vertically between the pedicle and the IVC. This exposes the dorsal portion of the right posterior pedicle, which may then be safely clamped and divided [18]. When individual isolation technique is done, it begins at the right lateral aspect of the hilum, with a meticulous individual dissection of the hepatic artery and portal vein posterior to the bile duct. The dissection continues until the right posterior hepatic artery and the right posterior portal vein are identified and isolated, which should include the direct visualization of the take-off of the right anterior and right posterior portal veins.

The approach to the right hepatic vein (RHV) is similarly critical to a successful RPS because most of bothersome bleeding occurs from the tributaries of hepatic veins. During the parenchymal transection, the branches of the right hepatic vein can be identified and traced posteriorly until reaching the trunk of the RHV. Special attention is needed to accurately identifying the true trunk of the RHV [12]. The RHV may also be identified at the lateral edge of the IVC after division of the hepatocaval ligament. Adequate preoperative imaging is critical to have an understanding of the hepatic vein anatomy, including the presence of a large right inferior hepatic vein inserting directly into the inferior vena cava. Intraoperative ultrasound is also a valuable tool that allows for visualization of the correct location of the RHV and its tributaries. To prevent undesirable venous bleeding, it is important to avoid excessive traction which can tear the veins, have full expose and appropriate length of vein before clipping or stapling, and avoid assumption and blind control, which can lead major bleeding from partially opened major vein or longitudinal opening of vein.

To minimize bleeding during parenchymal transection in hepatic resection, maintaining a low central venous pressure (CVP) is essential, usually below 5 mmHg. In case a central line is not placed, restriction of intravenous fluid, usually to less than 100 mL/h of crystalloid, is maintained until the parenchymal transection is completed. Colloids, unless necessary, are best reserved for after the transection is completed to prevent increase of CVP but is used afterward to allow euvolemia before the patient finishes the surgery. Effective communication with the anesthesiologist is crucial to maintain a safe operation while minimizing bleeding with low CVP.

Lesions of the right posterior section are considered technically demanding. The Louisville Statement on laparoscopic liver surgery and its subsequent Morioka revision state that laparoscopic surgery of the right posterior section should be performed by expert surgeons at high volume centers [19]. Despite advances in minimally invasive liver surgery, LRPS should be approached with caution only by those with extensive experience with laparoscopic hepatectomies.

Surgical Technique

The patient is positioned supine on the operating room table under general anesthesia. If performed open, access may be gained through a subcostal, hockey-stick, or chevron incision. In cases of laparoscopic approach, the patient is positioned in the French position, also known as split-leg, allowing for the primary surgeon to be positioned between the patients' legs. 15–30° left tilt with extra support under the patient's right side allows for increased ease of liver manipulation during right lobe mobilization. Additionally, hepatic vein tributaries becomes positioned more anterior (higher) to the IVC, which decrease the intravenous pressure and therefore less blood loss [20]. 10–15° revers Trendelenburg is also recommended since it can further lowers the intravenous pressure. In all cases, the patient should be secured to the table to allow wide range of motion in all directions.

Laparoscopic or Robotic Approach

In minimally invasive surgery (MIS) approaches, access is gained by optical trocar, insufflation needle, or standard cut-down techniques. Typically, five ports are placed in laparoscopic or robotic RPS. A 12-mm camera port is placed at the umbilicus. A flexible, three-dimensional scope can be useful for improved visualization. Four additional trocars are then placed under direct visualization. There are a variety of port placements, but our recommended approach for LRPS is shown in Fig. 26.1a. In case a 30° rigid

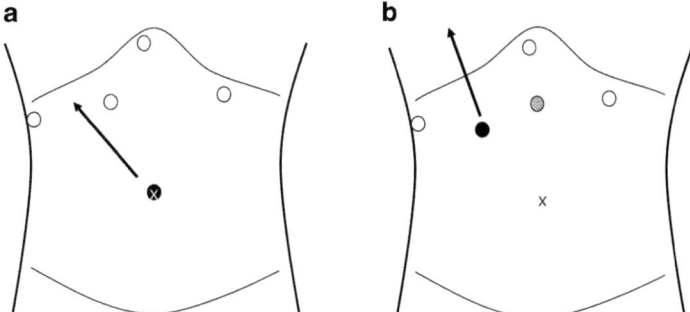

Fig. 26.1 Position of ports during right posterior sectionectomy. (**a**) With a flexible scope, the camera is inserted through the umbilical port (black) and positioned between right and medial port (arrow). (**b**) Position of ports using a rigid 30-degree scope. The camera port is placed close to the costal margin. The medial port (stipe) is placed medially to provide sufficient space between the ports

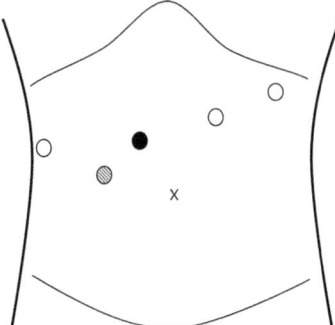

Fig. 26.2 Position of ports during robot-assisted right anterior, right posterior sectionectomy, and central hepatectomy. The camera is placed through arm 2 port (black), and the assistant's port (striped) is placed between arm 1 and arm 2

scope is used, the camera port should be placed closer to the costal margin to better visualize the superior area since range of visualization is limited compared to flexible scope (Fig. 26.1b). Figure 26.2 shows the port position during robot-assisted hepatectomy.

The falciform and round ligaments are dissected until the groove between the RHV and middle hepatic vein (MHV) is identified. The foramen of Winslow is then identified and preparations are made for performing a Pringle maneuver. The right lobe of the liver is then mobilized by releasing the lateral hepatic attachments including the right triangular and coronary ligaments. A snake retractor along with the gall bladder is used for retraction. "Right side up" tilt position of the patient helps drop the liver to the left using gravity. Once the right liver is fully mobilized, cholecystectomy is then performed.

Multiple methods for pedicle control exist as described in Sect. 2.1. If temporary control is preferred, then a laparoscopic bulldog clamp is introduced and placed over the right posterior pedicle. If individual dissection of Glissonian pedicle structures has been achieved, bulldog clamps can be separately applied to the right posterior portal vein and right posterior hepatic artery. If up-front permanent ligature is preferred, this is performed at this stage. These techniques will allow for demarcation of the ischemic segments 6 and 7, which will also represent the transection plane. The RHV, which lies along the plane can be identified with laparoscopic ultrasonography, and may also be used as a reference during transection.

Parenchymal transection then begins along the line of demarcation. Multiple techniques are available for parenchymal transection. The authors-preferred method involves utilizing an ultrasonic shears energy device (Harmonic™, Ethicon Endo Surgery, Inc., Johnson & Johnson Medical SPA, Somerville, NJ, USA, or Sonicision™, Covidien) for the superficial layers of the hepatic parenchyma (superficial 1–2 cm) and the laparoscopic CavitronUltrasonic Surgical Aspirator (CUSA; Integra LifeSciences, Princeton, NJ, USA) with the monopolar nosecone for the deeper layers . This is supported by a combination of bipolar forceps and the Aquamantys™ (Medtronic) device for appropriate hemostasis during parenchymal dissection. Small branches can be divided using ultrasonic shear, vessel sealer, or monopolar electrocautery, but larger branches greater than 2 mm are usually clipped and sharply divided. In most of the case of RPS, the plane of transection is kept on the lateral aspect of the RHV with the RHV preserved with the remnant liver. Conversely, in the cases RHV needs to be removed with the resected specimen like during living donation or when safe resection margin cannot be achieved without removal of the RHV, the plane of transection is kept on the medial aspect of the RHV. If TICGL technique is used, the parenchymal transection is continued until the right posterior pedicle is fully exposed, at which point it is encircled with an umbilical tape, retracted to the patients' left side (the remnant side) to prevent inadvertent stricture of the remaining structures, and then transected with a vascular staple load.

Parenchymal transection then continues until reaching the root of RHV. The major tributary branches of the RHV are then clipped and sharply divided or transected with a vascular staple load. Often, especially in large patients or when using robotic assisted, the final part of parenchyma lies too deep to be comfortably reached with instruments. Hanging maneuver can allow access to the deeper portion of the parenchyma. A tape is passed behind the right lobe and retracted toward the camera to bring the surgical plane closer. Placing new ports higher close to the costal margin or using the subxiphoid port instead of main working port can help reach the deep plane as well.

Once the transection of the parenchyma is completed, bolus of colloid and crystalloid is given as described previously to reach euvolemia. Hemostasis is performed and the abdomen is inspected for appropriate hemostasis and evidence of bile leak along the cut surface. The specimen is then brought out through a Pfannenstiel incision. After closure of the extraction site, the abdomen is re-insufflated for a re-evaluation of the cut surface for any bleeding site. While the CVP is low and abdomen is inflated causing positive intraabdominal pressure, bleeding from small injuries to the hepatic veins may not be evident due to pneumatic compression. Revisiting the surgical area after the patient has reached euvolemia and the abdomen has been deflated is important since there may be signs of bleeding from these minor injuries. An abdominal drain may be placed. The trocars are removed under direct visualization and closed in the standard fashion.

Open Approach

The open approach offers better tactile feedback. After incision is made, the liver is mobilized by freeing the falciform and round ligaments followed by the lateral attachments. A cholecystectomy is performed and the hilar dissection is begun. The author's preference is Glissonian approach but any techniques described above may be used to dissect, identify, and control the right posterior branches. Because the surgical plane of right posterior sectionectomy lies posteriorly, full mobilization of the right lobe should be done to bring the surgical plane anteriorly for better visualization. A couple of large pads placed behind the right lobe helps with good surgical field. Parenchymal transection continues along the line of demarcation until reaching the RHV. When the plane lies too deep, hanging maneuver, as described above, may be used to bring the surgical plane anteriorly for easier operation. The specimen is removed, and the abdomen is inspected for hemostasis and bile leak. The fascia, subcutaneous tissue, and skin are then closed in standard fashion.

Central Hepatectomy and Right Anterior Sectionectomy

The central hepatectomy (CH), also known as a mesohepatectomy, is a complex anatomic resection involving segments IV, V, and VIII. The right anterior sectionectomy (RAS) is similar but does not include the segment IV. Both techniques can be approached using similar method but are very complex and should only be performed by experienced liver surgeons. This approach is performed for any centrally located tumors that require removal of segment V, VIII or V, VIII, IV.

Pitfalls and Pearls

Central hepatectomy is the preferred approach for central lesions that are not amenable to trisectionectomy. While trisectionectomy is more commonly performed, when low functional liver remnant (FLR) is expected or when liver volume should be spared because the liver is not very healthy, such as after extensive chemotherapy, CH, or RAS is a reasonable approach. CH is particularly useful for tumors close to the hilar plate, or central tumors that are close to the left hepatic vein (LHV), as this approach will aid with exposure [21]. CH showed comparable outcomes to extended hepatectomy in terms of complication rates and overall survival rates. CH provides a balance between achieving complete tumor resection and preserving liver function or volume by selectively removing the affected central liver segments compared to right or left trisectionectomies. This increases the chance of successful repeat resection in cases of tumor recurrence or the need for subsequent liver surgeries such as in colorectal or neuroendocrine metastases where recurrence is observed more frequently [22, 23].

The hilar approach to the CH and RAS are similar in that Glissonian approach to control the right anterior branch may be preferred, just like in RPS, to allows clear demarcation of the resection plane [24]. Parenchymal-first approaches have been shown to have comparable outcomes, both in open and laparoscopic procedures, and may be easier for less experienced surgeons [25]. The authors prefer using the TICGL technique for CH or RAS [26]. Intraoperative ultrasonography is a valuable tool, as it allows for real-time visualization of the relationship of the tumor with the intrahepatic structures and the location of the right and left hepatic veins, which allows for confirmation of the correct anatomical resection plane. The choice of approach should prioritize surgeon comfort and prior experience in technique selection.

Control of Inflow and outflow plays a crucial role in the success of the operation. Randomized data from cirrhotic patients undergoing CH demonstrated that both intermittent hepatic inflow occlusion (the Pringle maneuver) and hemi-hepatic inflow occlusion were safe and effective, though hemi-hepatic or selective inflow occlusion might reduce blood loss [27]. Large series of patients also described hepatic outflow control through occlusion of the supra- and infra-hepatic IVC for total hepatic isolation, though this is often unnecessary [28]. While neither these approaches is mandatory for CH, surgeons must thoroughly assess the anatomical location of the tumor, the underlying liver quality and morphology, and their comfort or skill level during the careful planning of these maneuver.

As with the RPS, the CH may be done either open or through minimally invasive approaches. The MIS approaches have been shown to be safe when performed by experienced surgeons, though MIS may result in longer operative time [26]. Furthermore, various methods of laparoscopic transection have been described, providing choices to those who wish to pursue the less invasive option [25].

Despite the primary goal of parenchymal preservation, the CH may occasionally still be too extensive and resulting in a significant reduction in functional liver volume, which can cause increased morbidity or preclude resection in some cases. In certain cases, the limited central hepatectomy approach has been proposed depending on the location of tumor. This technique preserves the segment 8 dorsal Glissonean pedicle, and may also spare segment selective pedicles to segment IV or V. Although this technique is less standardized and more technically demanding, small series have shown comparable outcomes without increasing in local tumor recurrences [29].

Surgical Technique

Both the laparoscopic or robot-assisted and open approaches follow similar pathways, though the initial steps vary. In the laparoscopic approach, the patient is placed in the French (or supine, split-leg) position. Since the CH or RAS includes dissection of the parenchyma along the plane between right anterior and posterior section similar to RPS, a pad is inserted behind the right side of the patient to incline the patient 10–15° left decubitus. The surgeon stands between the patient's legs with the assistant and the assistant camera-operator both positioned to the patients left. In case a flexible scope is used, the 12-mm optical trocar is placed at the umbilicus, which will be used for the camera. We recommend using three-dimensional visualization. Four additional ports are placed under direct visualization. These may vary at surgeon preference, but a recommended position is shown in Fig. 26.3a. When a rigid 30° scope is used, the camera port should be placed closer to the costal rib (Fig. 26.3b). Figure 26.2 shows the port position

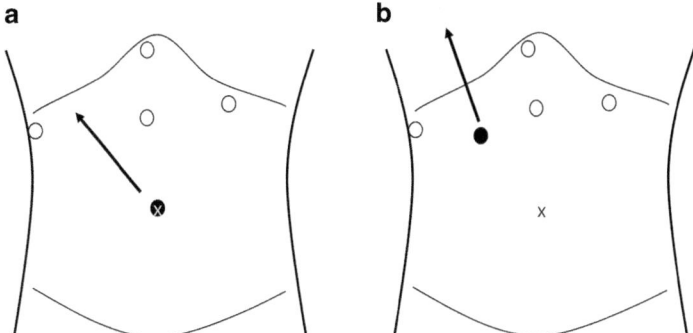

Fig. 26.3 Position of ports during central hepatectomy or right anterior sectionectomy. (**a**) With a flexible scope, the camera is inserted through the umbilical port (black) and positioned between right and medial port (arrow). (**b**) Position of ports using a rigid 30-degree scope. The camera port is placed close to the costal margin

during robot-assisted hepatectomy. In the open approach, a hockey stick or chevron incision is made.

The falciform and round ligaments are then dissected moving superiorly until the suprahepatic IVC is seen and the groove between the right and middle hepatic veins can be appreciated. The right lateral attachments of the liver may be incised for full mobilization of the right lobe. The foramen of Winslow is identified, and preparations are made for a Pringle maneuver using the surgeons' approach of preference. The cholecystectomy is then performed. It is important to be proficient in intra-operative ultrasonography, as this modality is utilized before the parenchymal transection is commenced to evaluate the intrahepatic location of the RHV, MHV, and LHV.

The right anterior Glissonian pedicle is identified using a combination of monopolar electrocautery and blunt dissection with bipolar forceps and a suction-irrigator device. Smaller branches from Glissonian pedicles may need to be divided to facilitate encircling the right anterior Glissonian pedicle. The exposed pedicle may be then either temporarily or permanently ligated. There are considerable variations noted in the course of the right anterior Glissonian pedicle, and it is imperative to have a clear understanding of the anatomy through preoperative imaging and intraoperative ultrasound [30]. After the pedicle is controlled, the ischemic margin of segments V and VIII is then noted and utilized as a guide for parenchymal transection. The demarcation line can be drawn on the surface of liver with monopolar electrocautery. Sometimes, access to the right anterior branch may not be easy, and it frequently is the case when there are anatomic variations of the portal structures such as trifurcation or branching of the right anterior branch from the left, since the right anterior pedicle lies deeper inside the parenchyma. In this situation, we can begin with the parenchymal transection of the left surgical plane first to facilitate the exposure and control of the right anterior pedicle. In CH, dissection is done along the falciform ligament and in RAS, between the right and left lobe, which is delineated by controlling the right pedicle. Also, left-side dissection is easier to obtain the correct surgical plane. For these reasons, the left side transection is done first before approaching the right plane.

Parenchymal dissection is begun on the superficial layer. Blind dissection using ultrasonic shear or bipolar device can be done up to 1–2 cm in depth. The deeper parenchymal transection is performed with the combination of CUSA, bipolar electrocautery, and Aquamantys™ until the right anterior pedicle is visualized. It is important to recognize the in-flow pedicles to segment IVa/b originating from the umbilical portion of the left Glissonian pedicle. The Glissonian pedicles supplying segment IV are identified and sequentially ligated as the parenchymal transection progresses. Special attention should be given to preserve the Glissonian pedicle inflows to the left lateral segment during the transection, particularly along the right of the falciform ligament. The right anterior branch can be controlled, either definitively or temporarily, using a bulldog clamp at this point if it has not been controlled previously. The dissection continues until the middle hepatic vein (MHV) is identified, but stapling the MHV is postponed until the right anterior pedicle is controlled and the right-side parenchymal transection is complete to preserve the outflow into the inferior vena cava (IVC) and prevent congestion of right anterior section.

After completion of the left-sided parenchymal transection, the right-side transection is performed. In case it is done by open approach, it is important to fully mobilize the right lobe to completely bring the transection plane anteriorly to provide safer and easier parenchymal dissection. During laparoscopic approach, tilting the patient left, such as in RPS, facilitates the traction of the liver leftward for better exposure of the transection plane. Additionally, the right hepatic vein rotates clockwise, positioning it not below the IVC but above it, which helps decrease blood loss by lowering the intravascular pressure [20].

Once sufficient parenchymal transection has been achieved to ensure proper exposure of the right anterior pedicle, it is divided with a stapler. It is important to staple closer to the specimen side while applying contralateral retraction to prevent unintended stricture of the remnant vascular or biliary structures. The transection proceeds along the ischemic margin, following the lateral/posterior aspect of segments V and VIII, while keeping the transection margin along the medial side of the right hepatic vein (RHV). The transection continues until the lateral side of the middle hepatic vein (MHV) is exposed at which point the MHV is stapled. The specimen is detached from the inferior vena cava (IVC) and the parenchymal transection is completed. Unless removal of part of the caudate lobe is needed to get a proper resection margin, it is not necessary nor recommended to expose the IVC since it may cause troublesome injury to the IVC and unnecessary bleeding. In case of RAS, the MHV is not controlled but only hepatic vein tributaries draining to MHV, such as V5 and V8, are controlled since the transection plane is kept on the right side of the MHV.

The specimen is removed through a Pfannenstiel incision. Like for any major liver resection with exposed large venous structures, it is important to close the main incision and re-insufflated to re-inspect the cut surface for any potential bleeding after the patient is at a euvolemic state. Minor bile leaks can often be found, which may be controlled with clips or sutures but should be cautious to not cause any stricture to remaining structures during this process. A drain is placed along the cut surface and abdomen is closed.

Conclusion

In conclusion, right posterior, right anterior, and central hepatectomy are complex procedures aimed at achieving negative margins through anatomic resection while preserving the functional liver remnant. The success of these operations depends on careful planning, considering tumor location, liver quality, and surgeon expertise. Minimally invasive and open approaches have demonstrated comparable outcomes. Inflow and outflow control are crucial in these procedures. Right posterior, right anterior, and central hepatectomy require careful consideration of patient-specific factors, precise surgical technique, and a multidisciplinary approach for optimal outcomes.

References

1. Ito H, et al. Effect of postoperative morbidity on long-term survival after hepatic resection for metastatic colorectal cancer. Ann Surg. 2008;247(6):994–1002.
2. Groeschl RT, et al. Hepatectomy for noncolorectal non-neuroendocrine metastatic cancer: a multi-institutional analysis. J Am Coll Surg. 2012;214(5):769–77.
3. Fisher SB, et al. A comparison of right posterior sectorectomy with formal right hepatectomy: a dual-institution study. HPB (Oxford). 2013;15(10):753–62.
4. Ho CM, et al. Total laparoscopic limited anatomical resection for centrally located hepatocellular carcinoma in cirrhotic liver. Surg Endosc. 2013;27(5):1820–5.
5. Eguchi S, et al. Comparison of the outcomes between an anatomical subsegmentectomy and a non-anatomical minor hepatectomy for single hepatocellular carcinomas based on a Japanese nationwide survey. Surgery. 2008;143(4):469–75.
6. Ivey GD, et al. Current surgical management strategies for colorectal cancer liver metastases. Cancers (Basel). 2022;14(4):1063.
7. D'Hondt M, et al. Laparoscopic right posterior sectionectomy: single-center experience and technical aspects. Langenbeck's Arch Surg. 2019;404(1):21–9.
8. Rhu J, et al. Laparoscopic versus open right posterior sectionectomy for hepatocellular carcinoma in a high-volume center: a propensity score matched analysis. World J Surg. 2018;42(9):2930–7.

9. Ferrero A, et al. Laparoscopic right posterior anatomic liver resections with Glissonean pedicle-first and venous craniocaudal approach. Surg Endosc. 2021;35(1):449–55.
10. Rhu J, et al. Laparoscopic right posterior sectionectomy versus laparoscopic right hemihepatectomy for hepatocellular carcinoma in posterior segments: propensity score matching analysis. Scand J Surg. 2019;108(1):23–9.
11. van der Heijde N, et al. Laparoscopic versus open right posterior sectionectomy: an international, multicenter, propensity score-matched evaluation. Surg Endosc. 2021;35(11):6139–49.
12. Wang MX, et al. The safety and feasibility of laparoscopic right posterior sectionectomy vs. open approach: a systematic review and meta-analysis. Front Surg. 2022;9:1019117.
13. Patriti A, et al. Robot-assisted versus open liver resection in the right posterior section. JSLS. 2014;18(3):e2014.00040.
14. Casciola L, et al. Robot-assisted parenchymal-sparing liver surgery including lesions located in the posterosuperior segments. Surg Endosc. 2011;25(12):3815–24.
15. Yamamoto M, et al. Glissonean pedicle transection method for liver surgery (with video). J Hepatobiliary Pancreat Sci. 2012;19(1):3–8.
16. Lee N, et al. Application of temporary inflow control of the Glissonean pedicle method provides a safe and easy technique for totally laparoscopic hemihepatectomy by Glissonean approach. Ann Surg Treat Res. 2017;92(5):383–6.
17. Machado MA, et al. The laparoscopic Glissonian approach is safe and efficient when compared with standard laparoscopic liver resection: results of an observational study over 7 years. Surgery. 2016;160(3):643–51.
18. Homma Y, et al. Pure laparoscopic right posterior sectionectomy using the caudate lobe-first approach. Surg Endosc. 2019;33(11):3851–7.
19. Buell JF, et al. The international position on laparoscopic liver surgery: the Louisville statement, 2008. Ann Surg. 2009;250(5):825–30.
20. Rhu J, et al. Laparoscopic versus open right posterior sectionectomy for hepatocellular carcinoma in a high-volume center: a propensity score matched analysis. World J Surg. 2018;42:2930.
21. Kogure M, et al. Parenchymal-sparing approaches for resection of tumors located in the paracaval portion of the caudate lobe of the liver-utility of limited resection and central hepatectomy. Langenbeck's Arch Surg. 2021;406(6):2099–106.
22. Lee SY. Central hepatectomy for centrally located malignant liver tumors: a systematic review. World J Hepatol. 2014;6(5):347–57.
23. Chouillard E, et al. Anatomical bi- and trisegmentectomies as alternatives to extensive liver resections. Ann Surg. 2003;238(1):29–34.

24. Maki H. Central hepatectomy using the hilar approach for removal of tumors in the paracaval portion of the caudate lobe. Surg Gastroenterol Oncol. 2019;24:203.
25. Zheng Z, et al. Laparoscopic central hepatectomy using a parenchymal-first approach: how we do it. Surg Endosc. 2022;36(11):8630–8.
26. Cho CW, et al. Short-term outcomes of totally laparoscopic central hepatectomy and right anterior sectionectomy for centrally located tumors: a case-matched study with propensity score matching. World J Surg. 2017;41(11):2838–46.
27. Wu CC, et al. Occlusion of hepatic blood inflow for complex central liver resections in cirrhotic patients: a randomized comparison of hemihepatic and total hepatic occlusion techniques. Arch Surg. 2002;137(12):1369–76.
28. Chen XP, et al. Mesohepatectomy for hepatocellular carcinoma: a study of 256 patients. Int J Color Dis. 2008;23(5):543–6.
29. Botea F, et al. Limited central hepatectomy for centrally located tumors under ultrasound-guidance: a feasible alternative to formal central hepatectomy. Int J Surg. 2020;75:S26–7.
30. Xu W, et al. Anatomical variation of the Glissonean pedicle of the right liver. Korean J Hepatobiliary Pancreat Surg. 2011;15(2):101–6.

Extended Hepatectomy 27

Peter J. Altshuler and Shareef M. Syed

Introduction

Historically, liver has been an organ of fascinating complexity. With its regenerative ability known since the myth of Prometheus, the first documented attempts to operate on the liver were performed in ancient Rome by Hippocrates, who described the drainage of pus from the liver through the skin. Medical advancements in the Renaissance era brought about a greater understanding of the internal structure of the liver, highlighted by Francis Glisson publishing the *Anatomia Hepatis* in 1664. It took more than 200, however, until the first successful formal liver resection was performed by Carl von Langenbuch, a German surgeon who removed a pedicled tumor from the left lobe of a 30-year-old female's liver. It took nearly 100 years from this point until liver resection would become an operation of acceptable risk. Over the past half-century, the field of liver surgery has undergone significant technical and technological developments, which, coupled with greater utilization of some of the unique anatomic and physiologic char-

P. J. Altshuler (✉) · S. M. Syed
Division of Transplant Surgery, Department of Surgery, University of California San Francisco, San Francisco, CA, USA
e-mail: Peter.Altshuler@ucsf.edu; Shareef.syed@ucsf.edu

© The Author(s), under exclusive license to Springer Nature Switzerland AG 2025
A. Alseidi et al. (eds.), *The SAGES Manual of Contemporary Indications and Management of Hepatic and Biliary Diseases*, https://doi.org/10.1007/978-3-032-04823-3_27

acteristics of the liver, have led to more extensive liver resections in a safe manner.

One classically accepted nomenclature of liver anatomy divides the organ into a left and right hemiliver, with each hemiliver subsequently divided into two sectors. Each of these four sectors contain two segments, named Couinad segments after French surgeon Claude Couinad. It was Couinad who in 1954 defined the extended hepatectomy [1], with Thomas Starzl further describing surgical techniques of extended hepatectomies in 1975 [2].

Indications

Indications for extended hepatectomy include both benign and malignant processes in which anatomic resection of more than four segments are required to achieve an adequate negative surgical margin. The most common indications for extended hepatectomy involve resection of malignant tumors of the liver and biliary tree, including cholangiocarcinoma, primary hepatocellular carcinoma, cancers with metastases to the liver, and other rarer malignancies of the liver. Additionally, extended hepatectomy may be warranted for large hepatic adenomas, hemangiomas, and other benign processes, as well as infectious processes such as large pyogenic abscesses if the disease encompasses a large enough portion of the liver such that anything less than extended hepatectomy would not achieve complete control of the disease.

Operative Planning

A thorough understanding of liver anatomy, including biliary and vascular structures, is critical to achieving a successful surgical outcome. This includes knowledge of conventional vascular and biliary ductal anatomy and recognition of potential anatomic variants that can exist. For a left extended hepatectomy, the left hemiliver is resected along with part of segment V or VIII with division/resection of the middle hepatic vein. For an extended right hepatectomy, the right hemiliver is resected along with part of segment IV with division/resection of the middle hepatic vein. Several imaging modalities exists to better delineate liver anatomy in both the preoperative and intraoperative contexts. These may be used in conjunction with one another so that the surgeon can create a complete road map of the hepatic vasculature and biliary ductal anatomy prior to performing the liver resection.

Identifying hepatic vasculature helps define inflow and outflow to the remnant liver and helps determine surgical resectability. This can be visualized through a combination of computed tomography (CT), magnetic resonance imaging (MRI), and ultrasound (US). A quadruple phase CT allows for visualization of the liver in the arterial, portal venous, systemic venous, and non-contrast phases and helps identify important extrahepatic manifestations of chronic liver disease such as the presence and location of varices and porto-mesenteric thromboses. MRI with contrast can be used in patients with renal insufficiency at risk of contrast-induced nephropathy. Doppler US can also be helpful preoperatively to quantify inflow and outflow by assessing for patency and flow within hepatic vasculature and can be a useful adjunct in the operating room to demarcate transection margins by identifying the course of critical vascular structures. Both arteriography and venography can also be utilized but are invasive and generally performed only if a preoperative vascular intervention be indicated.

Biliary anatomy can also be defined through various means. Preoperatively, MRI with and without contrast including magnetic resonance cholangiography (MRC) can be used to delineate the biliary tree to identify biliary drainage. Magnetic resonance imaging utilizing gadolinium-based, hepatocyte-specific contrast agents such as gadoxetate disodium can provide detailed visualization of biliary anatomy in delayed phases, allowing for hepatocyte uptake and excretion. Additionally, cholangiography can be performed preoperatively via endoscopic retrograde cholangiography (ERC) or percutaneous transhepatic cholangiography (PTC), as well as intraoperatively via ERC, PTC, or direct access cholangiography using a cholangiocatheter through a choledochotomy. Intraoperative cholangiography can be performed using radio-opaque contrast and by injecting air into the biliary system while clamping the distal common bile duct (air cholangiogram).

Another critical consideration during extended hepatectomy is the volume of liver that will remain following resection or the functional liver remnant (FLR). Inadequate FLR is associated with increases in morbidity related to liver failure and can significantly increase mortality [3]. Acceptable FLR is generally accepted at 20–25% for non-diseased livers, 30% for steatotic and 40% for cirrhotic livers [4, 5]. Advanced age, diabetes, obesity, prior chemotherapy, renal insufficiency, and malnutrition have also been identified as factors that may increase the risk for post-hepatectomy liver failure and require higher percentage FLR [6–8]. Calculating FLR can be done in several ways. Volumetric studies help predict remnant liver size, which in relation to patient total body surface area can help predict FLR adequacy. These studies can be performed using three-dimensional CT or MR volumetrics, or through retention and clearance of indocyanine green within the liver and biliary tree. Like indocyanine green clearance, hepatobiliary scintigraphy can assess for clearance of radiotracer within the liver and expected liver remnant.

In select patients who may have inadequate FLR to tolerate resection, preoperative modulative therapies such as portal vein embolization may be performed to induce hypertrophy of the FLR prior to resection. Radioembolization of tumors using Yttrium-90 has been demonstrated to induce significant growth of the contralateral hemiliver, with a kinetic growth rate of 0.5% per week following treatment and growth of 26–47% over a period of 8–40 weeks [9]. Portal vein embolization or ligation may also be useful, with kinetic growth rates exceeding 2% per week and degree of hypertrophy exceeding 10% [10]. One should consider these options after clearing the disease in the remnant or ensure low-volume disease with a preferential plan to address the disease in the remnant pre-procedure. Should embolization or ligation of the portal vein not induce sufficient hypertrophy of the FLR, liver venous deprivation can be attempted where the hepatic vein of the affected liver segment is embolized in a similar fashion to the portal vein. Associating liver partition and portal vein ligation for staged hepatectomy (ALPPS), a two-staged procedure may also be used in select circumstances for patients with inadequate FLR. In a small single center study comparing ALPPS ($n = 15$) and PVE ($n = 53$), ALPPS has shown to induce a degree of hypertrophy twice that of portal vein embolization, with a kinetic growth rate 10 times that of portal vein embolization. It is important to note that this bias toward ALPPS is based on the postoperative CT volumetric at a median follow-up time interval of 7 days (typical for ALPPS) [11]. The first stage of ALPPS involves division of the liver and ligation of portal inflow to the diseased liver segments—this allows for hypertrophy of the remnant liver, which once suitable to sustain liver function allows for the second stage in which the hepatectomy is performed.

Surgical Considerations

Incision

Access to the abdominal cavity can be approached through several incisions in an open approach. The choice of incision should factor in patient habitus, location and size of the liver lesion, and the ability to mobilize the liver safely and adequately. Common incisions include upper midline, upper midline with right transverse extension (Makuuchi), bilateral subcostal (Chevron), bilateral subcostal with midline extension (Mercedes Benz), or any variant of the previously mentioned.

Mobilization

Once the peritoneum has been safely accessed and the liver visualized, the round ligament is first identified and ligated. The falciform ligament should then be taken down until it splays into the coronary ligaments. Self-retaining retractors are then placed in the wound bed. Our preference is to use Thompson retractors that permit cephalad retraction to expose the dome of the liver and hepatic veins; however, any fixed retractor system that provides full exposure of the liver including its inflow and outflow can be used.

The left triangular ligament is divided, taking care to avoid injury to the underlying stomach and spleen. The lesser sac can then be entered by lifting on the pars flaccida, taking care to avoid injury to any potential replaced or accessory left hepatic artery. This allows for visualization of the IVC and caudate lobe from the left side, and aids in isolation of the hepatoduodenal ligament. The right side of the liver is mobilized by lifting the liver superiorly and taking attachments to the retroperitoneum using electrocautery. This dissection can continue until a plane is developed between the undersurface of the liver and the right adrenal gland and kidney. The right triangular ligament can then be divided as the liver is carefully rolled in a clockwise fashion, with dissection extending up until the lateral border of the right hepatic vein.

Dissection of the Porta Hepatis into the Hilar Plate

The porta hepatis provides hepatic arterial and portal venous inflow to the liver, as well as biliary outflow. With the liver adequately mobilized, the porta hepatis can be completely isolated through the Foramen of Winslow. Generally, the anatomic relation between the hepatic artery, common bile duct, and portal vein is such that the bile duct is anterolateral, hepatic artery is anteromedial, and portal vein is posterior. Aberrant anatomy may frequently exist such as the presence of a replaced or accessory right hepatic artery, which may arise from the superior mesenteric artery and courses along the lateral aspect of the porta hepatis. These anatomic variations should be identified preoperatively and can be confirmed intraoperatively through manual palpation as well as doppler ultrasonography.

Dissection of the porta hepatis begins by retracting the liver in a cephalad fashion and identifying the common bile duct. This can be done by carefully dissecting the anterolateral aspect of the porta until the bile duct is identified. Alternatively, a "dome down" cholecystectomy can be performed, and the cystic duct traced to the common bile duct. Once the bile duct is exposed, the proper hepatic artery can be identified. The surgeon can feel for a pulse on the anteromedial surface of the porta hepatis and can proceed with isolation of the hepatic artery in a similar fashion to the bile duct. Alternative means of exposure include identification of the gastroduodenal artery at the head of the pancreas and antegrade dissection along the common hepatic artery, or retrograde dissection whereby the common hepatic duct is traced toward the liver where, in most cases, the right hepatic artery can be identified coursing under the dissected common hepatic duct. This can then be traced back to the proper hepatic artery. The portal vein can then be isolated after clearing the porta hepatis of lateral lymphatic and nervous tissue that envelopes the three structures. Once the portal triad has been identified, each of the hepatic artery, portal vein, and bile duct can be dissected toward the hilar plate to their respective pedicles supplying or draining the remnant liver.

Hepatic arterial anatomy contains the greatest variation of any of the hepatic vascular and biliary structures as it occurs latest during embryogenesis. Aberrant arterial anatomy should be noted preoperatively to better understand the origin and course of the arterial pedicle supplying the remnant liver. Conventional Type I hepatic arterial anatomy exists in upward of 85% of patients, in which the common hepatic arises from the celiac artery, becoming the proper hepatic artery after the gastroduodenal artery and subsequently bifurcating into left and right hepatic arteries. Nine additional anatomic variants exist; however, all relating to the relationship of the hepatic arteries to the celiac, superior mesenteric, and left gastric arteries, as well as the presence of replaced or accessory arteries. For an extended right hepatectomy, the left hepatic artery serves as the pedicle supplying the remnant segments II and III. For an extended left hepatectomy, the posterior branch of the right hepatic artery supplies remnant segments VI and VII. The right or left hepatic artery should be dissected such that isolation of the arterial inflow is as specific as possible to assist in delineating transection margins.

The portal vein, despite having more consistent anatomy than the hepatic artery, still contains important variants. Approximately 80% of patients have "bifurcation type" portal anatomy, where the main portal vein bifurcates into the left portal vein and the right portal vein containing the right anterior and right posterior portal vein branches. In 10% of patients, a "trifurcation" type pattern exists where the left, right anterior, and right posterior pedicles branch off together at a common trunk. Finally, 10% of patients will have an early branching of the right lateral pedicle, with the right anterior and left portal vein pedicles branching downstream. Additional variants exist as well beyond these three most common phenotypes. For an extended right hepatectomy, the left portal vein will serve as the portal pedicle to the remnant, while the pedicle for an extended left hepatectomy is the right posterior portal vein.

Biliary ductal anatomy is more varied on the right than the left. In 97% of the population, a left hepatic duct exists, which lends more consistency to the biliary drainage of an extended right hepatectomy. In contrast, preserving biliary drainage of a left hepatectomy necessitates a thorough understanding of the variations that exist in right hepatic ductal anatomy. In general, the left hepatic duct serves as the biliary outflow for an extended right hepatectomy, while the right posterior branch of the right hepatic duct is the biliary drainage for an extended left hepatectomy.

Hepatic Vein Dissection

Dissection of the hepatic veins proceeds by identifying and preserving the vein(s) draining the remnant section. Conventional anatomy of the hepatic veins is defined by a dominant right hepatic vein and a middle and left hepatic vein that form a confluence before draining into the IVC. The right hepatic vein drains the right posterior sector (segments VI/VII) and may also include veins draining segments V/VIII. The middle hepatic vein drains segments IVA/B, V, and VIII. The left hepatic vein drains the left lateral sector (segments II/III) and segments IVA/B. Significant variability exists in hepatic venous drainage as well. For an extended right hepatectomy, dissection along the dome of the liver proceeds until the left or left/middle hepatic veins can be encircled; this is aided by inferomedial dissection in which the liver is rolled in a cephalad and lateral fashion to visualize the infrahepatic IVC and caudate lobe. For an extended left hepatectomy, identification and preservation of accessory right hepatic veins such as an inferior right or inferior middle hepatic veins is critical to preserving remnant liver function. Present in up to 70% of patients, inferior hepatic veins may drain segments VI and VII and sacrificing them may cause congestion of the remnant liver. These veins can be identified and preserved when mobilizing the liver medially and can be seen inserting directly on to the IVC. Like the left or left/middle hepatic veins, the right hepatic vein should be approached from above, below, and from the side, carefully creating a tunnel along the anterior surface of the IVC to isolate the vein. The hepatic venous drainage of segment IV should also be noted, particularly in extended right hepatectomies. Although the segment IV vein drains predominantly into the middle hepatic vein, it may also drain into the left hepatic vein, or into the confluence of the left and middle hepatic veins.

Parenchymal Transection

Once the vascular and biliary pedicles have been identified and isolated, clamps can be placed on the hepatic artery, portal vein, and if possible hepatic vein branches to be sacrificed to visualize the transection margin. The demarcation line for extended right hepatectomies should begin at the insertion of the left hepatic vein into the IVC and will generally follow just lateral to the falciform ligament anteriorly and down toward the cystic plate on the inferior surface of the liver. For an extended left hepatectomy, this margin begins at the medial edge of the right hepatic vein and courses over the dome of the liver anteriorly, and generally follows inferiorly lateral to the gallbladder fossa to the hepatic hilum. "Hanging the liver" is an additional technique that may help in both the elevation of the transection plane as well as hemostasis during the parenchymal transection. This classically involves slinging the liver with an atraumatic tape, such as a red rubber catheter, underneath the liver along the avascular plane between the liver and vena cava to exclude the inflow and outflow that is to supply and drain the remnant segments; however, the position of the tape can be modified depending on the resection being performed.

Parenchymal transection can be performed through several different techniques; however, the mainstay of resection should remain identifying the landmark hepatic vein at the transection margin that delineates resected specimen from remnant liver. Understanding its course allows for a parenchymal transection with minimal blood loss. Transection itself can be carried out using a clamp-crush technique, staplers, tissue sealing energy devices, monopolar or bipolar energy devices, ultrasonic aspirators, clips, or a combination of the above. Ultrasonic aspirators tend to allow for the most precise parenchymal transection. Large, transected veins and pedicles should be oversewn. A Pringle maneuver may also be performed to minimize blood loss, where the hepatoduodenal ligament is encircled and compressed to reduce inflow to the liver. This may be compressed for up to 15 min with 5-min intervals of decompression to prevent ischemic injury to the liver. Awareness of the size and quality of the remnant liver is critical in considering the Pringle maneuver. Selective inflow control can also be considered to reduce ischemia to the remnant liver.

Reconstruction

The parenchymal resection should be performed with an understanding of the vascular and biliary pedicles, which may need to be divided, and caution should be taken prior to encountering these larger structures. Depending on patient anatomy, the vascular and biliary structures may remain in continuity throughout the resection with branches divided. In these circumstances, no complex reconstruction is required. In certain circumstances, however, complete arterial, portal venous, or hepatic venous system disruption may be required to completely resect the diseased liver. The potential need for complex vascular or biliary reconstruction should be anticipated prior to the operation.

In general, vascular reconstruction should follow core principles of vascular anastomoses. Primary, tension-free end-to-end anastomosis of native vessels should first be considered. Should this not be feasible, transposition grafts (particularly for arterial reconstruction) can be used. Autologous interposition grafts can be utilized as well. Conduits can include internal jugular vein, reversed saphenous vein, left renal vein, gonadal vein, splenic vein, iliac vein, or even pericardium or peritoneum. ABO-compatible cadaveric allografts can also be utilized as conduits. Xenografts, such as bovine pericardium, may also be used. In general, the choice of conduit should most closely resemble the interposed vessels to achieve normal flow through the conduit. Synthetic grafts can be used as well; however, caution should be taken as the risk of bile leak after hepatectomy may result in these grafts becoming infected.

Hepatic Artery Reconstruction

Arterial reconstruction can present a challenge given the diminutive size of the arteries feeding the remnant liver. In considering arterial anatomy, it is important to note that "conventional" hepatic arterial anatomy exists in only 55% of patients.

For an extended right hepatectomy, the segment II/III artery off the left hepatic artery supplies the remnant liver. Aberrant left hepatic arterial anatomy can be favorable in these cases, as no arterial disruption to the left lateral segment is required during resection. Should arterial transection be necessary, proximal inflow options include using remnant proximal segment of the left hepatic artery, or if insufficient length the gastroduodenal artery, splenic artery, left gastric or gastroepiploic arteries can also be ligated distally and brought to the segment II/III artery. Interposition grafts, as described above, can also be used. These anastomoses will frequently have size mismatches, which can be overcome by spatulating or obliquely cutting the segment II/III artery to increase vessel circumference. After proximal and distal clamping, they can be sewn in an end-to-end fashion using small (6–0, 7–0, or 8–0), permanent, monofilament sutures placed in an interrupted or continuous fashion.

For an extended left hepatectomy, the right hepatic artery provides a posterior branch that feeds the remnant liver. Like the left, aberrant right hepatic arterial anatomy can be favorable and prevent the need for disrupting arterial flow to the remnant liver here as well. For both right and left hepatic arteries, should the previously mentioned options for transposition or interposition grafts be infeasible, a synthetic aorto- or ilio-hepatic graft may be used as well to provide arterial inflow.

Portal Vein Reconstruction

Portal venous inflow in an extended right hepatectomy arises from the left portal vein, which supplies branches to the lateral segments II/III. For an extended left hepatectomy, the right posterior branch of the right portal vein provides portal venous inflow. Again, preservation of native inflow is preferable when considering portal reconstruction; however, should this be infeasible, several options exist for reconstruction. The portal vein should first be fully mobilized to allow for maximal length on the vein. The coronary vein can be ligated in this circumstance as well should it tether the main portal vein. If the main portal vein can be sewn to the portal vein branch supplying the remnant liver with no tension, a primary anastomosis can be performed. Again, if necessary, the smaller segment of vein can be spatulated or everted to improve size matching. Interposition grafts can be used, with options including the left renal vein, splenic vein, internal jugular vein, iliac vein, or spiralized saphenous vein. Cadaveric vein grafts may be used as well. The anastomosis is typically performed using running 6–0 permanent, monofilament sutures, sewing the back wall first followed by the front wall. The suture can be tied with an air knot to serve as a growth factor once the portal vein clamps are released and portal flow re-initiated. For cases in which the portal vein may be anticipated to increase in size, as is the case in pediatric patients or in cases where substantial hypertrophy may be expected, the portal vein anastomosis can be performed using interrupted absorbable monofilament suture so that the anastomosis itself does not result in narrowing of the portal vein.

The lie of the reconstructed vessels is an important consideration in deciding to perform a primary anastomosis versus a venous extension. This is particularly relevant in right hepatectomies in which the native left portal vein can be sharply angulated and can predispose to stenosis or thrombus formation, even if native inflow is preserved. The right portal vein typically lies in a straighter orientation and is less prone to kinking.

Portal vein modulation may be required prior to performing a portal vein anastomosis should there be a portal vein thrombus or portosystemic shunt related to underlying liver disease. To perform a portal vein thromboendarterectomy, the portal vein should be dissected down toward the confluence of the splenic and superior mesenteric vein, and a vascular clamp should be applied as close as possible to this confluence. A Freer elevator can be used to endarterectomize as far down the vein as can safely be performed without injuring the vein, after which a Fogarty balloon can be passed into the splenic and mesenteric veins to perform a balloon thrombectomy. Should the flow in the portal vein be limited by presence of portosystemic collaterals, the collaterals can be identified and ligated to augment portal venous inflow. Doppler ultrasonography can be used to assess for flow rates through the portal vein to ensure adequacy of portal inflow.

Hepatic Vein Reconstruction

Ensuring adequate hepatic venous drainage is as essential to optimizing liver function as is preserving inflow. Again, a thorough understanding of the remnant liver's venous drainage is necessary to a successful operation. For an extended right hepatectomy, the left hepatic vein is preserved, and the middle and right hepatic veins sacrificed. While conventional hepatic venous anatomy permits resection of the middle hepatic vein, there exists an anatomic variant in which segment III drains into the middle, and not left hepatic vein. In this circumstance, the segment III branch must be reconstructed. Extended left hepatectomies generally rely upon drainage through right hepatic vein, although in up to 25% of the population there exists an inferior hepatic vein that drains segments VI/VII. In these circumstances, the right hepatic vein may be sacrificed with impunity.

Reconstruction of the hepatic veins can be technically challenging, as primary anastomosis or direct implantation are generally not possible due to the length and geometry of the defect. Total vascular isolation may be required to reconstruct hepatic venous drainage, and both inflow through the porta hepatis and outflow through a cuff of the remnant hepatic vein or suprahepatic vena cava should be controlled. Interposition grafts may be constructed using autologous vein, cadaveric vein, or can frequently be performed as well using cadaveric arterial grafts. Arterial conduits offer the benefit of maintaining luminal patency, whereas vein grafts, although anatomically similar to native hepatic vein, may compress and thrombose. Anastomoses here should be performed using a 5–0 or 6–0 permanent, monofilament suture.

Additionally, while there may not be a need to create an interposition graft, resection may include a cuff of hepatic vein, leaving a defect in the hepatic vein orifice. In this case, sewing a patch over the defect may be required to close the hepatic venotomy without narrowing its lumen. This can be done using autologous vein patch, pericardium or peritoneum, cadaveric vein, or xenograft (such as bovine pericardium).

Biliary Reconstruction

Biliary ductal transection generally occurs in an intrahepatic fashion during extended hepatectomy. Several anatomic variants exist in biliary ductal anatomy, and nontraditional anatomy is present in up to 40% of patients. An extended right hepatectomy preserves the bile ducts arising from the left hepatic duct draining segments II/III, while the right posterior sectoral ducts drain the remnant liver in an extended left hepatectomy. More than one duct may exist draining the remnant liver segments. Two options exist for reconstruction—duct-to-duct anastomosis and hepaticojejunostomy. A duct-to-duct anastomosis is rarely performed and requires the ability to approximate native ducts in a tension-free fashion. This can be performed using a combination of interrupted or running 6–0, 7–0, or 8–0 absorbable, non-braided suture; in our practice, the back wall is sewn first, and a plastic stent is placed in the bile duct. Once the stent traverses the anastomosis and ampulla, the front wall is then completed.

More commonly, a tension-free repair is not technically or oncologically feasible and a retrocolic Roux-en-Y hepaticojejunostomy can be performed. Here, the jejunum is transected 30–50 cm distal to the Ligament of Treitz, the distal cut edge of jejunum brought through an avascular opening in the transverse mesocolon and seated at the cut edge of the bile duct. An enterotomy is made on the jejunum and a hepaticojejunostomy is performed in the same fashion as in a duct-to-duct anastomosis. The jejunojejunostomy is either hand-sewn in two layers or stapled after ensuring at least 40 cm Roux-limb length.

Special Considerations

Minimally Invasive Surgery

The majority of extended hepatectomies are currently performed in an open fashion given the extent of resection and technical considerations in resection and reconstruction. Nonetheless, minimally invasive techniques, both laparoscopic and robotic, are more frequently utilized [12]. In both, intraoperative ultrasound can be easily utilized to delineate vascular and biliary anatomy intraoperatively. Advanced laparoscopic cameras as well as the robotic platform may offer additional delineation of anatomy through use of indocyanine green fluorescence, which will preferentially illuminate both tumors to assist in resection as well as the biliary tree to help identify biliary anatomy and potential bile leaks intraoperatively [13].

Ex Vivo Hepatectomy

Certain tumors or disease processes can be technically difficult or impossible to expose in situ, intimately involved with critical vascular structures, or may generate significant blood loss. In these circumstances, liver explant with ex vivo cold perfusion and backtable resection may be feasible. Derived from the core principles of liver transplantation, ex vivo hepatectomy with autotransplantation can allow for meticulous backtable dissection and complex vascular reconstruction in a bloodless setting [14].

Postoperative Management

Given the large surface of the cut edge of the liver as well as in cases requiring biliary reconstruction, our institutional practice is to place a closed suction drain in the postoperative wound bed.

Should a biliary anastomosis be performed with a small duct or a duct susceptible to ischemia, we will place a plastic stent. For cases in which arterial anastomoses are performed, it is our practice to place the patient on a daily aspirin to prevent neointimal hyperplasia. For patients with preoperative portal vein thrombosis, anticoagulation is resumed in the postoperative period when deemed safe from a bleeding perspective.

Complications

While technical refinements have reduced the morbidity of performing an extended hepatectomy, it nevertheless remains a complex operation with potential for significant morbidity and mortality. Given the vascularity and complex biliary tree within the parenchyma of the liver, the most common postoperative complications are related to bleeding, bile leak, and other postoperative fluid collections. These may be caused by infection in the postoperative setting or may result in infected fluid collections.

Another potentially serious complication in the postoperative setting is liver dysfunction. While the liver has regenerative potential, hepatic insufficiency may exist in the postoperative period. This can result in the development of post hepatectomy liver failure, which may manifest in cholestasis, coagulopathy, portal hypertension, and ascites. Additionally, infections in patients with insufficient synthetic liver function can be fatal given their resultant immunocompromised state [15].

Disclosures The authors have no conflicts of interest to disclose.

References

1. Couinad C. Lobes et segments hépatiques: notes sur l'architecture anatomiques et chirurgicale du foie [Liver lobes and segments: notes on the anatomical architecture and surgery of the liver]. Presse Med (1893). 1954;62(33):709–12.

2. Starzl TE, Bell RH, Beart RW, Putnam CW. Hepatic trisegmentectomy and other liver resections. Surg Gynecol Obstet. 1975;141(3):429–37.
3. Kishi Y, Abdalla EK, Chun YS, et al. Three hundred and one consecutive extended right hepatectomies: evaluation of outcome based on systematic liver volumetry. Ann Surg. 2009;250(4):540–8.
4. Vauthey JN, Chaoui A, Do KA, et al. Standardized measurement of the future liver remnant prior to extended liver resection: methodology and clinical associations. Surgery. 2000;127:512–9.
5. Shoup M, Gonen M, D'Angelica M, et al. Volumetric analysis predicts hepatic dysfunction in patients undergoing major liver resection. J Gastrointest Surg. 2003;7:325–30.
6. Guglielmi A, Ruzzenente A, Conci S, et al. How much remnant is enough in liver resection? Dig Surg. 2012;29:6–17.
7. Geisel D, Lüdemann L, Fröling V, et al. Imaging-based evaluation of liver function: comparison of 99mTc-mebrofenin hepatobiliary scintigraphy and Gd-EOB-DTPA-enhanced MRI. Eur Radiol. 2015;25:1384–91.
8. Makuuchi M, Takayasu K, Takuma T, et al. Preoperative transcatheter embolization of the portal venous branch for patients receiving extended lobectomy due to the bile duct carcinoma. J Jpn Pract Surg Soc. 1984;45:1558–64.
9. Teo JY, Allen JC Jr, Ng DC, et al. A systematic review of contralateral liver lobe hypertrophy after unilobar selective internal radiation therapy with Y90. HPB (Oxford). 2016;18(1):7–12.
10. Shindoh J, Truty MJ, Aloia TA, et al. Kinetic growth rate after portal vein embolization predicts posthepatectomy outcomes: toward zero liver-related mortality in patients with colorectal liver metastases and small future liver remnant. J Am Coll Surg. 2013;216(2):201–9.
11. Croome KP, Hernandez-Alejandro R, Parker M, Heimbach J, Rosen C, Nagorney DM. Is the liver kinetic growth rate in ALPPS unprecedented when compared with PVE and living donor liver transplant? A multicentre analysis. HPB (Oxford). 2015;17(6):477–84.
12. Pietrasz D, Fuks D, Subar D, et al. Laparoscopic extended liver resection: are postoperative outcomes different? Surg Endosc. 2018;32(12):4833–40.
13. Mehdorn AS, Beckmann JH, Braun F, Becker T, Egberts JH. Usability of Indocyanine green in robot-assisted hepatic surgery. J Clin Med. 2021;10(3):456.
14. Weiner J, Hemming A, Levi D, et al. Ex vivo liver resection and autotransplantation: should it be used more frequently? Ann Surg. 2022;276(5):854–9.
15. Capussotti L, Viganò L, Giuliante F, Ferrero A, Giovannini I, Nuzzo G. Liver dysfunction and sepsis determine operative mortality after liver resection. Br J Surg. 2009;96(1):88–94.

Part VIII
Biliary Procedures

Bile Duct Resection and Reconstruction

28

Caitlin A. McIntyre and Alice C. Wei

Introduction

Resection and reconstruction of the bile duct is a complex procedure that is performed independently or as a component of another hepatopancreatobiliary procedure. Indications for biliary resection and reconstruction include both benign and malignant entities, and the specific principles of perioperative and operative care are dependent on the indication. Herein, we will focus on the surgical principles of biliary resection and reconstruction, including surgical technique as well as preoperative and postoperative considerations.

C. A. McIntyre
Department of Surgery, Brigham and Women's Hospital, Boston, MA, USA

A. C. Wei (✉)
Department of Surgery, Hepatopancreatobiliary Service, Memorial Sloan Kettering Cancer Center, New York, NY, USA
e-mail: weia@mskcc.org

© The Author(s), under exclusive license to Springer Nature Switzerland AG 2025
A. Alseidi et al. (eds.), *The SAGES Manual of Contemporary Indications and Management of Hepatic and Biliary Diseases*, https://doi.org/10.1007/978-3-032-04823-3_28

Indications

Indications for biliary resection and/or reconstruction can be secondary to both benign and malignant etiologies. These include biliary strictures, which can be either malignant or benign, injury secondary to trauma or iatrogenic injury, or choledochoceles. Malignancy is another indication for biliary resection and/or reconstruction, which includes primary or metastatic cancers of the liver, bile ducts, head of pancreas, or ampulla. The majority of bile duct resections are performed concomitantly as part of another procedures (i.e., pancreatoduodenectomy, extended hepatectomy), while the primary indication for an isolated bile duct resection is common bile duct injury.

In a retrospective study using the Nationwide Inpatient Sample discharges between 2004 and 2011, which included 67,160 patients, more than one half of reconstructions were performed for nonmalignant indications while approximately 38% were performed in the setting of malignancy [1]. In the case of benign disease, 9.9% of biliary reconstructions were performed for biliary injuries, 2.5% for congenital anomalies, 2.3% for benign neoplasms, and 48% for other nonmalignant diseases [1].

Iatrogenic bile duct injury is the most common benign indication for biliary reconstruction. The incidence of bile duct injury following cholecystectomy is less than 1% overall, and has been quoted to be 0.4–1.0% after laparoscopic or robotic cholecystectomy and 0.2–0.5% after open cholecystectomy [2–5]. Early data suggested higher rates after laparoscopic cholecystectomy as compared to open, but now that the minimally invasive approach has been readily adopted, the incidence parallels that of open cholecystectomy, with a rate of 0.08% in modern series [6].

Preoperative Considerations

There are general considerations that should be taken into account on all patients, in order to be sure that patients are preoperatively optimized. For example, patient comorbidities need to be evaluated and patients optimized for general anesthesia. Specific anatomic considerations should be evaluated in each cases, and the operation planned accordingly. Preoperative anatomic mapping with MR cholangiography is prudent if biliary reconstruction is being performed. For bile duct injury, hepatic arterial and portal venous vasculature should be evaluated for concomitant injury.

Furthermore, additional considerations must be taken into account depending on the particular procedure being performed, many of which will be discussed in more depth later in this section as well as other chapters. In cases of biliary resection that include a partial hepatectomy, the extent of liver resection needs to be planned, future liver remnant (FLR) volume calculated, and augmentation of the FLR using techniques such as portal vein embolization (PVE) should be utilized as needed.

Workup

All patients undergoing biliary resection or reconstruction should have a thorough preoperative workup, including cross-sectional imaging, laboratory studies, and when appropriate, endoscopic evaluation. The specific workup is dependent on the underlying pathology, and should be tailored to the indication for the operation.

Basic laboratories obtained in the workup of biliary tract diseases include liver function tests, complete blood count and coagulation studies, which can provide information regarding the etiology and extent of biliary disease, as well as underlying liver disease. Tumor markers can also be obtained in cases where there is a concern for malignancy, including cancer antigen (CA) 19–9, carcinoembryonic antigen (CEA), and alpha-fetoprotein (AFP) levels. However, these are nonspecific and can be elevated in benign conditions including benign biliary obstruction or cholestasis, as well as in other non-hepatopancreatobiliary malignancies. Serum IgG4 should be sent if there is a biliary stricture without an associated malignant diagnosis to rule out an autoimmune cholangiopathy as the cause of the stricture.

Many patients will undergo an abdominal ultrasound early in the course of the disease process, as this is a common modality used in the initial evaluation of right upper quadrant pain. While ultrasound can detect gallstones and biliary ductal dilation, assessment of other underlying pathology requires additional workup.

Multiphasic computed tomography (CT) imaging is commonly used in the workup of biliary tract diseases, and is an important study for evaluating patients with concern for biliary obstruction. It can provide valuable information regarding the level of obstruction and can suggest the underlying etiology. A multiphasic CT of the abdomen and pelvis is the modality of choice to assess for possible malignancy of the biliary tree, liver, or pancreas, and should include non-contrast, arterial, portal venous, with or without delayed phases. The extent of the primary tumor can be adequately evaluated, including vascular involvement, as well as lymphadenopathy and possible distant metastasis, allowing for adequate treatment planning.

Magnetic resonance imaging/cholangiopancreatography (MRI/MRCP) is also used for the evaluation of biliary diseases and mapping of the biliary tract. Similar to CT, this can be used to evaluate the level of biliary obstruction, the presence of lymph node and distant metastases if a malignancy, and can provide additional information regarding the extent of involvement of the ductal system and hilar vasculature. The utility of MRCP in evaluating patients has been demonstrated in several studies and has shown to identify benign or malignant causes of biliary strictures with an accuracy of 90% [7].

Endoscopic intervention may be warranted in selected cases for diagnosis and/or treatment purposes. Endoscopic evaluation with endoscopic ultrasound (EUS) and endoscopic retrograde cholangiopancreatography (ERCP) with or without Spyglass should be used selectively. EUS allows for a more in-depth evaluation of a biliary stricture and may be useful as an adjunct modality if no mass lesion is seen on cross-sectional imaging. Endoscopic ultrasound can be used to better assess and obtain tissue biopsy for primary lesions or pathologic lymph nodes when present. ERCP is used for biliary stent placement for decompression of the biliary tree as discussed below, as well as can be used for tissue acquisition.

Spyglass, or endoscopic choledochoscopy, allows for direct visualization of the CBD lumen for any abnormalities. This is performed at the same time as ERCP, and therefore, tissue sampling as well as stent placement can be done concurrently. The utility of Spyglass has been demonstrated in several studies. In a retrospective series of 52 patients with indeterminate biliary strictures who underwent Spyglass with targeted biopsies, the sensitivity, specificity, and positive and negative predictive values of Spyglass were 88%, 94%, 96%, and 85%, respectively [8]. In patients who have indeterminate biliary strictures, the addition of Spyglass to ERCP and biopsy/brushings increases the sensitivity for detection of malignancy from 58% to 100% [9].

Preoperative Biliary Drainage

In cases of biliary obstruction, preoperative biliary drainage should be considered. Patients who present with cholangitis or those with biliary obstruction who are planned to receive neoadjuvant chemotherapy should undergo biliary drainage. However, the need for biliary drainage should be reviewed on an individualized basis as prior data evaluating preoperative drainage with surgical outcomes is mixed. Several studies have demonstrated decreased morbidity and mortality with the use of biliary stent placement, while others have showed an increased risk of complications, including surgical site infections and mortality. The decision for placement of a preoperative biliary stent is multifactorial, including considerations such as bilirubin level or anticipated FLR. For example, in cases of extended hepatectomy for hilar cholangiocarcinoma, preoperative biliary drainage is recommended when the anticipated FLR is <30% (as compared to those with an FLR >30%), as biliary drainage was associated with lower rates of postoperative liver failure and decreased mortality [10].

Biliary drainage can be performed endoscopically with ERCP and stent placement or through percutaneous drainage. In our practice, we favor ERCP with stent placement for obstructions below the bifurcation of the hepatic ducts and percutaneous transhepatic cholangiography (PTC), without transgression of the ampulla when the level of obstruction is at or above the bifurcation. A primary consideration when assessing methods of biliary drainage is to minimize the risk of colonization of the biliary tree and subsequent cholangitis. The incidence of cholangitis can be as high as 40% with ERCP, and even higher in patients who do not undergo successful drainage [11]. Furthermore, in cases of perihilar cholangiocarcinoma or other operations that involve hepatic resection, a priority should be optimal drainage of the FLR to ultimately preserve liver function.

Bile Duct Resection

Principles of Bile Duct Resection

Resection of the bile duct can be performed through an open or minimally invasive approach, and many principles are shared between the two methods. The decision to perform an open versus minimally invasive operation depends on the procedure being performed and the expertise of the surgeon. A biliary resection and reconstruction should be performed in the elective setting whenever possible. This allows for optimization of the patient, including resolution of cholangitis and improvement in jaundice.

Preoperative planning is of utmost importance and includes the evaluation of the anatomy, the level of biliary obstruction, or assessment of extent of disease if malignancy is present. Careful attention must be paid to the anatomy of portal structures, including variant or replaced arterial anatomy and sectoral branching of the portal vein and bile duct.

In cases of malignant disease, resection of the extrahepatic biliary tree is typically performed in conjunction with either a partial hepatectomy or pancreatoduodenectomy to ensure margin clearance. In instances of benign disease and select malignant disease, isolated resection of the extrahepatic bile duct can be completed. Indications for isolated bile duct resection are uncommon. The most common indications include injury to the common bile duct, benign bile duct stricture, or choledochocyst. The common bile duct should be resected to the suprapancreatic component;

however, in select cases, resection of the intrapancreatic common bile duct can be performed.

There are several considerations specific to biliary resection for malignancy. This includes obtaining adequate margins and performing an adequate portal lymphadenectomy when indicated. All tumors should be resected to negative margins as per AJCC standard definitions, and intraoperative frozen section can be utilized to confirm the presence of negative margins. A portal lymphadenectomy is indicated in cases of cholangiocarcinoma and gallbladder carcinoma, and care must be taken to decrease the risk of ischemia during this dissection. Furthermore, for malignant disease, several groups advocate for diagnostic laparoscopy at the time of the operation, as occult metastatic disease can be detected in up to 50% of patients [12].

Specifically in the case of bile duct injury, timing of repair can affect long-term outcomes. It is recommended that repair occurs either immediately after injury or delayed (>6 weeks), but repair between 2 and 6 weeks should be avoided. Prior studies have shown that repair during this intermediate time (2–6 weeks) is associated with increased morbidity, in particular, an increased rate of biliary stricture [13, 14].

Operation

The general operative steps are similar between open and minimally invasive approaches [15, 16]. Adequate exposure is an important consideration. Open resection is performed through an upper midline incision or a right subcostal incision. For minimally invasive biliary resection, patients are placed in right upper quadrant positioning. At our institution, a robotic approach is used with the patients in a split leg supine, 12–18° reverse Trendelenburg position. Four robotic ports are placed along the periumbilical line with a 12 mm assist port in the lower midline (Fig. 28.1).

The operation should begin with an extended Kocher maneuver and dissection of the hepatoduodenal ligament. During this portion of the operation, care must be taken to identify and preserve the hepatic arteries and portal vein, in order to maintain

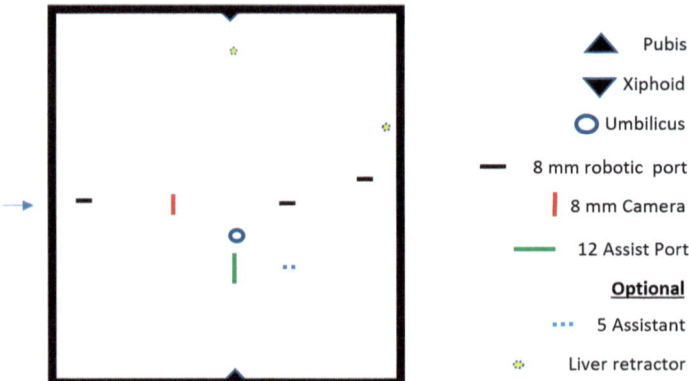

Supine split leg 12-18 degree reverse Trendelenberg position

Fig. 28.1 Patient position for robotic hepaticojejunostomy

blood supply to the remaining portion of the bile duct. In the case of biliary reconstruction following bile duct injury or prior surgery, adhesions may be present in the hepatoduodenal ligament and must be lysed to identify the proximal and distal biliary structures. The hilar plate may need to be lowered to access the proximal bile ducts.

Several techniques can be used to help delineate the bile duct and surrounding structures, and aid in resection. Direct cholangiography or indocyanine green fluorescence (ICG) cholangiography can be used to delineate the biliary system and/or vascular structures. Trans cystic catheters (e.g., pediatric feeding tubes or biliary Fogarty catheters) can be placed at the time of surgery or for patients who have preexisting biliary stents or PTC in place, and these tubes can be followed distally to assist in identification of the biliary structures. Intraoperative choledochoscopy can also be used. When a purported biliary structure is identified, it may be prudent to use a small gauge needle to confirm the presence of bile prior to entering the structure.

For resection of the bile duct, mobilization of the bile duct and early division of the distal extent can facilitate resection and minimize injury to other structures in the hepatoduodenal ligament.

For malignancies, proximal/distal and radial margin clearance must be considered, which may require multivisceral resections (i.e., liver resections or pancreaticoduodenectomy). Also, in such cases, regional lymphadenectomy should be performed including at minimum lymph node stations 8, 12 +/− 13. Frozen section margins of the bile duct should be considered when further margin clearance can be achieved. Following biliary resection, the distal portion of the common bile duct is oversewn, when present.

Reconstruction is then performed to restore continuity of the biliary tree and gastrointestinal tract. When performing resection, care must be taken to confirm that the bile duct remains well vascularized for the anticipated reconstruction. The entire common bile duct should be resected to the level of the common hepatic duct, as 70% of the blood flow to the bile duct comes from the hepatic arterial system on the liver side. This will ensure adequate vascularization for reconstruction.

Bile Duct Reconstruction

Principles of Bile Duct Reconstruction

A well-vascularized tension-free anastomosis is the key to a high-quality bile duct reconstruction. This can be achieved either with conventional open approach or a minimally invasive approach as long as meticulous surgical technique is used. Specific details of biliary reconstruction are dependent on the indication for reconstruction, extent of prior resection or injury, and other patient factors. In settings of bile duct resection for a benign or malignant indication, reconstruction is performed immediately following resection, whereas in cases of biliary injury, reconstruction can be either immediate or delayed. In operations for biliary injury, it is important to seek advice of an experienced hepatobiliary surgeon and consider referral to a tertiary center, as this has been shown to be associated with decreased morbidity.

There are several methods of biliary reconstruction, and the specific ductal-enteric anastomosis performed depends on the level of bile duct transection and any additional simultaneous resections. The most common reconstruction is a Roux-en-Y hepaticojejunostomy at the level of the common hepatic duct. This configuration ensures the biliary and enteric ends are optimally vascularized. Historically, other ductal-enteric anastomoses have been performed, such as a choledochojejunostomy; however, this reconstruction was associated with a high rate of strictures given that the blood supply to the bile duct comes from the liver side of the biliary tree. A choledochoduodenostomy can be performed in select cases depending on the anatomy and indications. Lastly, a primary repair or end-to-end repair should be avoided in all but very select cases due to high stricture rates.

The Roux limb of the hepaticojejunostomy is typically passed in a retro-colic fashion and should be approximately 40–60 cm in length [17, 18]. When performed in the context of a robotic pancreaticoduodenectomy, many prefer to use a retro-mesenteric, rather than a retro-colic neo-duodenal limb. The hepaticojejunostomy (HJ) can be performed in either a running or interrupted fashion using absorbable suture depending on the diameter of the bile duct and preference of the surgeon. Commonly, interrupted sutures are used for ducts that are small in diameter, whereas large ducts are more often done in a running fashion. Some groups will advocate for the use of trans-anastomotic stents, while others do not feel this is warranted [19]. In our practice, a running PDS-5-0 is used for open HJ reconstructions and a running barbed 4–0 V-loc is used for robotic reconstructions for bile ducts 5 mm or larger. For smaller ducts, an interrupted 5–0 PDS is used over a 5 French stent. Routine drainage following biliary reconstruction is not indicated and should be used selectively based on patient and operative risk factors.

There are special considerations that must be taken into account. If the bile duct is transected above the biliary confluence, multiple bile duct orifices are present. When possible, the biliary orifices should be incorporated into a single anastomosis by bringing together the mucosal edges between orifices with interrupted absorbable sutures. If the distance between orifices is too wide to permit this, then separate biliary-enteric anastomoses should be performed.

In cases of bile duct injury that involves less than one-third of the circumference of the duct for a short distance, primary repair with or without a T-tube may be considered if can done safely without compromising the bile duct lumen. In cases of biliary obstruction where resection is not indicated (i.e., metastatic cancer obstructing the distal bile duct), a side-to-side bypass can be performed.

Postoperative Considerations

An Enhanced Recovery After Surgery (ERAS) pathway to optimize patient recovery and decrease length of stay. Orogastric tubes can be removed immediately after surgery. Standard perioperative antibiotics are used for surgical site prophylaxis. Extended antibiotic coverage is not recommended for elective procedures. If drains are left at the time of resection, we practice early drain removal.

Complications

The most common morbidities associated with biliary resection and reconstruction include anastomotic stricture and leak, as well as other complications associated with abdominal operations, such as postoperative hemorrhage, surgical site infection, and difficulties from general anesthesia. The overall complication rate is dependent on indication for surgery and whether multivisceral resection was performed.

Anastomotic strictures occur in up to 13% of biliary reconstructions, and the incidence is dependent on the indication for reconstruction [20–22]. Patients who underwent preoperative biliary drainage and postoperative stenting were at an increased risk of stricture formation [20, 21]. Management of biliary strictures includes biliary stent placement, dilation, or in more severe cases, revision of the biliary-enteric anastomosis. Dilation can be performed endoscopically or using a percutaneous approach, with patency rates at 2 years following endoscopic balloon dilatation approaching 55–65% [23, 24].

Anastomotic leak is another complication associated with biliary reconstruction, occurring in up to 7% of cases [22, 25, 26]. Again, differences in rates of bile leak depend on the indication for resection, yet rates are similar between open and minimally invasive approaches. Initial management requires control of infection and percutaneous drain placement, and many of these will resolve with conservative management. In more severe cases, biliary stent placement or even reoperation may be required.

Conclusion

In conclusion, biliary resection is a commonly performed procedure for both benign and malignant indications, and most often this includes a multivisceral resection. Biliary reconstruction is performed following resection or in cases of injury to the bile duct. These are complex procedures that require the expertise of a high-volume hepatobiliary surgery center, and specific considerations must be evaluated in the context of the indication for the procedure as well as taking into account specific patient factors.

References

1. Eskander MF, Bliss LA, Yousafzai OK, et al. A nationwide assessment of outcomes after bile duct reconstruction. HPB (Oxford). 2015;17:753–62.
2. Gouma DJ, Go PM. Bile duct injury during laparoscopic and conventional cholecystectomy. J Am Coll Surg. 1994;178:229–33.
3. Morgenstern L, Wong L, Berci G. Twelve hundred open cholecystectomies before the laparoscopic era. A standard for comparison. Arch Surg. 1992;127:400–3.
4. Adamsen S, Hansen OH, Funch-Jensen P, et al. Bile duct injury during laparoscopic cholecystectomy: a prospective nationwide series. J Am Coll Surg. 1997;184:571–8.
5. Richardson MC, Bell G, Fullarton GM. Incidence and nature of bile duct injuries following laparoscopic cholecystectomy: an audit of 5913 cases. West of Scotland Laparoscopic Cholecystectomy Audit Group. Br J Surg. 1996;83:1356–60.

6. Halbert C, Pagkratis S, Yang J, et al. Beyond the learning curve: incidence of bile duct injuries following laparoscopic cholecystectomy normalize to open in the modern era. Surg Endosc. 2016;30:2239–43.
7. Suthar M, Purohit S, Bhargav V, et al. Role of MRCP in differentiation of benign and malignant causes of biliary obstruction. J Clin Diagn Res. 2015;9:TC08–12.
8. Manta R, Frazzoni M, Conigliaro R, et al. SpyGlass single-operator peroral cholangioscopy in the evaluation of indeterminate biliary lesions: a single-center, prospective, cohort study. Surg Endosc. 2013;27:1569–72.
9. Draganov PV, Chauhan S, Wagh MS, et al. Diagnostic accuracy of conventional and cholangioscopy-guided sampling of indeterminate biliary lesions at the time of ERCP: a prospective, long-term follow-up study. Gastrointest Endosc. 2012;75:347–53.
10. Kennedy TJ, Yopp A, Qin Y, et al. Role of preoperative biliary drainage of liver remnant prior to extended liver resection for hilar cholangiocarcinoma. HPB (Oxford). 2009;11:445–51.
11. Ipek S, Alper E, Cekic C, et al. Evaluation of the effectiveness of endoscopic retrograde cholangiopancreatography in patients with perihilar cholangiocarcinoma and its effect on development of cholangitis. Gastroenterol Res Pract. 2014;2014:508286.
12. Weber SM, DeMatteo RP, Fong Y, et al. Staging laparoscopy in patients with extrahepatic biliary carcinoma. Analysis of 100 patients. Ann Surg. 2002;235:392–9.
13. Sahajpal AK, Chow SC, Dixon E, et al. Bile duct injuries associated with laparoscopic cholecystectomy: timing of repair and long-term outcomes. Arch Surg. 2010;145:757–63.
14. Schreuder AM, Nunez Vas BC, Booij KAC, et al. Optimal timing for surgical reconstruction of bile duct injury: meta-analysis. BJS Open. 2020;4:776–86.
15. Wu J, Xiang Y, You G, et al. An essential technique for modern hepatopancreato-biliary surgery: minimally invasive biliary reconstruction. Expert Rev Gastroenterol Hepatol. 2021;15:243–54.
16. Marichez A, Adam JP, Laurent C, et al. Hepaticojejunostomy for bile duct injury: state of the art. Langenbeck's Arch Surg. 2023;408:108.
17. Lillemoe KD, Melton GB, Cameron JL, et al. Postoperative bile duct strictures: management and outcome in the 1990s. Ann Surg. 2000;232:430–41.
18. Stewart L. Iatrogenic biliary injuries: identification, classification, and management. Surg Clin North Am. 2014;94:297–310.
19. Mercado MA, Chan C, Orozco H, et al. To stent or not to stent bilioenteric anastomosis after iatrogenic injury: a dilemma not answered? Arch Surg. 2002;137:60–3.
20. Dimou FM, Adhikari D, Mehta HB, et al. Incidence of hepaticojejunostomy stricture after hepaticojejunostomy. Surgery. 2016;160:691–8.

21. House MG, Cameron JL, Schulick RD, et al. Incidence and outcome of biliary strictures after pancreaticoduodenectomy. Ann Surg. 2006;243:571–6. discussion 576-8
22. Bustos R, Fernandes E, Mangano A, et al. Robotic hepaticojejunostomy: surgical technique and risk factor analysis for anastomotic leak and stenosis. HPB (Oxford). 2020;22:1442–9.
23. Mizukawa S, Tsutsumi K, Kato H, et al. Endoscopic balloon dilatation for benign hepaticojejunostomy anastomotic stricture using short double-balloon enteroscopy in patients with a prior Whipple's procedure: a retrospective study. BMC Gastroenterol. 2018;18:14.
24. Mie T, Sasaki T, Okamoto T, et al. Risk factors for recurrent stenosis after balloon dilation for benign hepaticojejunostomy anastomotic stricture. Clin Endosc. 2024;57:253–62.
25. Farooqui W, Penninga L, Burgdorf SK, et al. Biliary leakage following pancreatoduodenectomy: experience from a high-volume center. J Pancreat Cancer. 2021;7:80–5.
26. Wang R, Jiang P, Chen Q, et al. Pancreatic fistula and biliary fistula after laparoscopic pancreatoduodenectomy: 500 patients at a single institution. J Minim Access Surg. 2023;19:28–34.

Radical Cholecystectomy

29

Elizabeth L. Carpenter
and Timothy E. Newhook

Introduction

Gallbladder cancer is the most common biliary tract malignancy [1]. However, while higher numbers may be seen internationally, gallbladder cancer is relatively rare in the United States with an overall incidence of 1.1 per 100,000 person-years according to a recent Surveillance, Epidemiology, and End Results (SEER) registry analysis of cases from 1973 to 2015 [1, 2]. Unfortunately, given the lack of early defined symptoms, the majority of patients present with locally advanced or metastatic disease [1].

The management of gallbladder cancer depends on pathologic factors. A simple cholecystectomy is sufficient for patients with tumors that do not invade the muscular layer (T1a) [3]. However, patients with resectable disease that invades the muscular layer (T1b) or through the muscular layer into the perimuscular connective tissue (T2) should undergo radical cholecystectomy, defined as resection of the gallbladder and gallbladder fossa with en bloc

E. L. Carpenter
San Antonio Military Medical Center, San Antonio, TX, USA

T. E. Newhook (✉)
Department of Surgical Oncology, The University of Texas MD Anderson Cancer Center, Houston, TX, USA
e-mail: TNewhook@mdanderson.org

© The Author(s), under exclusive license to Springer Nature Switzerland AG 2025
A. Alseidi et al. (eds.), *The SAGES Manual of Contemporary Indications and Management of Hepatic and Biliary Diseases*,
https://doi.org/10.1007/978-3-032-04823-3_29

partial hepatectomy, accompanied by portal lymphadenectomy [3, 4]. The surgical management of patients with T1b disease has been historically controversial, but radical cholecystectomy is associated with improved disease-specific survival in patients with T1b gallbladder cancer and is the recommended treatment per the 2015 American Hepato-Pancreato-Biliary Association (AHPBA) expert consensus statement [4, 5].

The extent of liver resection required for a radical cholecystectomy varies by literature source. Resection of adjacent liver parenchyma may be sufficient to obtain an R0 resection for lower stage tumors, whereas a formal IVb/V segmentectomy may be necessary for higher stage tumors [4]. Routine major hepatectomy and/or bile duct resection have been associated with worse patient outcomes without survival benefit and are therefore not recommended unless needed to obtain negative margins [3, 4, 6, 7].

This chapter will describe radical cholecystectomy with segment IVb/V resection as it pertains to the care of patients with known gallbladder cancer. The management of incidentally discovered gallbladder cancer after cholecystectomy has several notable differences from that of a gallbladder mass, which is the focus of this chapter, and will not be discussed. Oncologic extended resection, portal lymphadenectomy, and bile duct resection are the focus of other chapters.

Preoperative Planning

Preoperative imaging is not just a critical component of the workup and diagnosis of gallbladder cancer but also an invaluable tool for operative planning. When a gallbladder mass concerning for malignancy is identified, triple-phase contrasted CT is the initial imaging modality of choice to determine the extent of the disease and presence of metastasis, with a sensitivity of 85–100% and specificity of 67–83% for identification of resectable disease [8]. Meanwhile, MRI may be helpful for inspection of biliary ducts and the liver in the setting of steatosis or cirrhosis and assist with delineation of disease in close proximity to the hepatoduodenal ligament and/or portal vein [1, 4]. MRI may aid in the detection of suspicious lymph nodes. If in question, FDG-PET/CT as a complimentary study has an accuracy of up to 86% for identifying lymph node enlargement/involvement and is often used for staging purposes [1, 9].

Review of a patient's relevant anatomy is essential when planning the operation. Areas of particular focus should include whether the mass invades the perimuscular connective tissue on the peritoneal side versus hepatic side, which differentiates T2a from T2b disease, or extends into the liver or other adjacent organs (T3) [10]. A mass that invades the portal vein, hepatic artery, or ≥ 2 extrahepatic organs/structures defines T4 disease [3]. Invasion of extrahepatic structures and/or major vasculature seen in T3/T4 tumors may require a more extensive operation than described here, if warranted. Careful inspection should be undertaken of the hepatic artery, vein, and duct, noting their course, any aberrancy, and relationship to other structures (e.g., anterior or posterior positioning of right hepatic vein in relation to hepatic duct).

In addition to preoperative imaging, staging laparoscopy may be used to determine resectability. Simple laparoscopy can reveal peritoneal disease or metastatic liver surface deposits that preclude resection. Adjuncts, such as laparoscopic ultrasound, aortocaval lymph node sampling (especially if suspicious on MRI or PET/CT, as described above), or peritoneal washings, may reveal additional disease and/or lymph node metastasis on frozen section analysis. In one prospective study conducted between 2006 and 2011 for patients with radiographically resectable gallbladder cancer, the accuracy of staging laparoscopy was 94% for detectable lesions, such as peritoneal or liver surface metastasis, and 56% for unresectable disease overall. Subgroup analysis of this cohort determined that overall yield of staging laparoscopy was higher in patients with locally advanced cancer compared to early disease. However, there was no difference in accuracy between the two groups, which the authors suggest may underscore the importance of staging laparoscopy even in early gallbladder cancer [11]. For a mass detected on imaging, the National Comprehensive Cancer Network guidelines state that staging laparoscopy should be *considered* in determining resectability, whereas the AHPBA expert consensus statement *recommends* staging laparoscopy prior to laparotomy in cases of suspected disease without tissue diagnosis [3, 4].

Operative Approach

Minimally invasive surgery (MIS) has become the standard of care for routine cholecystectomy. Concerns, however, regarding cancer cell dissemination and inadequate oncologic resections due to complexity of a hepatectomy have hindered an MIS approach to gallbladder cancer [12–15]. Inferior nodal evaluation when using a minimally invasive technique has been observed in other biliary tract cancers, though in a retrospective analysis of the National Cancer Database comparing open versus MIS radical cholecystectomy for gallbladder cancer, lymph node yield was equivalent between the two groups [13, 16].

Given these concerns and in the absence of randomized data directly comparing approaches, MIS gallbladder resection for gallbladder cancer should be limited to specialized centers according to the most recent AHPBA consensus statement [4]. Technical expertise, experience of both the surgeon and facility, as well as individual patient factors, should all be carefully weighed when selecting an operative approach. Ultimately, a safe resection accompanied by sound oncologic principles is mandatory, regardless of the approach.

Perioperative Management

Patients should be evaluated for operative candidacy by assessing medical history, determining need of optimization of comorbid conditions or performance status, as well as prior abdominal and/or hepatobiliary surgery. Preoperative discussion with the anesthesia team regarding operative approach and management is critical. Particular attention must be paid to evaluation of hepatic reserve in the preparation for hepatectomy.

When considering preoperative antibiotic prophylaxis, coverage of skin flora is generally sufficient for resection of a gallbladder mass. If the patient has undergone preoperative biliary stenting, however, antibiotic prophylaxis should be extended to include intestinal flora coverage [17]. Deep venous thromboembolism mechanical and chemoprophylaxis should also be considered.

Open

Open surgery remains the gold standard of radical cholecystectomy [4, 14, 18]. All surgeons should be familiar with open resection, as the conversion rate from a minimally invasive (either laparoscopic or robotic) to open approach has been reported to be as high as 47% [13, 15, 18–20].

While a right subcostal "Kocher" incision is often described for access to the gallbladder and biliary tree, it is the authors' preference to utilize a midline laparotomy or inverted-L (modified "Makuuchi") incision (Fig. 29.1) to prevent need for crossing the midline for extension (seen in bilateral subcostal incisions) or xyphoid extension (seen in Mercedes/Hockey stick incisions) for an open radical cholecystectomy [17, 21, 22]. Xiphoid resection (optional) and placement of the Thompson retractor (Thompson Surgical Instruments, Inc., Traverse City, MI) with sidebars facilitates excellent exposure of the right upper quadrant (Fig. 29.2) [22]. For parenchymal transection of segment IVb and V, we recommend the use of the CUSA ultrasonic dissector (Integra LifeSciences, Princeton, NJ) as part of the "Two-Surgeon Technique," which is described in greater details later in the chapter [23, 24].

Laparoscopic

No randomized data exists to directly compare MIS to open radical cholecystectomy, but both retrospective and prospective cohort data demonstrate the safety of a laparoscopic approach, with com-

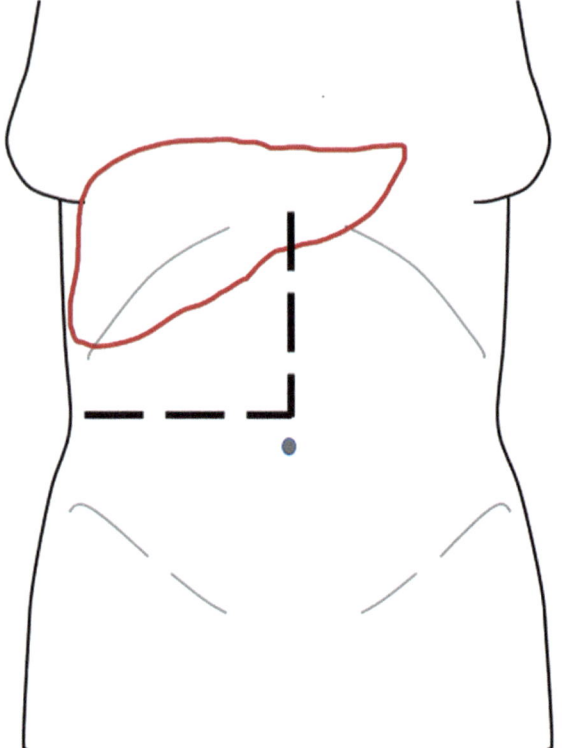

Fig. 29.1 Inverted L/modified "Makuuchi" incision

parable oncologic outcomes to open surgery [13, 25, 26]. Most importantly, laparoscopic resection is associated with earlier recovery and reduced readmission compared to an open approach [13, 27]. Additional advantages of the laparoscopic approach may include pneumoperitoneum assisting in tamponade of bleeding during liver parenchymal resection [28].

Patients may be positioned supine in mild reverse Trendelenburg. The operating surgeon may stand between the patient's legs or alternatively on the right side [25, 26, 28]. Port placement varies by surgeon. One set-up includes the camera 10 mm port placed in the supraumbilical position, a working

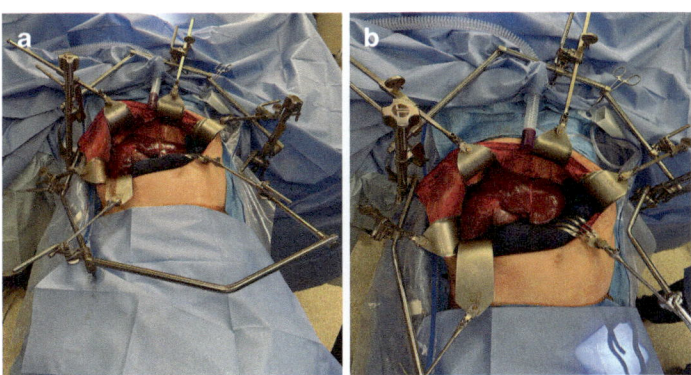

Fig. 29.2 Thompson retractor placement from end of operating table (**a**) and overhead (**b**) views

10 mm port in mid-clavicular left subcostal position with a 5 mm retractor port just below in anterior axillary line, another working 5 mm port in the mid-clavicular right subcostal position, and a 10 mm epigastric port (Fig. 29.3) [26].

Laparoscopic ultrasound should be used to identify surgical margins and relevant anatomy, including the segment IVb and V tributaries to the middle hepatic vein and portal triads of segments IVb and V [26]. Instruments of choice include the Harmonic Scalpel (Ethicon US, LLC, Cincinnati, OH) or monopolar diathermy to mark the dissection plane and incise Glisson's capsule. The Harmonic Scalpel, LigaSure (Medtronic, Minneapolis, MN), or bipolar device may be used for deep hepatic parenchymal dissection [25, 26, 28]. Further, the laparoscopic CUSA (Integra LifeSciences, Princeton, NJ) ultrasonic dissector may assist for parenchymal transection [23].

Robotic

Robotic-assisted surgery has become increasingly popular not only for a variety of common surgical procedures such as routine cholecystectomy but also for more complex cancer resections

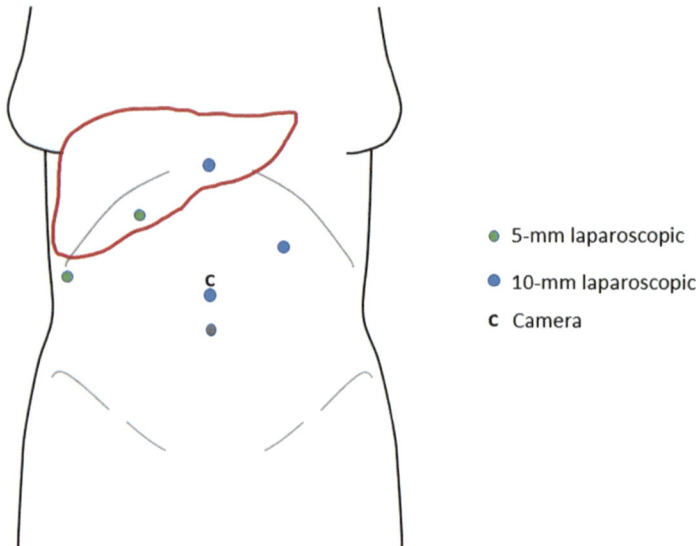

Fig. 29.3 Laparoscopic port placement

[29]. This platform combines the benefits of early recovery with an MIS approach with those seen exclusively in robotics, such as improved ergonomics and three-dimensional visualization [30]. Additionally, robotic resection may result in increased nodal harvest as compared to laparoscopic surgery and has been associated with reduced postoperative morbidity and blood loss when compared to open radical cholecystectomy [12, 18]. The use of indocyanine green (ICG) is not unique to robotics, but built-in fluorescence imaging may assist in defining anatomy during dissection, particularly in a reoperative field [31]. The costs of the robotic platform are a limitation of widespread implementation [12, 29].

Patients may be positioned supine in approximately 12–14° of reverse Trendelenburg. Recommended port placement using the DaVinci Xi platform (Intuitive Surgical Inc., Sunnyvale, CA) is

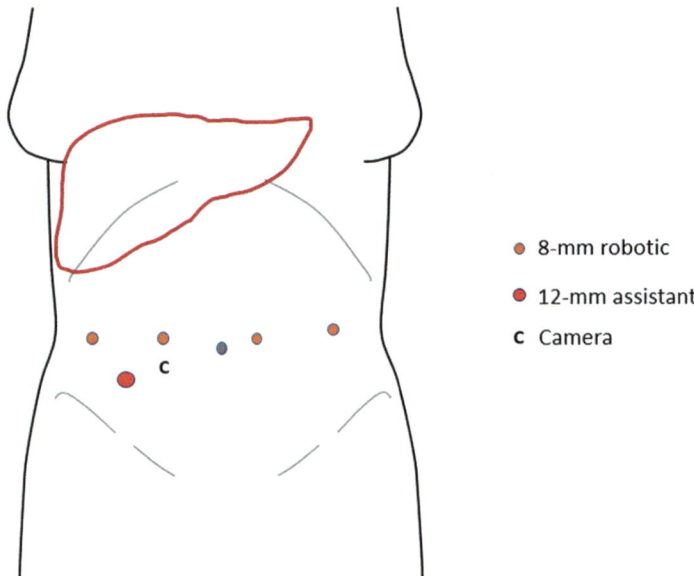

Fig. 29.4 Robotic port placement

demonstrated in Fig. 29.4. In Arm 1, the fenestrated bipolar with electrocautery is recommended, followed by the camera in Arm 2. In Arm 3, the authors recommend the cautery hook for portal dissection and vessel sealer for parenchymal transection via the clamp-crush technique. In Arm 4, either the Cadiere forceps or tip-up fenestrated grasper is typically used.

The set-up of each operative approach with positioning and instruments of choice are summarized in Table 29.1.

Table 29.1 Set-up by operative approach

Open	Laparoscopic	Robotic
Positioning: supine	*Positioning*: reverse Trendelenburg with left side down or low lithotomy	*Positioning*: supine in reverse Trendelenburg
Instruments: Thompson retractor	*Instruments*: Harmonic Scalpel, monopolar diathermy, Ligasure, bipolar diathermy	*Instruments*: Fenestrated bipolar (Arm 1), Camera (Arm 2), Hook/Vessel Sealer (Arm 3), Cadiere vs. Tip-up (Arm 4)

Key Steps

Here, we describe the essential steps required when performing a radical cholecystectomy, both from an open and robotic approach.

Open

1. Enter the abdomen via midline laparotomy or inverted-L incision (Fig. 29.1), with retractor set-up as shown in Fig. 29.2.
2. Carefully assess for evidence of metastasis on liver and peritoneal surfaces. Examine for celiac axis or aortocaval lymphadenopathy, which may prompt intraoperative frozen section prior to proceeding.
3. Divide the falciform ligament to facilitate exposure. This can later be used as a handle to assist with liver mobilization.
4. Perform an intraoperative ultrasound of the liver along the gallbladder and fossa to visualize extent of the tumor and its invasion, confirm planned margins, and evaluate relevant anatomy.
5. Divide the gastrohepatic ligament to expose the common hepatic artery and porta hepatis for examination. Here, the porta can be encircled for later Pringle maneuver with an umbilical tape for use as a Rommel tourniquet.

6. Complete the cholecystectomy. Ligate the cystic duct at its confluence with the common bile duct and send for frozen section analysis. If positive, consideration should be given to resect the hepatic and common bile duct, with reconstruction via Roux-en-Y hepaticojejunostomy. It is critical during this dissection to prevent rupture of the gallbladder and resultant bile spillage.
7. Begin the IVb/V segmentectomy. Mark Glisson's capsule with electrocautery, repeating an intraoperative ultrasound of the liver to confirm margins and again as needed throughout this portion of the operation. Parenchymal transection can be completed via a variety of techniques, to include clamp-crush, ultrasonic dissection, etc. Vessels may be ligated via clips, suture, or vascular staple load depending on size and surgeon preference. A Pringle maneuver is recommended to assist with hemostasis, if necessary.
8. At completion of hepatic resection, the transected parenchyma should be inspected for hemostasis and patency of biliary radicals. An air cholangiogram (described later in the text) is performed to evaluate for bile leak. Additional hemostatic agents, fibrin sealants, or electrocautery devices such as the Aquamantys (Medtronic, Minneapolis, MN) or argon beam coagulator may be used.
9. The abdomen is closed in the standard fashion. A drain is not routinely placed unless a biliary leakage is identified that cannot be repaired.

Robotic

1. (Laparoscopic) Access the abdomen via port positioning described above (Fig. 29.4).
2. (Laparoscopic) Start with a diagnostic laparoscopy, assessing for evidence of metastasis on peritoneal and liver surfaces or celiac axis/aortocaval lymphadenopathy requiring frozen section prior to proceeding.
3. (Laparoscopic) Divide the falciform ligament with electrocautery to expose the anterior surface of the liver.

4. (Laparoscopic) Perform an intraoperative ultrasound of the area of planned resection, confirming location of the tumor in relation to surrounding anatomy.
5. Dock the robot.
6. Divide the gastrohepatic ligament. Encircle the porta hepatis for later Pringle maneuver. Both extracorporeal and intracorporeal techniques for MIS Pringle maneuver have been described, but use a similar technique [32].
7. Perform a cholecystectomy, ligating the cystic duct at the confluence with the common bile duct. This should be sent for frozen analysis, as a positive margin may require resection of the hepatic and common bile duct with Roux-en-Y hepaticojejunostomy. Avoid rupture of the gallbladder or bile spillage.
8. The remaining steps of the procedure are performed as they would be in the open approach. In the MIS operation, ICG can be a useful adjunct to clarify anatomy, if needed. Parenchymal transection can be performed in a variety of fashions from a robotic approach. The authors prefer transecting the hepatic parenchyma using the Vessel Sealer (Intuitive Surgical Inc., Sunnyvale, CA) via a clamp-crush technique.
9. Once the resection is complete, the specimen is removed with an EndoCatch bag via an extension of a port site.
10. The robotic trocar sites are closed in the standard fashion.

Intraoperative Pitfalls and Postoperative Complications

Intraoperative pitfalls associated with any approach, whether open or MIS, can lead to complications that vary from troublesome to disastrous. A combination of dutiful preparation, excellent technique, and adherence to oncologic principles will assist in mitigating avoidable complications.

Undetected metastatic disease may be recognized on staging laparoscopy, as discussed earlier in the chapter, and with the use of adjuncts including laparoscopic ultrasound and aortocaval lymph node sampling [11]. A thorough investigation reduces the risk of a nontherapeutic operation. A positive margin, on the other hand, may be prevented via careful mapping prior to resection of anatomic landmarks with intraoperative liver ultrasound, which has a high sensitivity for detection of lesions deep in liver parenchyma [11].

Major bile duct and hepatic artery injury is a feared complication of any hepatectomy, potentially requiring further resection or even reconstruction. Good preoperative planning with an extensive study of the patient's anatomy is, in the authors' opinion, the best strategy to avoid iatrogenic injury. ICG is available for use in both laparoscopic and robotic cases, which may be especially helpful in delineating difficult anatomy in the setting of anatomic variations, as well as a reoperative field [33]. Venous tributaries to the main hepatic veins of segment IVb/V and further to the middle hepatic vein should be carefully identified and controlled.

Risk of postoperative bile leak may be reduced by several means. The air leak test, or air cholangiogram, is completed after parenchymal transection and following confirmation of a negative cystic duct margin. In this technique, a cholangiography catheter is placed within the cystic duct. The abdomen is filled with saline, and air is injected via this catheter while the distal common bile duct is occluded manually. Air bubbles may be seen in open bile ducts, which are thus identified and subsequently controlled. In its initial study conducted by Zimmitti et al., the air leak test led to a seven-fold higher rate of intraoperative leak detection and repair, with a reduction in both overall and severe postoperative bile leaks [34]. In regard to parenchymal transection, the "Two-Surgeon Technique" with saline-linked cautery and ultrasonic dissection is another means of reducing postoperative bile leak. This technique has also been shown to reduce inflow occlusion time, intraoperative blood loss, and total operating time [23, 24, 35].

Additional postoperative complications after radical cholecystectomy are similar to those seen after hepatectomy for other indications and are further described elsewhere in this book. Ischemic stricture of the common hepatic duct or common bile duct may be seen due to disruption of blood supply during portal lymphadenectomy [17, 36]. A summary of operative pitfalls and mitigation strategies are detailed in Table 29.2.

Table 29.2 Common pitfalls and mitigation strategies

Pitfall	Mitigation strategy
Unresectable disease	Staging laparoscopy, intraoperative ultrasound, and celiac/aortocaval lymph node sampling
Iatrogenic duct or vascular injury	Preoperative study of patient imaging, ICG (MIS)
Postoperative bile leak	Air leak test, "Two-Surgeon Technique"

Oncologic Outcomes and Follow-Up

Numerous studies have attempted to define specific regimens and elucidate benefit of adjuvant therapy in patients with gallbladder cancer. The BILCAP study, a multicenter phase III study of 44 hepatobiliary centers across the United Kingdom, aimed to determine the benefit of adjuvant capecitabine on overall survival (OS) in patients with histologically confirmed cholangiocarcinoma or gallbladder cancer undergoing curative intent resection. While the intention-to-treat (ITT) analysis failed to show benefit (51 mo vs. 36 mo, $p = 0.097$), a per-protocol (PP) analysis adjusted for nodal status, grade, and gender demonstrated a prolonged overall survival for those in the capecitabine group (53 mo vs. 36 mo, $p = 0.028$) [37]. Meanwhile, adjuvant S-1 therapy was investigated in an open-label, multicenter, randomized phase III trial (JCOG1202: ASCOT) between 2013 and 2018 in 38 Japanese hospitals for patients undergoing curative intent resection of biliary tract cancers. With a total of 440 patients enrolled, a 3-year OS was significantly prolonged in patients receiving S-1 adjuvant therapy compared to surgery alone (77.1% vs. 67.6%, $p = 0.008$) [38].

Despite the results of these two studies, other trials have failed to show a benefit of adjuvant therapy regimens in resectable disease. The phase III PRODIGE 12-ACCORD 18 trial conducted from 2009 to 2014 investigated patients receiving gemcitabine and oxaliplatin (GEMOX) versus surveillance, with no significant difference in the primary endpoint of recurrence-free survival

(30.4 mo vs. 18.5 mo, $p = 0.48$) or secondary endpoint of overall survival (75.8 mo vs. 50.8 mo, $p = 0.74$). Furthermore, in a planned subgroup analysis of patients with gallbladder cancer, those receiving GEMOX had significantly worse recurrence-free ($p = 0.034$) and overall survival ($p = 0.017$) than those in the surveillance arm [39].

Although multiple retrospective studies have attempted to clarify the role of adjuvant chemotherapy in resectable gallbladder cancer, more rigorous studies are needed [40–42]. However, achieving sufficient statistical power in prospective trials remains a significant challenge with the rarity of gallbladder cancer. The American Society of Clinical Oncology (ASCO) guidelines currently state that those patients with resectable biliary tract cancer should be offered 6 months of adjuvant capecitabine [43]. Regarding surveillance, patients should undergo periodic testing with a CT chest/abdomen/pelvis with or without CA 19–9 and CEA levels, though the optimal timing of such studies has yet to be determined [3, 4].

Conclusion

Although relatively rare in the United States, gallbladder cancer is the most common biliary tract malignancy. Most patients present with locally advanced or metastatic disease; however, those with resectable ≥T1b disease should undergo radical cholecystectomy with portal lymphadenectomy and en bloc liver resection [1, 3, 4]. Operative approaches may vary by experience; however, both open and MIS have been described for the surgical management of gallbladder cancer. The standard of care for resectable gallbladder cancer is surgery with chemotherapy, usually in the form of adjuvant capecitabine. With advances in systemic therapies for biliary tract malignancies, future studies will determine optimal perioperative treatment strategies, as well as optimal timing and selection of chemotherapy.

References

1. Misra S, Chaturvedi A, Misra NC, Sharma ID. Carcinoma of the gallbladder. Lancet Oncol. 2003;4(3):167–76. https://doi.org/10.1016/s1470-2045(03)01021-0.
2. Low SK, Giannis D, Thuong ND, et al. Trends in primary gallbladder cancer incidence and incidence-based mortality in the United States, 1973 to 2015. Am J Clin Oncol. 2022; https://doi.org/10.1097/coc.0000000000000918.
3. NCCN Clinical practice guidelines in oncology (NCCN guidelines®): hepatobiliary cancers. National Comprehensive Cancer Network. 2022. Accessed 20 June 2022. https://www.nccn.org/professionals/physician_gls/pdf/hepatobiliary.pdf
4. Aloia TA, Járufe N, Javle M, et al. Gallbladder cancer: expert consensus statement. HPB (Oxford). 2015;17(8):681–90. https://doi.org/10.1111/hpb.12444.
5. Hari DM, Howard JH, Leung AM, Chui CG, Sim MS, Bilchik AJ. A 21-year analysis of stage I gallbladder carcinoma: is cholecystectomy alone adequate? HPB (Oxford). 2013;15(1):40–8. https://doi.org/10.1111/j.1477-2574.2012.00559.x.
6. Fuks D, Regimbeau JM, Le Treut YP, et al. Incidental gallbladder cancer by the AFC-GBC-2009 Study Group. World J Surg. 2011;35(8):1887–97. https://doi.org/10.1007/s00268-011-1134-3.
7. D'Angelica M, Dalal KM, DeMatteo RP, Fong Y, Blumgart LH, Jarnagin WR. Analysis of the Extent of Resection for Adenocarcinoma of the Gallbladder. Ann Surg Oncol. 2008;16(4):806–16. https://doi.org/10.1245/s10434-008-0189-3.
8. Li B, Xu XX, Du Y, et al. Computed tomography for assessing resectability of gallbladder carcinoma: a systematic review and meta-analysis. Clin Imaging. 2013;37(2):327–33. https://doi.org/10.1016/j.clinimag.2012.05.009.
9. Ramos-Font C, Gómez-Rio M, Rodríguez-Fernández A, Jiménez-Heffernan A, Sánchez R, Llamas-Elvira JM. Ability of FDG-PET/CT in the detection of gallbladder cancer. J Surg Oncol. 2014;109(3):218–24. https://doi.org/10.1002/jso.23476.
10. Shindoh J, de Aretxabala X, Aloia TA, et al. Tumor location is a strong predictor of tumor progression and survival in T2 gallbladder cancer: an international multicenter study. Ann Surg. 2015;261(4):733–9. https://doi.org/10.1097/sla.0000000000000728.
11. Agarwal AK, Kalayarasan R, Javed A, Gupta N, Nag HH. The role of staging laparoscopy in primary gall bladder cancer—an analysis of 409 patients: a prospective study to evaluate the role of staging laparoscopy in the management of gallbladder cancer. Ann Surg. 2013;258(2):318–23. https://doi.org/10.1097/SLA.0b013e318271497e.

12. Jiayi W, Shelat VG. Robot-assisted radical cholecystectomy for gallbladder cancer: a review. J Clin Transl Res. 2022;8(2):103–9.
13. AlMasri S, Nassour I, Tohme S, et al. Long-term survival following minimally invasive extended cholecystectomy for gallbladder cancer: a 7-year experience from the National Cancer Database. J Surg Oncol. 2020; https://doi.org/10.1002/jso.26062.
14. Georgakis GV, Novak S, Bartlett DL, Zureikat AH, ZEH HJ III, Hogg ME. The emerging role of minimally-invasive surgery for gallbladder cancer: a comparison to open surgery. Conn Med. 2018;82(4)
15. Zimmitti G, Manzoni A, Guerini F, et al. Current role of minimally invasive radical cholecystectomy for gallbladder cancer. Gastroenterol Res Pract. 2016;2016:7684915. https://doi.org/10.1155/2016/7684915.
16. Shiraiwa DK, Carvalho P, Maeda CT, et al. The role of minimally invasive hepatectomy for hilar and intrahepatic cholangiocarcinoma: a systematic review of the literature. J Surg Oncol. 2020;121(5):863–72. https://doi.org/10.1002/jso.25821.
17. Bold RJ. Chap 3: radical cholecystectomy. In: Mulholland MW, editor. Operative techniques in surgery. Wolters Kluwer Health; 2015. p. 491–7.
18. Goel M, Khobragade K, Patkar S, Kanetkar A, Kurunkar S. Robotic surgery for gallbladder cancer: operative technique and early outcomes. J Surg Oncol. 2019;119(7):958–63. https://doi.org/10.1002/jso.25422.
19. Giulianotti PC, Bianco FM, Daskalaki D, Gonzalez-Ciccarelli LF, Kim J, Benedetti E. Robotic liver surgery: technical aspects and review of the literature. Hepatobiliary Surg Nutr. 2016;5(4):311.
20. Shen B-Y, Zhan Q, Deng X-X, et al. Radical resection of gallbladder cancer: could it be robotic? Surg Endosc. 2012;26(11):3245–50.
21. Jelinek LA, Jones MW. Surgical access incisions. In: StatPearls. StatPearls; 2022.
22. Chang SB, Palavecino M, Wray CJ, Kishi Y, Pisters PWT, Vauthey J-N. Modified Makuuchi incision for foregut procedures. Arch Surg. 2010;145(3):281–4. https://doi.org/10.1001/archsurg.2010.7.
23. Aloia TA, Zorzi D, Abdalla EK, Vauthey J-N. Two-surgeon technique for hepatic parenchymal transection of the noncirrhotic liver using saline-linked cautery and ultrasonic dissection. Ann Surg. 2005;242(2):172–7. https://doi.org/10.1097/01.sla.0000171300.62318.f4.
24. Palavecino M, Kishi Y, Chun YS, et al. Two-surgeon technique of parenchymal transection contributes to reduced transfusion rate in patients undergoing major hepatectomy: analysis of 1,557 consecutive liver resections. Surgery. 2010;147(1):40–8. https://doi.org/10.1016/j.surg.2009.06.027.
25. Piccolo G, Piozzi GN. Laparoscopic radical cholecystectomy for primary or incidental early gallbladder cancer: the new rules governing the treatment of gallbladder cancer. Gastroenterol Res Pract. 2017;2017:8570502. https://doi.org/10.1155/2017/8570502.

26. Palanisamy S, Patel N, Sabnis S, et al. Laparoscopic radical cholecystectomy for suspected early gall bladder carcinoma: thinking beyond convention. Surg Endosc. 2016;30(6):2442–8. https://doi.org/10.1007/s00464-015-4495-0.
27. D'Silva M, Han HS, Yoon YS, Cho JY. Comparative study of laparoscopic versus open liver resection in gallbladder cancer. J Laparoendosc Adv Surg Tech A. 2022;32(8):854–9. https://doi.org/10.1089/lap.2021.0670.
28. Gumbs AA, Jarufe N, Gayet B. Minimally invasive approaches to extrapancreatic cholangiocarcinoma. Surg Endosc. 2013;27(2):406–14. https://doi.org/10.1007/s00464-012-2489-8.
29. Sheetz KH, Claflin J, Dimick JB. Trends in the adoption of robotic surgery for common surgical procedures. JAMA Netw Open. 2020;3(1):e1918911. https://doi.org/10.1001/jamanetworkopen.2019.18911.
30. Byun Y, Choi YJ, Kang JS, et al. Early outcomes of robotic extended cholecystectomy for the treatment of gallbladder cancer. J Hepatobiliary Pancreat Sci. 2020;27(6):324–30. https://doi.org/10.1002/jhbp.717.
31. Newton AD, Newhook TE, Ikoma N, et al. Robotic completion radical cholecystectomy with fluorescence guidance. Ann Surg Oncol. 2021;28(11):6834. https://doi.org/10.1245/s10434-021-09819-w.
32. Piardi T, Lhuaire M, Memeo R, Pessaux P, Kianmanesh R, Sommacale D. Laparoscopic Pringle maneuver: how we do it? Hepatobiliary Surg Nutr. 2016;5(4):345–9. https://doi.org/10.21037/hbsn.2015.11.01.
33. Giulianotti PC, Bianco FM, Daskalaki D, Gonzalez-Ciccarelli LF, Kim J, Benedetti E. Robotic liver surgery: technical aspects and review of the literature. Hepatobiliary Surg Nutr. 2016;5(4):311–21. https://doi.org/10.21037/hbsn.2015.10.05.
34. Zimmitti G, Vauthey JN, Shindoh J, et al. Systematic use of an intraoperative air leak test at the time of major liver resection reduces the rate of postoperative biliary complications. J Am Coll Surg. 2013;217(6):1028–37. https://doi.org/10.1016/j.jamcollsurg.2013.07.392.
35. Takatsuki M, Eguchi S, Yamanouchi K, et al. Two-surgeon technique using saline-linked electric cautery and ultrasonic surgical aspirator in living donor hepatectomy: its safety and efficacy. Am J Surg. 2009;197(2):e25–7. https://doi.org/10.1016/j.amjsurg.2008.01.019.
36. Nishi T, Shimada H, Tokuyama M, et al. A case of severe biliary stenosis after cholecystectomy and hepatoduodenal ligament lymph node dissection for early gallbladder cancer. Ann Cancer Res Ther. 2011;19(2):34–6.
37. Primrose JN, Fox RP, Palmer DH, et al. Capecitabine compared with observation in resected biliary tract cancer (BILCAP): a randomised, controlled, multicentre, phase 3 study. Lancet Oncol. 2019;20(5):663–73. https://doi.org/10.1016/s1470-2045(18)30915-x.
38. Ikeda M, Nakachi K, Konishi M, et al. Adjuvant S-1 versus observation in curatively resected biliary tract cancer: a phase III trial (JCOG1202:

ASCOT). J Clin Oncol. 2022;40(4 Suppl):382. https://doi.org/10.1200/JCO.2022.40.4_suppl.382.
39. Edeline J, Benabdelghani M, Bertaut A, et al. Gemcitabine and oxaliplatin chemotherapy or surveillance in resected biliary tract cancer (PRODIGE 12-ACCORD 18-UNICANCER GI): a randomized phase III study. J Clin Oncol. 2019;37(8):658–67. https://doi.org/10.1200/jco.18.00050.
40. Kemp Bohan PM, Kirby DT, Chick RC, et al. Adjuvant chemotherapy in resectable gallbladder cancer is underutilized despite benefits in node-positive patients. Ann Surg Oncol. 2021;28(3):1466–80. https://doi.org/10.1245/s10434-020-08973-x.
41. Ozer M, Goksu SY, Sanford NN, et al. A propensity score analysis of chemotherapy use in patients with resectable gallbladder cancer. JAMA Netw Open. 2022;5(2):e2146912. https://doi.org/10.1001/jamanetworkopen.2021.46912.
42. Park Y, Kim K, Park HJ, Chun HJ, Choi D, Kim K. Role of adjuvant treatment in high-risk patients following resection for gallbladder cancer. In Vivo. 2022;36(2):961–8. https://doi.org/10.21873/invivo.12787.
43. Shroff RT, Kennedy EB, Bachini M, et al. Adjuvant therapy for resected biliary tract cancer: ASCO clinical practice guideline. J Clin Oncol. 2019;37(12):1015–27. https://doi.org/10.1200/jco.18.02178.

Portal Lymphadenectomy: Technical Pearls and Pitfalls

30

Hop S. Tran Cao, Reed I. Ayabe, and Ahad M. Azimuddin

Introduction

Portal lymphadenectomy is essential to the surgical management of biliary tract cancers. However, multiple studies demonstrate that this procedure is both underutilized and frequently inadequate when performed [1, 2]. The technical demands of portal lymph node dissection are not insignificant and may contribute to its suboptimal

---

H. S. Tran Cao (✉)
Department of Surgical Oncology, The University of Texas MD Anderson Cancer Center, Houston, TX, USA
e-mail: hstran@mdanderson.org

R. I. Ayabe
Division of Hepatobiliary and Pancreas Surgery, Department of Surgery, University of California Irvine, Irvine, CA, USA
e-mail: rayabe@hs.uci.edu

A. M. Azimuddin
Department of Surgical Oncology, The University of Texas MD Anderson Cancer Center, Houston, TX, USA

Division of Hepatobiliary and Pancreas Surgery, Department of Surgery, University of California Irvine, Irvine, CA, USA

Department of Surgery, Northwestern University Feinberg School of Medicine, Chicago, USA
e-mail: ahad.azimuddin@nm.org

© The Author(s), under exclusive license to Springer Nature Switzerland AG 2025
A. Alseidi et al. (eds.), *The SAGES Manual of Contemporary Indications and Management of Hepatic and Biliary Diseases*, https://doi.org/10.1007/978-3-032-04823-3_30

performance. A detailed discussion of the oncologic merits of portal lymphadenectomy for biliary tract cancers is beyond the scope of this chapter and is covered elsewhere. Instead, we herein describe our approach to portal lymphadenectomy for biliary tract cancer with a focus on the technical pearls and pitfalls of the operation.

Indications and Contraindications

Consensus guidelines from the American Joint Committee on Cancer (AJCC), the Americas Hepato-Pancreato-Biliary Association (AHPBA), and the National Comprehensive Cancer Network (NCCN) recommend routine performance of portal lymphadenectomy for all biliary tract cancers, including intrahepatic cholangiocarcinoma (iCCA), hilar cholangiocarcinoma (hCCA), distal cholangiocarcinoma (dCCA), and gallbladder cancer (GBC), that are stage T1b or higher [3–5]. Retrieval of six lymph nodes is recommended for iCCA and GBC, while the requisite number of nodes for hCCA and dCCA is unspecified [3]. Rarely, a more limited lymphadenectomy may be indicated for portal lymphadenopathy in the setting of liver metastases, most commonly from colorectal cancer.

Contraindications to portal lymphadenectomy are the same as those for primary tumor resection. Portal lymphadenectomy should not be conducted if the primary tumor itself cannot be safely removed, whether it be due to patient factors (e.g., medical comorbidities or poor performance status), tumor factors (e.g., locally advanced tumors), or liver-related factors (e.g., insufficient future liver remnant). Patients with distant metastatic disease, including those with lymph node involvement beyond the regional nodal basin, are not candidates for portal lymphadenectomy [6].

Rationale and Lymph Node Yield

Although the therapeutic benefit of portal lymphadenectomy remains a matter of debate, its role in staging and prognostication is unquestioned. A recent report including 6500 patients from the National Cancer Database who underwent intrahepatic cholangiocarcinoma resection found that prognostic accuracy was markedly improved if at least 6 nodes were retrieved [1]. The rationale for this 6-node threshold stems from a retrospective study from Memorial Sloan Kettering Cancer Center, which found that patients with ≥6 nodes retrieved and pN0 disease had significantly improved survival compared to those with <6 nodes removed and pN0 disease [7].

Anatomy

Portal lymphadenectomy includes the removal of all portal lymph nodes, which are contained in the fibrofatty tissues of the hepatoduodenal ligament. These correspond to Japanese Gastric Cancer Association stations 12a (proper hepatic artery), 12p (portal vein), and 12b (bile duct) (Fig. 30.1a) [8]. The cranial border of the portal nodes is the confluence of the right and left hepatic ducts while the caudal border is the head of the pancreas. This nodal tissue encases the hepatic artery, portal vein, and bile duct. A complete lymphadenectomy, therefore, requires dissection between and posterior to

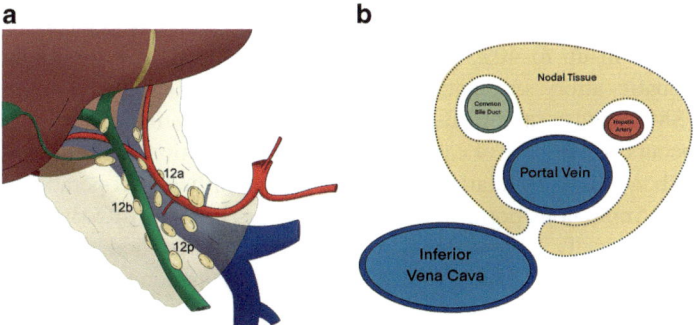

Fig. 30.1 Lymph nodes of the hepatoduodenal ligament. (**a**) Portal lymphadenectomy includes all nodal tissue in the hepatoduodenal ligament, including stations 12a (along the hepatic artery), 12b (along the bile duct), and 12p (behind the portal vein). (**b**) Nodal tissue encases the portal structures circumferentially. A complete lymphadenectomy requires retrieval nodes posterior to the portal vein and between the bile duct and portal vein

these structures, adding to the technical complexity of this operation (Fig. 30.1b).

It should be noted that in addition to the portal nodes, the peripancreatic and periduodenal nodes are included in the regional nodal basin for right-sided iCCA. For left-sided iCCA, regional nodes include the portal, inferior phrenic, and possibly the left gastric distributions.

Cross Sectional Imaging in Preoperative Preparation

High-quality cross-sectional imaging can be enormously helpful in surgical planning prior to portal dissection. Contrast-enhanced (triple-phase) computed tomography allows for the assessment of both lymphadenopathy and the anatomy of the hepatic artery and portal veins, of which there are many variants. The proper hepatic artery most commonly runs medial to the bile duct, while the portal vein courses posterior to both structures. The proper hepatic artery bifurcates into the left hepatic artery and right hepatic artery, the latter of which typically runs posterior to the common hepatic duct and gives off the cystic artery. It is critically important to identify anomalous hepatic arterial anatomy, which may be found in up to 40% of patients. A replaced or accessory right hepatic artery originating from the superior mesenteric artery (SMA) and coursing posterolateral to the portal vein and bile duct occurs in 10–12% of cases and can make dissection of the station 12b nodes particularly perilous if not identified preoperatively [9]. Anomalous portal vein anatomy occurs in up to 14% of cases but typically occurs distal to the hepatic hilum and does not impact the performance of portal lymphadenectomy to a large degree [10].

Biliary anatomy is best assessed with MRCP or MRI with Eovist in the delayed phase. Since most biliary anatomic variation occurs proximal to or at the hepatic duct confluence and is unlikely to affect the performance of the portal lymphadenectomy, we do not routinely obtain biliary-specific imaging. That said, one must keep in mind that drainage of the right posterior sectoral duct directly into the common hepatic duct near the cystic duct, although quite rare, can occur in up to 2% of cases.

It should be noted that lymphadenopathy detected on cross-sectional imaging may represent cN+ disease, which portends a very high risk of postoperative recurrence. In this setting, we and other groups are increasingly using neoadjuvant systemic therapy before curative-intent surgery. The main benefit of this approach is that it helps select patients who are most likely to benefit from an aggressive operation [11]. Neoadjuvant therapy may also be used as a conversion therapy to downsize tumors and allow for resection of initially unresectable tumors [12]. Neoadjuvant therapy may result in reduced nodal yield at the time of lymphadenectomy, as has been reported with other cancers, including pancreas, gastric, and rectal cancer, although this has not been well demonstrated in CCA. Nodal involvement beyond the regional portal nodal stations, such as celiac or para-aortic lymph nodes, should be considered a contraindication to surgery as this represents distant metastatic disease [6].

Type of Approach

Most available literature suggests that an open approach to portal lymphadenectomy provides a significantly higher lymph node yield compared to a laparoscopic approach [13, 14]. A meta-analysis from Guerrini et al. compares lymph node yield between open and laparoscopic liver resections for intrahepatic cholangiocarcinoma and found that while the laparoscopic approach achieved more rapid recovery and equivalent oncologic results, the total lymph node retrieval rate was significantly lower compared to the open approach [15]. Shiraiwa et al. conducted a systematic review of 25 studies comparing 129 open and 57 laparoscopic portal lymphadenectomies and found that lymph node yield was significantly lower in the laparoscopic group (OR, 0.46; 95% CI [− 0.87, = 0.06]; $P = 0.03$) [16]. Additionally, Martin et al. evaluated lymph node retrieval in 2309 intrahepatic cholangiocarcinoma via the National Cancer Database and found that minimally invasive lymphadenectomy is more likely to yield less than six lymph nodes compared to open lymphadenectomy (9% Laparoscopic, 15% Open, $p < 0.001$) [17]. Several factors have been proposed to account for the lower nodal yield via a laparoscopic approach. These include an overall reduced experience with laparoscopy in treating cholangiocarcinoma and the technically demanding nature of portal lymphadenectomy [18, 19]. The increasing use of the surgical robot may improve lymph node yield with minimally invasive portal dissection. In a cohort of 8612 patients undergoing hepatectomy for iCCA or GBC, laparoscopy was associated with a lower rate of obtaining ≥6 lymph nodes, while yield with the robotic and open approaches were comparable [20]. Improved lymph node yield with robotic surgery may reflect additional precision afforded by three-dimensional visualization, wristed instruments, and the availability of integrated fluorescence imaging to delineate vascular and biliary structures [21].

Operative Technique

Open Approach

1. Position and incision: Portal lymphadenectomy typically occurs at the time of primary tumor resection, with patient positioning and incision dictated by the latter. If portal lymphadenectomy is being performed in isolation, supine positioning with an upper midline incision is appropriate.
2. Kocherization of duodenum:
   - A wide Kocherization of the duodenum is performed to expose the posterior aspect of the duodenum and the head of the pancreas, a common place where 12b lymph nodes along the distal common bile duct are often nestled.
   - This maneuver also provides exposure of the inferior vena cava and aorta, where aortocaval nodes may be sampled for frozen analysis to rule out what would be considered distant metastatic disease.

- We will often perform this step first if preoperative imaging is suggestive of lymphadenopathy in the aortocaval space.
3. Common hepatic artery lymph node dissection:
   - The common hepatic artery lymph node marks the starting point of the portal lymphadenectomy. The pars flaccida is incised and the lesser omentum is divided to expose the caudate lobe of the liver and the common hepatic artery. Care must be taken to recognize and preserve any accessory or replaced left hepatic artery.
   - The hepatic artery lymph node is usually prominent, even when uninvolved by cancer. The tissue investing it is gently grasped, retracted, and lysed with cautery or bipolar energy. This avascular plane of dissection will lift the lymph node away from the underlying common hepatic artery and the superior border of the pancreas.
   - The dissection is extended in both directions. Nodal tissue is dissected back toward the hepatic artery origin to the right side of the celiac axis. Care must be taken to avoid traumatizing the coronary vein, which often drains into the portal vein in this region.
   - Continuing the dissection toward the liver reveals the gastroduodenal artery, which is preserved, and the right gastric artery. The right gastric artery may be divided with relative impunity to facilitate retrieval of the surrounding lymphatic tissue.
4. Proper hepatic artery and left-sided portal nodes:
   - The proper hepatic artery is skeletonized along its course toward the hepatic hilum. The left and right hepatic arteries are similarly identified and skeletonized. It is not uncommon to have separate hepatic artery branches to the left lateral liver (S2/3) and the left medial liver (S4). In general, the right hepatic artery runs posterior to the bile duct and additional dissection along this route is deferred to the subsequent steps. When the right hepatic artery runs anterior to the bile duct, continued skeletonization can be carried out along the exposed vessel.

- The left side of the portal vein is revealed during the dissection of the left hepatic artery branch(es). Nodal tissue to the left and behind the portal vein is also resected, following the vein's trajectory toward the caudate lobe.
- Looping the proper hepatic artery and retracting it to the left will expose the anterior surface of the portal vein and facilitate removal of nodal tissue in this location.

5. Bile duct nodes:
    - The pericholedochal tissue and lymph nodes are dissected starting distally, above the duodenum, and carried in a cranial direction to reveal the bile duct. A cholecystectomy is not necessarily required when performing portal lymphadenectomy for intrahepatic cholangiocarcinoma. However, in our practice, it is routinely done to facilitate the performance of the air leak test to rule out bile leakage during hepatectomy. In that scenario, we divide the cystic artery close to its origin with the right hepatic artery.
    - In the case of a completion radical cholecystectomy performed for incidental gallbladder cancer, we minimize direct manipulation of the surgical bed and carry our nodal dissection in a left-to-right direction, such that we identify the cystic duct at its junction with the common bile duct first and divide it there. We then dissect out the rest of the cystic duct stump and artery distally and remove it en bloc or separate from the gallbladder fossa (nonanatomic S4b/5 resection). If the cystic duct margin is affected grossly or by a frozen section, the bile duct is resected, and a Roux-en-Y hepaticojejunostomy is done.
    - It is important to retrieve nodal tissue between the bile duct and portal vein, which can be exposed by gently retracting the bile duct medially with a vein retractor or vessel loops.
    - Dissection continues up to the confluence of the right and left hepatic ducts, which marks the superior border of the portal lymphadenectomy. The right hepatic artery, which most often courses posterior to the common hepatic duct, is identified and preserved.

6. Anterior portal nodes:
    - Attention is focused on the triangle created by the upper border of the pancreas, the common bile duct, and the hepatic artery, with the artery and duct meeting at the triangle's apex. The dissection of the fibro-fatty tissue and lymph nodes in this triangle fully clears the anterior surface of the portal vein. The bile duct is gradually retracted to the patient's right and the hepatic artery to the patient's left, facilitating dissection of the tissue along the portal vein's anterior side to the hepatic hilum.
7. Retroportal, peripancreatic, and periduodenal nodes:
    - The fibro-fatty tissue and lymph nodes behind the pancreatic head and duodenum are removed starting caudally at the pancreatic head and progressing cranially along the portal vein toward the hepatic hilum. The vein of Belcher (posterosuperior pancreatoduodenal vein) may be encountered and can generally be preserved. Again, it is critical to recognize and preserve a replaced or accessory right hepatic artery running posterolateral to the portal vein in this area.
8. Dissection along the lesser curvature of the stomach:
    - For cholangiocarcinoma involving the left liver, especially in the presence of a replaced or accessory left hepatic artery, nodal dissection along this path is essential. We begin the nodal dissection along the aberrant artery and extend it back toward the origin of the left gastric artery at the celiac trunk.

Robotic Approach

1. Positioning and port placement:
    - The patient is positioned supine on the table with both arms out. They must be secured appropriately as the final position may have the bed in a reverse Trendelenberg position to 15° and the right side up to 5°, especially when the lymphadenectomy is performed along with hepatectomy for the primary tumor.

- *Trocar configuration*: The following description is for the Xi robot (Intuitive Surgical, Sunnyvale). Four 8-mm robotic trocars are placed across the abdomen, at a very slight angle, at the level of the apex of the insufflated abdominal wall. Our typical instrument lineup is as follows (Fig. 30.2):
  Arm 1: Fenestrated bipolar forceps.
  Arm 2: Camera.
  Arm 3: Dissection instrument—Maryland bipolar forceps, hook cautery, or vessel sealer may be used as needed.
  Arm 4: Cadiere forceps.
- A 12-mm assist trocar is placed in the suprapubic area or in the RLQ. This will serve as our specimen extraction site, and the choice of a 12-mm trocar aids in introducing gauze, a drop-in ultrasound probe, and needles if necessary. In the case a larger specimen is expected, the assist trocar will be incorporated into the planned Pfannenstiel incision.

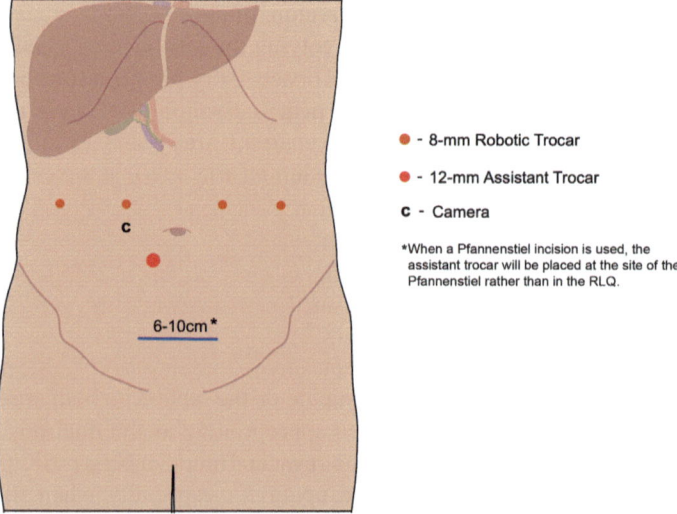

Fig. 30.2 Robotic trocar position for portal lymphadenectomy with specimen extraction site

2. The remaining steps of the procedure are the same as in open portal lymphadenectomy. Below we describe instruments and maneuvers that facilitate the previously described steps.
   (a) Kocherization of the duodenum: A rolled gauze is very useful to retract the duodenum medially in an atraumatic fashion.
   (b) Hepatic artery lymph node dissection:
      - The left lateral section of the liver can be retracted anteriorly using the shaft of a robotic instrument or a rolled gauze held by any blunt robotic graspers.
      - Our preference is to use the Maryland bipolar forceps for dissection of the vascular lymphatic tissue as this provides both precise dissection and hemostasis (Fig. 30.3a). A hook cautery or robotic shears may also be used. The fenestrated bipolar forceps can be used to both retract lymphatic tissue and obtain additional hemostasis as needed.
   (c) Proper hepatic artery and left portal nodes:
      - The gallbladder and/or falciform ligament can be used as "handles" to gently retract the liver superiorly to facilitate exposure of the hilum during this dissection.
      - If needed, the right gastric artery can be divided with hemoclips and the vessel sealer.
   (d) Bile duct nodes:
      - Gentle retraction of the bile duct can be accomplished using a rolled gauze or the side of a blunt robotic instrument (Fig. 30.3b). If additional retraction is needed, the bile duct can be encircled proximally and distally with vessel loops, which can be manipulated by either a robotic arm or the bedside assistant. The use of indocyanine green fluorescence can facilitate the visualization and safe dissection of the bile duct up to the confluence of the right and left hepatic ducts (Fig. 30.3c).
   (e) Retroportal, periduodenal, and peripancreatic nodes:
      - The nodes posterior to the portal vein should be accessible after a wide Kocher maneuver. If additional

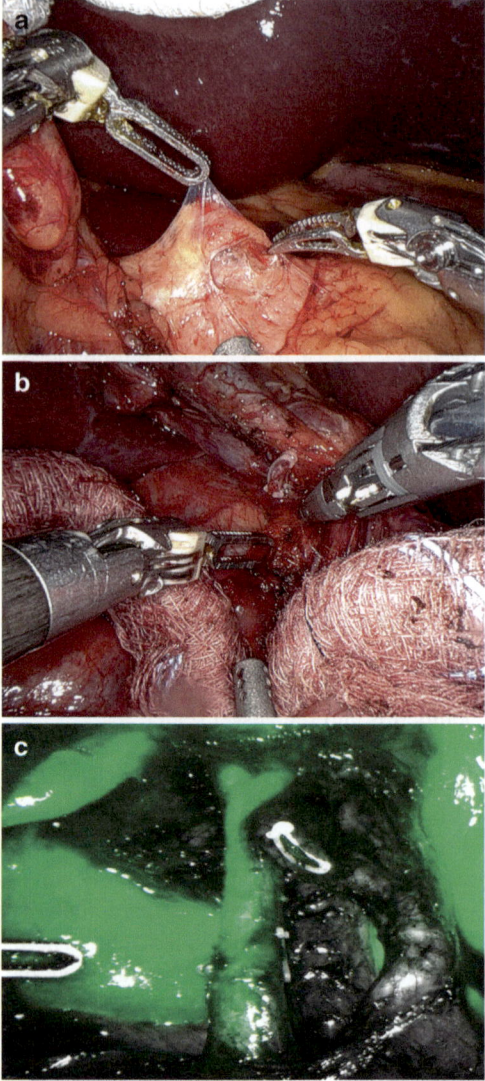

Fig. 30.3 Intraoperative images of robotic portal lymphadenectomy. (**a**) The first step of portal lymphadenectomy (robotic or open) is dissection of the common hepatic artery lymph node. (**b**) The blunt shaft of a robotic instrument is used to retract the portal structures medially to retrieve nodes posterior to the portal vein. (**c**) Integrated fluorescence imaging with indocyanine green helps to define the biliary anatomy

exposure of the retroportal space is needed, the portal vein can similarly be encircled with vessel loops for retraction.

Pearls & Pitfalls

Pearls

1. Although the therapeutic benefit of portal lymphadenectomy remains a matter of debate, its staging and prognostic values are well established. Therefore, we strongly recommend performing this procedure routinely when resecting biliary tract cancers.
2. It is essential to correctly identify the common bile duct, portal vein, and the common hepatic artery and its branches. A complete lymphadenectomy requires meticulous dissection between the bile duct and hepatic artery and skeletonization of these tissues.
3. The safest dissection plane is the avascular tissue investing the nodal tissue around these structures. Once lymph nodes are fractured, nuisance bleeding can obscure visualization and predispose to inadvertent vascular or biliary injury. For this reason, it is best to minimize direct manipulation of the lymph nodes themselves. This is particularly important when using the robotic platform, which lacks haptic feedback.
4. A Kocher maneuver will aid in the excision of lymph nodes that extend past the duodenal C-loop posterior to the common bile duct. Additionally, the dissection must encompass the nodes that extend medially along the common hepatic artery as it emerges from the celiac axis. These lymph nodes are in a groove between the common hepatic artery and the pancreatic upper border. The dissection is complete when the porta hepatis and hepatic artery down to the celiac axis have been skeletonized.
5. When dealing with completion surgery for incidental gallbladder cancer, we routinely re-excise the cystic duct stump to ensure negative margins. If this is positive, an extrahepatic bile duct excision with hepaticojejunostomy reconstruction will be necessary to achieve negative margins. This procedure will also substantially help the regional portal lymphadenectomy.

6. The portal triad structures should be skeletonized to ease the removal of all periportal nodal tissue. Studies have demonstrated that the lymphatic drainage of the liver is somewhat predictable, with the left lobe draining through the lesser omentum to the lymph nodes along the lesser curve and cardia of the stomach and the right lobe draining to the hepatoduodenal ligament and portocaval and retropancreatic lymph nodes. The lymph nodes along the main hepatic artery should be routinely excised, and subsequent lymphadenectomy should be customized based on the location of the primary intrahepatic cholangiocarcinoma and its concomitant draining lymph nodes [6].
7. The optimal lymphadenectomy should encompass all regional lymph node stations. All patients should have the lymph nodes of the hepatoduodenal ligament and the hepatic artery removed, as they are the first to be implicated in the metastatic process. For iCCA originating in the right hemiliver, the retropancreatic LNs, which are still regarded as first echelon nodes, may be implicated; hence, their regular excision is advised. Through the lesser omentum, another direct lymphatic channel is identified to run from the left hemiliver to the stomach. Therefore, in patients with iCCA originating from the left hemiliver, the lymph nodes around the cardiac section of the stomach and along the lesser curvature should also be removed for appropriate lymphadenectomy [22].

Pitfalls

1. A substantial portion of portal nodal tissue is located posterior to the common bile duct and in close proximity to the portal vein. Care must be taken while removing these lymph nodes to avoid damaging the portal vein or any aberrant right hepatic artery, which most often arises from the superior mesenteric artery (SMA) and travels along the lateral posterior portion of the hepatoduodenal ligament (type III anatomy). Preoperative imaging is therefore critical to ensuring safe surgery.

2. Because portal lymphadenectomy involves skeletonization of the portal structures, the potential exists for thermal injury to both the hepatic artery (with resultant pseudoaneurysmal damage) and the bile duct (with resultant bile duct stricture). Energy must be used with extreme caution around these structures.
3. When dissecting nodal tissue around the portal vein, blind use of the energy device can result in direct injury to the vein. Retraction of the nodal tissue away from the vein is critical.
4. Chyle leak can occur due to accidental injury of the cisterna chyli or the lymphatic channels running in the retropancreatic space. Prevention is key; lymphatic channels connecting to the retrieved lymph nodes should be clipped or tied to prevent chylous ascites and subsequent malnutrition.

Conclusion

Portal lymphadenectomy is indicated for the surgical management of biliary tract cancers, including intrahepatic cholangiocarcinoma, hilar cholangiocarcinoma, distal cholangiocarcinoma, and gallbladder cancer. Contraindications to portal lymphadenectomy are primarily those related to the inability to safely remove the primary tumor, such as patient health factors, advanced tumors, insufficient future liver remnant, and distant metastatic disease. Despite debates over its therapeutic benefit, the role of portal lymphadenectomy in staging and prognostication is well-established. Guidelines recommend a minimum retrieval of six lymph nodes for improved prognostic accuracy. Cross-sectional imaging helps in preoperative planning and understanding anatomical variations. Although the laparoscopic approach to portal lymphadenectomy has demonstrated benefits such as quicker recovery and equivalent oncologic results, studies suggest that the open approach yields significantly more lymph nodes. Advancements in robotic surgery might improve lymph node yield due to better visualization and precision, and emerging data point toward this promising potential of robotic assistance. The execution of the procedure, whether through an open or robotic approach, requires sound surgical technique and adherence to established protocols to ensure optimal outcomes. Meticulous dissection and skeletonization of critical structures, along with vigilant preoperative imaging review to avoid potential pitfalls such as thermal injuries, vascular and biliary damage, and chyle leaks, is necessary to ensure safe and effective treatment outcomes. Ultimately, mastering portal lymphadenectomy is vital for surgeons facing biliary tract cancers, promising improved prognostic accuracy and patient outcomes.

References

1. Moazzam Z, Alaimo L, Endo Y, Lima HA, Pawlik TM. Predictors, patterns, and impact of adequate lymphadenectomy in intrahepatic cholangiocarcinoma. Ann Surg Oncol. 2023;30(4):1966–77. https://doi.org/10.1245/s10434-022-13044-4.
2. Zhang XF, Xue F, Dong DH, et al. Number and station of lymph node metastasis after curative-intent resection of intrahepatic cholangiocarcinoma impact prognosis. Ann Surg. 2021;274(6):e1187–95. https://doi.org/10.1097/SLA.0000000000003788.
3. Chun YS, Pawlik TM, Vauthey J-N. 8th edition of the AJCC cancer staging manual: pancreas and hepatobiliary cancers. Ann Surg Oncol. 2018;25(4):845–7. https://doi.org/10.1245/s10434-017-6025-x.
4. Aloia TA, Járufe N, Javle M, et al. Gallbladder Cancer: expert consensus statement. HPB. 2015;17(8):681–90. https://doi.org/10.1111/hpb.12444.
5. NCCN Clinical practice guidelines in oncology: biliary tract cancers v1. 2023. (https://www.nccn.org/professionals/physician_gls/pdf/btc.pdf).
6. Squires MH, Cloyd JM, Dillhoff M, Schmidt C, Pawlik TM. Challenges of surgical management of intrahepatic cholangiocarcinoma. Expert Rev Gastroenterol Hepatol. 2018;12(7):671–81. In Eng. https://doi.org/10.1080/17474124.2018.1489229.
7. Ito H, Ito K, D'Angelica M, et al. Accurate staging for gallbladder cancer: implications for surgical therapy and pathological assessment. Ann Surg. 2011;254(2):320–5. https://doi.org/10.1097/SLA.0b013e31822238d8.
8. Japanese Gastric Cancer A. Japanese gastric cancer treatment guidelines 2021 (6th edition). Gastric Cancer. 2023;26(1):1–25. https://doi.org/10.1007/s10120-022-01331-8.

9. Hiatt JR, Gabbay J, Busuttil RW. Surgical anatomy of the hepatic arteries in 1000 cases. Ann Surg. 1994;220(1):50–2. https://doi.org/10.1097/00000658-199407000-00008.
10. Watanabe N, Ebata T, Yokoyama Y, et al. Anatomic features of independent right posterior portal vein variants: implications for left hepatic trisectionectomy. Surgery. 2017;161(2):347–54. https://doi.org/10.1016/j.surg.2016.08.024.
11. Ayabe RI, Paez-Arango N, Estrella JS, et al. Neoadjuvant chemotherapy for high-risk intrahepatic cholangiocarcinoma – does pathologic response mean better outcomes? HPB (Oxford). 2023; https://doi.org/10.1016/j.hpb.2023.01.011.
12. Fruscione M, Pickens RC, Baker EH, et al. Conversion therapy for intrahepatic cholangiocarcinoma and tumor downsizing to increase resection rates: a systematic review. Curr Probl Cancer. 2021;45(1):100614. https://doi.org/10.1016/j.currproblcancer.2020.100614.
13. Washington K, Rocha F. Approach to resectable biliary cancers. Curr Treat Options in Oncol. 2021;22(11):97. In eng. https://doi.org/10.1007/s11864-021-00896-3.
14. Ong CT, Leung K, Nussbaum DP, et al. Open versus laparoscopic portal lymphadenectomy in gallbladder cancer: is there a difference in lymph node yield? HPB. 2018;20(6):505–13. https://doi.org/10.1016/j.hpb.2017.10.015.
15. Guerrini GP, Esposito G, Tarantino G, et al. Laparoscopic versus open liver resection for intrahepatic cholangiocarcinoma: the first meta-analysis. Langenbeck's Arch Surg. 2020;405(3):265–75. https://doi.org/10.1007/s00423-020-01877-0.
16. Shiraiwa DK, Carvalho PFDC, Maeda CT, et al. The role of minimally invasive hepatectomy for hilar and intrahepatic cholangiocarcinoma: a systematic review of the literature. J Surg Oncol. 2020; https://doi.org/10.1002/jso.25821.
17. Martin SP, Drake J, Wach MM, et al. Laparoscopic approach to intrahepatic cholangiocarcinoma is associated with an exacerbation of inadequate nodal staging. Ann Surg Oncol. 2019;26(6):1851–7. https://doi.org/10.1245/s10434-019-07303-0.
18. Isetani M, Morise Z, Horiguchi A. Laparoscopic liver resection with lymph node dissection for gallbladder tumors suspected to be T1b/T2 carcinoma. Hepatoma Res. 2017;3(8):170. https://doi.org/10.20517/2394-5079.2017.17.
19. Sucandy I, Jabbar F, Syblis C, Crespo K, Ross S, Rosemurgy A. Robotic central hepatectomy for the treatment of gallbladder carcinoma. outcomes of minimally invasive approach. Am Surg. 2022;88(3):348–51. In eng. https://doi.org/10.1177/00031348211047457.

20. Kim BJ, Newhook TE, Tzeng CD, et al. Lymphadenectomy and margin-negative resection for biliary tract cancer surgery in the United States-differential technical performance by approach. J Surg Oncol. 2022;126(4):658–66. In eng. https://doi.org/10.1002/jso.26924.
21. Ayabe RI, Azimuddin A, Tran Cao HS. Robot-assisted liver resection: the real benefit so far. Langenbeck's Arch Surg. 2022;407(5):1779–87. https://doi.org/10.1007/s00423-022-02523-7.
22. Weber SM, Ribero D, O'Reilly EM, Kokudo N, Miyazaki M, Pawlik TM. Intrahepatic cholangiocarcinoma: expert consensus statement. HPB. 2015;17(8):669–80. https://doi.org/10.1111/hpb.12441.

Part IX

Locoregional Hepatic Therapies

Surgical Microwave Ablation of the Liver

31

Sushruta Nagarkatti, Aleksandr Kalabin, John B. Martinie, and David A. Iannitti

Introduction

The most commonly used ablative technologies in current clinical practice are radiofrequency ablation (RFA) and microwave ablation (MWA) [1, 2]. Both of these locoregional liver-directed therapies rely on the use of an energy source to cause local tissue destruction. The fundamental differences between them lie in the nature of the energy source, the mechanism of heat generation and its transfer within tissue [1, 2]. Of the two, surgical MWA in conjunction with the use of intraoperative ultrasound (IOUS) for targeting has emerged as a powerful tool in precise cancer care and is currently considered the modality of choice for many types of liver tumors.

The easiest way to think about the difference between RFA and MWA is that RFA produces thermal energy by passing a high fre-

S. Nagarkatti
University of Tennessee, Health Sciences Center, Memphis, TN, USA

A. Kalabin (✉) · J. B. Martinie · D. A. Iannitti
Atrium Health/Carolinas Medical Center, Charlotte, NC, USA
e-mail: Aleksandr.kalabin@atriumhealth.org;
John.martinie@atriumhealth.org; David.Iannitti@atriumhealth.org

quency electrical current through the patient, whereas MWA does not use a current, but rather "broadcasts" a microwave energy field from an antennae.

RFA involves the conduction of heat derived from the application of an alternating current (AC) within a closed circuit (within the patient) to an electrode placed directly in the tissue. The application of current between 375 and 480 kHz leads to high current density around the electrode resulting in heat generation and coagulative necrosis at temperatures above 50 °C [1, 2].

Since RFA relies on heat conduction to the local tissue as its primary mechanism of tissue destruction, the process is less efficient. It requires longer ablation times for heat generation and delivery with rapid heating that can lead to charring and tissue desiccation, which in turn impedes current, causing imprecise current conduction and resultant heat application [2].

MWA leads to tissue destruction by two mechanisms, active and passive heating. It primarily leads to coagulative necrosis of the local tissues from an active heating process. The active heating zone is generated when a nonionizing oscillating electromagnetic (EM) wave is applied through an ablation probe or antenna placed within the tissue [1]. The EM waves act on water molecules (dipole molecules) inducing high-frequency rotational movement that generates friction and heat-causing coagulative necrosis within the intended zone of ablation [1, 3]. This also leads to secondary passive heat that spreads beyond the zone of active heating by conduction leading to further tissue destruction. However, the passive heat effect is susceptible to a heat sink effect, and charring as with monopolar RFA, and is also more unpredictable in terms of size and pattern. The two frequencies of the microwave devices commonly used are 915 and 2450 MHz [1, 3]. Most of the commercially available MWA systems currently in use in the United States have generators that produce 2450 MHz (2.5 GHz), the main reason being higher power and shorter ablation times.

Compared with monopolar RFA, MWA is more efficient in producing higher temperatures in a larger ablation zone, in shorter time, with less heat sink effect. Furthermore, unlike RFA, MWA does not have an electrical current, and as such, the potential for a current sink is eliminated, something which can occur with RFA near larger blood vessels [1–3].

Indications and Contra Indications

MWA was initially utilized as liver-directed therapy in patients with either poor physiologic reserve from underlying medical comorbidities, or those with a large tumor burden requiring palliation. The indications have since expanded as a result of advances in both MWA and US technology. Development of both next-generation MWA generators and probes have led to more refined, consistent energy delivery. Coupled with improved IOUS image resolution, and advanced probes for laparoscopic targeting, the use of IOUS-guided MWA has become widespread.

Surgical MWA has advantages over both percutaneous MWA and resection. It allows a parenchyma sparing procedure in patients with underlying cirrhosis, poor underlying cardiopulmonary physiology, and those outside criteria for liver transplant. It can also be used in specific clinical scenarios such as ruptured hepatocellular carcinoma (HCC) alone or with transarterial chemoembolization (TACE) as an emergency salvage procedure. MWA can also be used in conjunction with hepatic resection as a complimentary modality to preserve future liver remnant (FLR) and improve margin negativity in patients with bilobar colorectal liver metastasis (CRLM). In patients with HCC tumors outside of Milan and UCSF criteria requiring transplant, it may be utilized as a downstaging modality. Other than this, MWA can be used as tumor debulking surgery in patients with GYN cancers and palliative technique for metastatic NET of GI tract.

One of the advantages over percutaneous MWA is that it allows for diagnostic laparoscopy, with accurate staging and assessment of occult peritoneal disease. Another advantage is that simultaneous surgical procedures (cholecystectomy, lymphadenectomy, liver biopsy) can be performed in the same setting. The use of intraoperative ultrasound increases the sensitivity and accuracy of liver tumor detection rates. Targeting of the liver lesion with IOUS is more precise, decreasing the chances of injury of intrahepatic structures, minimizing the risk of damaging of intraabdominal viscera. Periprocedural complications such as bleeding and hematoma formation can be detected at the same time with more appropriate and timely management.

MWA may therefore be used for, but not limited to:

1. Hepatocellular carcinoma (including ruptured HCC).
2. Colorectal liver metastasis.
3. Metastatic neuroendocrine tumors (NET) to the liver.
4. Benign liver pathology: bleeding or ruptured adenomas, symptomatic FNH, giant/symptomatic cavernous hemangiomas.
5. Metastatic of other cancers (non-colorectal–non-neuroendocrine tumors).

The use of MWA for any of these entities should be employed, of course after thoughtful discussions with the patient and a multidisciplinary team of disease-related specialist for each patient. For patients with primary or secondary liver tumors, all patients should be reviewed at a multidisciplinary tumor (MDT) conference, comprised of Hepatopancreatobiliary (HPB) and transplant surgeons, transplant hepatologists, interventional radiologists, medical and radiation oncologists, as well as care coordinators and nurse navigators. The risks/benefits and treatment options are all discussed as a team and subsequently presented to patients to maximize patient engagement in their medical decision-making whenever possible. This practice minimizes the inappropriate use of therapies (either surgical resection or MWA), which can often occur in healthcare settings that do not rely on the use of MDT conferences.

Although MWA for HCC is a viable option for patients with tumor burden in the setting of underlying cirrhosis, the selection of these patients must be thoughtful. The risk of hepatic decompensation must be factored into decision-making. Patients who are classified as Child-Pugh Class A and B have a relatively lower risk of hepatic decompensation and are more likely to tolerate the procedure. However, those with Childs C disease are at a much greater risk of decompensation. A good way to determine the physiologic reserve and risk of hepatic decompensation in a patient being considered for MWA is the assessment of their response to interventional transarterial liver-directed therapy (i.e., TACE or TARE).

There are certain clinical situations that preclude the use of MWA as a therapeutic option. Patients who have active decompensated cirrhosis, with vascular involvement of their tumors, or tumor burden more than 70% of liver volume are absolute contraindications to MWA.

Laparoscopic MWA of the Liver: Technical Considerations

Preoperative Planning

Preoperative planning is of utmost importance. Appropriate blood products should be available including platelets, plasma and packed red blood cells particularly for patients with underlying cirrhosis, liver dysfunction, or coagulopathies. Of particular concerns are patients with significant portal hypertension, encephalopathy, ascites, and jaundice. Intraoperative fluid resuscitation should be performed with albumin rather than crystalloid with close communication between the surgical and anesthesia teams.

Prior review of cross-sectional imaging is critical and must be readily available in the operating room. This allows for correlation with IOUS images for targeting purposes.

Anesthesia

All patients undergoing a laparoscopic ablation, whether RFA or MWA, are done under general anesthesia, which allows for paralysis, which is needed to establish and maintain pneumoperitoneum. This also virtually eliminates pain experienced by the patients *during the actual procedure*, although certainly patients often experience pain once awake, either at the trocar/port sites, needle entry points, or from irritation of the diaphragm. We believe this offers patients a significant advantage over percutaneous ablations performed in the IR suite by a radiologist, where the procedures are often performed under sedation and local anesthesia rather than General Endotracheal Anesthesia (GETA).

Positioning

The patient is positioned based on the location of the lesion to be targeted. Those located in the left lobe and the right anterior section allow the patient to be in supine position with both arms out. Those located in the right posterior section require the patient to be positioned at 45° with a break in the bed to facilitate exposure. Rolls are placed below the right side of the patient, which, in combination with bed rotation, allows the patient to attain up at a 45° angle. Alternatively, a "beanbag" type device can be place beneath the patient to help maintain the desired level of elevation of the right side. The right arm can either be positioned up and over to the left on an arm board fixed to the left side of the bed, or simply left along the right side of the body on several pillows, which is currently our preference (Fig. 31.1). The chest and legs are strapped into place, and the right chest is included in the sterile field.

Equipment and Room Setup

Appropriate monitor placement facilitates correlation between the laparoscopic and IOUS images. Of the two laparoscopic monitors, one is placed above the head of the patient, with the second on the patient's right side. The IOUS image monitor is placed adjacent to the right-sided laparoscopic monitor. Both sets are placed at or slightly below eye level. This setup is used since a large majority of the time, and the operating surgeon stands on the patient's left (Fig. 31.2).

The surgeon must have in-depth knowledge of both the IOUS and ablation equipment. This includes the ability to utilize both color and doppler modes, perform lesion measure-

31 Surgical Microwave Ablation of the Liver

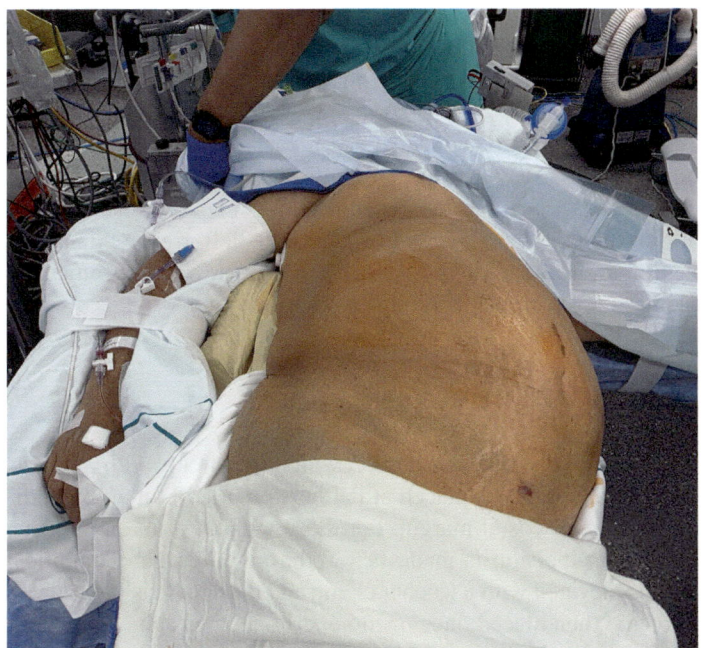

Fig. 31.1 Patient in left lateral recumbent position

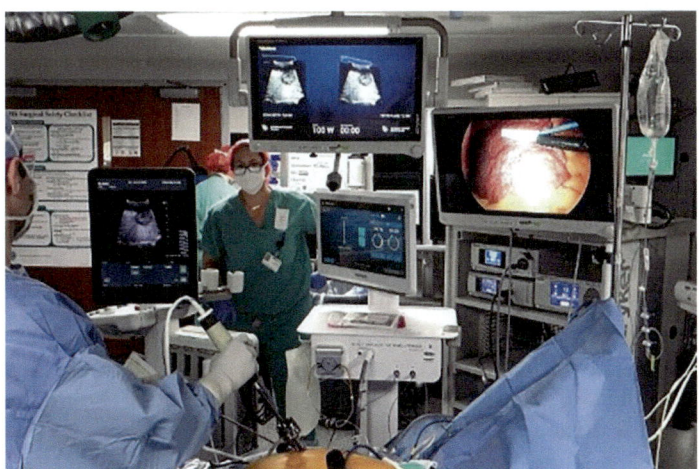

Fig. 31.2 Operating room set up

ment, invert images, and adjusting the depth, gain as well as time-gain compensation. They must also be familiar with and make it a practice to freeze, print, and store the images for medicolegal reasons.

The staff must be educated about each system and be able to efficiently assist with operating both IOUS and ablation system equipment. A flexible laparoscopic IOUS probe is used, which allows the use of both an "up–down" and "left–right" extension–flexion movement. In particular, the "up–down" movement is required for accurate targeting as described later.

Access and Port Placement

We prefer to use a Veress needle, which in patients with previous abdominal surgery is placed at Palmers point two finger breadths below the left costal margin. For those without prior surgeries, a small skin incision is made below the umbilicus, the umbilical stalk is elevated with a Kocher clamp and the needle is introduced. Ports are then placed once pneumoperitoneum is achieved.

Alternatively, the open, Hasson technique may be used, and depending on the planned location of the IOUS transducer, access is obtained in the periumbilical area.

Most procedures are performed using a single 12 mm port for the laparoscopic ultrasound probe, and two additional 5 mm ports. One 5 mm port is used for the camera, the other for an assistant port for suctioning, irrigation, and electrocautery as needed (Fig. 31.3). Port placement is dictated by both the individual patient body habitus, liver size, and the location of the liver lesions to be targeted, in addition to surgeon preference. For predominantly right-sided lesions, the 12 mm trocar is placed in the right mid-clavicular line at the level of the umbilicus. For left-sided lesions, this port is usually placed in the midline below the umbilicus. The 12 mm port is used for the IOUS probe. Preoperative imaging must be reviewed and used to guide placement of the additional 5 mm ports to triangulate toward the target lesions.

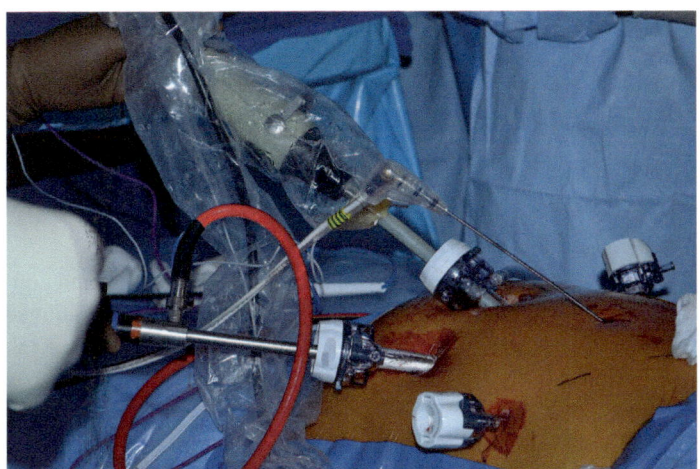

Fig. 31.3 Laparoscopic port placement with microvawe ablation antenna placed through the separate epigastric incision

Hand Positioning and IOUS Probe Placement

We use a laparoscopic IOUS transducer (BK Medical, Copenhagen, Denmark) that allows a "left–right" as we all as an "up–down" extension flexion movement. The "left–right" button is locked in neutral position, allowing the surgeon to use the "up–down" extension–flexion movement alone. This facilitates tissue apposition, and therefore delineates lesions more accurately for targeting. It also enables the surgeon to "scroll through" the lesions medially and laterally around the axis of the IOUS by performing continuous supination and pronation of the hand controlling the probe. The laparoscopic probe is introduced through the 12 mm port and held in the nondominant hand of the operating surgeon. The first step is to orient the laparoscopic probe and transducer with the desired laparoscopic image orientation. This is done by tapping the probe on the liver and looking at the IOUS image to make sure it is oriented the proper position.

The settings on the IOUS are then set to the appropriate image depth, which should allow the hyperechoic fat along the posterior edge of the liver to be seen during the initial scanning of the liver.

Ultrasound-Guided Targeting

The entire liver should be scanned thoroughly to identify and confirm the location of the lesions based on the information obtained from preoperative cross-sectional imaging. It is important to do so in order to identify any additional lesions that may not have been visualized with preoperative cross-sectional imaging, as well as to identify and change in the target lesions (growth). There are two primary techniques to scanning the liver:

- *Lawnmower technique*: This involves scanning the entire liver along the parenchymal surface in a back-and-forth, methodical fashion, from top to bottom, helping to build a three-dimensional mental image of the liver and any target lesions. This also includes building an image of the relationship between the portal pedicles and hepatic veins with their relationship to the lesions. This is further facilitated by reviewing preoperative imaging immediately prior to beginning the procedure.
- *Pedicle tracking technique*: This technique the surgeon follows the portal pedicles, left and right, proximally in the hilum, working their way out to the segmental branches, and identifying their relationship with the lesions. The relationship of the lesions to each portal pedicle is identified preoperatively and then confirmed by following the pedicle out during IOUS.

It is useful to have an ablation worksheet ready for use prior to beginning the targeting process. The circulator nurse or assistant should write down the number of lesions identified, their locations (which segments), and sizes. In addition, during the ablations, one should also have a system on the sheet for noting the size, the power used (Watts), and the time that each lesion was ablated.

Optimal and intuitive targeting occurs when the surgeon stands on the patient left, with the ablation probe advanced from the inferior abdomen toward the liver superiorly, caudal-to-cranial. This allows the needle trajectory to correspond with the targeted lesion from the surgeon perspective while matching the orientation of the needle visualized on the IOUS images and the laparoscopic images.

The lesion to be ablated is visualized so that it lies below the distal tip of the transducer, giving a two-dimensional view of the target that is correlated with the laparoscopic view. It is best to decrease the depth of the ultrasound to place the target lesion in the middle of the ultrasound image. (For lesions located in the first several centimeters of liver parenchyma, you do not want the ultrasound field set to depths of 8–10 cm, for example.) Continuous, short rotational supination and pronation hand movements at the level of the wrist in alternating fashion help to obtain a more three-dimensional position of the target and allow the surgeon to carefully guide the needle toward the lesion despite being off plane. This is referred to as "pill-rolling," in reference to the typical hand tremor seen in patients with Parkinson's disease.

The MWA needle is introduced into the abdomen through a small skin incision that is made 2–3 cm below the costal margin for an appropriate trajectory and avoid bending against or injuring the ribs. The MWA needle is introduced on the side that the lesion is located or lesions predominate. Right-sided lesions require the probe to be inserted below the right costal margin, leaving adequate space between the two. Those located in the posterior section require entry to be performed in the epigastric region. Left-sided lesions can be performed with the needle entering in the epigastrium or if needed, just below the left costal margin. The needle is advanced under direct laparoscopic vision while visualizing the projected IOUS image.

"In-plane" vs. "Step-off" Technique

When the ablation probe is in perfect alignment with the IOUS transducer, it is referred to as "in-plane." This trajectory and alignment with the transducer can be difficult to obtain given the limited freedom of movement, particularly once the MWA needle is introduced into the parenchyma. In order for the MWA needle to be perfectly "in-plane," it must be inserted directly over the laparoscopic ultrasound probe, which leads to awkward ergonomics for the surgeon and hand-collisions and interference. However, for those who prefer the "in-plane" technique, some of the ultrasound probes have an ablation needle guide to help keep the needle in-plane with the ultrasound.

We recommend the use of a "step-off" technique (Fig. 31.4). The IOUS transducer is shifted just slightly lateral to the path of the MWA needle and then rotated back to visualize the lesion. The length of the trajectory of the needle from its entry to the target should usually be a short distance. However, certain lesions

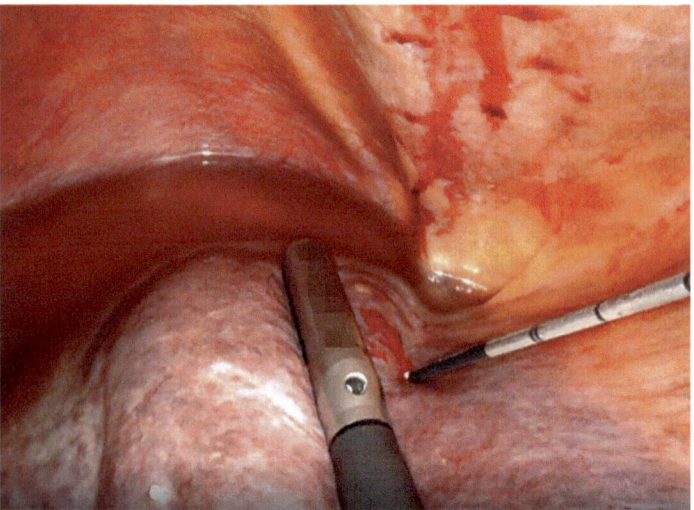

Fig. 31.4 Depiction of the "step-off" method for targeting with the IOUS probe lateral to the path of the ablation probe

located more superiorly or posteriorly have a longer distance to traverse before entering the IOUS image. In these cases, the IOUS must be used to ensure that no major vascular structures are crossed by the needle. It is during this time that the previously described alternating pronation and supination wrist rotations (pill-rolling) are required in order to guide the needle along its intended trajectory. The placement of the needle and its trajectory may be corrected at any point that it is felt to be inaccurate, and the steps may be repeated. Figures 31.4, 31.5, and 31.6 depict the placement of the MWA using this method of targeting.

The location of the MWA needle in relation to the lesion is based on the microwave field that is generated. This field is generated at the distal aspect of the needle, usually 1–2 cm from its tip, but is unique to each MWA design characteristics. It is critical to understand the technical aspects of each microwave needle (antennae) and the specific fields they are capable of producing, and where the ablation zone center is located along the needle as there are significant differences between systems. The tip of the needle should be placed closer to the far side of the lesion, toward the posterior or superior aspect so that the lesion lies within the center of the ablation zone. Several of the commercially available MWA systems have developed power/time curves, which can produce an

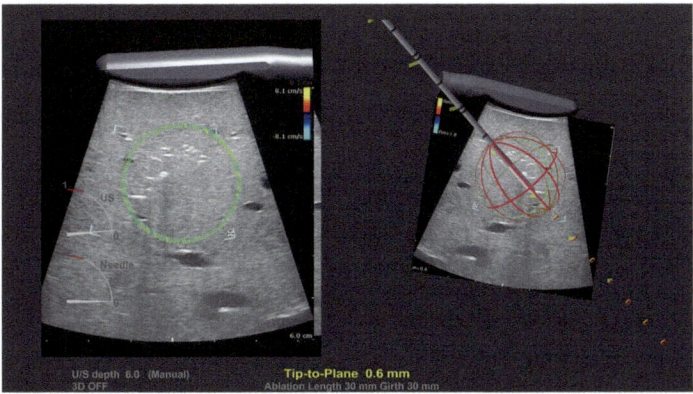

Fig. 31.5 Movement of the probe medially to visualize the lesion and probe

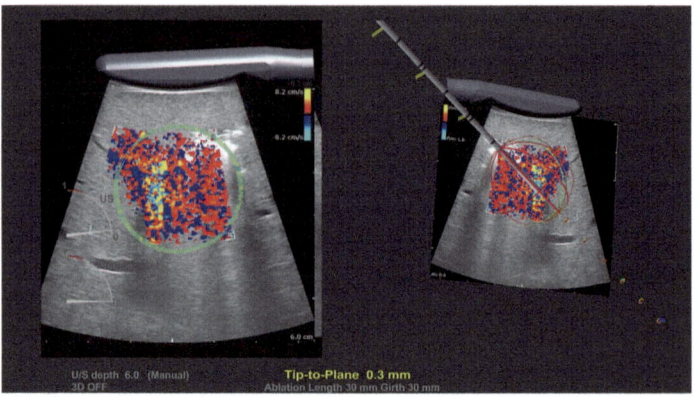

Fig. 31.6 Ultrasound images. The left image shows color doppler mapping of the target region. The right image shows instrument insertion, suggesting an interventional procedure

estimated volume or sphere of ablation zone, which can help the surgeon with estimating how much time is required to treat a specific target lesion (Fig. 31.5).

The number of lesions and their size also determines the placement of the needle. For a single lesion that can be addressed with one application, its center should be targeted. For larger lesions that require multiple ablations, ablation should be performed from deep to superficial. This is due to the fact that the ultrasound image characteristics are altered by gas bubbles formed in the tissue during the ablative process. Ablating the deeper aspect of a larger lesion therefore prevents the US images from being obscured. This principle should also be kept in mind when ablating multiple lesions.

At least a 5 mm margin is recommended, and this can be assessed using the color/Doppler mode on the ultrasound machine (Fig. 31.6). A fiduciary or metal clip is placed within the ablated lesion for identification and assessment of the lesion of follow-up imaging, as well as to make clear to radiologist reading subsequent imaging that an ablation had been performed. Track ablation should be performed once the lesion has been ablated in order to achieve hemostasis and prevent any tumor seeding. Should it be necessary, topical hemostatic agents may be injected along the track for additional hemostasis.

Postoperative Care and Discharge

Post-op Imaging Imaging with a triple phase CT scan of the liver is performed within 4–6 weeks of the ablation to detect any residual tumor, which, if present, constitutes an incomplete ablation. An incomplete ablation should be considered a technical failure on the part of the surgeon, rather than a failure on the modality of an ablation or the specific microwave system. This initial postprocedure CT scan serves as a baseline, with subsequent follow-up imaging performed as surveillance to determine local recurrence/regional recurrence. This imaging is usually based on the histological tumor type, as well as the institution. At our institution, this is followed every 4 months for first 2 years and every 6 months for the next 3–5 years. MRI is preferred over CT for longitudinal surveillance imaging for patients with chronic liver disease, cirrhosis, hepatocellular carcinoma, or adenomas.

Incomplete ablation and local recurrence may occur due to technical problems from targeting or inadequate thermal destruction of tumors, while regional and metastatic recurrence occur due to biology of the disease and its systemic nature.

Pitfalls

Prerequisites to performing safe ultrasound-guided MWA include appropriate and timely maintenance of the ultrasound machines, the laparoscopic ultrasound probes, and ablation probes as well as associated equipment. Operating room staff should be familiar with and receive prior training in the setup and use of the US and MWA device. Representatives from the respective device companies should be present in the operating room, or immediately available by phone, especially during the initial stages of the learning curve.

Appropriate preoperative preparation of the patients should include ready availability of blood on hold, particularly for cirrhotic patients with portal hypertension undergoing HCC ablation. Recanalized umbilical veins in this setting may lead to significant unexpected bleeding while obtaining access.

Thermal damage to surrounding vascular structures and adjacent organs remains a pitfall of the procedure. During mobilization of the liver, and while performing the ablation, protective sponges should be utilized in order to prevent injury to the stomach, hepatic flexure of the colon, duodenum, and the diaphragm.

Ablation time and amount of energy can be altered in order to perform ablations for tumors in close proximity to the hepatic veins or portal pedicles. A more predictable, uniform ablation field may be generated by using high-energy ablations for a shorter duration. Additionally, the use of systemic heparinization intraoperatively can decrease the risk of hepatic vein thrombosis.

The sequencing of multiple lesions or multiple ablations of a large single lesion requires adequate pre- and intraoperative planning. This is critical since ablating a lesion leads to a decrease in the visualization of hepatic parenchyma deep to the ablation zone. Utilizing preoperative imaging and IOUS together to help delineate a plan for optimal MWA probe placement for ablation provides adequate visualization in this setting.

A significant challenge occurs when there is discordance between preoperative imaging and IOUS findings. Lesions that are not visualized or have "disappeared" intraoperatively when the liver is imaged with US require ready access to recent preoperative triple phase CT or MRI in the operating room. The location of the lesion relative to the portal or hepatic veins can be used to determine the zone of ablation. However, rather than performing a blind ablation using these landmarks alone, our practice is to perform repeat cross-sectional imaging for disappearing lesions and attempt a second ablation if they are identified.

Complications

These may be a result of vascular, biliary, hollow viscus, or diaphragmatic injury. Postoperative liver dysfunction and infection of the ablation cavity may also occur.

Vascular complications include vascular injury with bleeding and/or thrombosis. Preventing vascular injury requires use of IOUS to assess the trajectory of the MWA probe prior to ablation. This helps to ensure that there are no major vascular pedicles within the trajectory at risk of injury. When a peripheral pedicle is injured, bleeding may be controlled with pressure or topical hemostatic products. In addition, performing track ablation may be used to control bleeding. In the event that these maneuvers are not able to control the bleeding, vascular embolization may be required. It is important to avoid placing a needle through or close to major pedicles, and certainly avoid applying energy that would cause thermal injury to these structures.

Vascular thrombosis is usually clinically occult, occurring in peripheral pedicles. However, anticoagulation may be required should there be propagation of a thrombus within a main portal pedicle.

MWA may rarely result in perforation of surrounding hollow viscus organs or the diaphragm. However, surgical MWA has advantages over percutaneous ablation in this regard. Surgical MWA allows mobilization of adhesions, local organs, and the liver from the diaphragm. Sponges soaked with saline may be used to protect these organs and diaphragm following mobilization of the liver and adhesions.

Patients with underlying cirrhosis are at risk of postoperative hepatic decompensation. This may be potentiated and occur due to portal vein thrombosis or infection within the ablation cavity. These factors must be considered, identified with a duplex US of the liver, or cross-sectional imaging and treated when present.

Rarely, a biliary stricture may occur. It is likely that these are underreported, given that most biliary injuries occur peripherally and do not manifest clinically. When recurrent cholangitis occurs due to a biliary stricture, it may be necessary to perform a segmental hepatectomy.

Infection within the ablation cavity occurs more commonly with percutaneous ablation. In a series of 1928 patients, the rate of infection was reported to be 0.2% [4].

Prophylactic antibiotics may be considered and used particularly when the patient has prior biliary enteric anastomosis.

Outcomes

MWA has emerged as a safe and effective first-line treatment option for patients with small (less than 3 cm) primary liver cancer, especially for those awaiting liver transplant or having advanced liver disease and are poor surgical candidates for liver resection (Child-Pugh score B). The European Society of Medical Oncology included thermal ablation as part of the treatment algorithm for patients with metastatic colorectal cancer [21]. Recent literature supports considering MWA for small, primary, and metastatic liver lesions for patients unsuitable for resection, having extensive surgical history, or in patients with insufficient future liver remnant.

Among the established thermal ablative techniques, MWA has become the preferred treatment modality due to its advanced technological profile allowing superior intralesional heating temperatures, larger ablation zones with reduced treatment times while maintaining high technical success rates and low rate of periprocedural complications.

Recent randomized controlled phase 2 trial evaluating technical success and local tumor progression of different thermal ablative modalities for liver tumors 1.5–4.0 cm observed no significant differences in rate of perioperative complications, median time to progression, and overall survival after 2-year follow-up [22]. Another systematic review/meta-analysis reported no significant difference between MWA and RFA in complete ablation rate, intrahepatic distant recurrence, and perioperative complication rate as well as comparable local tumor progression rates for liver tumors <3 cm [23].

Operative MWA approach with IOUS guidance has established its role in a variety of clinical scenarios in patients with primary and metastatic liver cancer, adding additional advantages of precise targeting, concomitant surgical staging, and minimizing periprocedural risks, especially for patients with minimal functional reserve or poor surgical candidates. Recently published studies concluded that operative MWA is both safe and effective first-line treatment modality with favorable perioperative and oncological outcomes in treatment of hepato-cellular carcinoma and metastatic colorectal cancer [5, 6]. Postoperative morbidity ranged between 7% and 54% [7–20], depending on the study; however, it should be noted that the vast majority of these were Clavien-Dindo grade 1 or 2 and associated with intrinsic liver disease rather than surgery itself. Again, perioperative mortality has been shown to be the highest in patients undergoing the procedure for HCC in the setting of underlying cirrhosis, supporting the fact that the majority of procedural complications are associated with liver dysfunction.

In terms of oncologic outcomes, the reported incidence of incomplete ablation and local recurrence ranges between 0.7% and 29.4% [7–20]. This may be related to a number of factors including differences in tumor biology and a steep learning curve associated with the procedure. Further, and more importantly, there is a lack of a standardization in both the interpretation and reporting of follow-up cross-sectional imaging performed. On the other hand, high local recurrence rates could reflect increasing size of tumors treated with MWA. Routine utilization of IOUS during surgical MWA and familiarity with operative MWA technique allows precise antenna placement/targeting and improves rates of complete ablation (confirmed on postoperative imaging) and thus long-term oncological outcomes, as well as to detect additional hepatic lessons not visible on preoperative imaging [10].

In our practice, minimally invasive IOUS-guided MWA is well tolerated by the majority of well-selected patients. In those with acceptable physiology and sufficient underlying liver reserve, it may be performed as an outpatient procedure with minimal perioperative morbidity. It is important to have an honest preoperative discussion that includes full disclosure of both potential short-term complications and oncological outcomes when compared with standard surgical approaches. Operative IOUS-guided MWA may be considered a rational first-line treatment option for patients with primary and metastatic liver tumors; however, further validation with prospective studies is warranted.

Summary

Surgical MWA ablation has recently become a first-line treatment option for variety of benign, primary, and metastatic liver tumors, especially in patients with cirrhosis and limited functional reserve. Modern microwave technology has many advantages over other energy-based thermal ablation modalities affecting perioperative and oncological outcomes. Utilizing high-frequency electromagnetic waves, it allows for more active heating with production of higher tissue temperatures in a shorter period of time and generate more predictable ablation zones with less susceptibility to heat-sink effect. Surgical ablation of liver tumors with IOUS guidance, on the other hand, allows for precise visualization, targeting minimization of periprocedural complications as well as enables to concomitantly perform oncological staging or other surgical procedures. We truly believe that recent improvements in microwave technology along with data supporting comparable short- and long-term outcomes of MWA treatment of hepatic tumors would facilitate increasing utilization of minimally invasive surgical ablative approaches as a locoregional treatment modality of choice.

References

1. Sastry A, Iannitti DA. Ablation therapy – percutaneous vs laparoscopic? Case for laparoscopic. In: Hepato-Pancreato-biliary and transplant surgery practical management of dilemmas. Beaux Books; 2018.
2. Swan R, Tsirline V, Sindram D, Martinie JB, Iannitti DA. Fundamentals of microwave physics: application to the hepatic ablation. J Microwave Surg. 2012:25–40.
3. Martin RCG, Rickert R. Chapter 96C: Microwave ablation and irreversible electroporation of liver tumors. In: Blumgart's surgery of the liver, biliary tract and pancreas. p. 1334–1358.e3.
4. Liang P, Wang Y, Yu X, et al. Malignant liver tumors: treatment with percutaneous microwave ablation–complications among cohort of 1136 patients. Radiology. 2009;251(3):933–40.
5. Ryu T, Takami Y, Wada Y, Saitsu H. Oncological outcomes of operative microwave ablation for intermediate stage hepatocellular carcinoma:

experience in 246 consecutive patients. J Gastrointest Surg. 2022;26(6):1178–86. https://doi.org/10.1007/s11605-022-05254-8. Epub 2022 Jan 21. PMID: 35064460

6. Wang T, Zhang XY, Lu X, Zhai B. Laparoscopic microwave ablation of hepatocellular carcinoma at liver surface: technique effectiveness and long-term outcomes. Technol Cancer Res Treat. 2019;18:1533033818824338. https://doi.org/10.1177/1533033818824338. PMID: 30803390; PMCID: PMC6378635

7. Tinguely P, Fusaglia M, Freedman J, et al. Laparoscopic image-based navigation for microwave ablation of liver tumors-a multi-center study. Surg Endosc. 2017;31(10):4315–24.

8. Pickens RC, Sulzer JK, Passeri MJ, Murphy K, Vrochides D, Martinie JB, Baker EH, Ocuin LM, McKillop IH, Iannitti DA. Operative microwave ablation for the multimodal treatment of neuroendocrine liver metastases. J Laparoendosc Adv Surg Tech A. 2021;31(8):917–25. https://doi.org/10.1089/lap.2020.0558. Epub 2020 Dec 8. PMID: 33296283

9. Abreu de Carvalho LF, Logghe B, Van Cleven S, et al. Local control of hepatocellular carcinoma and colorectal liver metastases after surgical microwave ablation without concomitant hepatectomy. Langenbeck's Arch Surg. 2021;406(8):2749–57.

10. Baker EH, Thompson K, McKillop IH, et al. Operative microwave ablation for hepatocellular carcinoma: a single center retrospective review of 219 patients. J Gastrointest Oncol. 2017;8(2):337–46.

11. Cillo U, Bertacco A, Fasolo E, et al. Videolaparoscopic microwave ablation in patients with HCC at a European high-volume center: results of 815 procedures. J Surg Oncol. 2019;120(6):956–65.

12. Correa-Gallego C, Fong Y, Gonen M, et al. A retrospective comparison of microwave ablation vs. radiofrequency ablation for colorectal cancer hepatic metastases. Ann Surg Oncol. 2014;21(13):4278–83.

13. Eng OS, Tsang AT, Moore D, et al. Outcomes of microwave ablation for colorectal cancer liver metastases: a single center experience. J Surg Oncol. 2015;111(4):410–3.

14. Groeschl RT, Pilgrim CH, Hanna EM, et al. Microwave ablation for hepatic malignancies: a multi-institutional analysis. Ann Surg. 2014;259(6):1195–200.

15. Leung U, Kuk D, D'Angelica MI, et al. Long-term outcomes following microwave ablation for liver malignancies. Br J Surg. 2015;102(1):85–91.

16. Martin RC, Scoggins CR, McMasters KM. Safety and efficacy of microwave ablation of hepatic tumors: a prospective review of a 5-year experience. Ann Surg Oncol. 2010;17(1):171–8.

17. McEachron KR, Ankeny JS, Robbins A, et al. Surgical microwave ablation of otherwise non-resectable colorectal cancer liver metastases: expanding opportunities for long term survival. Surg Oncol. 2021;36:61–4.
18. Swan RZ, Sindram D, Martinie JB, et al. Operative microwave ablation for hepatocellular carcinoma: complications, recurrence, and long-term outcomes. J Gastrointest Surg. 2013;17(4):719–29.
19. Takahashi H, Kahramangil B, Berber E. Local recurrence after microwave thermosphere ablation of malignant liver tumors: results of a surgical series. Surgery. 2018;163(4):709–13.
20. Takami Y, Ryu T, Wada Y, et al. Evaluation of intraoperative microwave coagulo-necrotic therapy (MCN) for hepatocellular carcinoma: a single center experience of 719 consecutive cases. J Hepatobiliary Pancreat Sci. 2013;20(3):332–41.
21. Van Cutsem E, et al. ESMO consensus guidelines for the management of patients with metastatic colorectal cancer. Ann Oncol. 2016;27:1386–422.
22. Radosevic A, Quesada R, Serlavos C, Sánchez J, Zugazaga A, Sierra A, Coll S, Busto M, Aguilar G, Flores D, Arce J, Maiques JM, Garcia-Retortillo M, Carrion JA, Visa L, Villamonte M, Pueyo E, Berjano E, Trujillo M, Sánchez-Velázquez P, Grande L, Burdio F. Microwave versus radiofrequency ablation for the treatment of liver malignancies: a randomized controlled phase 2 trial. Sci Rep. 2022;12(1):316.
23. Spiliotis AE, Gäbelein G, Holländer S, Scherber PR, Glanemann M, Patel B. Microwave ablation compared with radiofrequency ablation for the treatment of liver cancer: a systematic review and meta-analysis. Radiol Oncol. 2021;55(3):247–58.

Nonthermal Ablation

32

Yasmin Essaji, Christine Chung, Lauren M. Wancata, and Scott Helton

Percutaneous Ethanol Injection (PEI)

Percutaneous ethanol injection (PEI) involves the injection of medical grade ethanol (95%) and can be used for the treatment of encapsulated hepatocellular carcinoma (HCC). It has been used to treat other types of encapsulated hepatic tumors such as neuroendocrine tumors with some concern for its effectiveness. The use of PEI in treating HCC has become secondary to microwave and radiofrequency ablation because of their ability to more thoroughly treat larger tumors in a single setting. In addition, medical grade ethanol has become less available and prohibitively expensive. As with other forms of nonthermal ablation, PEI can be used to treat HCC in proximity to portal pedicles or hepatic veins. The efficacy of PEI depends on the uniform dispersion of ethanol throughout the tumor and requires the tumor to be well-

---

Y. Essaji
Department of Surgery, McMaster University, Hamilton, ON, Canada
e-mail: yasmin.essaji@medportal.ca; essajiy@mcmaster.ca

C. Chung · L. M. Wancata · S. Helton (✉)
Department of Surgery, Virginia Mason Franciscan Health, Seattle, WA, USA
e-mail: lauren.wancata@commonspirit.org;
scott.helton@commonspirit.org

encapsulated in order to prevent leakage of ethanol outside the tumor. It is most effective for tumors ≤3 cm, where tumor necrosis rate is 80%. It can also be used in repeated sessions for tumors ≥5 cm as tumor necrosis for a single treatment session is reported only to be 50% [1]. Many encapsulated HCCs have internal fibrous septations, which limit the uniform dispersion of ethanol throughout the tumor. Several strategies have been used to overcome this problem. This includes the placement of multiple injection needles into the tumor prior to injection or the injection of alcohol 1–2 weeks after transarterial hepatic artery embolization. The latter approach has been shown in studies to result in necrosis of the internal septations, which allows better dispersion of ethanol throughout the tumor and more uniform and thorough tumor necrosis [1] (Table 32.1).

PEI can be performed percutaneously in the interventional radiology suite or by laparoscopy or open surgery in the operating room under conscious sedation or general anesthesia. Targeting of the tumor and placement of the needle(s) is best facilitated by real-time ultrasound (US), and diffusion of ethanol within the tumor can be monitored as it creates an acoustical whiteout.

Table 32.1 Four main subtypes of nonthermal ablation

Chemical
Ethanol
Acetic acid
Epinephrine gel
Mechanical
Histotripsy
Irreversible electroporation (IRE)
Radiation
Intravascular Y-90
External beam (SBRT)
Biologic
Viruses
Adenovirus
Oncolytic viruses

PEI is best suited for small HCC (<3 cm) that are well encapsulated (confirmed by US, MRI, or CT prior to treatment). HCC associated with hepatitis B are more often encapsulated, whereas HCC associated with hepatitis C are more likely to be diffuse infiltrating type, which are not amenable to PEI. It is important to note that the injection of more than 15 cc of ethanol in a single session often results in significant abdominal pain and limits the amount that can be injected unless the patient is heavily sedated. Larger volumes of ethanol injection in a single session are best done under general anesthesia. Acetic acid injection has been shown to induce more thorough necrosis of HCC compared to ethanol, but has significant toxicity including renal failure, and hence not recommended.

Technique for large volume PEI under general anesthesia:

1. Perform thorough laparoscopy and US of the liver to identify lesion for targeting.
2. Target lesion with US; for small tumors <3 cm, a single needle can be placed; for tumors ≥3 cm, consider placing two to three needles spaced within the tumor to allow better diffusion of ethanol throughout the tumor.
3. Once ethanol is on the operative field, do not use any electrocautery as ethanol is extremely flammable. Intra-abdominal electrocautery can be used, if necessary, under CO_2 insufflation without concern for ignition.
4. Inject ethanol under US guidance using 10 mL syringes connected to each needle and use tactile feedback to avoid overfilling of the tumor to avoid reflux of alcohol into the portal system or tumor rupture.
5. Dilute any spilled ethanol with saline irrigation and aspiration to reduce peritoneal burn. This cannot be done percutaneously in the IR suite and limits the amount of ethanol that can be injected in a single session. Hence, when performed under conscious sedation, PEI usually requires multiple treatment sessions to effectively ablate a tumor; since this is not very convenient for the patient, we recommend a single session with larger volumes in the operating room.

Benefits of PEI in the OR with laparoscopy vs. IR suite:

- General anesthesia allows for injection of larger volumes of ethanol in a single session. Tumor targeting and placement of needles is facilitated by controlled ventilation and breath hold.
- Laparoscopically, the surgeon can use a suction irrigation system to dilute and aspirate spilled ethanol that leaks out of the tumor.
- Bleeding can be identified and easily controlled laparoscopically.
- Ability for breath hold allows for treatment of higher dome lesions, and the liver can also be mobilized laparoscopically.

Calculating the volume of ethanol to be injected:

- In general, up to 0.7 cc/kg or a maximum of 70 mL can be used in a single session.
- The goal is to provide enough ethanol to fill the entire volume of the tumor and to avoid excessive pressure so as to avoid tumor rupture.
- Tumor volume can be estimated based on the shape of the tumor (most commonly a sphere: $4/3\pi r^3$). It is advised to add 0.5 to the radius: $4/3\pi(r + 0.5)^3$ when calculating to account for spillage. Alternatively, tumor volume is more accurately measured using CT volumetry.

Complications:

- Portal vein (PV) thrombosis from ethanol reflux outside of the capsule.
- Tumor rupture.
- If done under conscious sedation, it may be painful from ethanol spillage into peritoneum.

- Alcohol intoxication and hangover (Toradol can be helpful in treatment of alcohol side effects).
- Platelet consumption and resultant thrombocytopenia (theorized to be a result of tumor necrosis).
- Segmental infarct if ethanol spills into another liver segment.
- Acute kidney injury (Figs. 32.1, 32.2, 32.3, and 32.4).

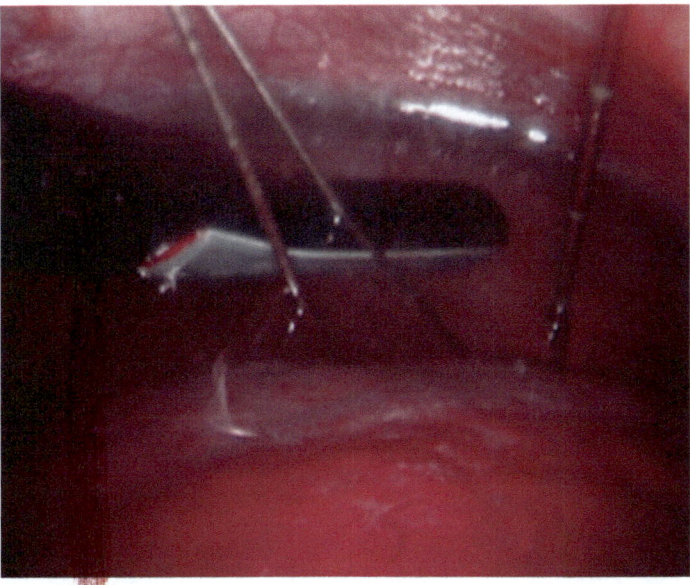

Fig. 32.1 Placing multiple injection needles into a large HCC under intraoperative laparoscopic US guidance using a standoff technique. (Picture courtesy of Dr. Scott Helton from Virginia Mason)

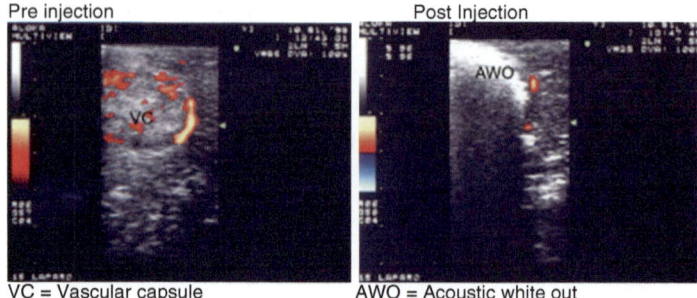

VC = Vascular capsule   AWO = Acoustic white out

Fig. 32.2 IOUS power doppler shows the effects of PEI on tumor vascularity and acoustical white out within minutes following injection of ethanol. (Picture courtesy of Dr. Scott Helton from Virginia Mason)

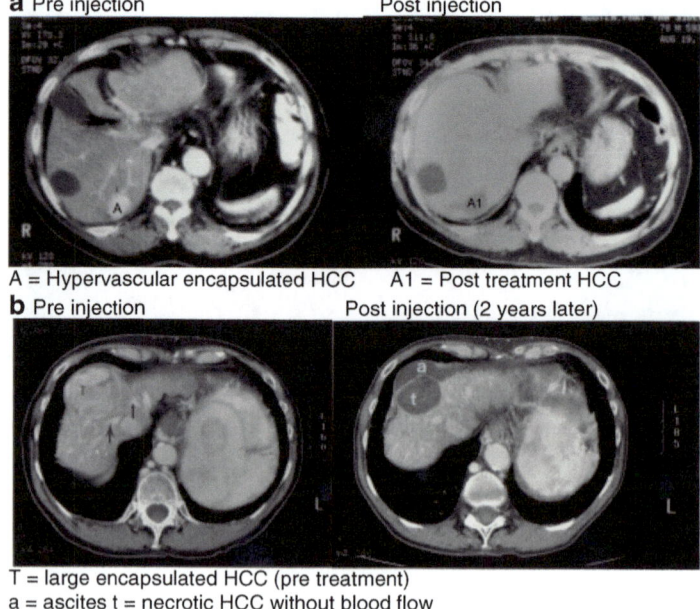

A = Hypervascular encapsulated HCC   A1 = Post treatment HCC

T = large encapsulated HCC (pre treatment)
a = ascites t = necrotic HCC without blood flow

Fig. 32.3 CT scans before and after PEI in a small (**a**) and large (**b**) encapsulated HCC. The lower panel shows a complete radiographic kill of tumor that has no arterial enhancement. (Picture courtesy of Dr. Scott Helton from Virginia Mason)

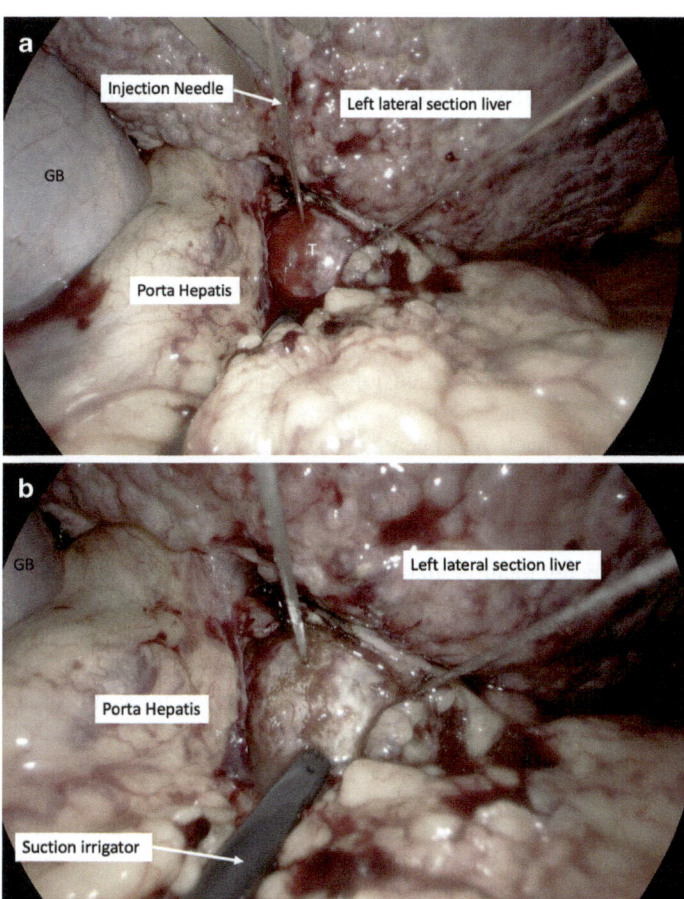

Fig. 32.4 Laparoscopic PEI of a 3 cm caudate lobe HCC in a patient with cirrhosis, portal hypertension, varices, trace ascites. Note the tumor abuts the porta hilum contraindicating the use of thermal ablation. A direct puncture of the tumor is made because it was not possible to traverse the liver with the needles. Note: the hypervascular tumor (**a**) becomes ischemic within minutes of PEI (**b**). (Picture courtesy of Dr. Scott Helton from Virginia Mason)

Irreversible Electroporation (IRE)

IRE is a technique in which electrical pulses are passed through cells causing "nanopores" in cell membranes and increasing the permeability of a cell membrane, which causes damage and apoptotic cell death. It can be used to ablate tumors without causing any thermal effect (no heat sink) or damage to nearby vascular or biliary structures, with real-time ultrasound imaging of ablated zones [2]. This technique is mainly used in hepatic or pancreatic masses that are unresectable or those that involve key vascular pedicles, but it is quite laborious as it requires precise placement of electrodes in three dimensions (precise spacing, precise depth, and appropriate bracketing of soft tissue) [3, 4]. While the percutaneous approach has been performed by a few interventional radiologists, experience to date is mostly seen with open laparotomy [5]. Additionally, because peritoneal disease can be found on diagnostic laparoscopy, the percutaneous approach is less ideal in that it may not identify metastatic disease in those who are thought to be IRE candidates. In some studies, IRE has demonstrated substantially prolonged survival when used in combination with conventional chemotherapy and radiation therapy, compared to historical controls [5]. In other studies, however, it has not shown to have a significant benefit in median survival [6].

Indications and inclusion criteria:

- Patient not considered a candidate for resection, transplant, or thermal ablation techniques.
- Tumor 3 cm or smaller.
- Patient has already received systemic therapy and disease has not progressed.

Exclusion criteria:

- Tumor >3 cm.
- Patients with pacemakers, with cardiac arrhythmias, extensive disease involvement outside of involved organ.
- Patients with uncorrectable coagulation disorders.

- Patients unable to undergo general anesthesia.
- Multifocal disease not amenable to complete ablation.
- Patients with metal in the region, such as metal stents.

NanoKnife IRE system:

- Footswitch, power cord, and line of single use disposable electrodes.
- Monopolar probes.
  - Single electrode.
  - 15 cm length or 25 cm length (obese patients).
  - 19-gauge needle with depth markings, and active electrode length adjustable in 0.5 cm increments from 0 to 4 cm, with a maximum insertion depth of 15 cm
  - Ideal spacing 1.5–2 cm between electrodes, with active tip 1–3 cm, all electrodes parallel to each other.
- Bipolar probes:
  - Two poles on the same needle separated by an insulated region with the ability to ablate larger areas.
- ECG Trigger Monitor (AccuSync 72):
  - Automatically detects the R wave (when IRE is delivered).
  - Provided with each generator.

Intraoperative procedure:

- Patient supine, under general anesthesia, and muscle paralysis.
- AccuSync system in place, with leads to anesthesia (requires five ECG buttons).
- ASA guidelines require a defibrillator to be readily available.
- Intraoperative ultrasound; ideally coupled with computer-generated guidance system for precise probe placement, NanoKnife generator, and electrodes.
- Determine lesion size and location.
- Use treatment planning computer software to determine correct electrode configuration.

Probe placement grid:

- 8 × 8 cm grid that displays selected probe array bracketing for a certain targeted ablation area
- Given that the majority of pancreatic neck tumors' longest axis is axial with infiltration of the celiac axis median (range 2–4 cm), it is not uncommon to have an anterior–posterior tumor maximum depth between 2.5 and 3.0 cm in size.

Targeted ablation area settings:

- Contains lesion zone, margin, target zone.
- Number electrodes [1–6].
- Determine and set electrode exposure (typically 1 cm maximum).
- Needles placed under direct US guidance to complete bracketing of the tumor.
- Confirm electrode spacing measurements.
  - 2.0 cm apart and 1 cm margin of normal soft tissue
- Update treatment planning software with true measurements and reposition and remeasure electrodes as needed.
- Connect electrodes to NanoKnife Generator.
- Review treatment parameters to ensure accuracy.
- Confirm 0/4 or 1/4 twitches.
- Physician delivers IRE energy.
- Standard default voltage of 1500 V/cm is initiated with planned delivery of 90 pulses and a pulse width of 70–90 μs.
- Monitor AccuSync display for saturation and/or double triggering, change lead pairs only if necessary.
- Sequential pullbacks are performed to obtain adequate margins both superiorly and inferiorly. Ablation of the tracks while probes are being removed can be performed.
- Postoperative CT imaging for complications, follow up imaging in 4 weeks, then every 3–6 months (Figs. 32.5, 32.6, 32.7, 32.8, 32.9, 32.10, 32.11, 32.12, and 32.13).

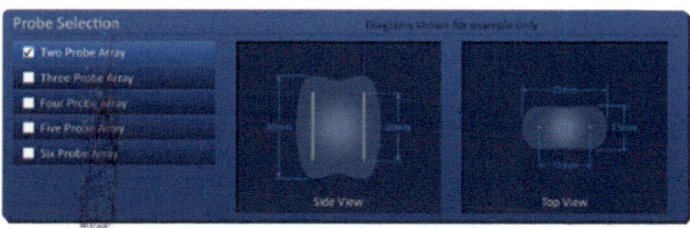

Fig. 32.5 Example of probe placement with width and depth orientation with two probes. (Image courtesy of AngioDynamics, Inc. and its affiliates)

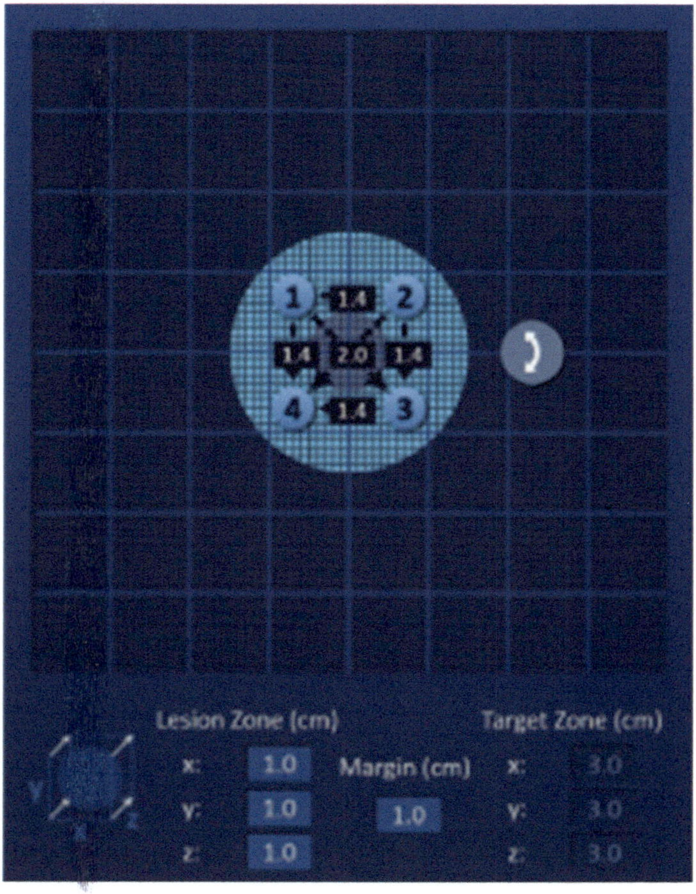

Fig. 32.6 Example of targeted ablation area setting and probe placement grid. (Image courtesy of AngioDynamics, Inc. and its affiliates)

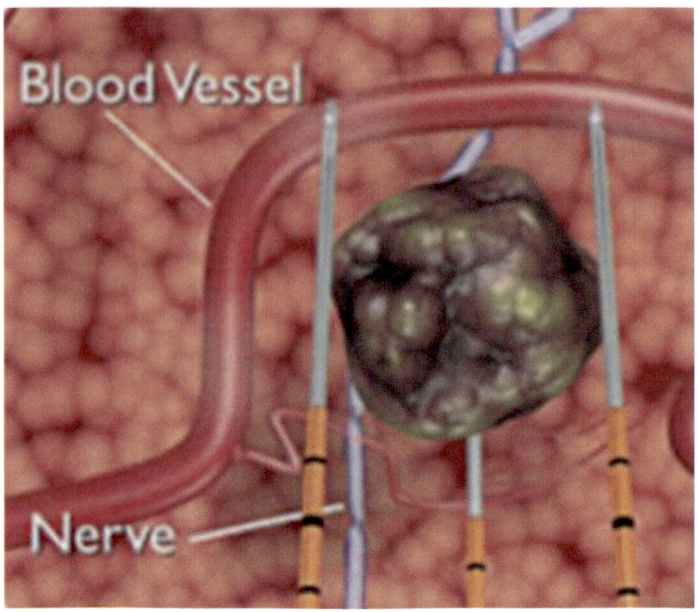

Fig. 32.7 Example of bracketing probes around a tumor. (Image courtesy of AngioDynamics, Inc. and its affiliates)

Key Point

Frequent findings are abdominal wall edema or ascites, sometimes narrowing or compression of vessel walls. Tumors often appear heterogeneous, because right after IRE the ablation zone may be bigger and hypodense. This will reduce over time and scarring will take place.

Key points:

- To reduce risk of tumor seeding, set probe exposure setting to 0 cm for each single electrode probe before removing from the patient.
- To reduce the risk of mechanical perforation during pulse delivery and subsequent thrombosis, probes should be placed parallel to critical structures.

Procedure Parameter Probe Spacing:	Setting
Minimum recommended spacing	1.0 cm
Maximum recommended spacing	2.0 cm
Typical range used	1.5-2.0 cm
Probe exposure Length	
Minimum recommended probe exposure	1.0 cm
Maximum recommended probe exposure	2.5 cm
Recommended starting point for most soft tissue	1.5 cm
Recommended starting point for high conductivity tissue (e.g. muscle)	1.0 cm
Recommended maximum probe exposure for high conductivity tissue	1.5 cm
Pulse Length	
Default system setting	90 μsec
Minimum recommended setting	70 μsec
Maximum system setting	100 μsec
Typical range used	70-90 μsec
Number of Pulses per probe pair	
Default system setting	70 pulses
Maximum system setting	100 pulses
Typical range used for this setting	70-90 pulses
Typical number of total pulses per probe pair (after multiple rounds)	140 pulses
Volts/cm:	
Default system setting	1500 volts/cm
Volts:	
Default system setting	The value for the default volts setting is based upon probe spacing, to achieve 1500 volts/cm
Minimum system setting	500 volts[1]
Maximum system setting	3000 volts
Probe pair current range	
Maximum current system will allow	50 amps
Typical current range target at conductivity test	20-35 amps [2]
Notes:	
1. During the conductivity test the system will deliver one pulse of approximately 400 volts 2. The current normally rises as pulses are delivered	

Fig. 32.8 Example procedure parameter settings. (Image courtesy of AngioDynamics, Inc. and its affiliates [7])

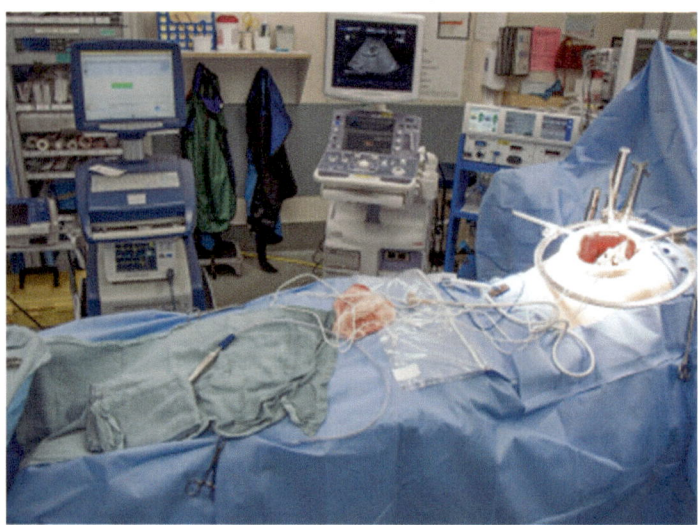

Fig. 32.9 General operating room setup. (Picture courtesy of Dr. Scott Helton from Virginia Mason)

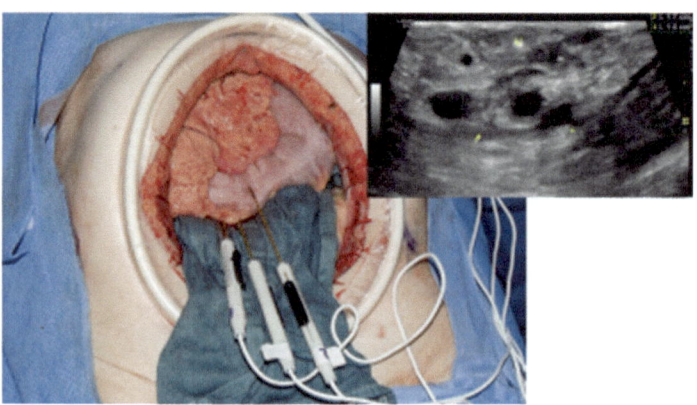

Fig. 32.10 Probes in place for pancreas mass using ultrasound guidance. (Picture courtesy of Dr. Scott Helton from Virginia Mason)

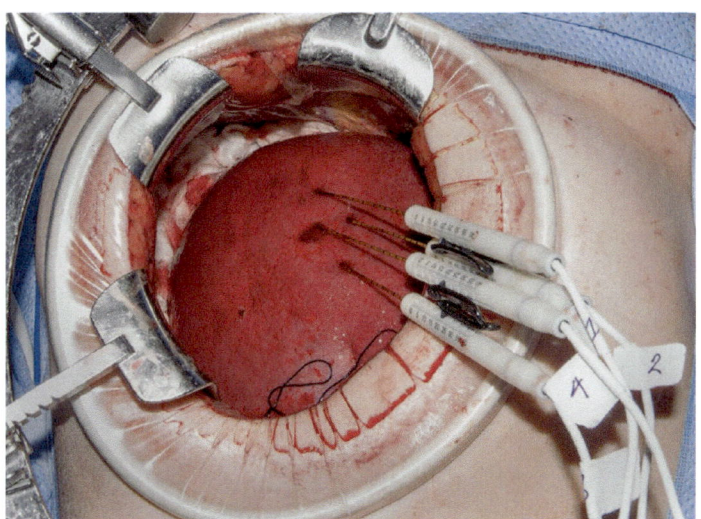

Fig. 32.11 Probes in place for liver mass using ultrasound guidance. (Picture courtesy of Dr. Scott Helton from Virginia Mason)

- For margin accentuation, perform IRE prior to complete dissection/transection, because there must be soft tissue in place for the IRE needle(s) insertion.

Complications:

- Transient elevation of transaminases and bilirubin for treated liver tumors.
- Transient ventricular arrhythmia, atrial fibrillation.
- Hepatic abscess or failure.
- Venous or arterial thrombosis.
- Pseudoaneurysm.
- Acute renal failure.
- Pneumothorax.
- Hemorrhage.
- Bowel perforation.
- Infection.
- Pancreatic fistula formation or abscess.

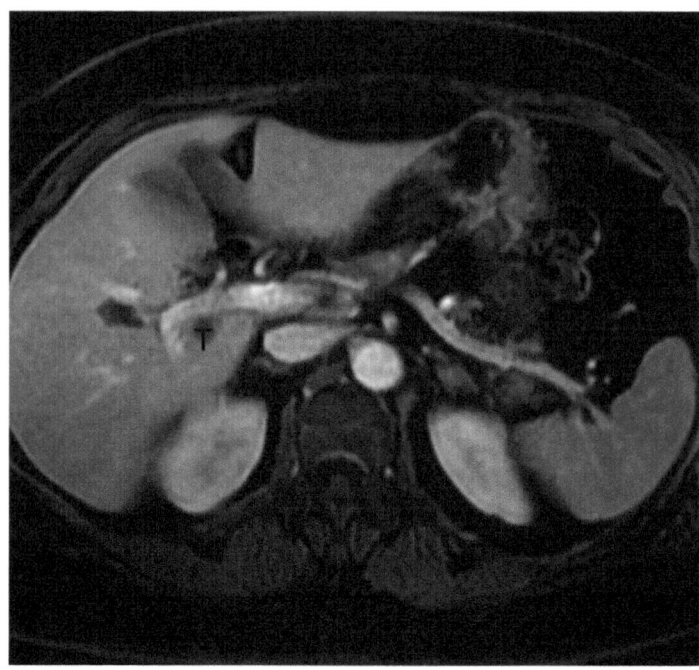

Fig. 32.12 T = tumor that is an IRE-candidate—within segment I abutting the right portal vein and not suitable for thermal ablation. (Picture courtesy of Dr. Scott Helton from Virginia Mason)

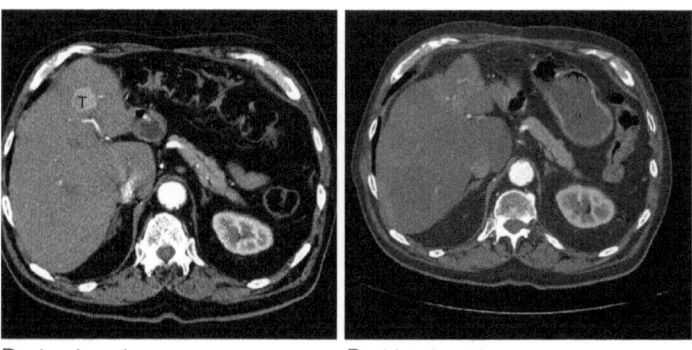

Pre treatment   Post treatment

Fig. 32.13 T = HCC tumor in umbilical fissure that would require hepatectomy if resected. (Picture courtesy of Dr. Scott Helton from Virginia Mason)

Histotripsy

Histotripsy is an emerging technology of noninvasive and nonthermal ablation with many applications including the destruction of liver tumors. Histotripsy utilizes ultrasound to create cavitation: a process of generation, oscillation, and collapse of microbubbles within the tissue that leads to tissue destruction. The tissue is then subsequently absorbed by the body over time.

Due to the fact that different tissues have different thresholds for histotripsy-induced damage, this property can be utilized to target certain tissues while preserving others. For example, in the liver, tumor tissue can be destroyed while adjacent bile ducts and large vessels are preserved. Additionally, lesions can be targeted within millimeters. This precise selective destruction of tumors has important advantages over thermal ablation, which should not be used to treat tumors that are adjacent to key vascular and biliary pedicles because of collateral damage.

There have been multiple studies evaluating the feasibility of histotripsy in animal models and it has been tested in several organs including the liver, prostate, kidney, breast, pancreas, and blood vessels. These animal studies have demonstrated the feasibility and efficacy of selective tissue destruction [8, 9].

A feasibility clinical trial evaluating the use of histotripsy for liver tumors in eight humans was reported in 2024. The trial (THERESA trial) utilized histotripsy for hepatocellular carcinoma and other metastases [10]. The study demonstrated the ability of histotripsy to accurately ablate and shrink tumors with minimal complications. This study was followed by a prospective, multi-institutional, international single arm trial (#HOPE4LIVER US; clinical trials.gov: *NCT04572633*) designed to assess the efficacy and safety of histotripsy in treating primary and metastatic liver tumors in 44 patients in Europe, England, and the United States. Technical success was observed in 42 of 44 treated tumors (95%), and procedure-related major complications were reported in three of 44 participants (7%): both meeting the performance goal [11]. A subsequent larger international study reported on 295 patients who underwent histotripsy for 510 tumors at 18 centers

[12]. Histotripsy was well tolerated, with few overall complications and rare serious complications, indicating a safety profile that compares favorably with that of other liver-directed therapies for the treatment of liver tumors. Long-term follow-up data and oncologic outcomes have not yet been reported.

The setup for histotripsy is quite complex (Figs. 32.1 and 32.2) and includes an investigational device (VORTX Rx, HistoSonics, Inc., Ann Arbor, MI), an operator (typically a radiologist or a surgeon), general anesthesia, and a special ultrasound therapy transducer. The device delivers ultrasound pulses (700 kHz) of microsecond (<20 us) duration to induce controlled inertial acoustic cavitation at a known focal zone (bubble cloud). The bubble cloud produces complete mechanical cellular destruction at the focal point. The therapy transducer contains a coaxially aligned diagnostic ultrasound probe allowing real-time tumor targeting, bubble cloud visualization, histotripsy monitoring, and immediate post-histotripsy verification. The therapy transducer is attached to a software-controlled micro-positioning system, enabling fully automated treatment of a preplanned ablation volume. The system requires coupling the therapy transducer to the patient's skin with cooled degassed water that is held in a special drape attached to the skin surface. The length of treatment is based on the tissue/disease and volume of tumor to be treated.

Histotripsy is completely noninvasive and provides highly selective tissue destruction while sparing collateral damage to adjacent anatomical structures that need to be preserved. Limitations include inability to treat areas that may be obscured by overlying bone or gas. The HistoSonics system is currently the only FDA-approved histotripsy device in the United States. Long-term outcome studies have yet to be published. The results of ongoing current and future clinical trials are awaited. For further details on this system, the interested reader is encouraged to visit https://histosonics.com/ (Figs. 32.14 and 32.15).

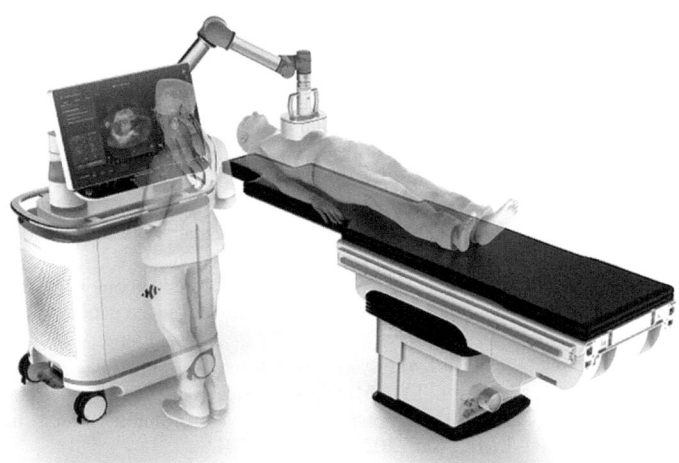

Fig. 32.14 The HistoSonics system. (Photos courtesy of Joshua King, HistoSonics)

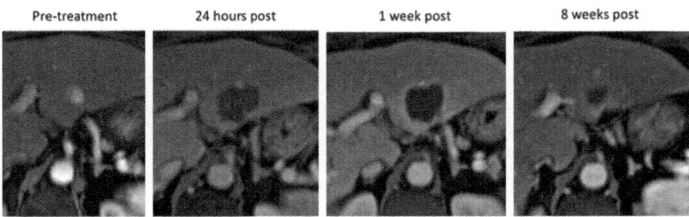

Fig. 32.15 Evolution of tumor treated with histotripsy and evolution of treatment zone. (Courtesy of Joshua King, HistoSonics)

References

1. Chao-Sheng L, Kuo-Ching Y, Ming-Fang Y, et al. Prognosis of small hepatocellular carcinoma treated by percutaneous ethanol injection and transcatheter arterial chemoembolization. J Clin Epidemiol. 2002;55(11):1095–104. https://doi.org/10.1016/s0895-4356(02)00487-0.
2. Narayanan G, Froud T, Suthar R, et al. Irreversible electroporation of hepatic malignancy. Semin Intervent Radiol. 2013;30(1):67–73.

3. Meijerink MR, Ruarus AH, Vroomen LGPH, et al. Irreversible electroporation to treat unresectable colorectal liver metastases (COLDFIRE-2): a phase II, two-center, single-arm clinical trial. Radiology. 2021;299(2):470–80.
4. Kingham TP, Karkar AM, D'Angelica MI, et al. Ablation of perivascular hepatic malignant tumors with irreversible electroporation. J Am Coll Surg. 2012;215(3):379–87.
5. Martin R, Kwon D, Chalikonda S, et al. Treatment of 200 locally advanced (stage III) pancreatic adenocarcinoma patients with irreversible electroporation. Ann Surg. 2015;262(3):486–94.
6. Månsson C, Brahmstaedt R, Nygren P, et al. Percutaneous irreversible electroporation as first-line treatment of locally advanced pancreatic cancer. Anticancer Res. 2019;39(5):2509–12.
7. Angiodynamics. NanoKnife system user manual version 3.0.
8. Worlikar T, Mendiratta-Lala M, Vlaisavljevich E, et al. Effects of histotripsy on local tumor progression in an in vivo orthotopic rodent liver tumor model. BME Front. 2020;2020:9830304.
9. Vlaisavljevich E, Kim Y, Allen S, et al. Image-guided non-invasive ultrasound liver ablation using histotripsy: feasibility study in an in vivo porcine model. Ultrasound Med Biol. 2013;39:1398–409.
10. Vidl-Jove J, Serres X, Vlaisavljevich E, et al. First-in-man histotripsy of hepatic tumors: the THERESA trial, a feasibility study. Int J Hyperth. 2022;39:1115–23.
11. Mendiratta-Lala M, Wiggermann P, Pech M, et al. The #HOPE4LIVER single-arm pivotal trial for histotripsy of primary and metastatic liver tumors. Radiology. 2024;312(3):e233051.
12. Wehrle C, Burns K, Ong E, et al. The first international experience with histotripsy: a safety analysis of 230 cases. J Gastrointest Surg. 2025;29(4):102000.

Hepatic Artery Infusion Pump: Open and Robotic Techniques for Placement

33

Mengyuan Liu and T. Peter Kingham

Introduction

Regional liver-directed chemotherapy is not a novel concept. Nitrogen mustard gas was injected directly into the hepatic artery in the 1950s [1]. Since then, the rationale for hepatic artery infusion chemotherapy (HAIC) was strengthened by the discovery that liver metastases derive their blood supply from the hepatic artery while hepatic tissue is supplied by the portal vein [2]. Furthermore, fluorodeoxyuridine (FUDR) supplanted other agents due to its high hepatic extraction rate of 94–99%, while an implantable metal hepatic artery infusion pump (HAIP) allowed for continuous infusion of HAIC [3].

When it was first introduced, HAIP was placed via laparotomy, either as a stand-alone procedure or as part of combined liver resection or colorectal surgery. Minimally invasive techniques for HAIP placement emerged with laparoscopic surgery [4, 5], but shifted to robotic surgery because the platform allowed for fine motor control during vascular work [6]. Specifically, the rationale for robotic HAIP includes faster recovery [7, 8]: earlier initiation

M. Liu · T. P. Kingham (✉)
Department of Surgery, Memorial Sloan Kettering Cancer Center, New York, NY, USA
e-mail: kinghamp@mskcc.org

of HAIC and decreased adhesions for future liver surgery. Robotic HAIP can also be safely combined with liver resections or colorectal surgery [9].

Perioperative Considerations

Considerations for HAIC should be made in conjunction with a medical oncologist experienced in its administration and side effects. Currently, HAIC is used in colorectal liver metastases in the setting of adjuvant therapy [10], conversion therapy for unresectable disease [11], or palliative therapy for liver-dominant disease that has failed systemic therapy [12]. There is also evidence for HAIC in unresectable intrahepatic cholangiocarcinoma [13]. Contraindications to HAIC include multiple sites of extrahepatic disease, extensive hepatic replacement by tumor, or impaired liver function (bilirubin >3), with evidence of portal hypertension. A diagnostic laparoscopy is typically performed first to exclude any extrahepatic disease that would abort the operation.

Most commonly, HAIC is used in the adjuvant setting for colorectal liver metastases (CLM) to prevent hepatic recurrences. Half of recurrences after complete resection of CLM are in the liver, arguing for limiting the liver disease. Multiple randomized trials have demonstrated that HAIC can curb hepatic recurrences [14], for example at 2 years, the hepatic recurrence was reduced from 40% to 10% with HAIC . This response is durable with long-term follow-up, showing improved median 10-year hepatic recurrence-free survival (not reached vs. 32.5 months, $p < 0.01$) and 10-year overall survival (41% vs. 27%, $p = 0.1$) [10]. HAIC can also be used in CLM patients who are not upfront resectable, with 52% of patients able to undergo resection after response to HAIC [11]. Similarly, it has been used in unresectable cholangiocarcinoma, with 58% having a radiologic response and 20% converting to resection [13].

The HAIP catheter is placed in the gastroduodenal artery (GDA) and infuses chemotherapy to the liver via the hepatic artery (Fig. 33.1). Accessory or replaced hepatic arteries are ligated and flow to that lobe occurs through cross perfusion.

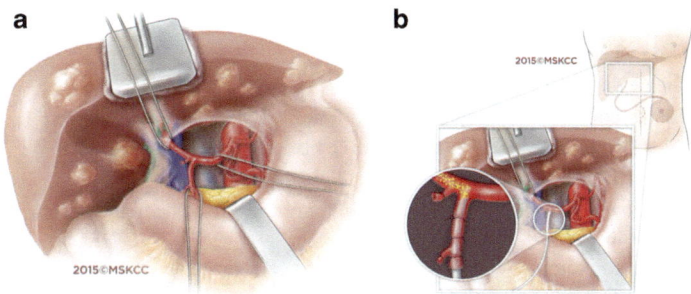

Fig. 33.1 (**a**) Hepatic artery anatomy for placement of hepatic artery infusion pump with common hepatic artery, proper hepatic artery, and gastroduodenal artery encircled. From Ref. [8] (Elsevier). (**b**) Placement of catheter into gastroduodenal artery at the confluence with common hepatic artery

Placement of the HAIP into an artery other than the GDA incurs more complications and a higher incidence of extrahepatic perfusion [16]. Preoperatively, the hepatic anatomy should be carefully defined with a high-quality CT angiogram as the need for complex vascular reconstruction is a relative contraindication to the robotic technique.

Principles

The aim of the operation is to isolate the common hepatic artery, proper hepatic artery, and GDA without damage. The arteries should be free of excessive tissue for 2 cm to allow space for a bulldog clamp and to ensure extraneous branches that permit extrahepatic perfusion are tied. Accessory or replaced hepatic arteries are identified but ligated at the end of the operation once successful cannulation of GDA is confirmed. Cannulation of the replaced hepatic artery or splenic artery is possible if the GDA is inadvertently damaged [16].

Extrahepatic perfusion can be avoided by reviewing the CT angiogram for any aberrant hepatic anatomy and carefully isolating the arteries from collateral branches. There is often a supra-

Table 33.1 Sequence of cannulation. GDA, gastroduodenal artery

Sequence of cannulation
Ligate distal GDA with silk suture
Clamp common and proper hepatic arteries with bulldog
Pass 3 silk sutures, hockey stick and 11-blade into the abdomen
Pass silk suture behind the proximal GDA
Pull down on distal GDA, make arteriotomy with 11-blade, remove 11-blade
Dilate arteriotomy with hockey stick, insert catheter
Assistant stabilizes catheter while the proximal silk suture is tied on GDA
Secure catheter in the GDA with 2 additional ties

duodenal artery that arises from the GDA and failure to ligate it will result in perfusion of the duodenum.

The sequence of cannulation should be well-rehearsed (Table 33.1). The catheter tip should be comfortably within reach and all equipment should be prepared in advance. The first assistant or the robotic bedside assistant should be knowledgeable about the sequence of cannulation as injury to the arterial wall or false passage with the catheter can result in a dissection that renders the artery unusable for HAIP. For minimally invasive approaches, a plan for open conversion, though rare (4–17%), should be discussed with all team members at the start of the operation [5, 7].

Setup and Port Placement

For open procedures, the patient is placed supine with arms out. A self-retaining body wall retractor is used for exposure. Typically, a midline incision is used but can be flexible if concomitant liver surgery requires an alternative incision. The 7 × 7 cm HAIP pocket is marked and should reside two to three fingerbreadth below the costal margin and above the anterior superior iliac spine (Fig. 33.2). In obese patients, the pocket can be moved to the chest wall where less subcutaneous fat prevents the pump from migrating or flipping [17].

Fig. 33.2 Schematic of pump pocket and port placement. Triangle represents the xiphoid and circle represents umbilicus. Port 3 is typically the camera port (**c**). A 12 mm assistant resides between ports 2 and 3 (**a**)

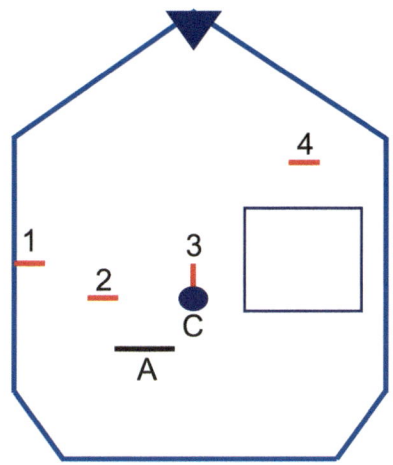

For robotic procedures, the patient is placed supine on a robotic operating table, often the legs are split to allow space for an assistant, especially during combined liver or colon surgeries. The arms are tucked and the feet are secured to minimize movement in a reverse Trendelenburg position. The HAIP pocket is marked prior to incision, so ports are not placed in that area.

Four robotic ports and one 12 mm assistant port are placed (Fig. 33.2). Ports can be adjusted in concomitant liver or colon surgery but in general triangulate toward the porta hepatis. The patient is placed in 20° of steep reverse Trendelenburg and the robot is docked from the patient's right side. After insufflation and port placement, the liver is retracted with a Nathanson and the assistant gently provides caudal tension on the stomach to maximize the porta hepatis exposure. If indocyanine green (ICG) is used to visualize the bile duct, it should be given at the beginning of the case.

Techniques

The HAIP takes approximately 30 min to prime and should be prepared whenever the surgeon is committed to pump placement, typically after a negative diagnostic laparoscopy or confirmation of favorable arterial anatomy.

Dissection of the porta hepatis starts with entry into pars flaccida and identification of the common hepatic artery lymph node. After this lymph node is removed, the common hepatic artery should be within view. The dissection continues toward the proper hepatic artery, and right gastric artery is typically ligated to visualize the GDA.

The GDA should be skeletonized for 2 cm and all collateral branches are tied with silk sutures so as to not interfere with the cannulation. The proper hepatic artery should be dissected until its bifurcation and the common bile duct is visible to its right and portal vein is seen posteriorly. Accessory or replaced hepatic arteries are also identified at this time. After dissection, the common hepatic artery, proper hepatic artery, and GDA should appear as in Fig. 33.3. Papaverine can be used to dilate the GDA if its lumen appears small.

A cholecystectomy is performed because HAIC induces cholecystitis [1]. The pump pocket is prepared by extending the incision down to fascia and to the marked edges of the pocket. The catheter is inserted into the abdomen under direct visualization and then is beveled just beyond the first bead. Four sutures anchor the corners of the HAIP to the fascia.

Sequence of cannulation (Table 33.1) begins by ligating the distal GDA with a silk tie. This tie is used for gentle caudal retraction on the GDA (Fig. 33.4a). Next, the common hepatic artery, proper hepatic artery, and accessory/replaced hepatic artery are clamped with a bulldog or vessel loop. A silk tie is passed under the proximal GDA to be used later to secure the catheter. During an open procedure, the arteriotomy is made with a 11-blade to encompass two-thirds of the GDA. One person dilates and elevates the arteriotomy while another passes the catheter into the

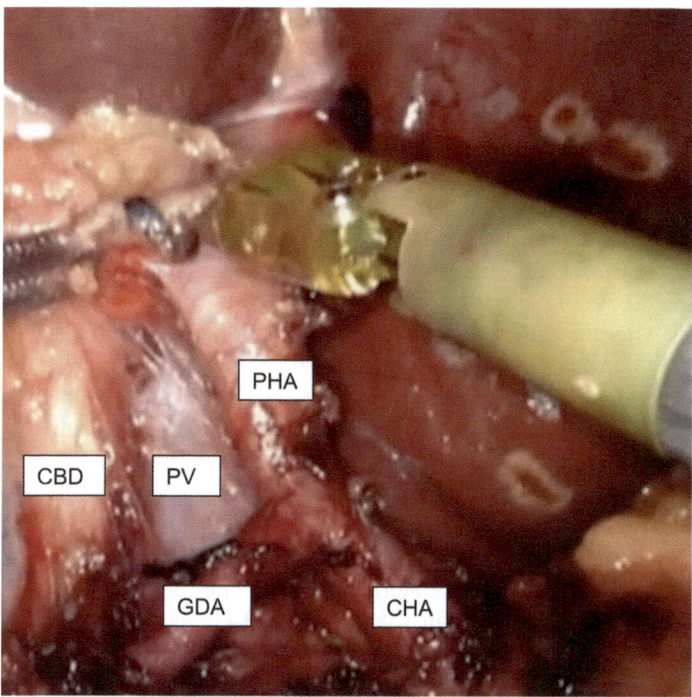

Fig. 33.3 Exposure of the hepatic artery anatomy prior to cannulation with at least 2 cm of common hepatic artery, proper hepatic artery, and gastroduodenal isolated

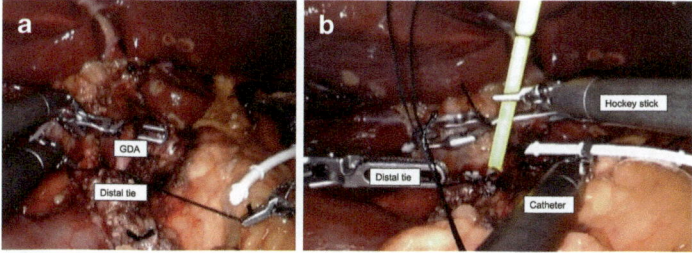

Fig. 33.4 (**a**) Sequence of cannulation starts with tying the gastroduodenal artery distally. (**b**) The distal tie is used for gentle caudal retraction on the GDA. After arteriotomy, the hockey stick is used to dilate and lift the artery to allow for catheter insertion

GDA; careful not to push with undue tension as it may cause a false passage and an arterial dissection.

On the robot, the assistant passes through the assistant port the hockey stick, the 11-blade, and the silk sutures. Arm 1 provides caudal tension on the GDA while the assistant pushes down on the distal stomach for visualization. The 11-blade makes an arteriotomy and then is quickly removed from the abdomen by the assistant. Arm 4 dilates the arteriotomy with the hockey stick and lifts it up while Arm 2 inserts the catheter into the GDA (Fig. 33.4b).

After the catheter is in the correct position at the confluence of the GDA and common hepatic artery, the assistant stabilizes the catheter while the proximal silk tie is secured just behind the first bead. After each knot, the catheter should be flushed to ensure that the knot is not too taut. The catheter is secured with two additional silk ties, one behind the second bead and one in between the two beads.

The falciform ligament should be completely taken down and ligated to prevent collateral flow to the abdominal wall. Methylene blue is then instilled into the HAIP and bilobar perfusion is assessed (Fig. 33.5). The absence of bilobar perfusion

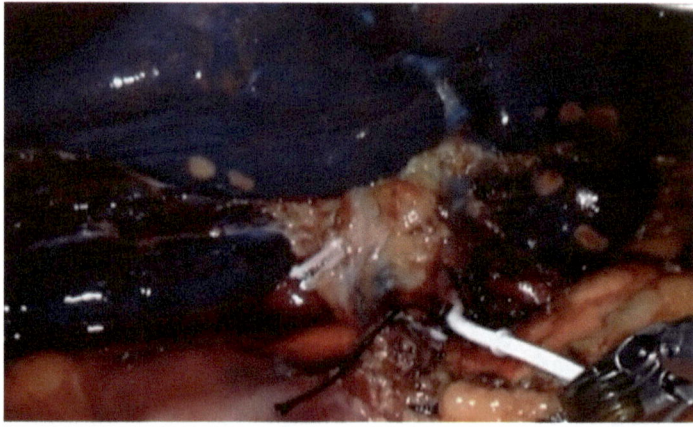

Fig. 33.5 Successful methylene blue test shows bilobar liver perfusion and absence of extrahepatic perfusion

suggests an accessory or replaced hepatic artery is nonoccluded, which should be identified and addressed. There should be no blue dye outside the liver in the stomach, duodenum, or pancreas. If there is extrahepatic perfusion, likely collateral vessels still need to be identified and ligated. After the methylene blue perfusion test is complete, the clamped accessory/replaced hepatic arteries can be ligated formally. The HAIP is then flushed one final time.

The catheter should sit in the abdomen free of tension. If there is concomitant colon surgery, the catheter should be moved far away from the colorectal operative field to avoid contamination and the pump pocket is closed prior to the colorectal operation.

Postoperative Consideration

A nuclear medicine study is performed to confirm bilobar liver perfusion, which can occur as soon as the first postoperative day after minimally invasive surgery. For open HAIP placement, the study can be performed as soon as the patient is mobile with adequate pain control. If the study shows extrahepatic perfusion, additional angiography and embolization are required before the HAIP can be used for chemotherapy.

Complications related to this procedure are either due to HAIC or HAIP [18]. The hepatic artery also supplies the bile ducts and the high doses of chemotherapy delivered to them can cause biliary damage. Liver function should be carefully monitored and elevations in enzymes require FUDR dose reductions and filling the pump with dexamethasone. Rarely, the damage can progress to biliary sclerosis and cholangitis. Complications related to HAIP include pump pocket (hematomas, infections), catheter (dislodgements, erosions), or those related to the vasculature (arterial dissection, pseudoaneurysms). Early pump complications are salvageable [16], but those relating to catheter or vessel damage may require embolization or stenting across the GDA, which render the HAIP unusable.

Conclusion

HAIP provides regional liver-directed chemotherapy and is a valuable tool in the management of colorectal liver metastases, especially in converting more patients to complete resections or limiting the liver disease in the setting of progression on systemic therapy. The outcomes of open versus minimally invasive surgery for HAIP are equivalent [5, 7, 8].

Robotic HAIP placement is a safe procedure and allows for quicker recovery to initiation of pump chemotherapy. Given the degree of vessel work involved, it should be performed by surgeons proficient in gentle and meticulous tissue handling on the robot.

Disclosure No relevant disclosures.

References

1. Anteby R, et al. Getting chemotherapy directly to the liver: the historical evolution of hepatic artery chemotherapy. J Am Coll Surg. 2021;232(3):332–8.
2. Ackerman NB. The blood supply of experimental liver metastases. IV. Changes in vascularity with increasing tumor growth. Surgery. 1974;75(4):589–96.
3. Ensminger WD, Gyves JW. Clinical pharmacology of hepatic arterial chemotherapy. Semin Oncol. 1983;10(2):176–82.
4. Franklin MNR Jr, Stubbs R. Laparoscopic approach for regional hepatic chemotherapy in the treatment of primary or metastatic malignancy. Minimal Access Surg Oncol. 1995:153–7.
5. Franklin ME Jr, Gonzalez JJ Jr. Laparoscopic placement of hepatic artery catheter for regional chemotherapy infusion: technique, benefits, and complications. Surg Laparosc Endosc Percutan Tech. 2002;12(6):398–407.
6. Hellan M, Pigazzi A. Robotic-assisted placement of a hepatic artery infusion catheter for regional chemotherapy. Surg Endosc. 2008;22(2):548–51.
7. Dhir M, et al. Robotic assisted placement of hepatic artery infusion pump is a safe and feasible approach. J Surg Oncol. 2016;114(3):342–7.

8. Qadan M, et al. Robotic hepatic arterial infusion pump placement. HPB (Oxford). 2017;19(5):429–35.
9. Creasy JM, et al. Implementation of a hepatic artery infusion program: initial patient selection and perioperative outcomes of concurrent hepatic artery infusion and systemic chemotherapy for colorectal liver metastases. Ann Surg Oncol. 2020;27(13):5086–95.
10. Kemeny N, et al. Hepatic arterial infusion of chemotherapy after resection of hepatic metastases from colorectal cancer. N Engl J Med. 1999;341(27):2039–48.
11. D'Angelica MI, et al. Phase II trial of hepatic artery infusional and systemic chemotherapy for patients with unresectable hepatic metastases from colorectal cancer: conversion to resection and long-term outcomes. Ann Surg. 2015;261(2):353–60.
12. Ammori JB, et al. Hepatic artery infusional chemotherapy in patients with unresectable colorectal liver metastases and extrahepatic disease. J Surg Oncol. 2012;106(8):953–8.
13. Cercek A, et al. Assessment of hepatic arterial infusion of floxuridine in combination with systemic gemcitabine and oxaliplatin in patients with unresectable intrahepatic cholangiocarcinoma: a phase 2 clinical trial. JAMA Oncol. 2020;6(1):60–7.
14. Kingham TP, D'Angelica M, Kemeny NE. Role of intra-arterial hepatic chemotherapy in the treatment of colorectal cancer metastases. J Surg Oncol. 2010;102(8):988–95.
15. Kemeny N, et al. Intrahepatic or systemic infusion of fluorodeoxyuridine in patients with liver metastases from colorectal carcinoma. A randomized trial. Ann Intern Med. 1987;107(4):459–65.
16. Allen PJ, et al. Technical complications and durability of hepatic artery infusion pumps for unresectable colorectal liver metastases: an institutional experience of 544 consecutive cases. J Am Coll Surg. 2005;201(1):57–65.
17. Shin PJ, Kingham TP. Minimally invasive approaches to hepatic arterial infusion pump placement in metastatic colorectal cancer. Laparosc Surg. 2019:4.
18. Sharib JM, et al. Hepatic artery infusion pumps: a surgical toolkit for intraoperative decision-making and management of hepatic artery infusion-specific complications. Ann Surg. 2022;276(6):943–56.

Index

A
ABC-02 trial, 21, 25, 78, 100
Abdominal access, 487
Abdominal cavity, 485
Ablation, 156–163, 169, 201–203
ABO-compatible cadaveric allografts, 571
Active heating zone, 636
Acute normovolemic hemodilution (ANH), 353
Adenocarcinoma, 237–240, 245
Adenomatous polyps, 36
Adequate lymphadenectomy, 18
Adjuvant external beam radiation therapy, 24
Adjuvant radiotherapy, 21
Adrenocortical carcinoma (ACC), 221–223
Air bubbles, 607
Air cholangiogram, 528
Air leak test, 528
Alpha-fetoprotein (AFP), 583
Alternating current (AC), 636
American Association for the Study of Liver Diseases (AASLD) liver biopsy, 472–475
American Joint Committee on Cancer (AJCC)/Union for International Cancer Control (UICC) TNM staging system, 91–92
Anastomotic leak, 592
Anatomic metastasectomy/segmentectomy, 496
  anatomical segmentectomy, 500, 501
  pre-operative considerations
    chemotherapy induced hepatotoxicity, 496
    hepatocellular carcinoma and cholangiocarcinoma, 497, 498
    imaging, 498, 499
    operative steps, 499, 500
    synchronous colon cancer primary and liver metastases, 496, 497
Anatomic resection (AR), 164, 498
Anatomical artery variants, 337
Anatomical liver resection, 481
Angiogenic switch, 220
Anterior portal nodes, 623
Anterior superior iliac spine (ASIS), 521
Anterior-inferior liver segments, 482, 487
Antibiotics, 651
Antifibrinolytics effect, 353
Antimicrobial prophylaxis, 166
Aquamantys™ (Medtronic), 317

Argon beam, 507
Argon beam coagulator (ABC) system, 320, 321, 486
Arterial reconstruction, 571
Associating liver partition and portal vein ligation for staged hepatectomy (ALPPS), 301, 384, 564
Autotransfusion, 352

B
Balloon dilation, 452
Basket retrieval, 452
BCAT phase III trial, 101
B-catenin mutated HCA, 118
BCLC staging system, 136–140
  advanced stage, 140
  early stage, 138, 139
  end stage, 140
  intermediate stage, 139
  very early stage, 138
Bilateral subcostal incision (Chevron incision), 278
Bilateral subcostal incision with midline cephalad extension (Mercedes incision), 278
BILCAP phase III randomized control trial, 21, 77, 101
Bile duct, 447, 581
Bile duct exploration, 446
Bile duct injury (BDI), 440
Bile duct nodes, 622, 625
Bile duct reconstruction
  complications, 591, 592
  indications, 582
  postoperative considerations, 591
  preoperative considerations, 582, 583
    preoperative biliary drainage, 585, 586
    work up, 583–585
  principles of, 589–591
Bile duct resection, 52
  indications, 582
  operation, 587–589
  preoperative considerations, 582, 583
    preoperative biliary drainage, 585, 586
    work up, 583–585
  principles of, 586, 587
Bile leak, prevention of, 527–529
Bile stasis, 72
Biliary anatomy, 563
Biliary bypass, 104
Biliary drainage, 585, 586
Biliary ductal anatomy, 568
Biliary ductal transection, 574
Biliary epithelium, 72
Biliary intraepithelial neoplasms (BilIN), 7, 39, 40
Biliary obstruction, 89, 93, 96, 97, 104, 585
Biliary resection, 582, 586, 587
Biliostasis, 319, 326–327
Biopsy, 452
Bipolar sealing devices, 315
Bismuth type I and II lesions, 99
Bismuth type III lesions, 99
Bismuth type IV lesions, 99
Bismuth-Corlette classification system, 90–92
Blood loss, 349–358, 361
Blood transfusion, 349
Blumgart pre-surgical clinical T staging system, 92–93
BRAF V600E alterations, 154
Breast cancer, 223, 225
Breast cancer liver metastasis (BCLM), 223–225
Bubbles, 528

C
CA 19-9, 609
Cadaveric vein grafts, 572
Cannulation, 680, 682
Capecitabine, 609
Carbonic anhydrase 19-9 (CA 19-9), 93

Carcinoembryonic antigen (CEA), 93, 583
Caroli's disease, 72
Cavitron ultrasound surgical aspirator (CUSA), 312–318, 321, 326, 401
Central hepatectomy and right anterior sectionectomy, 552
   pitfalls and pearls, 552–554
   surgical technique, 554–557
Central venous pressure (CVP), 547
Chemotherapy Induced hepatotoxicity, 496
Child-Pugh Class B liver function, 498
Child-Pugh classification system, 375, 517
Cholangiocarcinoma, 497–498, 623
Cholangiogram, 451
Cholangiogram catheter, 442
Cholecystectomy, 36–41, 45–47, 49, 50, 526, 622, 682
Cholecystocholangiography, 446
Choledochal cysts, 72
Choledochal stones, 452
Choledochoceles, 582
Choledochoscopy, 446, 447, 450, 451
   equipment, 448
   robotic-assisted operations, considerations in, 453, 454
   technique, 448–452
      access/cannulation of biliary tree, 449
      accessory channel, further interventions through, 451, 452
      advance choledochoscope, 449, 450
      closure of, 452
      trajectory of, 448
      tips and troubleshooting, 452, 453

Cholelithiasis, 6, 440
Chronic biliary infection, 6
Chronic cholecystitis, 13
Cirrhosis, 663
Cirrhotic livers, 307
Clamp-crushing technique, 311–312
CLARINET trial, 205
Classic bile duct anatomy, 337
Clinical Risk Score (CRS), 152, 154, 156
Clonorchis sinensis, 88
Coagulopathy, 484
Colorectal cancer, 495
Colorectal liver metastases (CRLM), 497, 637, 678
   adjuncts to surgical treatment
      ablation, 156–163
      cryoablation, 158, 159
      hepatic artery infusion therapy, 161
      irreversible electroporation, 159, 160
      SBRT, 160
      systemic chemotherapy, 162–163
   clinical risk score models, 152–153
   determining resectability, 149–151
   epidemiology, 147
   imaging, 148–151
   metachronous, 148
   perioperative management
      antimicrobial prophylaxis, 166
      minimizing blood loss, 165–166
      venous thromboembolism prophylaxis, 166
   postoperative management
      electrolyte abnormalities, 166
      fluid resuscitation, 166–167
      liver function, 167
   prognostic factors, 151–156

Colorectal liver metastases (CRLM) (*cont.*)
   surgical management
      disappearing liver metastases, 171–172
      HAI therapy, 168
      open versus minimally invasive approach, 169–170
      resection margin, 168
      resection versus ablation, 169
      synchronous CRLM, 172, 173
      transplantation, 170–171
   surgical therapy, 163–165
   surveillance, 167
   synchronous, 147
Common bile duct (CBD), 440
Contrast-enhanced IOUS (CE-IOUS), 164
Contrast-enhanced ultrasound (CEUS), 12, 396
Control method, 390
Couinaud scheme, 501
Couinaud's segments, 164, 481
Cryoablation, 157, 158
CryoSeal Fibrin Selant System™, 323
Cryotherapy, 156
Cystic duct lymph node positivity, 11
Cystic duct resection margin, 11
Cystic ductotomy, 442
Cystic lymph node, 11
Cystic plate cholecystectomy, 399
Cytoreductive surgery, 235

D
D1 lymph node stations, 12
D2 lymph node stations, 12
Da Vinci Xi robotic platform, 338, 489
Degree of hypertrophy (DoH), 382
Depth, 423
Device-assisted techniques, 312
Digitoclasy, 311
Direct cholangiography, 95
   bile duct resection, 588
Direct liver suturing, 357–358
Disappearing liver metastases (DLM), 171, 172
Doppler ultrasound, 427, 573
Duct-to-duct anastomosis, 574
Dysplastic focus, 116
Dysplastic nodules, 116–117

E
Electrocautery, 486
Electrolyte abnormalities, 166
Electromagnetic (EM) wave, 636
Electrosurgical hemostasis, 477
Embolization techniques
   hepatic vein embolization, 380–382
   portal vein embolization, 380
Endometrial cancer, 225–226
Endoscopic choledochoscopy, 585
Endoscopic liver biopsy, 470
Endoscopic retrieval bag, 471
Endoscopic retrograde cholangiography (ERC), 563
Endoscopic retrograde cholangiopancreatography (ERCP), 95, 96, 447, 584
Endoscopic ultrasound (EUS), 584
Enhanced Recovery After Surgery (ERAS), 591
Epigenome-wide association study, 9
Epithelial ovarian cancer, 235, 237
Esophageal cancer, 226, 227
Ethanol, 659
Everolimus, 205
Evicel™, 323
Ex vivo hepatectomy, extended hepatectomy, 575

Extended hepatectomy, 561
  complications, 576
  ex vivo hepatectomy, 575
  hepatic artery reconstruction, 571, 572
  hepatic vein reconstruction, 573, 574
  indications, 562
  minimally invasive surgery, 575
  operative planning, 562–565
  portal vein reconstruction, 572, 573
  postoperative management, 575
  surgical considerations
    hepatic vein dissection, 568, 569
    incision, 565
    mobilization, 565, 566
    parenchymal transection, 569, 570
    porta hepatis dissection, 566–568
    reconstruction, 570, 571
Extended radical lymphadenectomy, 52
Extent of lymphadenectomy, 18
Extracorporeal Satinsky clamp, 436
Extracorporeal techniques, Rummel tourniquet technique, 434, 435
Extrafascial approach, 391
Extrahepatic cholangiocarcinomas (ECC), 71, 72
  anatomic classification, 90
  clinical presentation, 89
  diagnostic workup, 93–96
  etiology, 87
  histology, 89
  incidence, 87, 88
  operative strategies, 98–100
  pathophysiology, 88
  preoperative evaluation, 96–98
  prognosis, 88
  risk factor, 88
  staging, 92, 93
  systemic treatment, 100–104

F

Falciform and round ligaments, 555
Falciform ligament, 414, 499, 565, 684
FDG-PET/CT, 597
FGFR genetic aberration, 79
Fibrin sealants (FS), 322, 323
FibroSure, 469
Fibrous scarring, 395
FIGHT-202 phase II trial, 79
Finger-fracture technique, *see* Digitoclasy
Flat/non-tumoral forming dysplasia, 39–40
FloSeal Hemostatic Matrix™, 323
Fluid resuscitation, 166–167
Fluorescence intensity color map, 456
Fluorescent cholangiography (FC), 454–458
  equipment, 455
  fluorescence imaging, 455
  robotic-assisted operations, 458
  technique, 455–456
    fluorescence imaging activation, 456
    ICG injection, 455, 456
    tips and troubleshooting, 456, 458
Focus, 424
Fong score, 154
Frequency, 423
Future liver remnant (FLR), 372–373, 516, 564, 583

G

Gain, 423
Gallbladder adenomatous polyps, 5
Gallbladder cancer (GBC), 595
  adjuvant treatment, 21–24
  clinical presentation, 9–15

Gallbladder cancer (GBC) (*cont.*)
    incidental GBC, 10–12
    intraoperative discovery, 14–15
    suspected before surgery or non-incidental gallbladder cancer, 12–14
  diagnosis, 4
  epidemiology, 3, 4
  genetics, 7–9
  immunology, 9
  immunotherapy (PD-L1 inhibitors), 24–25
  incidence, 3
  management of, 595
  mapping, 10
  minimally invasive techniques and indications, 20
  OER, 15
    adequate lymphadenectomy, 18
    hepatic spread, 17
    inadequate lymphadenectomy, 18
    overall and progression-free survival, 17
    prognostic factors after, 18–19
    recurrence risk, change in, 20
    residual cancer or residual disease impact, 19
    stage T1b, 15
    stage T2, 15, 16
    stage T2b, 16
    surveillance after, 19–20
  palliative treatment, 25
  pathogenesis, 9
  risk factors, 5, 7
    chronic biliary infection, 6
    gallbladder adenomatous polyps, 5
    gallbladder stones, 6
    obesity, 5, 6
    tobacco smoking, 6
    type 2 diabetes, 6

Gallbladder carcinoma histology patterns, 8
Gallbladder epithelium, 7
Gallbladder polyps (GP), 3, 5
  definition, 36
  diagnostic modalities, 36
  management, 37
  polyp size, 37
  pseudopolyps, 36, 37
  size, 39
  symptomatic patient, 38
  transabdominal ultrasound, 36
  true polyps, 36
Gallbladder stones, 5, 6
Gallstones, 3, 6
Gastric cancer, 227, 228
  loco-regional modalities, 229
  resection vs. no resection, 228
Gastric cancer liver metastases (GCLM), 227–229
Gastroduodenal artery (GDA), 678, 680
Gastrointestinal stromal tumors (GISTs), 217, 229–232, 243
Gates, 392
Gelatin matrix topical hemostatic agents, 322
Gemcitabine/cisplatin/durvalumab (GCD) therapy, 100, 104
Genetic biomarkers, 155–156
Genetic syndromes, 193
Genome-wide association study, 8
Genomics, 68
Glissonean approach, 397, 400
  ICG-guided robot-assisted left hepatectomy with, 402, 403
  ICG-guided robot-assisted S3 segmentectomy with, 403, 404
Glissonean pedicles, 391, 400, 545, 550
Glissonean/Walaeus sheath, 391, 546

Glucagon, 445
Guidewire, 451

H
Harmonic Scalpel (HS), 313, 314
Hematogenous metastasis, 236
Hemihepatectomy, 515
Hemorrhage control
  laprscopic surgery
    compression and perihepatic packing, 358
    exposure and visualization, 359
    increasing pneumoperitoneum, 358
    low CVP, 358
    open conversion, 360
    Pringle manuever, 359
    quick stitches, 359
  non-operative techniques, 351–354
    autotransfusion, 352–353
    cell-salvage, 352–353
    low central venous pressure anesthesia, 351–352
    pharmacologic agents, 353–354
  open surgery
    direct liver suturing, 357–358
    manual compression, 357
    perihepatic packing, 357
    Pringle maneuver, 357
  pre-operative care and planning, 350–351
  vascular occlusion, 354
    intraoperative ultrasound, 354–355
    parenchymal transection, 355
    remnant surface management, 355
    topical hemostatic agents, 355, 356
Hemostasis, 319, 326–327, 551
  laprscopic surgery
    compression and perihepatic packing, 358
    exposure and visualization, 359
    increasing pneumoperitoneum, 358
    low CVP, 358
    open conversion, 360
    Pringle manuever, 359
    quick stitches, 359
  left lateral sectionectomy, 507
  non-operative techniques, 351–354
    autotransfusion, 352–353
    cell-salvage, 352–353
    low central venous pressure anesthesia, 351–352
    pharmacologic agents, 353–354
  open surgery
    direct liver suturing, 357–358
    manual compression, 357
    perihepatic packing, 357
    Pringle maneuver, 357
  pre-operative care and planning, 350–351
  vascular occlusion, 354
    intraoperative ultrasound, 354–355
    parenchymal transection, 355
    remnant surface management, 355
    topical hemostatic agents, 355, 356
Hemostatic agents, 321–323
Hemostatic fibrin, 486
HepaScore, 469
Hepatectomy, 515, 596
  degree of hypertrophy, 382
  embolization techniques
    hepatic vein embolization, 380–382
    portal vein embolization, 376–382
  future liver remnant, 372–373

Hepatectomy (*cont.*)
  inadequate growth of FLR, 384
  kinetic growth rate, 383
  open right and left, 515, 516
    anatomy, 516
    incisions and exposure, 520, 521
    portal vein embolization and hepatic vein embolization, 519, 520
    postoperative liver function, determinants of, 517, 518
  optimal FLR Volumes, 373–376
  preoperative imaging, 368–372
    MDCT, 369–370
    MRI, 370–372
    ultrasound, 368, 369
Hepatic and biliary diseases, 543, 561
  central hepatectomy and right anterior sectionectomy, 552
    pitfalls and pearls, 552–554
    surgical technique, 554–557
  right posterior sectionectomy
    laparoscopic/robotic approach, 548, 550, 551
    open approach, 551, 552
    pitfalls and pearls, 544–548
    surgical technique, 548
Hepatic arterial anatomy, 303, 567
Hepatic arterial infusion (HAI) therapy, 76, 78, 161, 168
Hepatic artery, 625
  anatomy, 302
Hepatic artery infusion chemotherapy (HAIC), 677
Hepatic artery infusion pump (HAIP), 161, 172
  perioperative considerations, 678, 679
  postoperative consideration, 685
  principles, 679, 680
  set up and port placement, 680, 681
  techniques, 682, 685
Hepatic artery infusion therapy, 161
Hepatic artery lymph node dissection, 621, 625
Hepatic artery reconstruction, 571, 572
Hepatic premalignant lesions
  dysplastic foci, 116
  dysplastic nodules, 116–117
  hepatocarcinogenesis
    molecular (genetic and epigenetic) changes, 114
    morphologically distinguishable hepatocyte alterations, 115–116
  hepatocellular adenoma, 118
  imaging, 119
  surveillance, 118, 120
  treatment, 120–121
Hepatic resection, 495, 499
Hepatic vascular anatomy, 350
Hepatic vasculature, 563
Hepatic vein dissection, 568, 569
Hepatic vein embolization (HVE), 148, 150, 380, 381, 519–520
Hepatic vein reconstruction, 573, 574
Hepatic vein tributaries, 548, 557
Hepaticojejunostomy (HJ), 574, 590
Hepatitis B (HBV) infection, 129
Hepatitis C (HCV) infection, 129
Hepatitis D (HDV) infection, 129
Hepatitis infection, 129
Hepatocarcinogenesis, 113–116
  molecular (genetic and epigenetic) changes, 114
  morphologically distinguishable hepatocyte alterations, 115–116
Hepatocellular adenomas (HCAs), 118, 119, 121
Hepatocellular carcinoma (HCC), 497–498

BCLC staging system, 136–140
  advanced stage, 140
  early stage, 138, 139
  end stage, 140
  intermediate stage, 139
  very early stage, 138
  hepatitis infection, 129
  imaging, 130
  liver transplantation, 133–134
  radiotherapy, 134–135
  risk factors, 128, 129
  screening, 130
  serum markers, 130
  surgical resection, 132–133
  systemic therapies, 136
  transarterial therapies, 135–136
  treatment options, 131–132
  tumor ablation, 134
Hepatocyte nuclear factor-1 alpha (HNF1a) mutated HCA, 118
Hepatoduodenal ligament, 402, 434
  lymph nodes of, 617
Hepatolithiasis, 63
Hepatopancreatobiliary (HPB) surgery, 14, 15, 440, 533
High-grade dysplastic nodules (HGDNs), 116, 117, 119, 120
Hilar dissection, 389, 390
  ICG-guided robot-assisted left hepatectomy with Glissonean approach, 402, 403
  ICG-guided robot-assisted S3 segmentectomy with Glissonean approach, 403, 404
  intrafascial approach, 390, 391
  minimally invasive surgery, 397
    laparoscopy, 397–400
    robot-assisted liver surgery, 400–402
  open surgery, 395, 396
  pre-op and preparation pearls, 392–394
HistoSonics system, 675
Histotripsy, 673–675
Horizontal limb, 413
Hydro-Jet® (ERBE), 317–318
Hypertrophy of contralateral liver segments, 519
Hypervascular neoplasms, 370

I

Iatrogenic bile duct injury, 582
ICG-guided robot-assisted left hepatectomy, with Glissonean approach, 402, 403
ICG-guided robot-assisted S3 segmentectomy, with Glissonean approach, 403, 404
Immunosuppressive microenvironment, 9
Immunotherapy (PD-L1 inhibitors), 24–25
Inadequate lymphadenectomy, 18
Incidental gallbladder carcinoma
  bile duct resection, 52
  clinical evaluation, 49
  intraoperative management, 46–49
  minimally invasive techniques, 53
  multivisceral resection, 52
  muscularis mucosa, 51
  occult port site metastasis, 53
  pathologic evaluation, 49, 50
  port site and peritoneal metastasis, 53
  postoperative pathologic diagnosis, 46, 49–52
  radical cholecystectomy, 51, 52
  re-resection, 53, 54
  staging laparoscopy, 53
Index cholecystectomy, 14

Indocyanine green fluorescence (ICG) cholangiography, 588
Inferior partial hepatectomy
  laparoscopic surgery, 486–488
  open approach, 485, 486
  preoperative imaging, 482–484
  robotic surgery, 489
  surgical approach/preoperative preparation, 484
  transthoracic approach, 490
Inferior right hepatic vein (IRHV), 304, 483
Inferior vena cava (IVC) ligament, 390
Inflammatory HCA, 118
Inflow occlusion, 306, 309–312, 317, 324–325
Initial hypotheses, 218–219
In-plane technique, 646–648
Interventional transarterial liver directed therapy, 639
Intra-abdominal electrocautery, 659
Intra-arterial therapy, 203–205
Intracholecystic papillary neoplasms (ICPN), 40
Intracorporeal bulldog clamp, 436
Intracorporeal techniques, 325
  Huang Loop, 435, 436
  vascular clamp techniques, 436
Intraductal Papillary Mucinous Neoplasms of the pancreas (IPMNs), 62
Intraductal papillary neoplasm of the bile duct (IPNB)
  cholangioscopy-derived biopsy, mucin or bile samples, 68
  classification, 62–63
  definition, 62
  diagnostics, 64
  epidemiology, 63
  genomics, 68
  management, 64–65
  molecular profiling, 67
  prognosis, 65–67
  radiologic subtypes, 64
  risk factors, 63
  subtypes, grading, and long-term outcomes, 66–67
Intrahepatic cholangiocarcinoma (iCCA), 8, 71, 76, 79, 368, 498
  diagnosis and staging, 73–75
  epidemiology, 71–72
  growth pattern, 73
  pathophysiology, 72, 73
  patient management, 76
  resectable disease, 75–78
  risk factors, 72
  staging, 75
  unresectable disease, 78–80
Intraoperative cell salvage (ICS), 353
Intraoperative cholangiograms (IOC), 440, 445
  equipment, 441
  practice guidelines, 440
  robotic-assisted operations, 446
  technique, 441–444
    access/cannulation of biliary tree, 441–443
    closure of biliary access, 444
    contrast injection, 443
    interpretation, 444
    intraoperative image capture, 443
  tips and trouble shooting, 444, 445
Intraoperative ultrasound, 163, 164, 171, 307–308, 399, 402, 412, 499
  anatomical landmarks, 424, 426
  evaluating liver parenchyma, 424
  setup and settings, 423, 424
Inverted L-modified "Makuuchi" incision, 600
Irreversible electroporation (IRE), 157, 159–160, 203
  non-thermal ablation, 664

exclusion criteria, 664, 665
indications and inclusion criteria, 664
intraoperative procedure, 665
probe placement grid, 666
targeted ablation area setting and probe placement grid, 667
targeted ablation area settings, 666
Ischemic demarcation, 338

J
J-shaped incision (Makuuchi incision), 278

K
KEYNOTE-966 trial, 78
Kinetic growth rate (KGR), 383, 384, 519
Kocher clamp, 642
Kocher incision, 599
Kocher maneuver, 627

L
Laparoscopic approach
  patient positioning
    lateral decubitus, 282–283
    supine position, 281–282
  radical cholecystectomy, 599
  trocars placement, 283–288
    left-sided segments, 285
    posterior segments, 286–288
    right-sided segments, 285–286
Laparoscopic cholecystectomy, 12
Laparoscopic common bile duct exploration (LCBDE), 447, 452
Laparoscopic left liver mobilization, 419
Laparoscopic liver resections (LLRs), 323, 324, 400
Laparoscopic mobilization
  laparoscopic left liver mobilization, 419
  laparoscopic right liver mobilization, 418, 419
  positioning and port placement, 417
Laparoscopic MWA of liver
  "in-plane" vs. "step-off" technique, 646–648
  access and port placement, 642
  anesthesia, 639, 640
  complications, 650, 651
  equipment and room setup, 640, 642
  hand positioning and IOUS probe placement, 643, 644
  outcomes, 652, 653
  pitfalls, 649, 650
  positioning, 640
  post op imaging, 649
  pre-operative planning, 639
  ultrasound guided targeting, 644, 645
Laparoscopic or robotic approach, 548, 550, 551
Laparoscopic port placement, 418
Laparoscopic right liver mobilization, 418–419
Laparoscopic surgery, inferior partial hepatectomy and superior partial hepatectomy, 486–488
Laparoscopic ultrasonography, 487
Laparoscopic ultrasound
  liver mobilization, 427–429
  radical cholecystectomy, 601
Laparoscopy, 397–400, 504, 597
Large cell change (LCC), 115–117
Laser ablation (LA), 201–203
Lawnmower technique, 644
Left hepatic vein (LHV), 303, 304

Left lateral sectionectomy, 496, 504
  anatomical segmentectomy, 500, 501
  hepatocellular carcinoma and cholangiocarcinoma, 497, 498
  imaging, 498, 499
  operative steps, 499, 500
    continuous assessment, 505
    hemostasis, 507
    mobilization, 506
    patient positioning and access, 505
    transection, 507
  pre-operative considerations, chemotherapy induced hepatotoxicity, 496
  synchronous colon cancer primary and liver metastases, 496, 497
Left liver mobilization, 417
Left superficial vein (LSV), 304
Left triangular ligament, 566
Leiomyosarcomas (LMS), 243
Lesser curvature of the stomach, 623
LigaSure (LS), 315
Liver biopsy, 465
Liver core needle biopsies, 465
  alternatives, 469
  complication, 471, 472
  contraindications, 468
  indications, 466, 467
  limitations, 468
  techniques, 469–471
Liver elastography, 469
Liver function, 167
Liver Imaging Reporting and Data system (LI-RADS), 131
Liver mobilization, 342, 411
  intraoperative ultrasound, 412
    anatomical landmarks, 424, 426
    evaluating liver parenchyma, 424
    setup and settings, 423, 424
  laparoscopic mobilization
    laparoscopic left liver mobilization, 419
    laparoscopic right liver mobilization, 418, 419
    positioning and port placement, 417
  open liver mobilization
    left liver mobilization, 417
    right liver mobilization, 412, 413, 415, 416
  robotic mobilization of the liver
    positioning and port placement, 420
    robotic left liver mobilization, 422
    robotic right liver mobilization, 420, 421
  ultrasound in minimally invasive approaches
    laparoscopic ultrasound, 427–429
    robatic ultrasound, 429
Liver parenchyma, 489
Liver Reporting and Data System (CT/MRI LI-RADS), 120
Liver resection, 497, 562, 596
Liver transplantation (LT), 133–134, 206–207
Liver venous deprivation (LVD), 519
Livers, cirrhotic, 307
Local ablative therapies, 157
Low-grade nodules (LGDNs), 116, 117
Lung cancer, 232, 233
Lymph node yield, portal lymphadenectomy, 616

M

Magnetic resonance cholangiography (MRC), 563, 583, 584
Magnetic resonance imaging (MRI), 370–373, 584
Makuuchi's ligament, 421
Malignancy, 582

Mammalian target of rapamycin (mTOR) inhibitor, 205
Manual compression, 357
Marginal zones, 483
Maximizing parenchymal preservation, 164–165
Melanoma, 233–235
Mesohepatectomy, 552
Metastasectomy, for gastric cancer, 229
Metastatic small bowel adenocarcinoma, 245, 246
Microfibrillar collagen (MC), 321
Microwave ablation (MWA), 157, 159, 201, 202, 635, 636, 638
Middle hepatic vein (MHV), 303, 304, 318
Middle right hepatic vein (MRHV), 304
Midline incision, 278
Midline laparotomy, 520
Midline vertical limb, 413
Minimally invasive anatomical liver resection (MIALR), 397
Minimally invasive approaches, ultrasound in
  laparoscopic ultrasound, 427–429
  robatic ultrasound, 429
Minimally invasive Pringle maneuvers, 433, 434
  extracorporeal techniques, Rummel tourniquet technique, 434, 435
  intracorporeal techniques
    Huang Loop, 435, 436
    vascular clamp techniques, 436
Minimally invasive surgery (MIS), 394, 533, 598
  extended hepatectomy, 575
  hilar dissection, 397
  laparoscopy, 397–400
  robot-assisted liver surgery, 400–402
Minimally-invasive transthoracic liver resection (MITTLR), 490
MIS left hepatectomy, 533
  caudal approach, 537, 539
  challenges, 541
  contraindications, 535
  hepatic pedicle, intermittent clamping of, 535
  inflow control, 540
  instruments, 536
  laparoscopy, 537
  long-term outcomes, 534
  parenchymal division, 540
  pertinent imaging, 534
  pneumoperitoneum, 535, 536
  robotic, 539
  surgery, 537
MIS right hepatectomy, 533
  caudal approach, 537, 539
  challenges, 541
  contraindications, 535
  hepatic pedicle, intermittent clamping of, 535
  inflow control, 540
  instruments, 536
  laparoscopy, 537
  long-term outcomes, 534
  parenchymal division, 540
  pertinent imaging, 534
  pneumoperitoneum, 535, 536
  robotic, 539
  surgery, 537
Model for end-stage liver disease (MELD) score, 375
Molecular profiling, 67, 79
Multidetector computed tomography (MDCT), 369, 370
Multidisciplinary tumor (MDT), 638
Multiphasic computed tomography (CT) imaging, 584
Multiple injection needles, 661
Multivisceral resection, 52
Muscularis mucosa, 51

N

Nanoknife IRE system, 665
Neoadjuvant therapy, 97, 100, 619
Neuroendocrine tumors (NET)
  ablation, 201–203
  endoscopic assessment, 195
  grading, 194
  imaging, 195
  incidence, 193
  intra-arterial therapy, 203–205
  nonsurgical and multimodal
      treatment strategies, 194
  resection and cytoreductive
      approach, 197–201
    evolving trends, 197–200
    recurrence and progression,
        200–201
    tackling extrahepatic disease,
        200
  symptoms and biochemical
      characterization, 194
  systemic therapy, 205–206
  transplantation, 206–207
  treatment strategies, 196–197
Nodular tumors, 89
Non-alcoholic steatohepatitis
    (NASH), 127–129
Nonalcoholic steatohepatitis-related
    hepatocellular carcinoma,
    403
Non-anatomic hepatectomy, 545
Non-anatomic resection (NAR), 164
Non-colorectal non-endocrine liver
    metastases
    (NCRNNELMs)
  adrenal, 221–223
  biology
    immunology, 220–221
    initial hypotheses, 218–219
    mechanical and
        hemodynamic properties
        of liver, 219–220
    pathophysiology and
        molecular basis, 220
  breast cancer, 223, 225
  endometrial, 225–226
  epidemiology, 216–218
  esophageal cancer, 226
  gastric cancer, 227, 228
    loco-regional modalities, 229
    resection vs. no resection,
        228
  GISTs, 229, 231, 232
  lung cancer, 232, 233
  melanoma, 233–235
  ovarian cancer, 235, 237
  pancreatic ductal
      adenocarcinoma, 237
    metachronous, 240
    synchronous, 238–240
  RCC, 241, 242
  small bowel, 245–246
  soft-tissue sarcomas, 243, 245
  testicular cancer, 247–248
  thyroid cancer, 248–249
  urothelial cancers, 249–250
Non-incidental GBC, 12
Nonseminoma tumor, 247
Non-thermal ablation
  bracketing probes, 668
  complications, 671
  histotripsy, 673–675
  irreversible electroporation, 664
    exclusion criteria, 664, 665
    indications and inclusion
        criteria, 664
    intraoperative procedure, 665
    probe placement grid, 666
    targeted ablation area setting
        and probe placement grid,
        667
    targeted ablation area
        settings, 666
  liver mass using ultrasound
      guidance, 671
  operating room setup, 670
  pancreas mass using ultrasound
      guidance, 670
  percutaneous ethanol injection,
      657–659
    benefits, 660
    complications, 660, 661

CT scans, 662
  lobe HCC, 663
  technique, 659
  volume calculation, 660
 procedure parameter, 669
 subtypes of, 658
 umbilical fissure, HCC tumor in, 672
Nontriadal artery, 117, 119

O

Obesity, 5
Occult biliary leaks, 486
Occult port site metastasis, 53
Omnitract, 280
Oncologic extended resection (OER), 11, 12, 14–16, 18–20, 26
 adequate lymphadenectomy, 18
 hepatic spread, 17
 inadequate lymphadenectomy, 18
 overall and progression-free survival, 17
 prognostic factors after, 18–19
 recurrence risk, change in, 20
 residual cancer or residual disease impact, 19
 stage T1b, 15
 stage T2, 15, 16
 stage T2b, 16
 surveillance after, 19–20
Oncology Thompson retractor, 521
Open approach
 access, 277–280
  incision, 277–278
  retractors, 279–280
  surgical field, 277
 advantages, 275
 disadvantages, 275
 hepatic and biliary diseases, 551, 552
 patient positioning, 276–277
 radical cholecystectomy, 604, 605
Open liver mobilization, 414
 left liver mobilization, 417
 right liver mobilization, 412, 413, 415, 416
Open right and left hepatectomy, 515, 516, 521–527
 anatomy, 516
 incisions and exposure, 520, 521
 portal vein embolization and hepatic vein embolization, 519, 520
 postoperative liver function, determinants of, 517, 518
Open surgery, hilar dissection, 395, 396
Opisthorchis viverrini endemicis, 88
Optimal exposure, 521
Optimal hepatic cytoreduction, 236
Optimal lymphadenectomy, 628
Orthotopic liver transplantation (OLT), 99, 100
Ovarian cancer, 217, 220, 235, 236
Oxidized cellulose topical hemostatic agents, 321–322

P

Palliation, 104, 105
Pancreatic ductal adenocarcinoma (PDAC), 237–240
 metachronous, 240
 synchronous, 238–240
Papillary tumors, 90
Parenchyma, 507
Parenchymal division, 540
Parenchymal transection, 325–326, 403, 550, 569, 570
 anatomical variants, 302–304
 Aquamantys, 317
 biliostasis, 319, 326–327
 Cavitron Ultrasound Surgical Aspirator, 314–315
 clamp-crushing technique, 311–312
 device-assisted techniques, 312

Parenchymal transection (*cont.*)
digitoclasy technique, 311
Harmonic Scalpel, 313
hemostasis, 319, 326–327
hemostatic agents, 321–323
hemostatic devices, 320–321
Hydro-Jet® (ERBE), 317–318
inflow occlusion, 309–310, 324–325
intraoperative ultrasound, 307–308
laparoscopic liver resection, 323, 324
LigaSure (Valleylab), 315
MHV, 318
parenchymal vascular demarcation, 308, 309
preoperative imaging, 300–301
principles, 306
sharp dissection, 311
stapling technique, 312
techniques for, 310–312
3D reconstruction, 305–306
Thunderbeat, 314
TissueLink, 316–317
transection plane, 324
Parenchymal vascular demarcation, 308, 309
Parenchymal-sparing resection, 164
Pedicle tracking technique, 644
Peptide receptor radionuclide therapy (PRRT), 205, 206
Percutaneous core needle biopsies, 470
Percutaneous ethanol injection (PEI), 657–659
benefits, 660
complications, 660, 661
CT scans, 662
lobe HCC, 663
technique, 659
volume calculation, 660
Percutaneous liver biopsy, 469
Percutaneous transhepatic cholangiography (PTC), 95, 563, 585
Pericholedochal tissue, 622
Periduodenal nodes, 623
Perihepatic packing, 357
Perihilar cholangiocarcinoma, 368
Perihilar extrahepatic cholangiocarcinoma, 90–92
Peripancreatic nodes, 623
Peripheral liver lesion, 476
Peripheral-to-central technique, 325
Peritoneal dissemination (PD), 235
Peritoneal metastases, 53, 236
Pharmacologic agents, 350, 353
PlasmaJet, 320
Platinum-based chemotherapy, 235, 236
Pneumoperitoneum, 535
Porcelain gallbladder, 12, 41
Port site metastasis, 53
Porta hepatis, 489, 566
Porta hepatis dissection, 566–568
Portal hypertension, 663
Portal lymphadenectomy, 615
anatomy, 617, 618
indications and contraindications, 616
operative technique
open approach, 620–623
robotic approach, 623–625, 627
pearls, 627, 628
pitfalls, 628, 629
preoperative preparation, cross sectional imaging in, 618, 619
rationale and lymph node yield, 616
robotic trocar position for, 624
type of approach, 619, 620
Portal triad, 628
Portal vein (PV), 500, 567
anatomy, 337
modulation, 573
reconstruction, 572, 573
Portal vein embolization (PVE), 98, 148, 150, 151, 301, 376, 377, 379–384, 519–520
Portal venous inflow, 572

Post op imaging, laparoscopic
  MWA of liver, 649
Posterior-superior segments, of
  liver, 482
Postoperative bile leaks, 527–529
Postoperative liver failure, 338
Pre-malignant gallbladder lesions
  dysplastic precursors of, 39
    flat/non-tumoral forming
      dysplasia, 39–40
    tumoral forming dysplasia,
      40–41
  gallbladder polyps
    definition, 36
    diagnostic modalities, 36
    management, 37
    Polyp size, 37
    pseudopolyps, 36, 37
    size, 39
    symptomatic patient, 38
    transabdominal ultrasound,
      36
    true polyps, 36
  porcelain gallbladder, 41
Pre-operative autologous blood
  (PABD), 352, 353
Preoperative delineation, 350
Primary sclerosing cholangitis, 5,
  72, 73
Primary small bowel malignancy,
  245
Pringle maneuver, 300, 309, 312,
  313, 324, 325, 357, 359,
  434, 485
Pro-angiogenic factors, 220
Procoagulant agents, 354
PRODIGE 12-ACCORD
  18-UNICANCER GI
  phase III trial, 101
PRODIGE trial, 21
Prophylactic cholecystectomy, 12
Pseudopolyps, 36, 37
Purified plant starch topical
  hemostatic agents, 321

Q
Quadruple-phase MDCT, 369
Quadruple-phase contrast helical
  computed tomography
  (CT), 498
Quick stitches, 359

R
Radical cholecystectomy, 51, 52,
  595
  intraoperative pitfalls and
    post-operative
    complications, 606, 607
  oncologic outcomes and
    follow-up, 608, 609
  open, 604, 605
  operative approach, 598
    laparoscopic, 599
    laparoscopic ultrasound, 601
    open surgery, 599
    perioperative management,
      598
    robotic-assisted surgery,
      601–603
  pre-operative planning, 596–598
  robotic, 605, 606
  set-up by operative approach,
    604
Radioembolization (RE), 203, 204
Radiofrequency ablation (RFA),
  157–160, 201, 202, 635
Radiofrequency devices (RFD),
  315, 316
Radiological Simultaneous
  Portohepatic Vein
  Embolization (RASPE),
  519
Radiotherapy, 134–135
Receiver operating characteristic
  (ROC) curve, 383
Reconstruction, 570, 571
Recothrom™ (ZymoGenetics)
  recombinant thrombin, 323

Regenerative nodules, 117
Regional liver-directed chemotherapy, 677
Regional lymphadenectomy, 65
Remnant liver ischemia (RLI), 397
Remnant surface management, 355
Renal cell carcinoma (RCC), 241–243
Replaced/accessory artery, 337
Resection and cytoreductive approach, 197–201
  evolving trends, 197–200
  recurrence and progression, 200–201
  tackling extrahepatic disease, 200
Retrohepatic IVC, 416
Retroperitoneal leyomeiosarcoma, 244
Retroportal nodes, 623
Reverse L incision, 521
Reverse Trendelenburg, 505
Right anterior sectionectomy (RAS), 552
Right hepatic vein (RHV), 303, 304, 390, 547
Right liver mobilization, 412–416, 418
Right subcostal incision (Kocher incision), 278
Right superficial vein (RSV), 304
Robot-assisted liver surgery, 400–404
Robotic approach
  advantages, 288
  patient positioning and operating room configuration, 288–290
  portal lymphadenectomy, 623–625, 627
  radical cholecystectomy, 605, 606
  trocars placement, 290–294
    left-sided segments, 291–292
    posterior segments, 293–294
    right-sided segments, 292–293
Robotic hepatic resection
  anatomic evaluation, 336–338
  liver mobilization, 342
  parenchymal transection, 343–344
  set up, 339–341
    assistant setup and instrumentation, 341
    initial incisions and diagnostic laparoscopy, 340
    patient positioning and anesthesia, 339
    preoperative preparations, 339
    Pringle maneuver and hilar dissection, 342–343
    robotic system docking, 341
    robotic system setup, 340
    trocar placement, 340, 341
    ultrasonographic examination, 341
  suitability of, 338
  surgical instruments, 339
Robotic hepaticojejunostomy, patient position for, 588
Robotic left liver mobilization, 422
Robotic liver resections (RLRs), 400
Robotic liver surgery, 402
Robotic mobilization of the liver, 421
  positioning and port placement, 420
  robotic left liver mobilization, 422
  robotic right liver mobilization, 420, 421
Robotic port placement, 603
Robotic portal lymphadenectomy, 626
Robotic right liver mobilization, 420–422
Robotic surgery, inferior partial hepatectomy and superior partial hepatectomy, 489

Robotic trocar position, for portal lymphadenectomy, 624
Robotic ultrasound, 429
Robotic-assisted surgery, radical cholecystectomy, 601–603
Rochard retractor, 279
Rouviere's sulcus, 546
Roux limb of the hepaticojejunostomy, 590
Rummel tourniquet technique, 435

S

SABR-COMET trial, 160
Sclerosing tumors, 89
Selective internal radiotherapy, 203
Self-retaining retractors, 565
Seminomas tumor, 247
Serum carbohydrate antigen (CA) 19-9, 14
Serum IgG4, 583
Sessile polyp, 5
Sharp dissection, 311
Sinusoidal capillarization, 119
Small bowel, 245–246
Small cell change (SCC), 115–117
Small retrohepatic caval branches, 522
Small-bowel adenocarcinoma, 245
Soft-tissue sarcomas (STSs), 243, 245
Somatostatin analogues (SSA), 205
Spyglass, 585
Staging laparoscopy, 53
Staining technique, 501
Standard abdominal ultrasound, 12
Standard upper midline laparotomy incision, 485
Stapling technique, 312
Stent-based biliary decompression, 104
Step-off technique, 646–649
Stereotactic body radiotherapy (SBRT), 76, 78, 79, 157, 160

Stone clearance, 453
Stone fragmentation, 452
Stones, 452
Substantial hypertrophy, 572
Superficial transection, 404
Superior partial hepatectomy
  laparoscopic surgery, 486–488
  open approach, 485, 486
  preoperative imaging, 482–484
  robotic surgery, 489
  surgical approach/preoperative preparation, 484
  transthoracic approach, 490
Supine straight split-leg position, 505
Suprahepatic inferior vena cava, 425
Surgical liver biopsy, 470
Surgical microwave ablation of liver, 635–639
Surgical resection, 132–133
Surgiflo™, 323
Surveillance, Epidemiology, and End Results (SEER), 595
SWOG S0809 trial, 101
Synchronous colon cancer primary and liver metastases, 496–497
Synchronous colorectal liver metastases, 172, 173
Systemic chemotherapy, 162–163
Systemic therapies, 136
Systemic therapy, 205–206

T

Tagasako/Ulrich retractor, 279
Takasaki's concept, 398
T-cell dysfunction, 9
Temporary inflow control of the Glisson (TICGL) technique, 546
Tension-free repair, 574
Testicular cancer, 247–248
Thermal damage, 650
Thompson retractor, 280, 601
3D reconstruction, 305–306

Thrombin-based agents, 486
Thunderbeat (TB), 314
Thyroid cancer, 248–249
Tisseel™, 323
TissueLink (TL), 313, 316–318
Ton That Tung approach, 391
TOPAZ-1 trial, 78
Topical hemostatic agents, 355, 356
Topical thrombin (TT), 323
Total hepatic isolation (THI), 310
Total liver volume (TLV), 518
Total transthoracic hepatectomies, 287–288
Total vascular isolation, 573
Trace ascites, 663
Trans cystic catheters, 588
Transarterial (bland) embolization (TAE), 128, 133, 135, 136, 203
Transarterial chemoembolization (TACE), 76, 78, 128, 133, 135, 136, 203, 204, 637
Transarterial radio embolization (TARE), 76, 78, 128, 133, 135, 136, 139
Transarterial therapies, 135–136
Transcholedochal choledochoscopy, 450
Transcholedochal/transbiliary cholangiogram, 446
Transdiaphragmatic ultrasound, 288
Transection, left lateral sectionectomy, 507
Transection plane, 324
Transjugular liver biopsies, 470
Transplenic access, 379
Transthoracic approach, inferior partial hepatectomy and superior partial hepatectomy, 490
Triple-phase MDCT, 369
True polyps, 36
T staging system, 93
Tumor ablation, 134
Tumoral forming dysplasia, 40–41
Two-step air leak test, 527–529
Two-surgeon technique, 523

Type 2 diabetes, 6

U

Ultrasonic devices, 313–315
Ultrasound, in minimally invasive approaches
    laparoscopic ultrasound, 427–429
    robatic ultrasound, 429
Unclassified HCA, 118
Urothelial cancers, 249–250
Uterine cancer, 225

V

Vascular anatomy, 350, 351, 355
Vascular clamp techniques, 436
Vascular occlusion, 300, 309, 311, 324, 326, 354
    intraoperative ultrasound, 354–355
    parenchymal transection, 355
    remnant surface management, 355
    topical hemostatic agents, 355, 356
Vascular thrombosis, 651
Venous thromboembolism prophylaxis, 166
Venous tributaries, 607
Veress technique, 283, 290, 642

W

Walaeus sheath, 391
Waterjet, 401

X

Xanthogranulomatous cholecystitis, 13
Xenografts, 571

Z

Z-type pattern, 337